Mastering the Techniques of LASIK, EPILASIK and LASEK (Techniques and Technology)

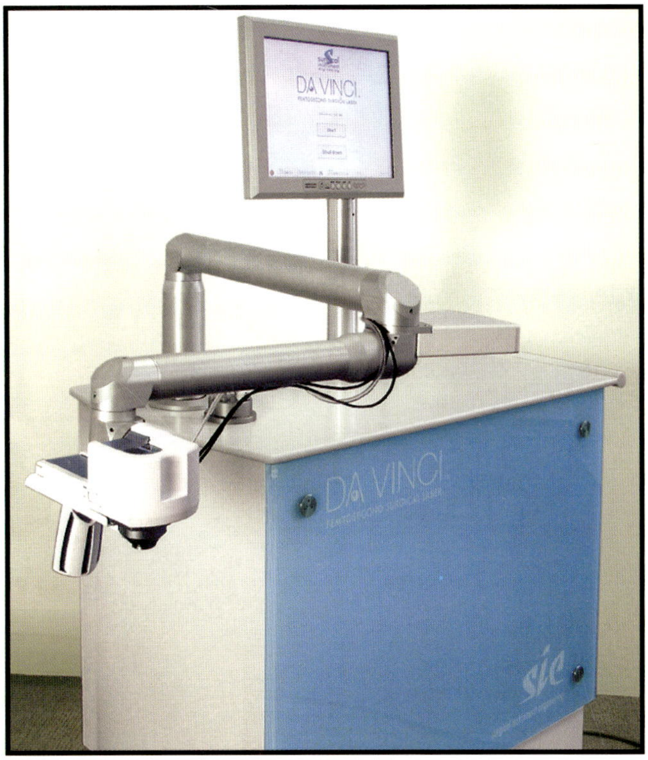

System requirement:

- **Windows XP or above**
- **Power DVD player (Software)**
- **Windows media player version 10.0 or above**
- **Quick time player version 6.5 or above**

Accompanying DVD ROM is playable only in Computer and not in DVD player.

Kindly wait for few seconds for DVD to autorun. If it does not autorun then please follow the steps:

- Click on my computer
- Click the **DVD drive labelled JAYPEE** and after opening the drive, kindly double click the file **Jaypee**

DVD Contents

Mastering the Techniques of LASIK, EPILASIK and LASEK (Techniques and Technology)

Editors

Ashok Garg
MS PhD FIAO (Bel) FRSM ADM FAIMS FICA
International and National Gold Medalist
Chairman and Medical Director
Garg Eye Institute and Research Centre
235-Model Town, Dabra Chowk
Hisar 125005, India

Jorge L Alió MD PhD
Chairman and Professor of Ophthalmology
Instituto Oftalmologico De Alicante
Avda. Denia 111, 03015
Alicante, Spain

Bojan Pajic MD
Chief of the Cornea and Refractive Surgery Department
Klinik Pallas, Louis Giroud-Str. 20
4600 Olten, Switzerland

Cyres K Mehta
MS FAGE FSVH FNRERF FSEC
Director and Consultant Ophthalmic Surgeon
The Mehta International Eye Institute
and Colaba Eye Hospital
Seaside, 147, Colaba Road
Mumbai 400005, India

Foreword
Ioannis G Pallikaris

JAYPEE BROTHERS
MEDICAL PUBLISHERS (P) LTD

Wolters Kluwer Health | Lippincott Williams & Wilkins

First published in India in 2007 by
Jaypee Brothers Medical Publishers (P) Ltd, New Delhi, India.
EMCA House, 23/23B Ansari Road, Daryaganj, New Delhi 110 002, India
Phones: +91-11-23272143, +91-11-23272703, +91-11-23282021, +91-11-23245672
Fax: +91-11-23276490, +91-11-23245683
e-mail: jaypee@jaypeebrothers.com, Visit our website: www.jaypeebrothers.com

First published in USA by The Lippincott Williams & Wilkins, 530 Walnut Street, Philadelphia, PA 19106, USA. Exclusively worldwide distributor except South East Asia (India, Nepal, Sri Lanka, Bhutan, Pakistan, Bangladesh).

ISBN 978-0-7817-9125-0

To

- *My Respected Param Pujya Guru Sant Gurmeet Ram Rahim Singh Ji for his blessings and motivation.*
- *My Respected parents, teachers, my wife Dr Aruna Garg, son Abhishek and daughter Anshul for their constant support and patience during all these days of hard work.*
- *My dear friend Dr Amar Agarwal, a renowned International Ophthalmologist for his constant support, guidance and expertise.*

Ashok Garg

- *To Mayca, Jorge, Fernando and Maria Lucia and most especially to my beloved wife Maria, for the hours that were taken from our family life to make this book possible.*

Jorge L Alió

- *To my son Valentin Aleksandar.*

Bojan Pajic

- *My parents for everything*
- *To Vini my Best friend*

Cyres K Mehta

Contributors

Amar Agarwal MS FRCS FRC Ophth
Consultant
Dr Agarwal's Eye Hospital
19, Cathedral Road
Chennai 600086, India

Anand Shroff MS
Shroff Eye Hospital
222, SV Road, Bandra (W)
Mumbai-400050, India

Antonio Calossi MD
Via 2 Giugno 52
50053, Certaldo (FI)
Italy

Ariadna Silva-Lepe MD
Terranova NO 676-101
Col. Providencia
Guadalajara, Jal
Mexico, CP 44630

Arthur Cheng MD
Department of Ophthalmology
and Visual Sciences
The Chinese University of
Hong Kong
C/o Prince of Wales Hospital
7B, Staff Quarters
Shatin, NT, Hong Kong SAR
PRC

Arun C Gulani MD MS
Director
Gulani Vision Institute
4500 Salisbury Rd Suite 160
Jacksonville, Florida, USA

Ashish Doshi MS
Dr Agarwal's Eye Hospital
19, Cathedral Road
Chennai-600086, India

Ashok Garg
MS PhD FIAO (Bel) FRSM ADM FAIMS FICA
International and
National Gold Medalist
Chairman and Medical Director
Garg Eye Institute and
Research Centre, 235-Model Town,
Dabra Chowk, Hisar 125005, India

Athiya Agarwal MD DO FRSH
Consultant
Dr Agarwal's Eye Hospital
19, Cathedral Road
Chennai-600086, India

Barbara Kusa MD
Centre Microchirurgia
Ambulatoriale, Via Donizetti, 24,
20052—Monza, Italy

Bojan Pajic MD
Chief of the Cornea and
Refractive Surgery Department
Klinik Pallas, Louis Giroud-Str. 20
4600 Olten, Switzerland

C Feinbaum MD
Instituto Oftalmologico
De Alicante
Avda. Denia 111, 03015, Alicante,
Spain

Chaitra Jayadev MS
Aditya Jyot Eye Hospital
Pvt. Ltd., Plot No. 153, Road No.9
Major Parmeshwaran Road
Opp SIWS College, Gate No.3
Wadala, Mumbai-400031, India

Chris P Lohmann MD PhD
Universitats—Augenklinik
Franz-Josef-Strau B-Allee
D-93042, Regensburg, Germany

Cyres K Mehta
MS FAGE FSVH FNRERF FSEC
Director and Consultant
Ophthalmic Surgeon
The Mehta International Eye
Institute and Colaba Eye Hospital
Seaside, 147, Colaba Road
Mumbai 400005, India

Dan Davis MD
Chu Vision Institute
Edina, Minn
USA

David Pinero MD
Instituto Oftalmologico
De Alicante
Avda. Denia 111, 03015
Alicante, Spain

David T Vroman MD
Magill Research Centre for Vision
Correction, Storm Eye Institute-
MUSC, 167, Ashley Avenue,
Charleston, South Carolina
29425, USA

Dennis SC Lam MD
Department of Ophthalmology
and Visual Sciences
The Chinese University of
Hong Kong, 3/F, Hong Kong
Eye Hospital, 147-L, Argyle Street,
Kowloon, HK SAR, PRC

Dipan Desai MS
Director
Desai Eye Hospital and Laser
Center, 2nd Floor Anand Complex
Opp. Shilp, CG Road
Near Navrang Pura
Ahmedabad-380009, India

Dipti N Shah MS
Doctor Eye Institute
Spenta Mansion, 1st Floor
SV Road, Andheri (West)
Mumbai-400058, India

Erik L Mertens MD FEBO
Medical Director
Antwerp Eye Center
Kapelstraat 8
B-2660 Antwerp
Belgium

Fabrizio I Camesasca MD
Department of Ophthalmology
Istituto Clinico Humanitas
Rozzano, Milano, Italy

Fernando Rodriquez Mier MD
Instituto Oftalmologico Hoyos
Rambla de Sabadell 62 1°
08201 Sabadell,
Barcelona, Spain

Francisco Arnalich MD
Instituto Oftalmologico
De Alicante
Avda. Denia 111, 03015
Alicante, Spain

Francisco Sánchez León MD
Instituto Nova Vision
Medical Director
Cornea, Refractive and
Anterior Segment Clinic
Cd de Mexico, Acapulco
Mexico

Frederic Hehn MD
Centre de La Vision
Nations - Vision
23, Boulevard de l'europe
54500, Vandoeuvre
France

Guillermo Avalos-Urzua MD
Terranova NO. 676-101
Col. Providencia
Guadalajara, Jal, Mexico
CP 44630

Hermann Anhalm PhD
Senior Optometrist
Depatment of Ophthalmology
Klinik Pallas, Louis Giroud-Str. 20
4600 Olten, Switzerland

Hijab Mehta MS DOMS FCPS
Aditya Jyot Eye Hospital Pvt. Ltd.
Wadala, Mumbai-400031, India

Hitendra Mehta MS
Aditya Jyot Eye Hospital Pvt. Ltd.
Wadala, Mumbai-400031, India

Ioannis G Pallikaris MD PhD
Professor and Head
Department of Ophthalmology
University of Crete
Heraklion, Crete
Greece

Jairo E Hoyos MD PhD
Instituto Oftalmologico Hoyos
Rambla de Sabadell 62 1°
08201 Sabadell
Barcelona, Spain

Jairo E Hoyos-Chacón MD
Instituto Oftalmologico Hoyos
Rambla de Sabadell 62 1°
08201 Sabadell
Barcelona, Spain

Jessica Matsumoto MD
Chu Vision Institute
Edina, Minn
USA

Jörg Müller MS
Department of Ophthalmology
Klinik Pallas, Louis Giroud-Str. 20
4600 Olten, Switzerland

Jorge L Alió MD PhD
Chairman and Professor of
Ophthalmology
Instituto Oftalmologico
De Alicante
Avda. Denia 111, 03015
Alicante, Spain

Joseph Colin MD
Hôpital Pellegrin-Tripode-
Service d' Ophthalmologie Place
Amilie Raba-Léon-33076
Bordeauxcedex, France

JT Lin PhD
Photon Data Inc.
7055, University Blvd,Winter
Park, Florida, USA

Jutta Horwath-Winter MD PhD
Department of Ophthalmology
Medical University Graz
Auenbruggerplatz 4
8036 Graz, Austria

Keiki R Mehta MS DO FIOS
Chairman and Medical Director
Mehta International Eye Institute
147, Shahid Bhagat Singh Road
Colaba Road, Mumbai-400005
India

Kerry D Solomon MD
Magill Research Centre for Vision,
Correction, Storm Eye Institute-
MUSC, 167, Ashley Avenue
Charleston, South Carolina, 29425
USA

Kumar J Doctor MS DNB
Director
Doctor Eye Institute
Spenta Mansion, 1st Floor
SV Road, Andheri (West)
Mumbai-400058, India

Luis E Fernández de Castro MD
Magill Research Centre for Vision Correction, Storm Eye Institute-MUSC, 167, Ashley Avenue,
Charleston, South Carolina,
29425, USA

Maeve O'Doherty PhD
Mater Hospital, Eccles st,
Dublin 7, UK

Maria C Arbelaez MD
Al Wattiyah, Romaila Building
106, El-Maghraby Eye and
Ear Centre,
PO Box 513, PC 112 Rwui,
Muscat, Sultanate of Oman

Maria I Kalyvianaki MD
Department of Ophthalmology
University of Crete
Heraklion, Crete, Greece

Massimo Camellin MD
Rovigo, Italy

Matteo Piovella MD
Centro Microchirurgia
Ambulatoriale
Via Donizetti 24,
20052, Monza, Italy

Melania Cigales - Jirout MD
Instituto Oftalmologico Hoyos
Sabadell (Barcelona), Spain

Michael C Knorz MD
Klinikum Mannheim
Theodor Kutzer Ufer 1-3
Mannheim, Germany

Nilesh Kanjiani MS
Consultant
Dr Agarwal's Eye Hospital Pvt Ltd
19, Cathedral Road
Chennai-86, India

Paul Karpecki MD
Director of Research
Moyes Eye Center
Kansas City, USA

Rishi Mohan MD DNB FRCS
Director
MM EyeTec, 29 Link Road
Lajpat Nagar-III
New Delhi-24, India

Robert Montes-Micó MD
Instituto Oftalmologico
De Alicante
Avda Denia 111, 03015
Alicante, Spain

Roberto Pinelli MD
Director
Instituto Laser Microchirurgia
Oculare, Crystal Palace
Via Cefalonia, 70
25124 Brescia, Italy

S Natarajan MS
Chairman and Medical Director
Aditya Jyot Eye Hospital Pvt Ltd
Plot No. 153, Road No. 9
Major Parmeshwaran Road
Opp. SIWS College, Gate No. 3
Wadala, Mumbai-400031, India

Sanjay Chaudhary
New Delhi, India

Sonika Doshi MS
Dr Agarwal's Eye Hospital
19, Cathedral Road
Chennai-600086, India

Soosan Jacob MD DNB FERC
Dr Agarwal's Eye Hospital
19, Cathedral Road
Chennai-600086, India

Srinivas K Rao MD
Department of Ophthalmology
and Visual Sciences
The Chinese University of
Hong Kong
3/F, Hong Kong Eye Hospital
147-L, Argyle Street, Kowloon
HKSAR, PRC

Sunita Agarwal MS DO PSVH
Dr Agarwal's Eye Hospital,
19, Cathedral Road,
Chennai-600086, India
15, Eagle Street, Langford Town,
Bangalore, India

Tahira Agarwal FICS DO FORCE
Dr Agarwal's Eye Hospital
19, Cathedral Road
Chennai-600006, Tamil Nadu
India

Vikentia J Katsanevaki MD PhD
Vardinoyannion Eye Institute
University of Crete, Greece

Vivek Kadambi MD DOMS
Director
Kadambi Laser Vision Clinic and
Research Foundation Pvt. Ltd.
157, Defence Colony
4th Main Road, Indira Nagar
Bangalore-560038, India

Y Ralph Chu MD
Medical Director
Chu Vision Institute
Edina, Minn, USA

Foreword

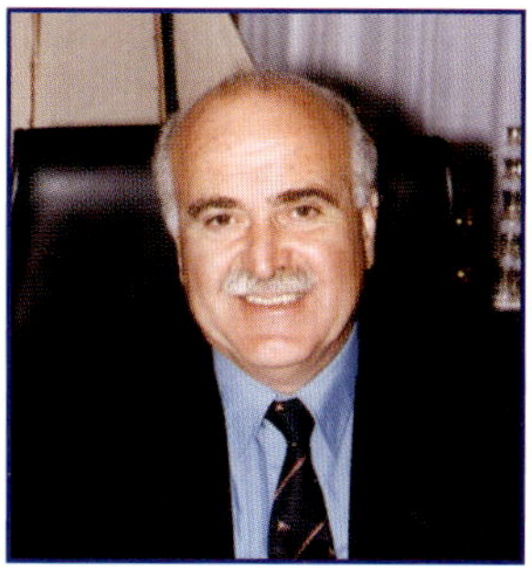

Refractive surgery is a subspecialty of ophthalmology gaining worldwise acceptance rapidly. The introduction of laser in situ keratomileusis (LASIK) in the field of refractive surgery, with the impressive final outcomes (such as quick visual rehabilitation, minimal postoperative discomfort, and the ability to correct high degrees of myopia without postoperative corneal haze) in comparison with previously used techniques, contributed to further acceptance of refractive surgery among patients and doctors.

With accumulated experience and with the application of more sophisticated techniques, the safety and efficacy of refractive surgery has considerably increased during the recent years. In addition, patients' satisfaction and complaints together with the doctor's clinical suggestions are being long-term investigated in order to determine the maximum efficacy after refractive surgery. The initial enthusiasm is replaced by a more systematic approach, which contributes to better results leading to increasing patients' satisfaction and physicians' confidence.

In this concept, this book is timely and concise on the many interesting entities of LASIK technique while the large collection of esteemed authors and chapters stimulate the reader to search in the literature for additional contents. It is thoroughly researched and easy to read. **I would like to congratulate Dr. Garg and the co-editors for their successful work with this book which further contributes in the evolution of the refractive surgery.**

Prof. Ioannis G Pallikaris
Chairman
University of Crete - School of Health Sciences
Institute of Vision and Optics (IVO)
Vardinoyiannion Eye Institute of Crete (VEIC)
GR 71 003 Voutes, Heraklion
Crete - Greece
Tel: +30 2810 392450
Fax: +30 2810 542094
e-mail : pallikar@med.uoc.gr
http://www.ivo.gr

Preface

Rapid strides have been made in the field of Corneal Refractive Surgery in the relatively short span of the last decade. With the advent of new laser machines and techniques a new paradigm shift in ophthalmology was introduced regarding refractive surgery. Excimer Laser Surgery provides an accurate tool to reshape the cornea to correct refractive errors in a successful manner. Ten years ago only Excimer Lasers were available but now Broad beam, Slit beam, Spot Lasers and Solid State Laser have revolutinized the Corneal Refractive Surgery Treatment. The leading factors that have influenced the changing phase of Corneal Refractive Surgery have been knowledge gained from the experience and improvements in technology that have implemented that knowledge. New Wavefront and Topography guided Lasik systems, Epilasik and Lasek techniques that have evolved in recent years have not only helped design better ablation profiles for individual patients but also provided a more objective means of measuring outcome resulting in improved algorithms for future treatments.

This International book contains 46 chapters covering all aspects of practical Lasik, Epilasik and Lasek techniques. A galaxy of top International Lasik Experts have shared their experiences in form of chapters for the benefit of those ophthalmologists who wants to start these techniques in their practice. A video DVD Rom is being given with this book showing latest Lasik, Epilasik and Lasek techniques by International Masters of this field.

Our special gratitude to M/s Jaypee Brothers Medical Publishers Pvt. Ltd. specially Shri Jitendar P Vij (CEO), Mr. Tarun Duneja (General Manager – Publishing) and all staff members who worked hard to publish this book in a short span of time.

As the clinical practice of Lasik, Epilasik and Lasek is on the rise worldwide, we are hopeful that this book shall provide useful practical tips and guidance to every interested ophthalmologist.

Editors

Contents

SECTION I: PREOPERATIVE EVALUATION AND MACHINES DYNAMICS

SECTION II: LASIK, EPILASIK AND LASEK SURGICAL TECHNIQUES

SECTION III: COMPLICATIONS AND THEIR MANAGEMENT

SECTION IV: RECENT ADVANCES AND FUTURE PROSPECTS

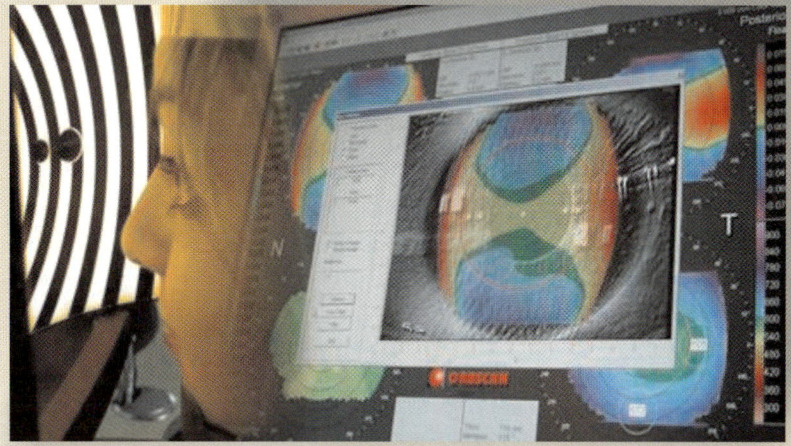

Preoperative Evaluation and Machines Dynamics

SECTION ONE

Fundamentals in Corneal Topography

1

FRANCISCO ARNALICH, DAVID PIÑERO, JORGE L ALIÓ (SPAIN)

INTRODUCTION TO CORNEAL TOPOGRAPHY

Corneal topography is a noninvasive imaging technique for mapping the anterior surface of the cornea. Taking into account that the cornea is responsible for over two thirds of the total eye's refractive power, its shape is of critical importance in determining the quality of the ocular optical system and therefore the quality of vision. Very small changes in corneal shape resulting from surgery or disease can have a dramatic effect on the focus of the retinal image. For this reason, understanding and quantifying corneal contour has become an essential preoperative measurement for designing surgical intervention in refractive surgery, for assessing the outcomes of keratoplasty, as well as corneal transplantation, or for evaluating the optical performance of the eye. Different methods for measuring corneal topography have been developed along several centuries, depending on the incoming advances of technology.

Different features used to characterize optical properties of the cornea must be introduced in advance:

Height or Elevation

Distance of each point of a surface from a reference surface (Fig. 1.1). Fine details of the cornea can be obtained by taking the sphere as the reference surface.

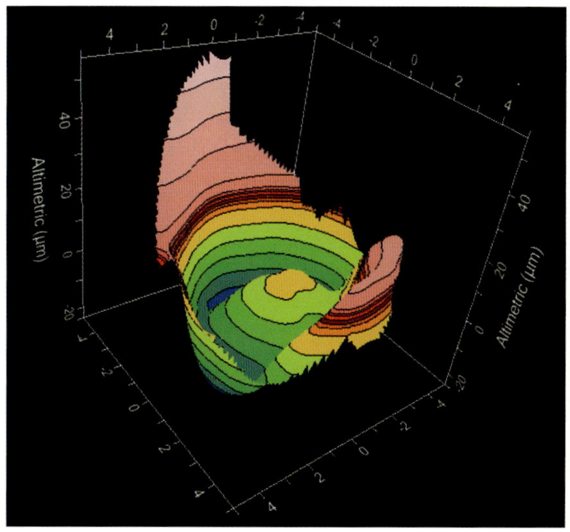

Fig. 1.1: Elevation of the anterior surface of a cornea from a perfect sphere

Once the shape of the corneal surface has been expressed in terms of height, other parameters such as slope, curvature and power can be calculated from it.

Radius of Curvature

The radius of curvature is usually expressed in millimeters and it is a way of characterizing the curvature of the anterior surface of the cornea. Corneas with a steep surface slope have a small radius of curvature while those with a flatter surface slope have a larger radius of curvature.

Power

The power is an optical property expressed in diopters (D) that depends on the shape of the surfaces and the variation of refractive index between both sides of the surface. The keratometric diopter is calculated using the radius of curvature and the standard keratometric index of refraction (SKI = 1.3375), an approximation derived from some assumptions. We can express this relation with the following formula:

$$P(D) = \frac{SKI - 1}{r} = \frac{337{,}5}{r(mm)}$$

The evolution of the quantitative assessment of the anterior corneal curvature has been progressive and its range of measurement has been extended from the four points a few millimeters apart measured by keratometers to a grid of thousands of points covering almost the entire cornea measured by computerized corneal topography.

Corneal Shape

The cornea is an optical structure of the eye characterized by its transparency and it is formed by two surfaces. The average anterior and posterior corneal power are + 48.6 D and - 6.8 D respectively. To simplify this model in clinical practice, we consider only one refractive surface with a resulting corneal power of about 42-44 keratometric diopters.

Normal corneas have some interesting features:

- Viewed from the front, the cornea is slightly oval with vertical and horizontal diameters of approximately 11 and 12 mm respectively.
- It has an average apical radius of curvature of about 7.8 mm, with a normal range of 7-8.5 mm.
- The average corneal keratometry profile changes little with age. It has been stated that the cornea flattens about 0.5 D by the age of 30 years and it steepens about 1 D by the age of 70 years. During adulthood, the horizontal radius is usually 0.05-0.25 mm flatter than the vertical, which contributes to higher incidence of with the rule astigmatism in young adults. This difference between curvatures of vertical and horizontal meridians decreases with age, finally disappearing at the age of 70 years. The higher incidence of against the rule astigmatisms at advanced ages is mainly explained by the lenticular changes.
- The normal cornea flattens progressively from the center to the periphery by 2-4 D (Fig. 1.2), with a more pronounced flattening of the nasal area than the temporal area. This gives to the anterior corneal surface an aspherical configuration and it

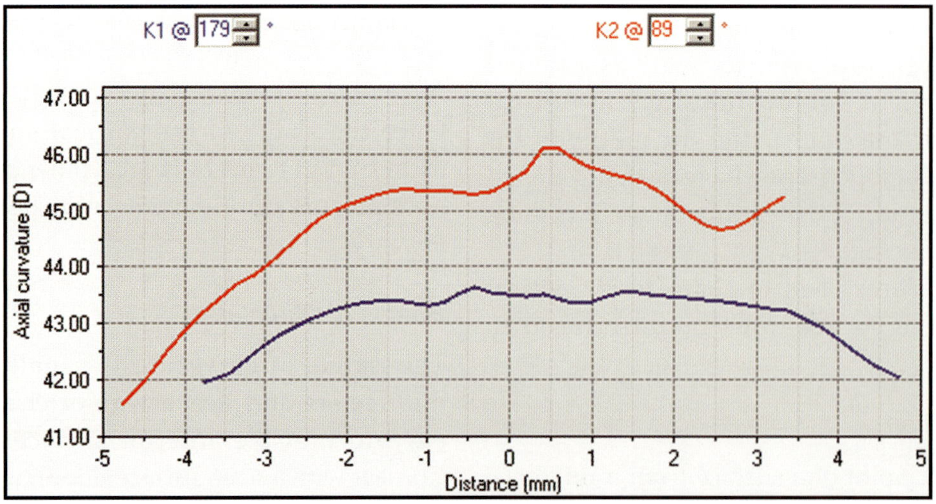

Fig. 1.2: Profile of the steepest and flattest meridian of a cornea (progressive flattening toward the periphery)

is assumed to have a conic section. This model could be represented by means of this equation:

$$X^2 + Y^2 + (1+Q)Z^2 - 2RZ = 0,$$

where the Z axis is the axis of revolution of the conic, R is the radius at the corneal apex, and Q is the asphericity, a parameter used to specify the type of conicoid. This parameter (Q) can take different values giving the following different kind of configurations (Fig. 1.3):

- $Q = 0$: Perfect spherical surface
- $Q > 0$: Oblate surface, ellipsoid with major axis in X-Y plane
- $(-1) < Q < 0$: Prolate surface, ellipsoid with major axis in Z direction
- $Q = -1$: Paraboloid configuration
- $Q < -1$: Hyperboloid configuration

Several studies have checked that the anterior corneal configuration tends to be prolate. This means negative asphericity values, ranging normal values from -0.26 to -0.11, depending on the study considered.

In a map with a color-coded power scale (corneal topographic map), we can see how the dioptric power declines towards the periphery (Fig. 1.4). Depending on how the dioptric power declines, we can recognise five different normal topographic patterns. The approximate distribution of keratographic patterns described in normal eyes includes the following:

- Round: 23% (Fig. 1.5)
- Oval: 21% (Fig. 1.6)
- Symmetric bow tie: 18%
- Asymmetric bow tie: 32% (Fig. 1.7)
- Irregular: 7% (Fig. 1.8)

The bow tie configuration represents the existence of corneal astigmatism. The localization of the steepest axis defines against-the-rule astigmatism (horizontal axis) (Fig. 1.9), with-the-rule astigmatism (vertical axis) (Fig. 1.10), or oblique astigmatism (near meridian angle 45° or 135°) (Fig. 1.11).

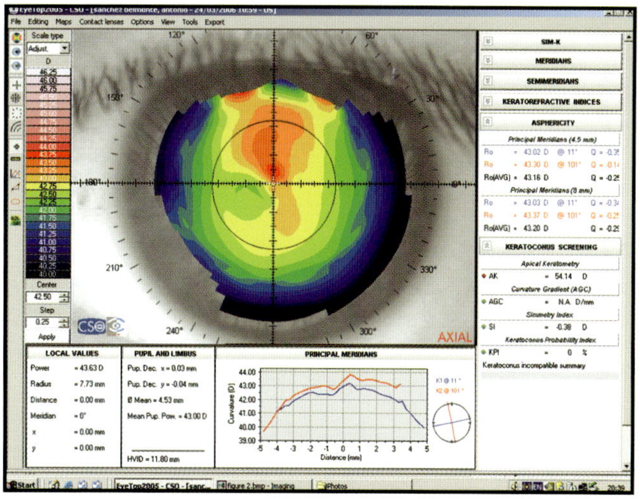

Fig. 1.4: Topographic pattern of a normal cornea, a prolate cornea

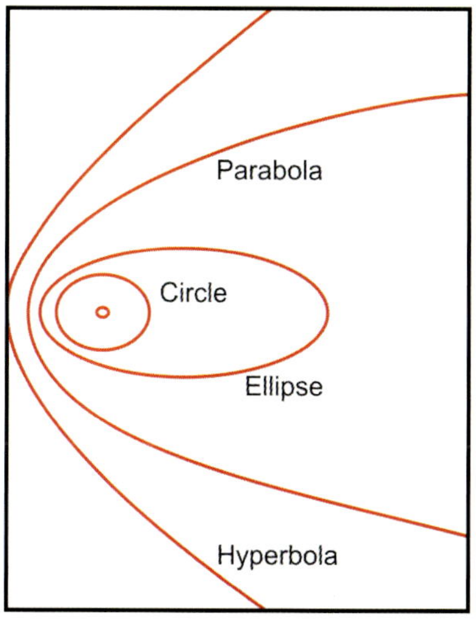

Fig. 1.3: Different kind of configurations of a surface

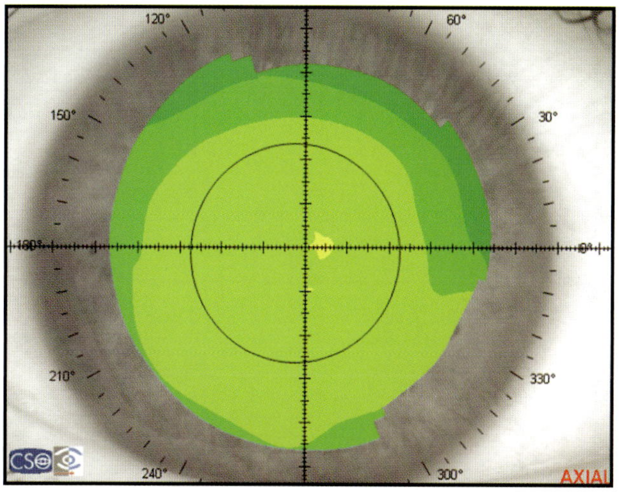

Fig. 1.5: Round topographic pattern

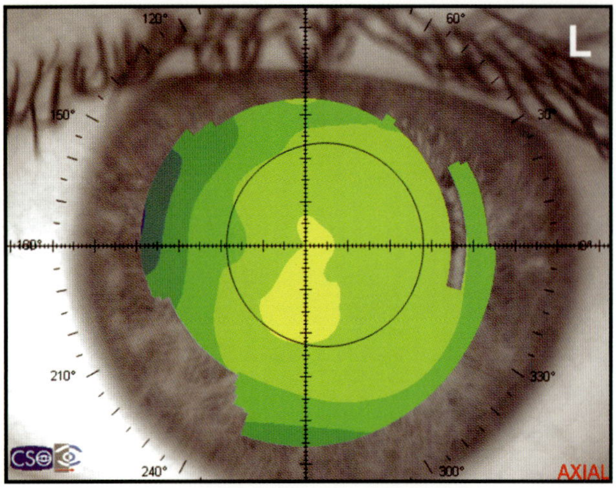

Fig. 1.6: Oval topographic pattern

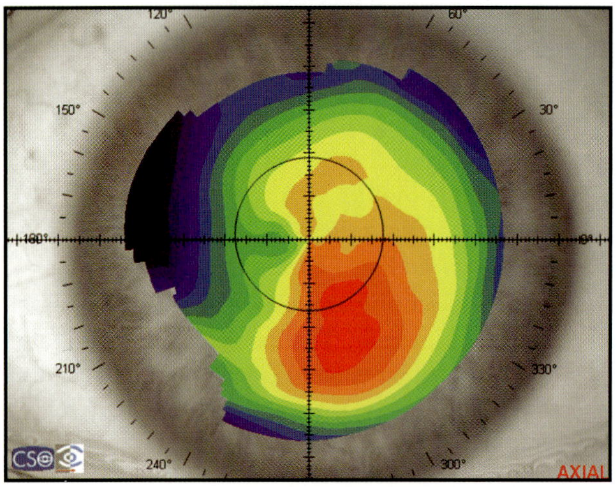

Fig. 1.7: Asymmetric bow tie topographic pattern

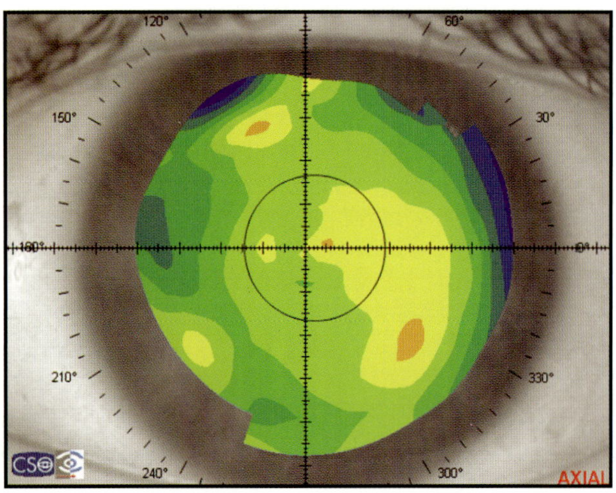

Fig. 1.8: Irregular topographic pattern

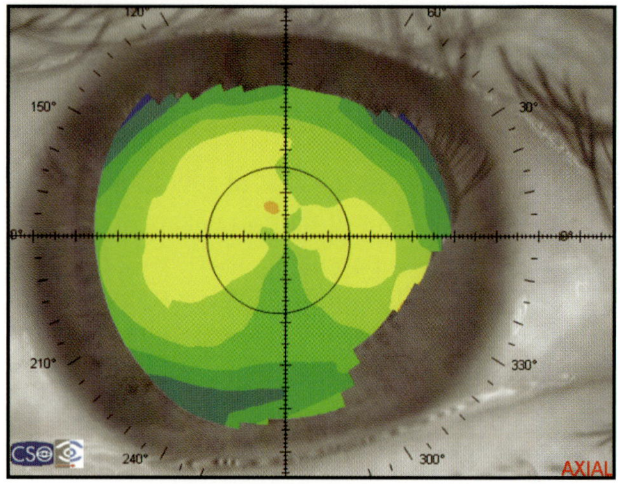

Fig. 1.9: Symmetric bow tie, showing an against-the-rule astigmatism

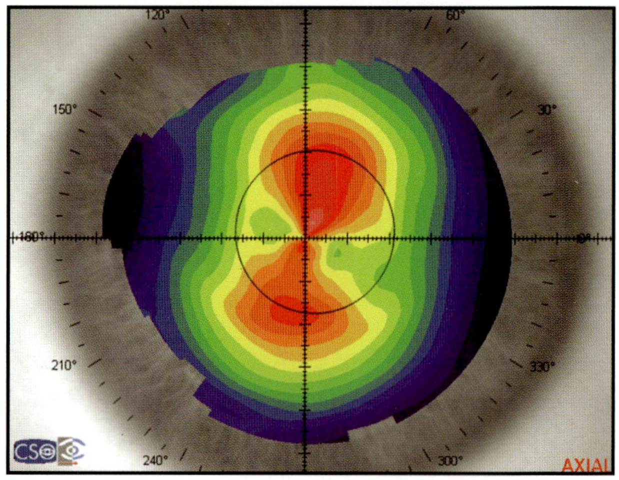

Fig. 1.10: Symmetric bow tie, showing a with-the-rule astigmatism

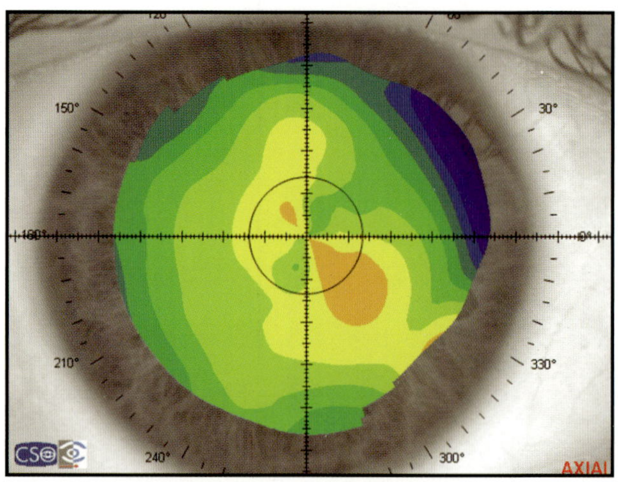

Fig. 1.11: Symmetric bow tie, showing an oblique astigmatism

Corneal Topography Technology: Evolution

Corneal topography has been used to measure the anterior surface of the human cornea to detect and diagnose pathological conditions, plan refractive surgery, and fit contact lenses.

Scheiner in 1619 was the first in analysing corneal curvature by matching the image of a window frame reflected from a subject's cornea with that produced by one of his calibrated spheres.

Following this basis and using the ability of the anterior corneal surface to behave as a convex mirror, in 1854 Helmholtz created the first true keratometer, also called ophthalmometer. Before this, some authors (Mandell, Ramsden, Kohlrausch) had tried to developed an apparatus for determining corneal curvature, creating some kind of prototypes. The Helmholtz keratometer projects four points onto the cornea, creating a reflected image, which can be analysed and converted to corneal radius data by using an equation that considers distance from mire to cornea, image and mire size. In 1881, Javal and Schiotz improved Helmholtz laboratory apparatus and built an ophthalmometer designed for clinical use (Fig. 1.12). Although keratometers are still used commonly in clinical practice, it has important limitations:

- It performs measurements of the central 3 mm, accounting only for 6% of the corneal surface.
- It assumes that the cornea has a perfect spherocylindrical shape, which is not true.
- Information from periphery is not provided.
- It gives no information of the central zone inside the four points measured.

The keratoscope let us examine a much greater area of the cornea. Clinical keratoscopy has been used since 1870, when Placido studied the corneal surface by observing the corneal reflections of a series of illuminated concentric rings (known as Placido's rings) (Fig. 1.13). In 1896 Allvar Gullstrand incorporated the disk in a self-developed instrument for examining photographs of the cornea by a means of a microscope and calculating corneal curvature by means of a numerical algorithm. Depending on the distance between the concentric rings, the examiner can evaluate qualitatively the corneal shape. A steep area of the cornea causes a crowding of the mires at this area, while a flat cornea makes the opposite effect. Irregularity of the surface is seen as mire distortion.

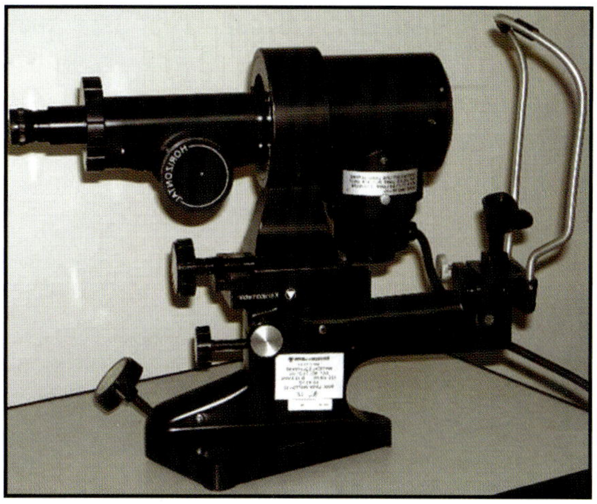

Fig. 1.12: Nowadays available keratometer

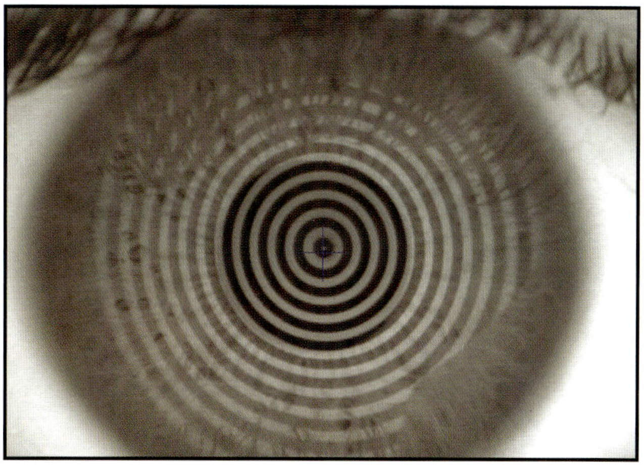

Fig. 1.13: Projection of Placido rings

In the 1980s, photographs of the projected images were hand-digitalized and then analysed by a computer. However, the automation of process and the image capture by a digital camera became soon a reality. Advances in video and personal computer technology made it possible to instantaneously acquire and analyze high quality images. These improvements made quantitative keratoscopy practical for routine clinical use. The Corneal Modeling System (CMS) produced by Computed Anatomy became the first widely used computerized videokeratoscope.

In an effort to improve accuracy and avoid the assumptions necessary for computerized videokeratoscopy, new technologies (projection systems) have appeared commercially in the last years, such as rastereography, laser interferometry, Moiré interference and slit-scan systems (Fig. 1.14). These systems directly measure the true shape of the anterior corneal surface in terms of height, not from curvature. From these measurements slope, curvature and power can be calculated.

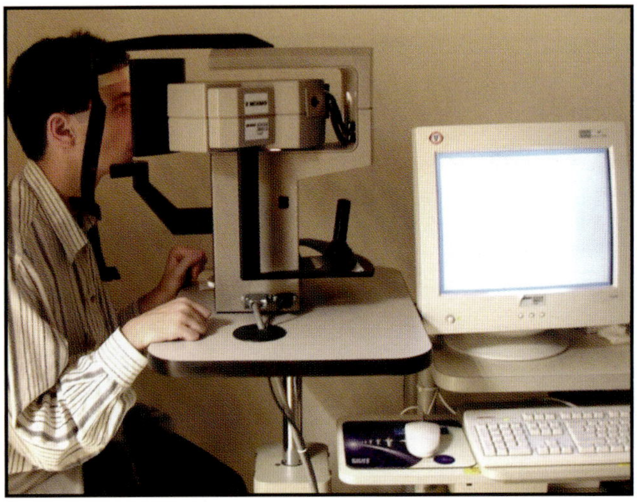

Fig. 1.14: A slit-scan system: Orbscan II

Measurement Procedure

Corneal topography is a noninvasive method for determining the shape of the cornea. Each one of the commercially available devices has a specific method of operation, although some aspects are common.

Placido-based Systems

The Placido-based systems require an intact epithelial surface and tear film in order to obtain accurate and reliable measurements. The patient is sat facing a bowl containing the projected pattern which is focused on the anterior surface of the patient's cornea. The pattern reflected off from the cornea is analysed by a computer that provides data about the geometric configuration of the cornea in different kind of numerical and graphical formats.

Some of the errors that examiner can make using a Placido-based system are the following: focusing errors (Fig. 1.15), alignment (Fig. 1.16) and fixation errors (that could induce wrong levels of astigmatisms), wrong calculation of the position of the center from the small central rings, increased inaccuracy toward the periphery due to the lack of accuracy of the preceding points. We can conclude that critical points for a precise measurement are accurate alignment, centring and focusing. These issues depend on the ability of the examiner to take a good measurement.

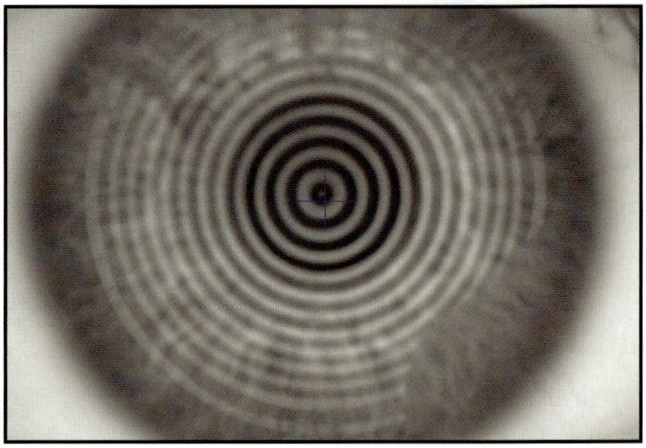

Fig. 1.15: Lack of focus of the Placido rings image

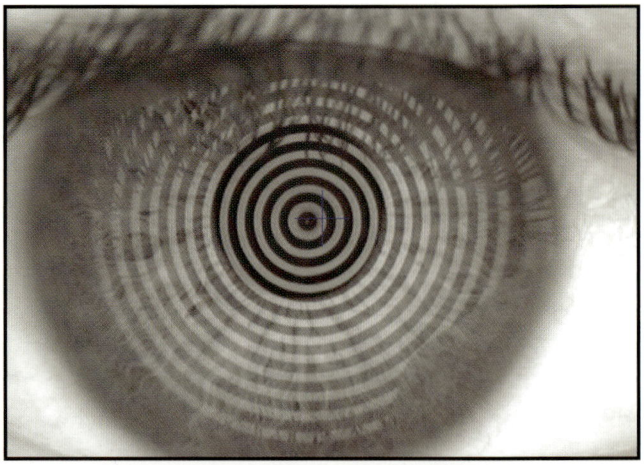

Fig. 1.16: Alignment error during corneal topography examination

There is another potential source of errors. It is essential for obtaining a good exam that the tear film forms a smooth layer over the irregular corneal epithelium. Tear film break-up causes mistracking of the mires and artifacts in the corneal map that appears as irregularity areas or false irregular astigmatism. For example, a dry patch could be associated with an area of focal flattening in the corneal map (Fig. 1.17). In order to avoid disturbing of the tear film, corneal topography should be performed before giving dilating drops and taking intraocular pressures.

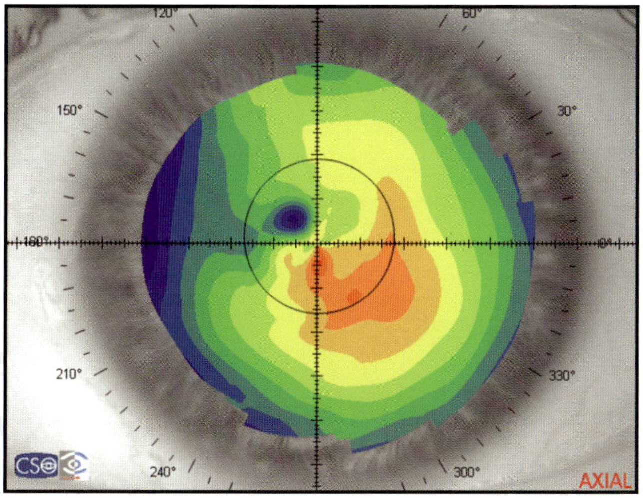

Fig. 1.17: Dry patch associated with an area of focal flattening

In addition, there are a variety of complex surfaces that are very difficult to characterize. Errors greater than 4 D may occur in very steep or flat corneas, keratoconus with local steepening, sharp transition zones after uncomplicated refractive surgeries, diffusely irregular surfaces after penetrating keratoplasty, and complex surfaces after decentered ablations in refractive surgery or central islands. These complex cases may be easily identified on the raw image of the Placido rings projected onto the cornea. When there are abnormalities in tear film break up, the raw image is also very valuable.

The presence of areas which are not analysed on the corneal maps may be due to the configuration of the nose or the position of the eyelids (Fig. 1.18). To avoid these artifacts, it is important to instruct the patient to keep the eyes wide open and to maintain a good position and fixation.

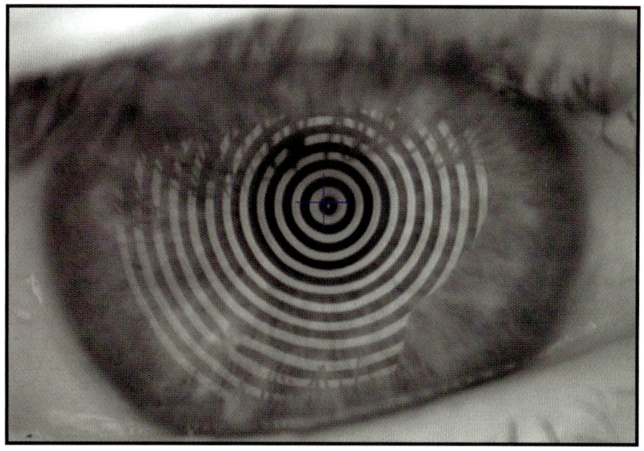

Fig. 1.18: Incomplete corneal image due to the position of the eyelids (not wide opened)

Non Placido-based Systems

The accuracy and reproducibility of rastereography system is in the range of Placido-based system, but the advantage is that the former do not require an intact epithelial surface. A rastereography system projects a grid of known geometry onto the cornea through a cobalt blue filter. Topical fluorescein is used to stain the tear film. Then, the system calculates elevation or height by evaluating the distortion of the grid lines. From elevation data obtained across the full corneal surface, curvature data is derived by means of a specific algorithm.

In the slit-scan systems, a slit is projected sequentially onto the cornea at different angles. This is the basis used by the Orbscan corneal topography system. A high-resolution video camera captures 40 light slits projected onto the cornea. The diffuse reflection is obtained from the cornea, iris, and lens. By triangulation, data is obtained from the anterior and posterior surfaces of the cornea and from other structures. These issues permits this instruments to calculate anterior chamber depth or full pachymetry of the cornea. The accuracy and repeatability of this instrument is reported to be below 10 μ and it is significantly dependent on many factors, such as movement of the patient's eye, stability of tear film, ability of patients to keep the eyes wide open, corneal transparency, and the presence of corneal abnormalities. One of the limitations of slit-scan system is the longer time of image acquisition in comparison with any of the other commercially available instruments. In the other hand, it brings the possibility to characterize the posterior corneal surface. This issue is important for the detection of incipient keratoconus conditions.

ANALYSIS OF THE CORNEAL TOPOGRAPHY DATA: CORNEAL MAPS, DESCRIPTORS AND INDEXES

Corneal topography provides a great amount of information regarding the corneal surface. By representing this data as a colour-coded map, an experienced clinician can quickly evaluate corneal shape and other features closely associated with shape. A corneal map has a color scale that assigns particular color to certain keratometric dioptric range. Steep areas normally are represented by warm colors (red and orange) while flat areas are represented by cool colors (green and blue) (Fig. 1.19).

Before examining the color-coded map, it is critical to check the raw image of Placido rings projected on the cornea. It is important to confirm that the unprocessed data is reliable, as further analysis is

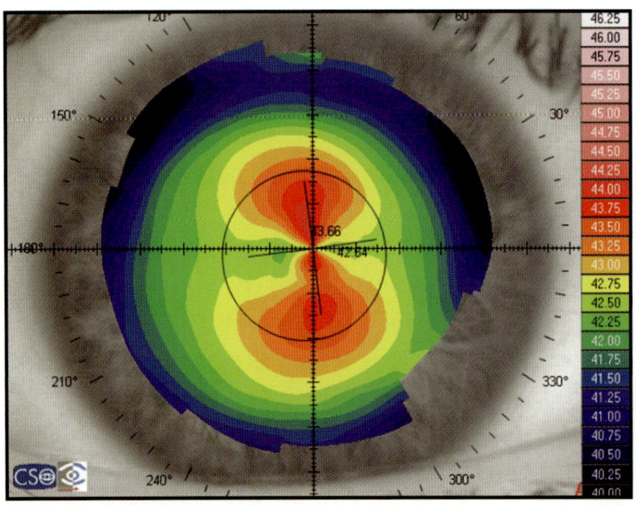

Fig. 1.19: Corneal map with color scale

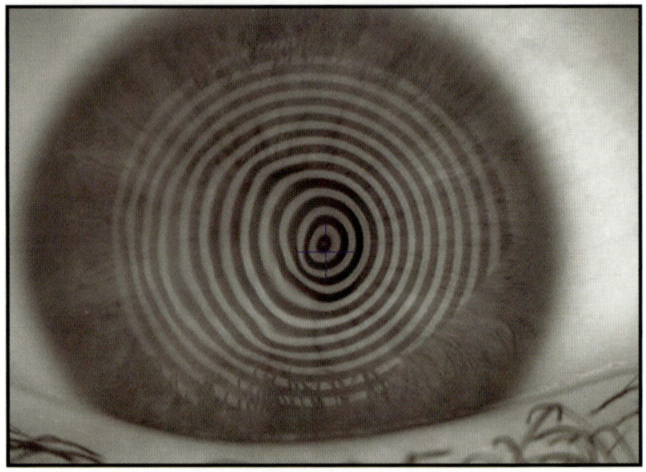

Fig. 1.20: Irregular videokeratoscope image due to the presence of a leukoma

based on these data (Fig. 1.20). If an irregular videokeratoscope image is present, it can lead to wrong interpretation of the corneal map. Therefore it is necessary to find out the causes of this special corneal configuration to avoid misleading information.

Topographic Displays: Corneal Maps

There are different kinds of maps that provide different data from the same corneal shape. Each one of them has its own indications and limitations:

- *Axial or sagital map (Fig. 1.21A)*: Despite its limitations, it remains the most widely recognized map because it is easy to understand. Colors visually correspond to flatness and steepness. The axial map measures the radius of curvature supposing a center of rotation on the axis of the videokeratoscope (the center of curvature of all the points of the particular surface lies on the same axis). It provides a general view of the curvature profile of the cornea, but the localized changes in curvature and peripheral data are poorly represented.
- *Instantaneous or tangential map (Fig. 1.21B)*: It is more sensitive and represents local changes and peripheral data much better than axial maps do. The radius of curvature is calculated by referring to its neighbouring points, not to the axis of the

videokeratoscope. These maps best identify corneal pathology such as ectatic disorders or surgically induced changes.

- *Refractive map (Fig. 1.21C)*: It is useful when assessing the visual performance of a patient, for example after refractive surgery. It is calculated based on Snell's law of refraction, assuming optical infinity.
- *Elevation or height map (Fig. 1.21D)*: It displays corneal height or elevation relative to a reference plane with a presumed assumption of the shape, which may be the best-fit sphere, best-fit asphere, average corneal shape, or even based on preoperative data. The same surface may appear different when it is mapped against different reference surfaces. Points above the reference surface are positive (hot colors) and points below the reference surface are negative (cool colors). It is very useful in detecting local irregularities, corneal ectatic diseases, or surgically induced changes.
- Irregularity map: It is similar to an elevation map, but it uses the best fit toric surface as reference.
- Difference map: It shows the change in curvature or any other parameter between two maps (Fig. 1.22).

Depending on the kind of software associated to the videokeratocope, several other displays may be available as three dimensional maps (Fig. 1.23), relative maps, numerical views, profile views, etc.

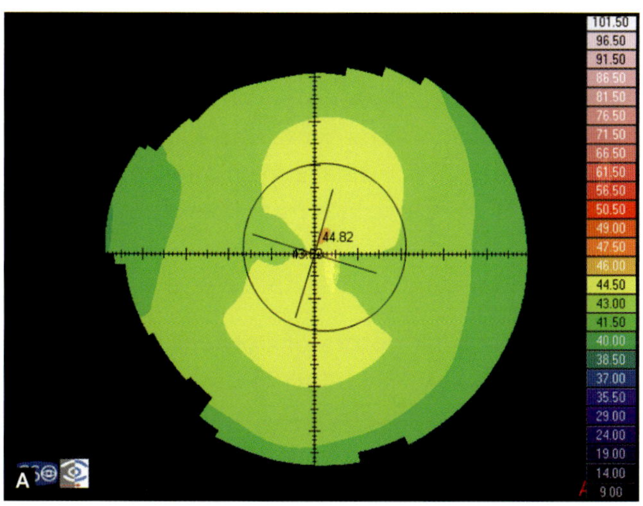

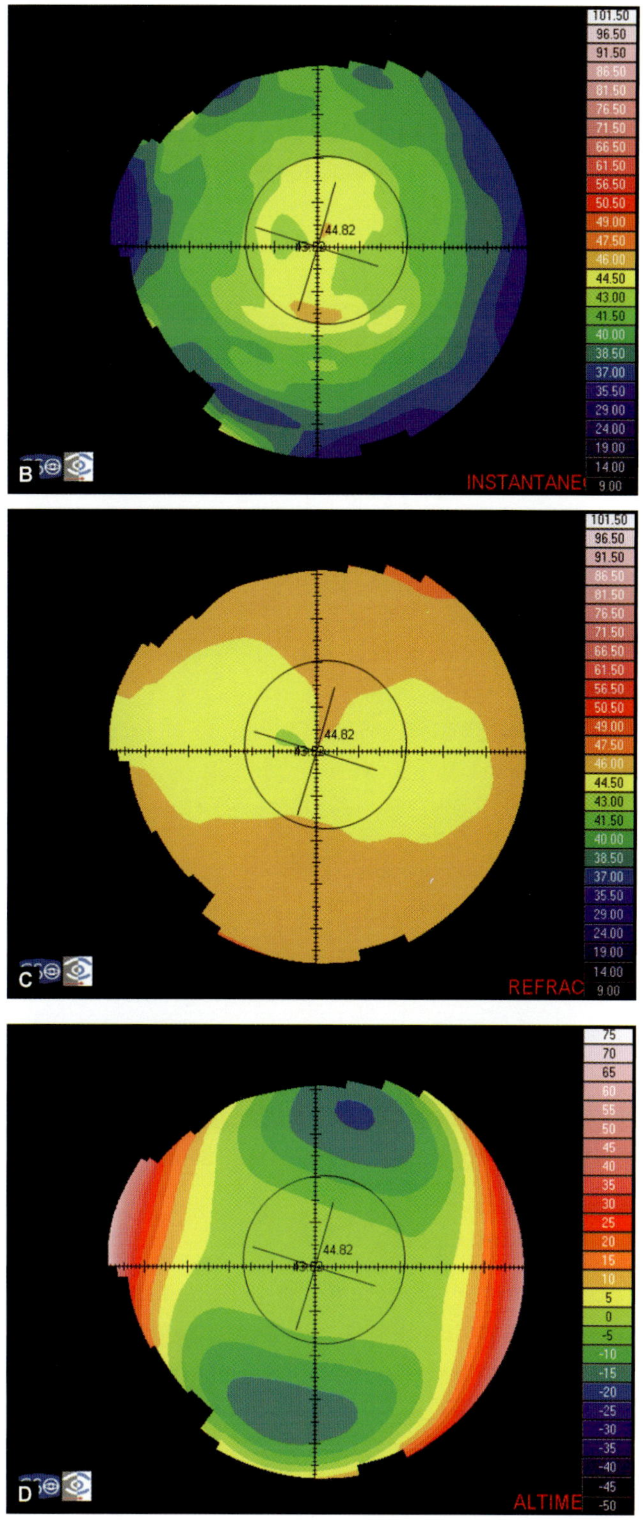

Figs 1.22A to D: Corneal topography analysed using different kind of maps: (A) Axial map, (B) Instantaneous map, (C) Refractive map, and (D) Elevation map

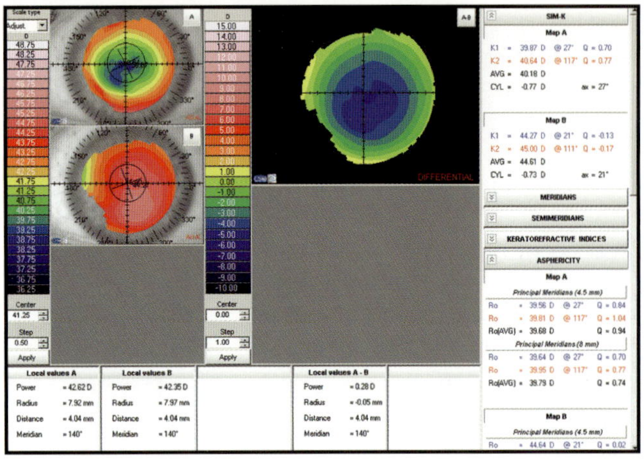

Fig. 1.22: Difference map showing the effect of a myopic LASIK treatment

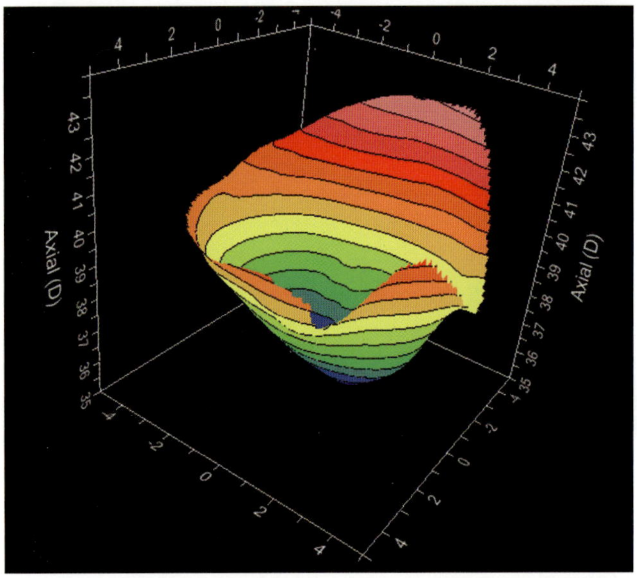

Fig. 1.23: Three dimensional map

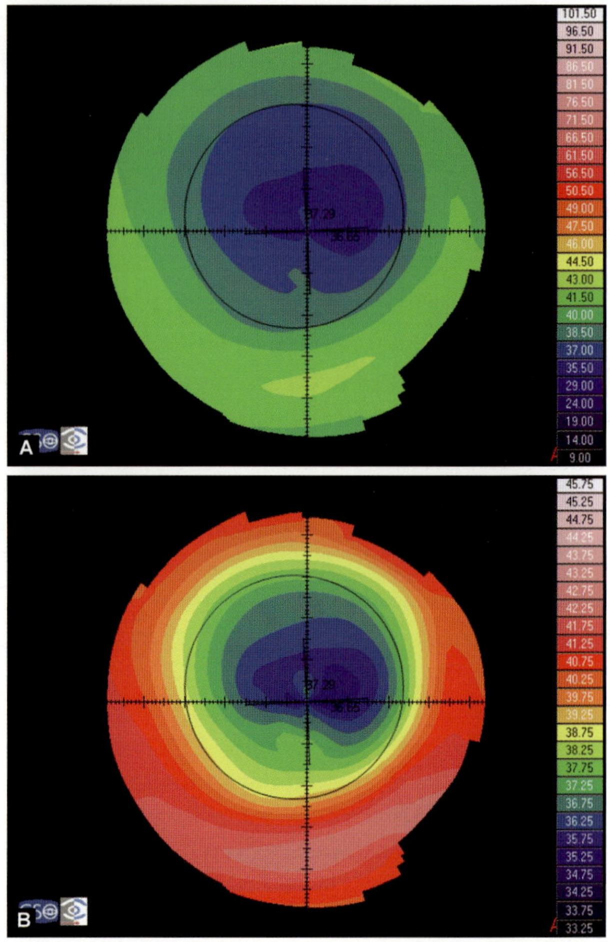

Figs 1.24A and B: Axial map of a post-myopic LASIK using: (A) an absoluted or fixed scale, and (B) a normalized or variable scale

Color-Coded Scales

It is important when reading a corneal map to take into consideration the type of scale used. We cannot compare maps with different scales because it could lead us to a wrong clinical decision.

Absolute or fixed scale (Fig. 1.24A) uses the same color for the same curvature or elevation no matter what eye is examined. These maps allow direct comparison of two different maps buy it does not discriminate subtle changes of curvature.

Normalized or variable scale (Fig. 1.24B) uses a given color for different curvatures or elevations on each cornea analysed, depending on the range for that particular cornea, determined by its flattest and steepest values. Maps with this scale cannot be compared directly and have to be interpreted based on the keratometric values from their different color scales. An advantage of this kind of scale is that it shows a more detailed description of the surface.

Quantitative Descriptors of Corneal Topography: Corneal Indexes

Computerized topography systems provide also a variety of numerical descriptors, usually called corneal indexes. These indexes are used to describe quantitatively different features of corneal topography. The most important ones are described below:

Simulated keratometry (SimK): It characterizes corneal curvature in the central area, correlating well with the measurements provided by the classic keratometer. It calculates the power and axis of the steepest meridian (K1) and the flattest meridian (K2), as well as the cylinder value (difference between K1 and K2).

Average corneal power: It is an area-corrected average of corneal power and it could be useful in the calculation of the appropriate intraocular lens.

Corneal asphericity (Q): It represents how much the curvature varies from the centre to the periphery of the cornea. A normal cornea tends to be prolate (becomes flatter toward the periphery). A prolate surface corresponds with negative Q values, whereas an oblate surface is represented by positive values of Q.

Shape factor (SF): It is another way of calculating corneal asphericity. It is calculated with the square of the value of the eccentricity, which can be obtained from the equation of the mathematical description of anterior corneal surface. The normal value ranges from 0.13 to 0.35 and it results negative after a myopic keratorefractive procedure.

Eccentricity This parameter has different names depending on the instrument considered. It characterizes the shape of the anterior corneal surface: a positive value is for prolate corneas, negative for oblates corneas, and zero for an ideal perfect spherical cornea. Average value in normal corneas is around 0.5.

There are some indexes that are specific of some kind of commercially available instruments. These indexes can be used in clinical practice as different mathematical estimates of the visual disturbance that can be expected to be caused by the amount of irregularities of the anterior corneal surface. Below we list some of them:

Surface regularity index (SRI): It is a measurement of the regularity of the corneal surface and it is higher as irregularity increases. Normal values are below one.

Potential visual acuity (PVA): It is an estimation of the expected visual acuity that is achievable based on corneal topography data.

Surface asymmetry index (SAI): It measures the difference between points located 180^a apart in a great number of equally space meridians. The more asymmetric the cornea is, the more SAI differs from zero.

Indexes for the detection of keratoconus: Several mathematical algorithms have been developed to aid detecting different states of keratoconus condition with high sensitivity and specificity. Some of them are the I-S value, the Differential Sector Index (DSI), the Opposite Sector Index (OSI), the Irregular Astigmatism Index (IAI), etc.

CLINICAL APPLICATIONS OF CORNEAL TOPOGRAPHY

The Assessment of the Refractive Patient

Corneal topography is mandatory in a refractive surgery setting:

a. Preoperatively, to screen for irregular astigmatism, ectatic corneal disorders, and other abnormalities, and to monitor topographic stability following discontinuation of contact lens wear.
b. Operatively, to determine surgical parameters (e.g., microkeratome settings) and to perform customized corneal ablations using topographic data.
c. Postoperatively, to monitor and assess the surgical outcomes, detect the causes of visual complaints such as blurred vision, glare, or diplopia, and to assist the surgeon in correcting undesirable postoperative results when planning retreatment, as in decentered ablations, asymmetric healing, etc. However, recent studies show that corneal wavefront-guided procedures may provide better outcomes.

Preoperative Evaluation

Detecting Irregular Astigmatism

Irregular astigmatism occurs when the principal meridians are not orthogonal or perpendicular to each other or when there are other rotational asymmetries that are not correctable with the conventional sphero-cylindrical lenses (Fig. 1.25). Corneal topography, especially photokeratoscope view and tangential map, plays a critical role in the detection of preoperative corneal irregular astigmatism.

Common causes of corneal irregular astigmatism include dry eye, corneal scars, ectatic corneal degenerations, trauma, pterygium, and surgery. Some causes of corneal irregularity may be discovered just with careful inspection of the photokeratoscope view showing irregular mires as in poor quality of tear film, subtle corneal scar, or epithelial basement membrane degeneration. The latter is a risk factor for corneal ecstasies after refractive surgery.

Minor degrees of irregular astigmatism are not uncommon and would not contraindicate standard refractive surgery. However, significant amount of irregular astigmatism can limit surgical outcomes due to poor predictability. Surgeons should be especially aware when dealing with rigid contact lens wearers who expect final uncorrected visual acuity to be similar to their previous best corrected visual acuity, as well as in patients who state that their vision with rigid lenses is significantly better than with spectacles.

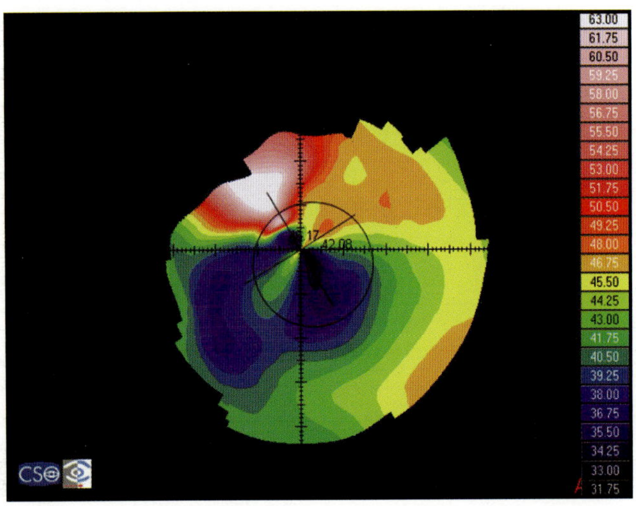

Fig. 1.25: Irregular astigmatism

Ensuring Refractive and Topographic Stability following Discontinuation of Contact Lens Wear

Corneal topography is essential for monitoring corneal topographic changes after discontinuation of contact lens wear to ensure stability before surgery. Contact lens should be discontinued prior to the topographic and refractive examination for the following durations: 5-7 days for standard soft lenses, 10-14 days for toric soft lenses, 2 weeks for rigid gas permeable lenses (RGP), and at least 1 month for polymethylmethacrylate lenses (PMMA). It is well understood that corneal refractive procedures should be deferred until the cornea returns to its baseline topographic state.

Contact lens wear can alter the shape of the cornea and induce corneal warpage (Fig. 1.26). Corneal warpage occurs more frequently in wearers of hard PMMA contact lenses or RGP contact lenses as a result of the mechanical pressure exerted by the lens, and corneal hypoxia.

There are at least four different forms of noticeable topographic changes that usually occur mixed with one or more of the other forms:

1. *Peripheral steepening*. Surgeons must be aware of inferior corneal steepening (*pseudokeratoconus*) that resembles keratoconus. It is caused by a superiorly riding contact lens. In corneal warpage, the shape indexes do not indicate any keratoconic condition, and the flat K is not as steep as in keratoconus.

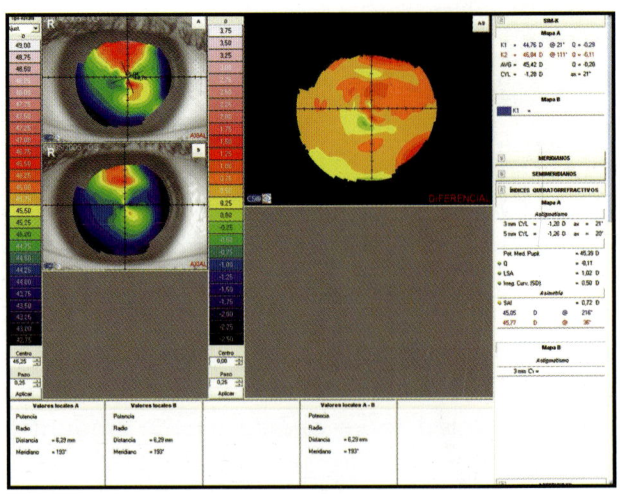

Fig. 1.26: Difference map showing a general flattening induced by a RGP contact lens

2. *Central flattening*, that may be overlooked because the topography tends to look normal and symmetrical. Improper focusing can simulate central flattening, so checking photokeratoscope view seems necessary.
3. *Furrow depression*, because of flattening under the edge of the contact lens. It is best seen with decentred rigid or hard lenses where the lens rides high or low in the stable resting position.
4. *Central molding or central irregularity*. It is seen as a steepening under the region covered by the centre of the lens, and it is always irregular or patchy in appearance.

Ruling out Keratoconus and Other Ectatic Corneal Disorders

Ectatic corneal disorders, such as keratoconus (Fig. 1.27), pellucid marginal degeneration (Fig. 1.28), and keratoglobus, are considered contraindications to corneal refractive surgery. Corneal topography is of great importance in detecting these disorders.

Although keratoconus can be detected by qualitative methods, early or subclinical keratoconus are usually missed. Modern corneal topographers usually include software to predict the presence of keratoconus by quantitative methods in a more sensitive and specific way. Special effort is made in seeking for early keratoconus or "forme fruste keratoconus", considered a contraindication to LASIK due to possible evolution into clinically significant keratoconus within months or years after the surgery.

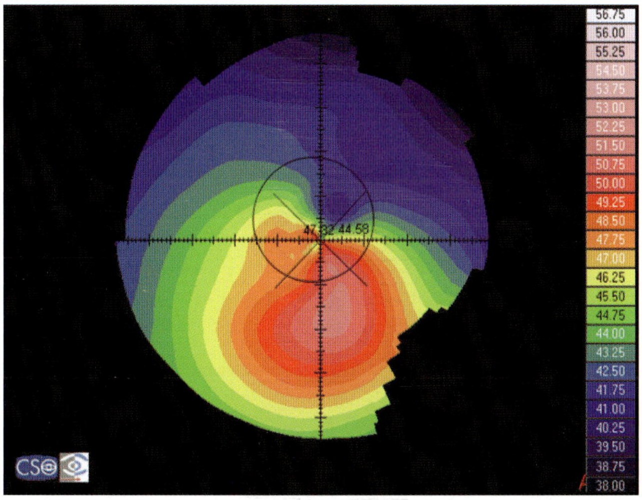

Fig. 1.27: Corneal topography in keratoconus

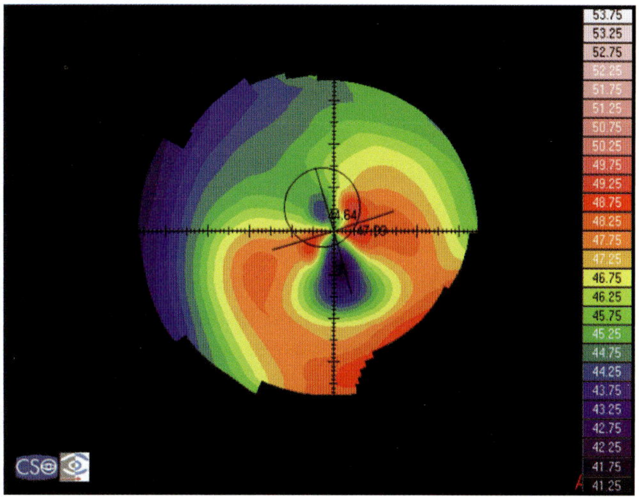

Fig. 1.28: Corneal topography in pellucid marginal degeneration

Rabinowitz and Mc Donnell developed the first numerical method for detecting keratoconus using only topographic data. They established three criteria to determine whether the patient has keratoconus or not:

- The I-S value, which measures the differences between the superior and inferior paracentral corneal regions(3 mm above or below the corneal center).
- The maximum central corneal power (Max K)
- The power difference between both eyes.

They obtained the following results:

- Keratoconus suspect: Central corneal power > 47.2 D or I-S > 1.4.
- Clinical Keratoconus: Central corneal power > 47.8 D or I-S > 1.9.
- Normal subjects had a power difference between the two eyes < 0.5 D

However, using only these simple measurements for keratoconus diagnosis presents specificity problems.

To solve the specificity problem, the new strategy must be able to detect and consider the unique characteristics of keratoconus maps, such as local abnormal elevations. The **Keratoconus Prediction Index**, developed by Maeda et al, is calculated from the Differential Sector Index (DSI), the Opposite Sector Index (OSI), the Centre/Surround Index (CSI), the SAI, the Irregular Astigmatism Index (IAI), and the percent Analyzed Area (AA). This method partially overcomes the specificity limitation.

Maeda et al also developed the **neural network model**, based on artificial intelligence. It is a much more sophisticated method for classifying corneal topography and detecting different corneal topographic abnormalities; it employs indexes that were empirically found to capture specific characteristics of the different corneal pathologies, including keratoconus. Further modifications in neural network approach developed by Smolek and Klyce supposedly produce 100% accuracy, specificity and sensitivity in diagnosing keratoconus.

Newer approaches for detecting early keratoconus (Fig. 1.29) and increased risk of ectasia after refractive surgery include patterns and indices based on the anterior or posterior elevation best fit sphere maps, obtained from Orbscan®. However, further studies are needed to assess the performance of the topography elevation criteria in detecting keratoconus. It is known that the cone of the keratoconic cornea appears as an area of increased elevation surrounded by concentric zones of decreasing elevation. Two indices have been

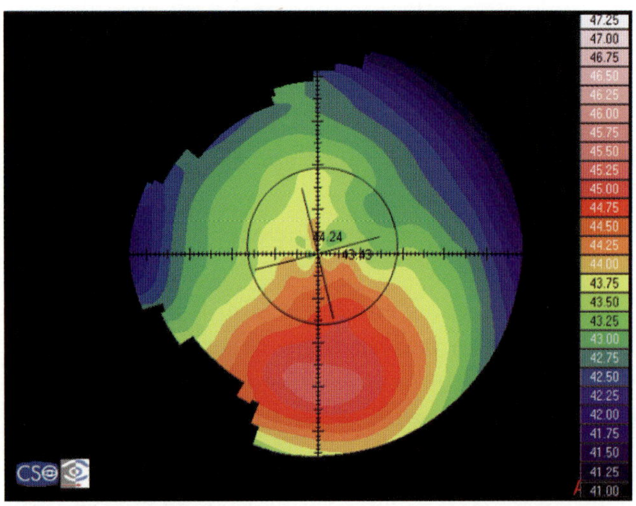

Fig. 1.29: Keratoconus suspect

proposed to screen keratoconic corneas based on the Orbscan system:

1. Maps with posterior elevation greater than 40 μm between patient cornea and best-fit sphere. Posterior corneal elevation may be the earliest sign of "forme frustre keratoconus"
2. Maps with four or more colors within the central 3-mm area are judged abnormal in screening using the 10- and 20-μ interval color scales for the anterior and posterior elevation maps of the scanning slit topography, respectively.

Keratoconic eyes exhibit significantly more ocular higher-order aberrations due to an increase of corneal higher-order aberrations compared to normal eyes. Coma-like aberrations were dominant compared with spherical-like aberrations in keratoconic eyes (Fig. 1.30), although both were significantly higher than in normal subjects. Wavefront sensing could also help to differentiate keratoconic eyes from normal eyes by analyzing the characteristics of the higher-order aberrations. The corneal wavefront aberration, which is the component of the total ocular wavefront

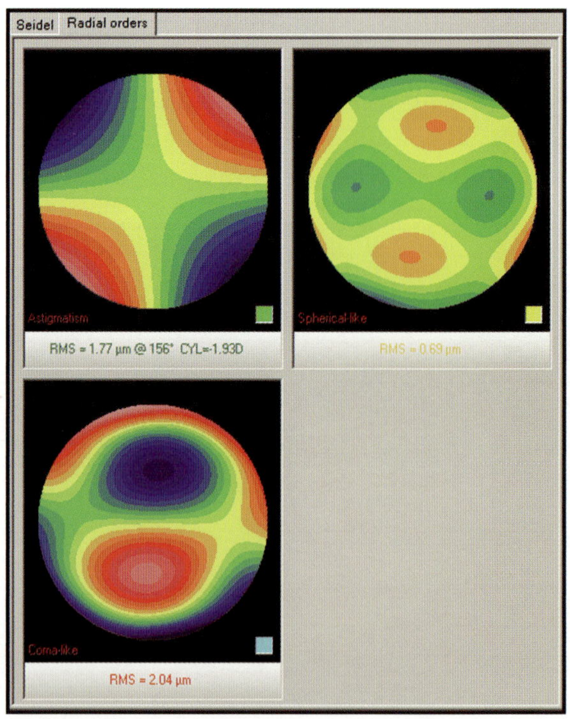

Fig. 1.30: Corneal aberrations in a keratoconus eye. Coma-like aberrations are dominant

aberration attributed to the cornea, can be derived from the corneal topographic height data. Specifically, the calculation of wavefront aberrations is performed by expanding the anterior corneal height data into the set of orthogonal Zernike polynomials.

To summarize, corneas with" forme fruste keratoconus" or other ectatic disorders have increased risk of post-LASIK ectasia. Clinicians may employ one of the several methods noted above. However, it is important to remember that there is no approach that guarantees correct discrimination of all normal and ectatic corneas. Therefore, if an ectatic disorder is suspected, LASIK will not be safely performed.

Operative Evaluation

Currently, the vast majority of interest and research surrounding customized corneal ablation centers on utilizing the wavefront data and/or a combination of wavefront and topographic data. The corneal wavefront aberration, which is the component of the total ocular wavefront aberration attributed to the cornea, can be derived from the corneal topographic height data (Fig. 1.31). Specifically, the calculation of wavefront aberrations is performed by expanding the anterior corneal height data into the set of orthogonal Zernike polynomials.

Postoperative Evaluation

Although Corneal Topography is an excellent tool in assessing quality of the surgery and optical performance, its main indication after refractive surgery is to determine the cause of visual complaints including visual impairment.

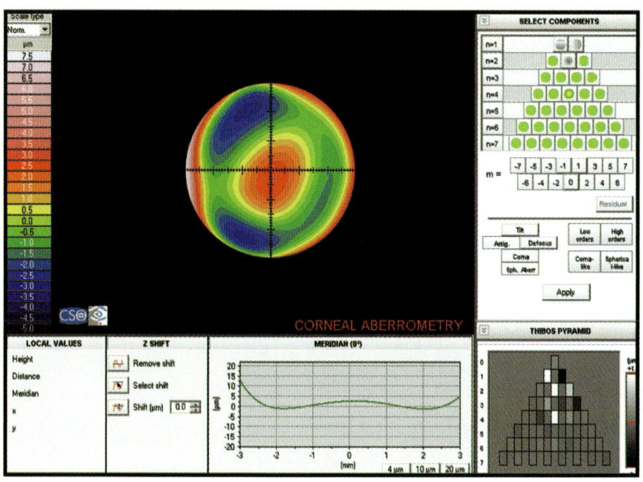

Fig. 1.31: Corneal aberrometry

When evaluating postoperative topographic maps, it is useful to examine several different kinds of maps:

a. The axial map is useful because the patterns are familiar and abnormal patterns are readily detectable.
b. The tangential map provides more precise information when evaluating local irregularities.
c. The elevation map may reveal local variations in height that may suggest asymmetry that can contribute to loss of quality of vision.
d. The difference map is used to assess the accuracy of centration.

Normal Topographic Changes after Refractive Surgery

Keratorefractive procedures attempt to alter the curvature of the central and mid-peripheral cornea, and usually have a minimal effect on the corneal periphery. The area in which the curvature is modified is called the *optical zone*. This tends to be surrounded by a small zone of altered curvature before normal cornea is reached at the periphery.

Postradial Keratotomy (RK)

Radial keratotomy (RK) is used to correct myopia by placing multiple deep radial incisions in the midperiphery and leaving a central clear zone (optical zone). These incisions cause a flattening of the central cornea, surrounded by a bulging ring of steepening called the paracentral knee or inflection zone that is situated at the 7 mm zone. This increases asphericity and corneal irregularity.

A very typical finding in these corneas is a topographic pattern with a polygonal shape (Fig. 1.32), which is seen in over a half of them. The polygons include squares, hexagons and octagons, depending on the number of incisions. The angles of the polygons correspond closely to the central ends of these incisions.

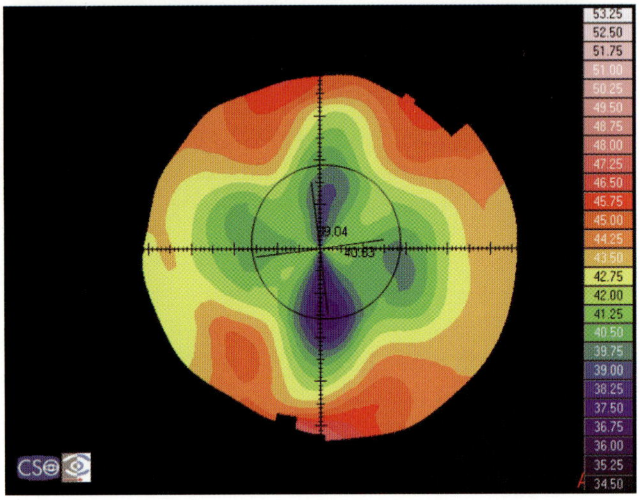

Fig. 1.32: Polygonal shape in radial keratotomy

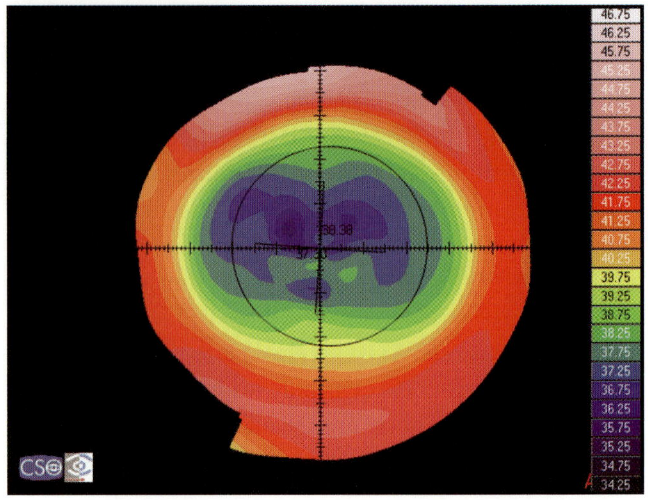

Fig. 1.33: Post-myopic PRK corneal topography

Postastigmatic Keratotomy (AK)

This technique is a simple modification of the radial keratotomy that is used to correct astigmatism. Instead of placing incisions radially on the cornea, incisions are strategically placed on the steepest meridian. The incisions induce a flattening in that meridian, but provoke steepening in the perpendicular meridian, in a process called coupling. The astigmatic change achieved is the sum of the flattening in one meridian and the steepening in its perpendicular meridian.

Postphotorefractive Keratotomy (PRK)

Photorefractive keratotomy (PRK) is a procedure that uses a kind of laser (excimer laser, a cool pulsing beam of ultraviolet light) to reshape the cornea. To correct myopia, the excimer laser flattens the central cornea by removing tissue in that area. To correct hyperopia, the optical zone needs to be steepened by removing an annulus of tissue from the mid-periphery of the cornea. Regular astigmatism is corrected by differential ablation of tissue in the steeper meridian.

The topographic pattern in myopic corrections shows an oblate profile, with flattening of the central cornea (Fig. 1.33). The treatment zone is usually well delineated by the close proximity of adjacent contours at its edge, especially in the next days following the procedure during the first period of overcorrection. Later on, wound healing partially fills the ablated area. Hyperopic corrections have a pattern of central steepening surrounded by a ring of relative flattening at the edge of the treatment zone (more prolate profile). In astigmatic treatments, the treatment zone is oval.

Postlaser In Situ Keratomileusis (LASIK)

LASIK is an excimer laser procedure like PRK, but instead of superficial ablation, the cornea is ablated under a superficial corneal flap in order to minimize the influence of the epithelium and to enable stromal wound healing in a more predicted fashion. The topographic patterns for myopic (Fig. 1.34) and hyperopic (Fig. 1.35) corrections are the same as in PRK. However, overcorrection is not as large, and topographic stability is obtained earlier.

Postlaser Thermal Keratoplasty (LTK)

In laser thermal keratoplasty (LTK), a Holmium laser is used to heat stromal collagen in a ring around the outside of the pupil. The heat causes the tissue to shrink, producing a zone of localized flattening centered on the spot, and a surrounding zone of steepening. This bulging effect of the central cornea makes it possible to correct hyperopy (Fig. 1.36). The typical topographic pattern shows the central corneal steepening and a ring of flattening overlying the spots.

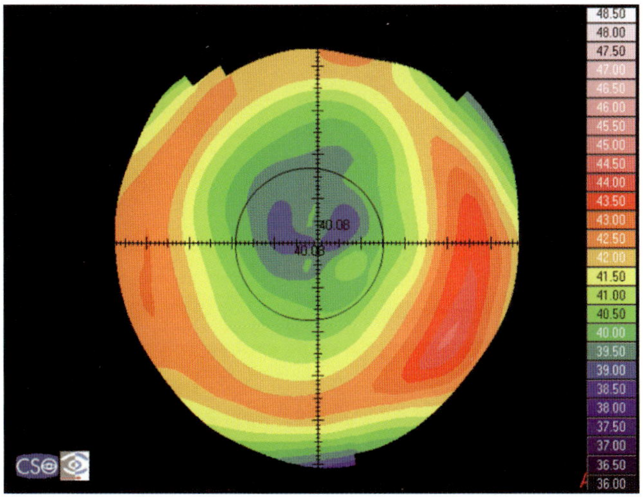

Fig. 1.34: Post-myopic LASIK corneal topography

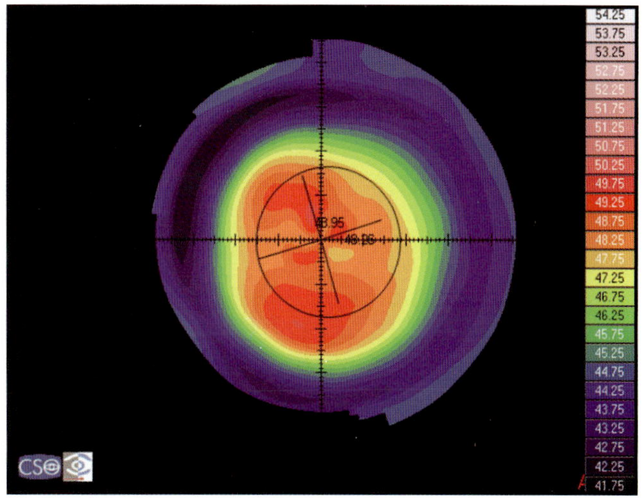

Fig. 1.35: Post-hyperopic LASIK corneal topography

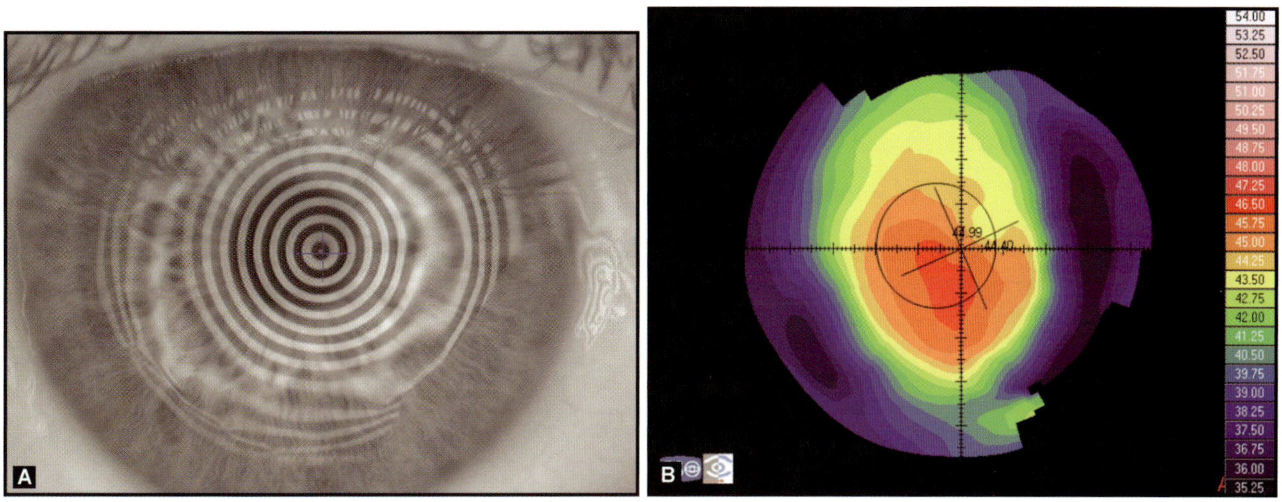

Figs 1.36A and B: Post-LTK corneal topography examination: (A) raw videokeratoscope image; (B) axial map

Abnormal Topographic Patterns after Refractive Surgery: Complications

Visual complaints after refractive surgery may be due to surface anomalies, which are too subtle to be detected on biomicroscopic examination, but can be revealed by corneal topography.

a. **Decentrations** can be identified by the relatively asymmetric localization of the treatment area (Fig. 1.37). It is a shift of the centre of the ablation pattern form the pupil or visual axis to a more eccentric location. To be clinically significant, decentrations of current large diameter (6 mm) optical zones, have to be over 1 mm, unless the patient has relatively large pupils. Decentrations should be differentiated from irregular wound healing, because the former shows a decentred zone on early corneal topography.
b. **Central island** shows a central area of relatively less flattening measuring >1.0 mm in diameter and >1.0 diopter in power, and not extending to the periphery (Fig. 1.38). The central island is surrounded around its entire periphery by areas of greater power diminution. This area of underablation causes blurred vision, halos, and decreases corrected and uncorrected visual acuity.

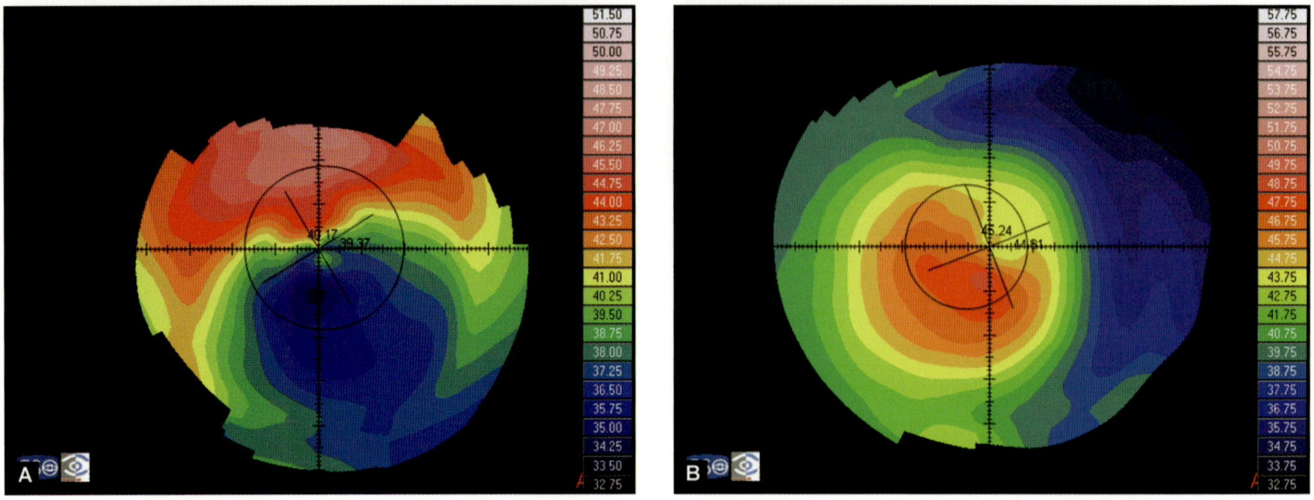

Figs 1.37A and B: Decentered LASIK profiles. (A) Myopic treatment, (B) Hyperopic treatment

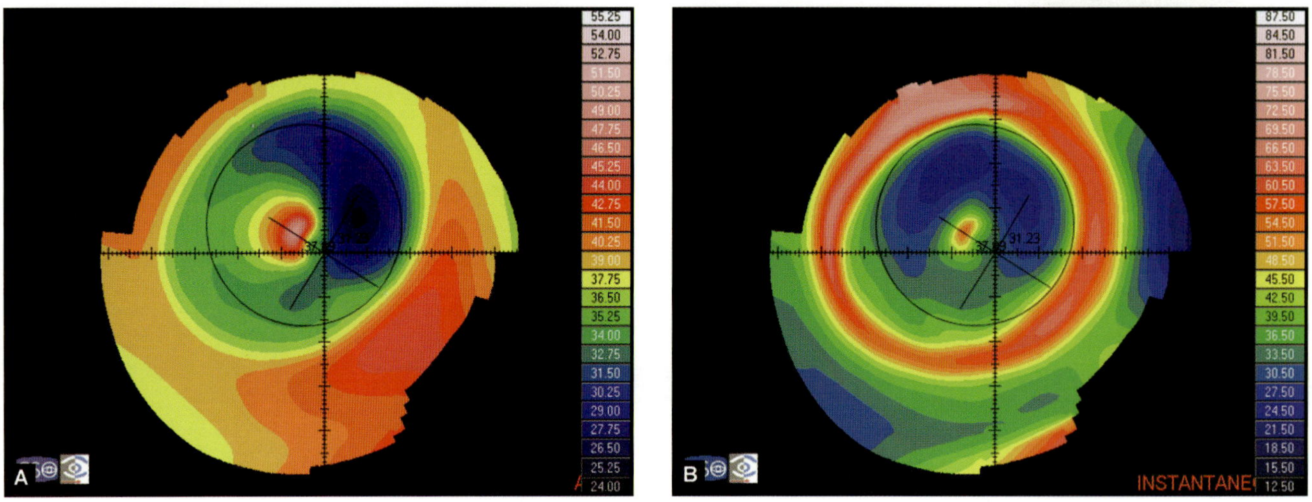

Figs 1.38A and B: Central island in myopic treatment. (A) Axial map; (B) Instantaneous map

c. **Keyhole** shows topographic regions, quantitatively measuring >1.0 mm in size and 1.0 diopter of relatively less flattening, extending in from the periphery of the ablation zone in one meridian.

d. **Focal irregularities or irregular astigmatism**, refers to irregularities in the cornea surface that do not follow the regular "bow tie" pattern of astigmatism (Fig. 1.39). Most of the times they are produced by an inhomogeneous laser beam or an irregular process of corneal healing.

e. **Corneal ectasia**. Topography shows irregular astigmatism often with inferior steepening of the cornea (Fig. 1.40), and posterior corneal ectasia on the posterior surface elevation map.

f. **Epithelial in-growth** at the periphery of the flap-stromal interface produces an area of steepening surrounded by an area of marked flattening making the corneal surface more irregular (Fig. 1.41). This is seen in LASIK procedures.

Preoperative and Postoperative Assessment of Intrastromal Corneal Rings

Corneal topography is also very valuable in the assessment of intrastromal corneal ring implantation.

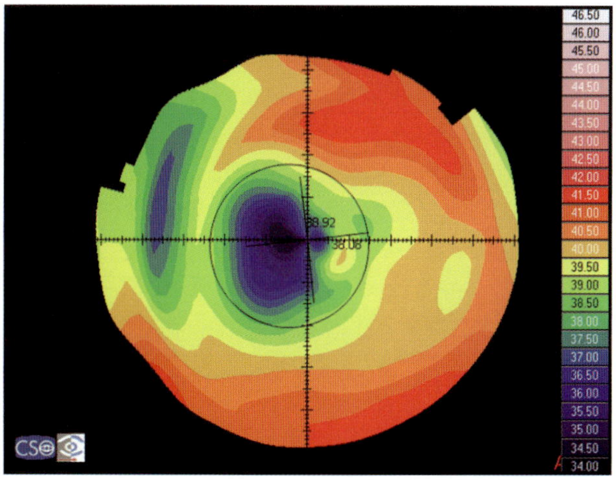

Fig. 1.39: Central corneal irregularity after LASIK for myopia and astigmatism

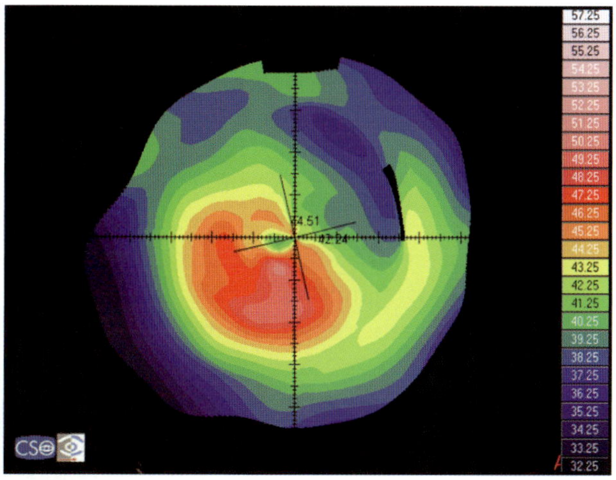

Fig. 1.40: Corneal ectasia after LASIK treatment

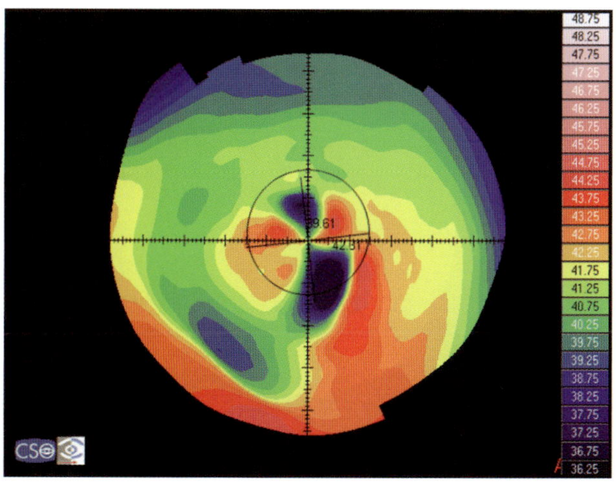

Fig. 1.41: Irregular astigmatism induced by an inferior epithelial ingrowth

The intrastromal corneal ring inserts act as passive spacing elements that shorten the arc length of the anterior corneal surface and therefore flatten the cornea. Corneal topography demonstrate that general flattening of the central cornea occurs after placement of ring and ring segments, but the normal positive asphericity of the cornea is maintained. The ring itself can be identified in the topographic map as a peripheral annulus of local steepening, surrounding, as already mentioned, a flattened central cornea (Figs 1.42A and B).

According to the FDA, intrastromal corneal rings are intended for the reduction or elimination of mild myopia (-1.00 to -3.00 D spherical equivalent at the spectacle plane) and they may now be used to reduce

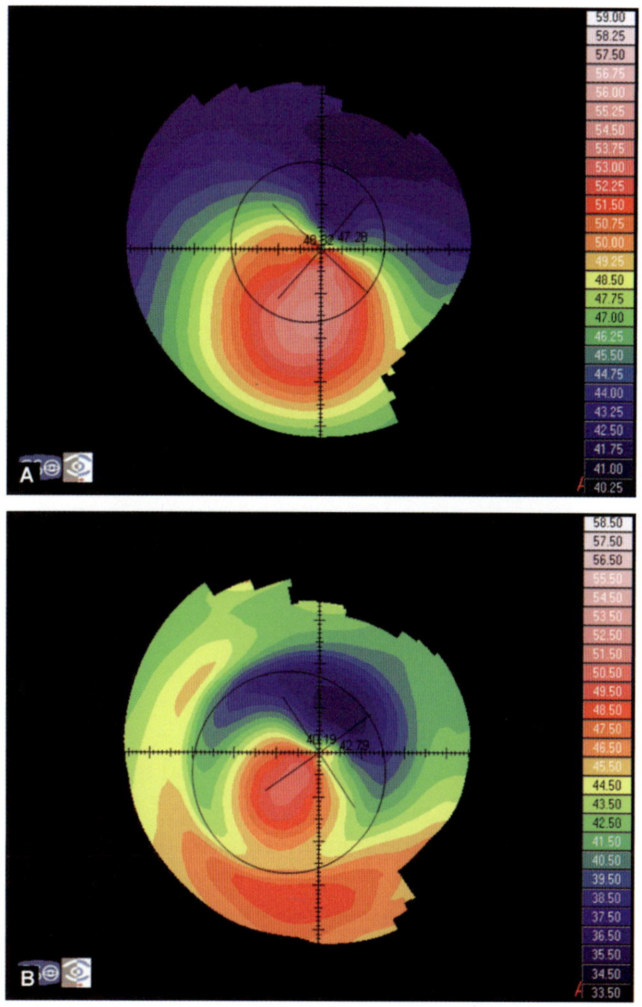

Fig. 1.42: Intracorneal rings implantation in a keratoconus eye. (A) preoperative axial map; (B) postoperative axial map

irregular steepening (irregular astigmatism) caused by keratoconus. Therefore, intrastromal corneal rings are also intended for patients with keratoconus who are no longer able to achieve adequate vision using contact lenses or glasses and for whom corneal transplantation is the only remaining option.

In a recent study, Intacs (a model of intracorneal ring), provided better results in visual acuity and corneal topography quality and significantly reduced the spherical equivalent in eyes with keratoconus with relatively low mean K values (< or = 53 D) and a relatively low spherical equivalent. In contrast, when performing the procedure in advanced keratoconus (mean K-reading > or = 55 D), poor results can be anticipated.

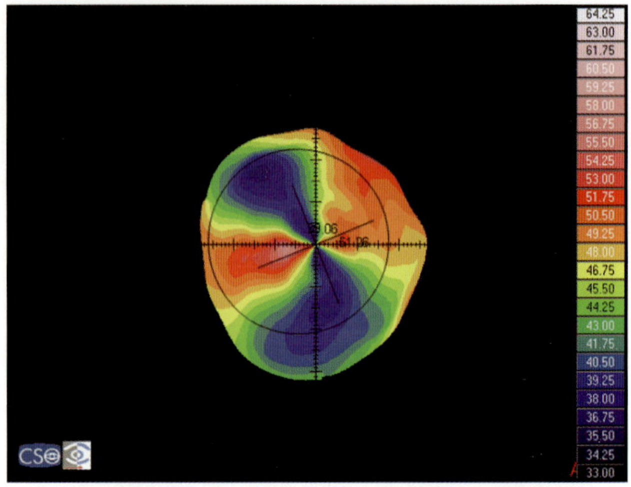

Fig. 1.43: Corneal topography after penetrating keratoplasty, showing a bow tie configuration

The Assessment of the Corneal Astigmatism after Keratoplasty

Corneal topography is helpful in evaluating and managing patients following penetrating keratoplasty. Its main indications are:

- Evaluating unexplained decreased visual acuity after keratoplasty.
- Planning how to reduce high astigmatism after surgery. Different options are arcuate incisions in the highest power meridian, compression sutures in the lower power meridian, or refractive surgery with LASIK or PRK.
- Guiding selective suture removal to reduce astigmatism in graft patients.

Different patterns of corneal shape result after penetrating keratoplasty, the most frequently seen are:

a. *Homogeneous*, in corneas with less than 1.25 D of topographic astigmatism.
b. *Orthogonal symmetric toric bow tie (Fig. 1.43)*, showing an astigmatic pattern equal to or greater than 1.25 D, with equal slopes (less than 1D of difference) of the hemimeridians along a single meridian.
c. *Orthogonal asymmetric toric bow tie*, showing an astigmatic pattern equal to or greater than 1.25 D with unequal slopes (more than 1D of difference) of the hemimeridians along a single meridian.
d. *Nonorthogonal toric bow tie*, showing that the principal meridian's half bow ties are misaligned by more than 10° from 180°.
e. *Steep and flat*, showing a cornea that is steeper on one side and progressively flattens toward the other side.
f. *Irregularly irregular*, showing multifocal patterns of steepening or flattening not meeting the specific criteria of any other pattern previously described.

Although we have mentioned penetrating keratoplasty, the same patterns can be seen in lamellar keratoplasty, such as in deep anterior lamellar keratoplasty. Deep endothelial lamellar keratoplasty does not generate postsurgical astigmatism (Fig. 1.44).

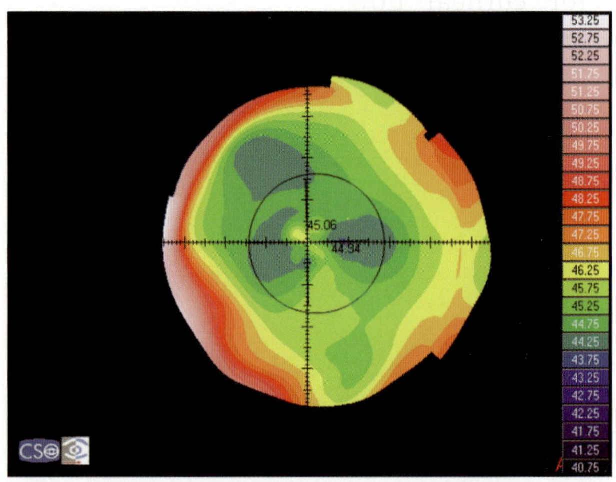

Fig. 1.44: Corneal topography after lamellar keratoplasty

Applications in Cataract Surgery

Corneal topography has become a useful tool when pursuing excellence in the outcomes of cataract surgery:

- To plan the place of the incision in phacoemulsification, in order to reduce postsurgical astigmatism, or even to correct preoperative astigmatism.
  For instance, it is known that an incision between 9 and 12 o'clock generates less astigmatism than 12 o'clock incisions. It is also well understood that to prevent astigmatism postoperatively, the incision should be placed at the steepest meridian in eyes with preoperative astigmatism greater than 0.5 D.
- To evaluate and plan the surgical approach in postoperative astigmatism.
- To predict corneal power in eyes with prior keratorefractive surgery.
  In eyes that have undergone previous keratorefractive surgery, accurate IOL power calculation remains a challenge due to inaccurate estimation of corneal power since standard keratometry or simulated keratometric values from topography cannot accurately measure the corneal curvature. Various methods have been developed to improve the accuracy of corneal power estimation. The clinical history method has been shown in general to be an accurate method for corneal power calculation; however, unacceptably large refractive surprises have still occurred. Also, historical data are mandatory in this method. Newer, more promising approaches involve calculating corneal refractive power from certain corneal topographic displays.

Evaluation of Irregular Astigmatism

The condition of irregular astigmatism is variously defined. To give a simple definition, irregular astigmatism is an astigmatic state not correctable by a sphero-cylindrical lens.

With the advent of computerized topographic systems, it is possible to distinguish two different types:

- *Regularly irregular* with either unequal slopes of the hemimeridians along a single meridian (the "asymmetric bow-tie") or hemimeridians of equal slope but not aligned with each other (the "angled bow-tie" or nonorthogonal astigmatism). A combination of both patterns usually occurs.
- *Irregularly irregular* state is seen when even computerized topography cannot demonstrate a recognizable pattern, and the corneal surface can only be described as rough or uneven.
  Modern videokeratoscopy may define approximately 40% of normal corneas with a toric refractive error as possessing primary irregular astigmatism. Although some of these primary cases may have decreased best corrected visual acuity, clinically, the secondary forms of irregular astigmatism are more invalidating. Corneal topography has been used to evaluate the state and progression and to plan treatment of the following secondary forms:
- For visual impairment in corneal dystrophies and bullous keratopathy.
- To follow up corneal ulceration or abscess, and to determine the shape of the cornea after healing and scarring.
- To evaluate the visual effect of posttraumatic scarring, cause by incisions, excisions, burns, etc.
- To study postsurgical irregular astigmatism that may present after trabeculectomy, extracapsular lens extraction, keratoplasty, PRK, LASIK, LASEK, radial keratotomy, scleral encirclement, among others.

Diagnosis of Surface and Ectatic Diseases

Keratoconus

Keratoconus is characterized by a localized conical protrusion of the cornea associated with an area of noninflammatory corneal stromal thinning, especially at the apex of the cone (Fig. 1.27). The condition usually occurs in the second or third decade of life resulting in a moderate to marked decrease in visual acuity secondary to irregular astigmatism and corneal scarring.

The typical associated topographic pattern is the presence of an inferior area of steepening usually in the temporal quadrant. In advanced cases, the dioptric power at the apex is at or above 55 D (Fig. 1.42A). The superior-nasal quadrant of the cornea is commonly the last to be affected, and thus an "island" of normal corneal topography often remains in this area even in the more advanced stages of the condition. In a small group of patients, the topographic alterations may be centred at the central cornea, showing an asymmetric bow tie configuration with the inferior loop normally larger than the superior loop (Fig. 1.45).

Keratoconic Corneas have three common characteristics that are not present in normal corneas:

- An area of increased corneal power surrounded by concentric areas of decreasing power,
- A inferior-superior power asymmetry,
- A skewing of the steepest radial axes above and below the horizontal meridian.

Pellucid Marginal Degeneration

Pellucid marginal degeneration is a bilateral, non-inflammatory, peripheral corneal thinning disorder, characterized by inferior corneal protrusion, above a narrow band of clear, thinned corneal stroma that is concentric to the limbus. In this disease the position of the ectasia is extremely peripheral and it presents a crescent-shaped morphology.

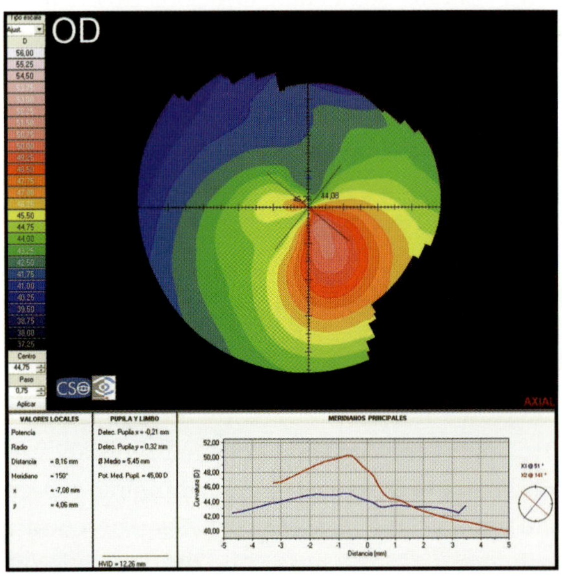

Fig. 1.45: Keratoconus, showing an asymmetric bow tie configuration with the inferior loop normally larger than the superior loop

The videokeratographic pattern has a classic butterfly appearance that results in a flattening of the vertical meridian and a marked against-the-rule irregular astigmatism (Fig. 1.28).

Keratoglobus

Keratoglobus is a rare bilateral disorder in which the entire cornea is thinned most markedly near the corneal limbus, in contrast to the localized central or paracentral thinning of keratoconus. It is very difficult to obtain reliable and reproducible measurements in these cases due to the high level of irregularity and the poor quality of the associated tear film. Reliable topographic exams show an arc of peripheral increase in corneal power (steepening) and a very asymmetrical bow tie configuration.

Terrien's Marginal Degeneration

In Terrien´s marginal degeneration there is a flattening over the areas of peripheral thinning. When thinning is restricted to the superior and/or inferior areas of the peripheral cornea, a high against-the-rule or oblique astigmatism is seen. If the area of thinning is small or if the disorder extends around the entire 360º, central cornea may remain relatively spared with a spherical configuration.

Pterygium

It is a winglike mass of fibrovascular tissue extending from the conjunctiva to the cornea, usually are found more commonly nasally than temporally. When the growth of this pathological tissue is enough a flattening of the cornea at the axis of the lesion occurs causing a marked with-the-rule astigmatism, even of more than 4 D (Figs 1.46A and B). The wider the extension of the lesion and of the optical zone interested by it, the more marked this astigmatism. Corneal topography can monitor the evolution of the pathology and evaluate the surgical outcome.

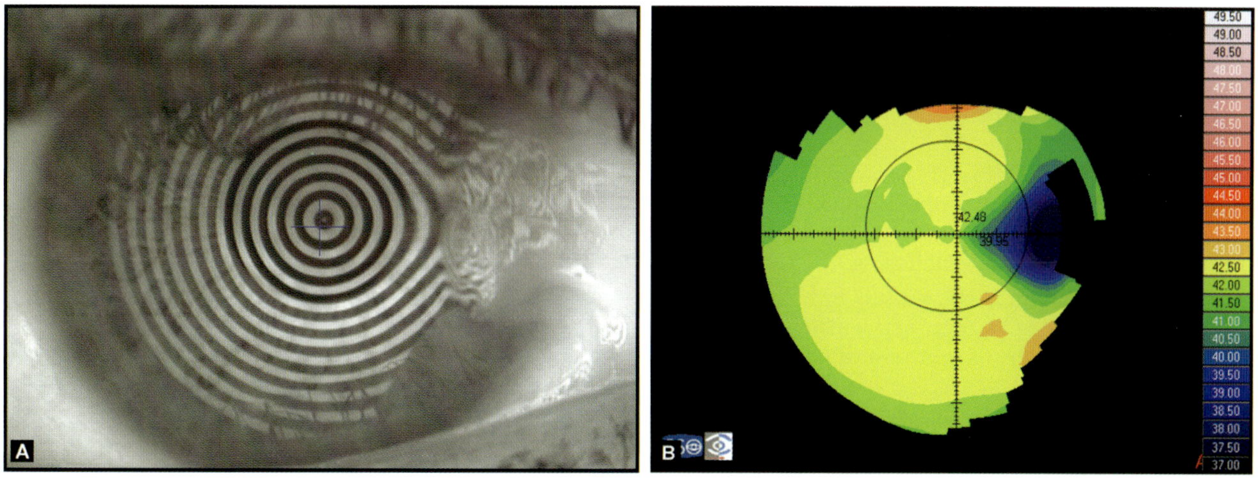

Figs 1.46A and B: Corneal topography in pterygium. A—raw videokeratoscope image; B—axial map

Other types of corneal pathology such as epithelial dysplasia and epithelial basement membrane disease can also be evaluated using corneal topography.

Contact Lens Fitting

Most corneal topographers provide software that can design an appropriate contact lens based upon the topography (Fig. 1.47). The information corneal topography provides can greatly enhance the ability to manage complex contact lens fits and increase the overall success rate. It is practically mandatory when fitting contact lenses in patients with irregular astigmatism, for example after penetrating keratoplasty, after keratorefractive procedures, after corneal rings implantation or in advanced keratoconus, to locate precisely the corneal apex. Other uses are for refitting warped corneas, and in orthokeratology.

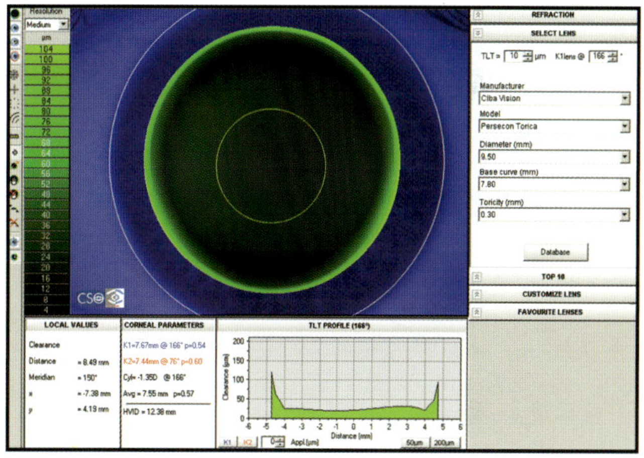

Fig. 1.47: Contact lens fitting option from the CSO corneal topography system

Evaluation of Tear Film Quality

High-speed videotopography provides the possibility of quantitative measurement of tear-film dynamics and may have clinical value in the management of ocular surface disorders that present with tear film abnormalities such as dry eye.

BIBLIOGRAPHY

1. Alio JL, Shabayek MH. Corneal higher order aberrations: A method to grade keratoconus. J Refract Surg 2006;22:539-45.
2. Alio JL, Shabayek MH, Belda JI, Correas P, Feijoo ED. Analysis of results related to good and bad outcomes of Intacs implantation for keratoconus correction. J Cataract Refract Surg 2006;32:756-61.
3. Bogan SJ, Waring GO, Ibrahim O, Drews C, Curtis L. Classification of normal corneal topography based on computer-assisted videokeratography. Arch Ophthalmol 1990;108:945-49.
4. Boyd BF, Agarwal A, Alio JL, Krueger RR, Wilson SE, editors. Wavefront analysis, aberrometers and corneal topography, Highlights of Ophthalmology, 2003.
5. Cairns G, McGhee CNJ. Orbscan computerized topography: Attributes, applications, and limitations. J Cataract Refract Surg 2005;31:205-20.
6. Corbett M, O'Brart D, Rosen E, Stevenson R. Corneal topography: Principles and applications. BMJ Publishing Group, 1999.

7. Corneal Topography. American Academy of Ophthalmology. Ophthalmology 1999;106:1628-38.
8. Courville CB, Smolek MK, Klyce SD. Contribution of ocular surface to visual optics. Exp Eye Res 2004;78: 417-25.
9. Dabezies OH, Holladay JT. Measurement of corneal curvature: keratometer(ophthalmometer). In Contact lenses: the CLAO guide to basic science and clinical practice, Kendall/Hunt Publishing Co, 1995;253-89.
10. Demers PE, Steinert RF, Gould EM. Topographic analysis of corneal regularity after penetrating keratoplasty. Invest Ophthalmol Vis Sci 2002;43: 1783-90.
11. Goggin M, Alpins N, Schmid LM. Management of Irregular Astigmatism. Curr Opin Ophthalmol. 2000;11:260-66.
12. Goto E, Yagi Y, Matsumoto Y, Tsubota K. Impaired functional visual acuity of dry eye patients. Am J Ophthalmol 2002;133:181-86.
13. Joslin CE, Wu SM, McMahon TT, Shahidi M. Higher-order wavefront aberrations in corneal refractive therapy. Optom Vis Sci. 2003;80:805-11.
14. Karabatsas CH, Cook SD. Topographic analysis in pellucid marginal corneal degeneration and keratoglobus. Eye 1996;10:451-55.
15. Kaufman H, Barron B, McDonald M, Kaufman S. Companion handbook to the cornea. Butterworth Heinemann, 1999.
16. Klyce SD. Corneal topography and the new wave. Cornea 2000;19:723-29.
17. Krachmer JH, Mannis MJ, Holland EJ, editors. Cornea. Surgery of cornea and conjunctiva. Elsevier-Mosby, 2005.
18. Maeda N, Klyce SD, Smolek MK. Neural network classification of corneal topography. Preliminary demonstration. Invest Ophthalmol Vis Sci 1995;36: 1327-35.
19. Mejía-Barbosa Y, Malacara-Hernández, D. A review of methods for measuring corneal topography. Optom Vis Sci 2001;78:240-53.
20. Miller D, Greiner JV. Corneal measurements and tests. In Principles and practice of ophthalmology, WB Saunders Co, 1994;7.
21. Nemeth J, Erdelyi B, Csakany B, Gaspar P, Soumelidis A, Kahlesz F, Lang Z. High-speed videotopographic measurement of tear film build-up time. Invest Ophthalmol Vis Sci 2002;43:1783-90.
22. Rabinowitz YS. Keratoconus. Surv Ophthalmol. 1998;42:297-319.
23. Rabinowitz YS, Nesburn AB, McDonnell PJ. Videokeratography of the fellow eye in unilateral keratoconus. Ophthalmology 1993;100:181-86.
24. Rao SK, Padmanabhan P. Understanding corneal topography. Curr Opin Ophthalmol 2000;11:248-59.
25. Tanabe T, Oshika T, Tomidokoro A, Amano S, Tanaka S, Kuroda T, Maeda N, Tokunaga T, Miyata K. Standardized color-coded scales for anterior and posterior elevation maps of scanning slit corneal topography. Ophthalmology 2002;109:1298-302.
26. Wang L, Koch DD. Corneal Topography and its integration into refractive surgery. Comp Ophthalmol Update 2005;6:73-81.
27. Wilson SE, Ambrosio R. Computerized corneal topography and its importance to wavefront technology. Cornea 2001;20:441-54.
28. Wilson SE, Klyce SD. Advances in the analysis of corneal topography. Surv Ophthalmol 1991;35:269-77.
29. Wilson SE, Lin DT, Klyce SD, Insler MS. Terrien's marginal degeneration: Corneal topography. Refract Corneal Surg 1990;6:15-20.

Principles of Scanning Lasers for Customized LASIK

2

JT Lin (USA)

INTRODUCTION

Scanning (flying-spot) laser has been widely used in almost (except VISX system) all of the LASIK procedures. However, it has been over 10 years since the first system called scanning Mini-Excimer was designed, invented and patented by JT Lin (US Pat 5,144,630; 5,520,679). It also took over 20 years after the first ArF excimer laser ablation of organic tissue reported by Taboada and the IBM patent. The major milestone of the development of refractive surgery lasers may be summarized as follows:

- 1981-82 ArF excimer laser ablation of organic tissue (Taboada, Seinivasan)
- 1983 Excimer laser (broad beam) PRK patented (L'Espearnce, Troke)
- 1992-93 Scanning laser for PRK patented (Lin/LaserSight)
  UV-213 solid state for PRK (Lin/LaserSight, Lai/Novatec)
- 1995 FDA approval for PRK and PTK (Summit, VisX)
- 1996 Computer simulation of customized ablation (Lin)

It should be emphasized that customized LASIK guided by topography would not be possible without the invention of the small-spot scanning method which provides both accuracy and flexibility of the ablating profiles. The invention of eye-tracking (by Lai) further improved the reliability of scanning lasers. Greater details of other technologies developed for vision corrections are shown in Table 2.1 and 2.2 including the use of IOL, LTK, DTK, CK and methods for presbyopia treatment using SEB, ACS and LPT, etc.

Comparison for methods for hyperopia correction is shown in Table 2.3, where Ho:LTK (made by Sunrise) with FDA approval was not accepted by the market due to the major regression. The DTK method using diode laser is in clinical trials. DTK-Plus is a revised system proposed by Lin (patent pending) for maximal penetration depth and more stable outcome. The CK (conductive keratoplasty) method was FDA approved for both hyperopia and pseudo-accommodation (presbyopia, monovision). Various phakic IOLs are also developed for both hyperopia and myopia, particularly for high-power correction and for eyes after cataracts. Greater details of IOL may be found in a book edited by Garg and Lin: Mastering IOLs: Principles and Innovations (Jaypee Brothers, New Delhi, India, 2006).

Table 2.4 compares presbyopia correction methods including the sclera expansion band (SEB, patented by Schachar), anterior ciliary sclerotomy (proposed by Thornton), SEP (by Fukusaku) and laser method (by Lin) of LASA, LACA and LATK. All of these methods are in clinical trial stages. The recently developed accommodating IOL such as 1CU (made

Table 2.1: The milestones of vision correction technology and representing pioneers (or inventors) and manufacturers

Year	*Technology*	*WHO*
1890's	Thermal lesions of rabbit cornea	Lans
1950's	Fordable PC IOL in aphakia	Ridley
	Minus AC IOL in phakia	Strampeli, Barraquer
1970's	RK for myopia correction	Fedorov
1980's	Radio frequency (RF) for hyperopia	Rowsey
	Ho:YAG thermal keratoplasty	Sand
	ALK for myopia	Barraquer
	ArF tissue ablation	Sriaivasan/IBM
	Data of excimer ablation	Tsuboda
	ArF excimer laser for PRK	L'Esperance/VisX
1990's	LTK using Ho:YAG, clinical results	Sunrise
	DTK using CW diode laser	ProLaser, Inc.
	CK (conductive keratoplasty)	Refractec, Inc.
	PRK clinical and FDA approval	VisX, Summit, Inc.
	Solid-state Nd::YAG laser for IRK	Phoenix, Inc.
	Pico-second Nd:YAG laser for IRK	ISL, Inc.
	Solid-state UV laser for PRK	Lin/LaserSight
	Mini-Excimer scanning laser	Lin/LaserSight
	Solid-state UV laser with eye tracking	Lai/Novatek
	Mid-IR OPO-laser for PRK	Lin/Photon Data
2000's	Microkeratome device for LASIK	Moria, Inc.
	Scanning laser for customized LASIK	Lin
	Elevation map (Orbscan)	Bausch and Lomb
	Topography-guided LASIK	Meditec, WaveLight
	Presbyopia correction by SEB	Schachar
	ACS with silicone expansion plug	Fukasaku
	ACS using diamond knife	Thornton
	Laser sclera ablation (IR), LASA	Lin/SurgiLight
	Laser sclera ablation (UV), LASA	Lin/New Vision
	Laser ciliary-body ablation	Lin/New Vision
	DTK-plus for hyperopia/presbyopia	Lin/New Vision
	Phakic IOL	CIBA Vision, Bausch and Lomb
	Accommodative IOL (AIOL)	HumanOptics, C&C Vision
	Smartscan AIOL	Medennium
	Wavefront for customized LASIK	Alcon, Topcon, Tracey, Bausch and Lomb, Nidek

by HumanOptics) may be the alternative for presbyopia. Excimer laser (LASIK) bifocal reshaping also provides pseudo-accommodation for presbyopia in addition to the use of CK or DTK for monovision treatments.

Engineering and Clinical Correlation

Clinical issues of LASIK include patient centration, operative eye motion, corneal haze, night halo and power regression effects, pain, wound healing (re-epithelizlization time), and procedure time. These clinical issues are directly correlated to engineering aspects that involve laser parameters (beam energy/pulse, spot size, homogeneity, and fluence on the ablated corneal surface) and delivery methods (diaphragm, scanning, mask, fiber). In addition, non-excimer solid-state lasers without fluorine gas may be preferred for their ease of operation and low maintenance.

Table 2.2: Summary of technologies for vision corrections (laser and non-laser methods)

Method	*Features*
1 PRK, LASEK	Corneal surface ablation with epithelium removed preserved; suitable for low diopter corrections (< 3.5 D).
2. LASIK	Stroma ablation by laser after a "flap" is prepared by microkeratome.
3. LASA, LACA	Presbyopia treatment by laser scleral ablation (LASA) to increase accommodation via ciliary body contraction; combining effects of lens curvature change and anterior chamber shift. Efficiency may be improved by deeper laser ciliary-body ablation (LACA).
4. LZT, LCT	Laser zonules thermal (LZT) stimulation for presbyopia; noninvasive method using gona lens and focused laser. Laser ciliary-body thermal shrinkage (LCT) for presbyopia.
5. SEB	Scleral expansion band implanted in scleral layer: major regression.
6. ACS	Anterior ciliary sclerotomy by diamond knife incision; major regression which may be reduced by silicon expansion plug.
7. CK	Conductive keratoplasty using radio frequency wave for monovision correction; treated eye to see near but losing its far vision.
8. LTK and DTK	Laser thermal keratoplasty (LTK) using Ho:YAG (at 2.1 um) or diode laser (1.45 to 2.1 micron) (DTK).
9. BFCR	Bifocal corneal reshaping by excimer LASIK for pseudo-accommodation.
10. AIOL	Accommodative IOL implanted to lens capsule; forward movement for accommodation; could be single or dualoptics IOL.
11. Phakic IOL	IOL implanted in the anterior, posterior chamber, or lens capsular bag.
12. MIOL	Multifocal IOL implanted for patient with high refraction errors.
13. ICRS	Intracorneal ring segments for low myopia and astigmatism.
14. Advanced CL	Advanced contact lens having multifocal or designed for the correction of high-order aberration.
15. Super Vision	Customized LASIK combined with wavefront technology; flying-spot scanning laser with eye tracking is required for customized and irregular corneal reshaping.

*Major technologies (inventors): Broad beam excimer (L'Esperance, Blum, Tsuboda); LTK (Sand); SEB (Schachar); Flying-spot LASIK (Lin); LAPR & LACA (Lin), LZT (Lin, Martinez); Eye-tracking (Lai); Solid-state UV Laser for LASIK (Lin, Lai); BFCR (Ruitz). Most of the above technologies have been patented (1988-2004) and greater details may be found in US pat. No: 4718418, 5484432, 5520679, 5144630, 6263879, 6258082, 5533997, 5354331.

Table 2.3: Comparison of technologies for hyperopia correction

Method	*Features*
LASIK	ArF excimer laser corneal surface ablation
Ho:LTK	Ho:YAG laser (at 2.1 micron) nonfocused beam, shallow penetration
DTK	Diode-laser (at 1.88 micron), focused CW beam
DTK-Plus	Diode-laser (at 1.4 to 1.9 micron), optimal focused beam
CK	Penetration depth controlled by electrode length
IOL	Phakic IOL implant (plus lens)

Table 2.4: Comparison of presbyopia correction methods and the mechanisms

Method	*Technique description*	*Mechanism*
SEB (1)	Scleral expansion band	Lens equatorial diameter expansion with increased zonules tension for accommodation.
ACS (2)	Radial incision of sclera	Scleral tissue incision for the expansion of "crowding" chamber and lens
SEP (3)	Silicon expansion plugs	Same as ACS but with implant for reduced regression
SCI (4)	Band implanted in ciliary body	Based on Helmholtz theory that lens diameter decreases with zonules relaxation
LASA (5)	IR or UV laser sclera ablation	Based on 'Elastic theory" of Lin-Kadambi hypothesis, where the laser-ablated scleral gap is filled with subconjunctival tissue with increased elasticity for effective accommodation. Regression caused by tissue healing may be minimized.
LACA (6)	Laser ciliary body ablation	Deeper ablation for greater efficacy and stability
LATK (7)	Laser thermal keratoplasty	Thermal shrinkage deep into the choroids or ciliary body combined with LTK (DTK)

Notes: (1) method first proposed by R. Schachar; (2) first proposed by Cramer in 1860, see also S. Thornton ; (3) first proposed by H. Fukasaku in Japan; (4) method proposed by G. Baikoff in France; (5) method proposed in 1998 and patented by JT Lin in 2001; (6), (7) Lin, US pending patents, 2005.

As summarized in Table 2.1, the milestone of the vision correction technologies in the major areas of IOL, AIOL, LASIK, LTK, DTK, CK and more recently, the ACS, SEB, LASA, LPT procedures for presbyopia corrections. Advanced microkeratomes and wavefront device are also developed in the recent few years. Several specialized topic books have been published to cover the detailed technologies and clinical outcome. They include:

a. Refractive Surgery, ed. by Agarwal et al (Jaypee Brothers, New Delhi, India, 2000);
b. Presbyopia: A surgical textbook, ed. by Agarwal et al (SLACK, NJ, 2002);
c. Mastering the techniques of corneal refractive surgery, ed. by Garg et al (Jaypee Brothers, New Delhi, India, 2005);
d. Intraocular lens power calculation, ed. by Shammas HJ (SLACK, NJ, 2004);
e. Phakic intraocular lens, ed. by Hexlton DR et al. (SLACK, NJ, 2004);
f. Wavefront customized vision correction, ed. by Krueger RR et al. (SLACK, NJ, 2004).
g. Mastering IOLs: Principles and Innovations, ed. by Garg A and Lin JT. (Jaypee Brothers, New Delhi, India, 2006)

The above references, except (g), are all mainly dealing with clinical aspects and lack of principles or mathematical formulas which would be emphasized in this chapter.

In this chapter we shall first review the current status of refractive surgical lasers (including excimer and nonexcimer). The correlation of engineering parameters and clinical requirements with optimal considerations are presented. The fundamentals of corneal reshaping with formulas for both spherical and aspherical ablation profiles and the advantages of the multizone method are discussed. We shall also present updated information on the scanning laser system with an emphasis on customized ablation.

TECHNOLOGY SUMMARY

Lasers in UV, visible and IR spectrum have been widely used in various ophthalmic applications such as glaucoma, cataract (or phaco emuleification) aged-related macular degeneration (AMD) and most importantly, for refractive corrections as summarized in Tables 2.1 and 2.2.

Refractive surgical lasers (RSL) have been used to correct the refractive errors including myopia (nearsighted), hyperopia (farsightedness), astigmatism and presbyopia (aging eye). These corneal reshaping procedures can be performed via several mechanisms including:

1. Corneal surface ablation (PRK, LASEK),
2. Cornea stroma ablation (LASIK),
3. Corneal collagen tissue thermal shrinkage (LTK, DTK).

Prior to laser refractive surgeries, at least two major techniques were performed for vision corrections: Radial keratotomy (RK) and automatic lamellar keratomileusis (ALK). The advantages of RK over RSL are smaller investment (in cost and maintenance) and faster refractive outcome. RK procedures, however, suffer major disadvantages including slow healing, corneal weakening, low success rate, and instability. RK procedures also depend very much on the doctor's experience, limited to low (-3.0 diopter) myopic corrections and not for hyperopia.

The earlier RSL procedure known as photorefractive keratectomy (PRK) using an argon fluoride (ArF) excimer laser (at the 193-nm UV wavelength) and for large area corneal surface ablation. During 1990s, PRK has been the only procedure recognized as having a high clinical success rate and predictable diopter corrections for myopia, astigmatism, and hyperopia. Alternative methods such as intrastroma photorefractive keratectomy (IPK, using Nd:YLF and doubled YAG), conductive keratoplasty (CK) and laser thermo keratoplasty (LTK using Ho:YAG or diode-laser DTK at 1.4 to 2.1 micron) have also been proposed.

The more recent procedure called laser in situ keratomileusis (LASIK) has replaced the PRK with advantages such as no epithelial removal, minimal corneal would healing, reduced haze and regression, and quicker recovery of vision. LASIK, however, requires investments in a microkeratome and also in doctor training. An alternative procedure called LASEK, similar to PRK without the use of microkeratome, has been used for thin cornea or low-diopter correction.

The success of RSL procedures of LASIK using UV lasers (either excimer or solid-state lasers) is mainly attributed from the following unique features:

1. Minimal tissue thermal damage due to the short wavelength used;
2. Tissue bond-breaking of corneal collagen by high photon energy;
3. Precise corneal tissue surface ablation (on the order of 0.2 to 0.4 um per pulse) achieved by using small laser fluence of 150 to 200 mJ per centimeter square;
4. Use of computer programmed algorithm for ablation profile control;
5. Use of eye tracking to minimize off-center ablation caused by eye movement;
6. Use of flying spot scanning for customized ablation;
7. Use of advanced topography device and wavefront technology for supervision, where high order surface aberration may be minimized. New UV RSL lasers were also been explored (during 1992–1998) as potential substitutes for the first-generation ArF excimer lasers, which can be bulky, heavy, and high in gas and maintenance costs. These new UV lasers include:
   a. the Laser-Harmonic-1 (flash-lamp pumped) using the fifth harmonic of and Nd:YAG at 213 nm, and the LaserHarmonic-2 diode-pumped Nd:YLG (or YLF) at 213 (or 209) nm, both patented by JT Lin;
   b. the Ti:sapphire (fourth-harmonic) UV solid-state laser at 208 nm, made by Novatec (California); and
   c. The compact mini-excimer made by lasersight (patented by Lin). At the 1991 ARVO and 1992 SPIE conferences, Lin reported the first flash-lamp pumped, solid-state UV (at 213 nm) PRK laser where tissue ablation was performed in collaboration with groups at Emory University and the University of Miami. At the 1993 SPIE Biomedical Optics Meeting (Los Angeles,

California), Lin reported the first diode-pumped UV solid-state laser (at 209 nm). At the 1992 American Academy of Ophthalmology (AAO) meeting, Lin introduced the first Mini-Excimer laser for PRK.

In contrast to the first-generation broad-beam technology, which used industrial-type, high-power (about 300 mJ from the laser or 30 mJ on the corneal surface) excimer lasers, the recent generation excimer systems use high-repetition-rate excimer laser operated at a much smaller beam spot size of 0.8 to 1.5 mm in a scanning mode. It only requires a laser energy per pulse of only 0.8 to 2.0 mJ on the corneal surface to achieve the same range of fluence (or energy per unit area) (160 to 200 mJ/cm^2) as that of the high-power broad-beam excimers which require about 35 mJ per pulse.

Ultra-short-pulse lasers were also proposed for LASIK procedures. They include picosecond and femto-second Ti:sapphire, Nd:YLF, or Nd:YAG lasers, in which the wavelengths are not required to be in the UV range. A "plasma-assisted" ablation mechanism occurs in these short-pulse lasers. A mid-IR laser generated from optical parametric oscillation (OPO) and Er:YAG was also proposed for LASIK procedures. (Lin, US Patent, 2001). Various beam delivery devices have been used, as shown in Fig. 2.1 including the broadbeam laser with diaphragm and the small beam laser with computer controlled scanning mirrors. Fig. 2.2 shows the rotating scanning

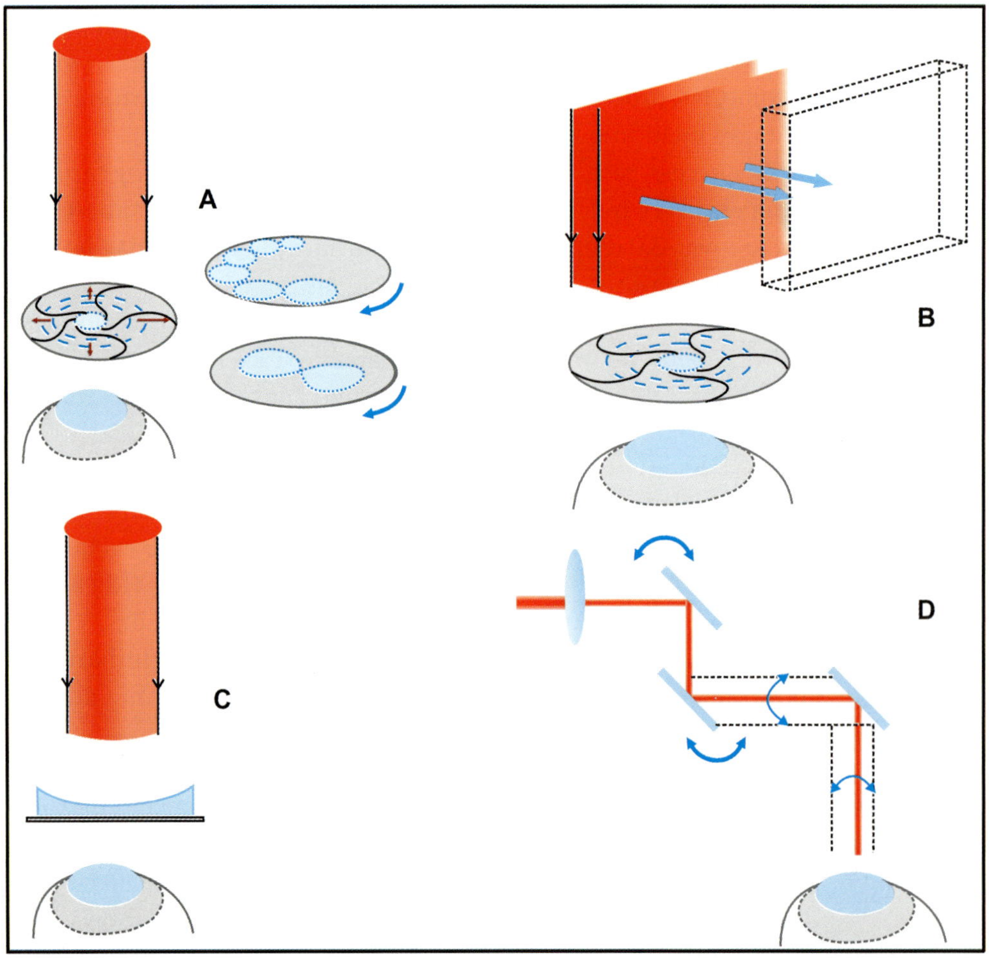

Fig. 2.1: Various beam delivery devices used in refractive surgery laser systems: (A) broad-beam system using diaphragm/iris (Visx, Summit) or rotating mask (Meditec), (B) line-beam scanning over iris (Nidek), (C) broad-beam using erodable mask (Summit), and (D) flying spot scanning (PDI, SurgiLight, LaserSight, Autonomous and Chiron-217)

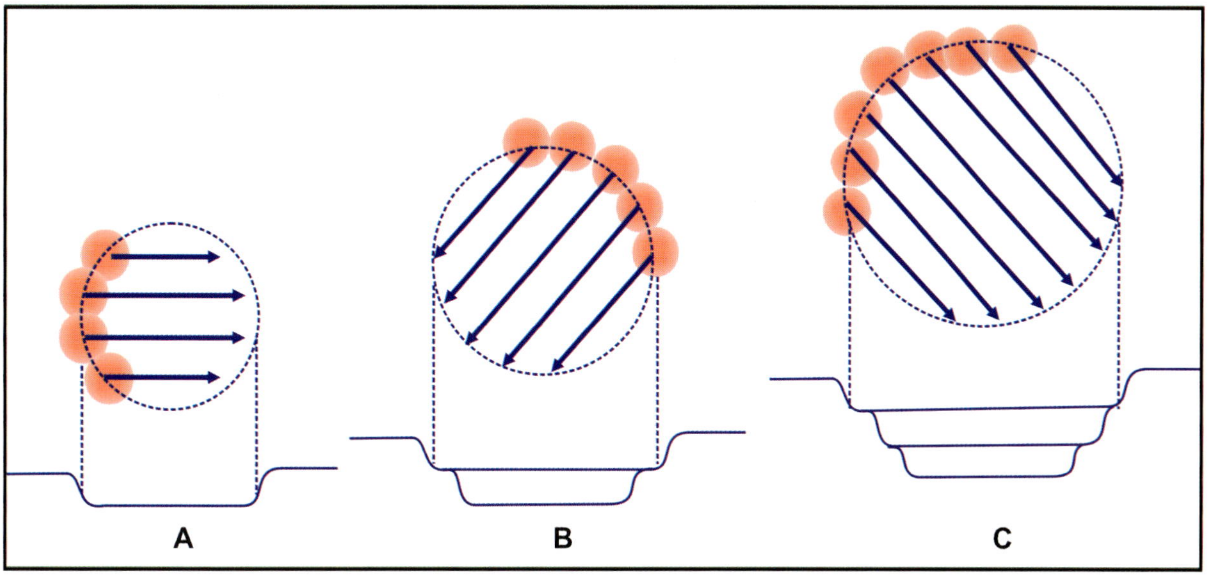

Fig. 2.2: Shows the schematics for flying spot scanning used in system made by PDI and LaserSight, where each scanning layers are rotated when the circle is expanded to achieve a smooth overlapping surface. The end result of the scanning layers is a smooth profile as shown in the figure

for smooth surface which is also shown in Fig. 2.3 for myopic profile.

LASIK PRINCIPLES

LASIK consists of 3 steps: (1) microkeratome device is used to prepare a corneal flap (about 8 to 9 mm in diameter and 130 to 180 micron in thickness); (2) UV laser (excimer or nonexcimer) is used to ablate the corneal stroma under the lifted flap; and (3) The flap is then put back into place. A single-zone method was used at the early stage and was improved to multi-zone to reduce the amount of tissue removed by the laser, a condition required for high diopter corrections and for safety reason.

Single-Zone Method

For an ablation zone diameter of W (in mm) and given the nominal radius of corneal curvature R about (7.8 mm), the binominal expansion of the corneal surface profile (assumed to be spherical) gives an approximate myopic (with D< 0) correction profile (within 5% accuracy) as follows;

$$M(x) = h + 4D X^2/3 \quad (1)$$

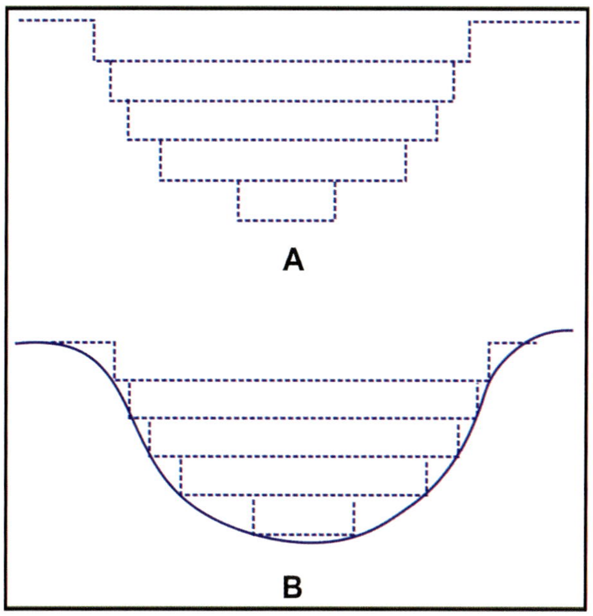

Fig. 2.3: (Solid curve) for the case of myopic correction, in comparison to the step-like rough profile as is generally found in the broad-beam system using an iris (as shown by the dashed curves)

where the center ablation depth h is related to the diopter power D and the ablation zone diameter W by

$$h = -DW^2/3 \quad (2)$$

Similarly, the hyperopic ablation profile is given by

$$H(x) = 4DX^2/3 \quad (3)$$

where the correction power (D) is a negative (positive) value for myopic (hyperopic) corrections.

The proceeding equations are good for spherical corrections, i.e., x is the position from the center of ablated corneal. For cylinder corrections such as astigmatism or compound (toric cylinder), the ablation profile is given by h(x) + h(y), with different value of D assigned in Eq. (1). Based on the proceeding basic equations, we are able to summarize some of the important LASIK clinical issues:

a. Given a given refractive correction D, the central depth of the ablated corneal surface is proportional to the square of the ablation zone size W. Therefore W = 6.5 to 7.0 mm is typically used in myopic LASIK to avoid major haze (caused by large ablation depths) but still keep minimal night halo (caused by small zones).
b. Given an ablation zone W, the central depth is proportional to the correction power D, and the myopic ablation depths (in microns) per diopter are calculated to be 12.0 and 14.1 micron for ablation zone W of 6 and 6.5 mm. Given an error of 1 um in ablation depth, the error caused is less than 0.1 diopter. However, a small error in W will cause a big diopter correction error. For example, a 10% error in W (or from 6.0 mm to 6.6 mm) will cause a diopter correction of 20% reduction, from – 5.0 to – 4.1 diopters, at a given programmed central ablation depth of 60 μm.
c. To avoid significant haze effects caused by deep ablations for high diopter corrections, e.g. h=120 μm for D= -10 correction at an ablation zone of 6 mm, a multizone method has been commonly used to replace the above single-zone method. See the following for greater details.

Multizone Method

As shown by Fig. 2.4, the purpose of multizone ablation (MZA) is to reduce the center ablation depth of the single-zone method, while the overall ablation zone size can be increased by using a smaller inner zone (at full correction) and expanding to larger zone size (the outer zone) but with partial correction. The center depth of an MZA may be reduced to 64% of that of the single zone by a 20% reduced size in the inner zone, or 80% that of the single-zone size. For example, MZA preferred design for a D = – 10 myopic correction at a zone size W of 6.5 mm is as follows. Each zone diameter is defined as W1, W2, W3 for the inner, second and outer zone, respectively and outer zone W3=W (size of single-zone).

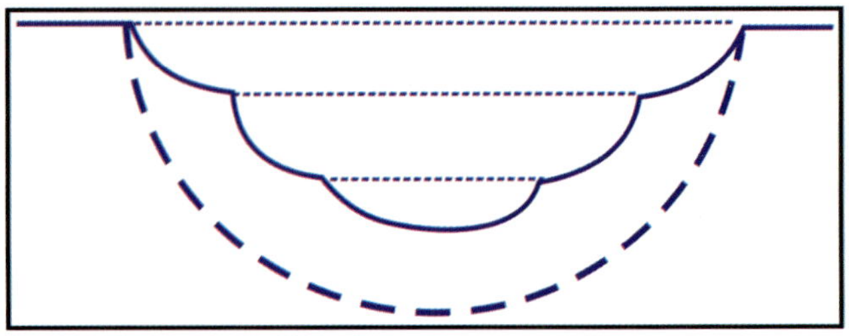

Fig. 2.4: Schematics of single zone and three zone

Zone	W1	W2	W3
zone size	5.2	6.0	6.5 (mm)
correction	– 10.0	– 5.0	– 3.0 (diopter)

In above example, the central ablation depth of single zone is k1 = 10 × (6.5 × 6.5)/3 = 140.8 (micron) which is reduced by a factor of square of (W1/W3), or square of (5.2/6.5) = 0.64 in a 3-zone method. An alternative method using the super-position of three profiles (each at 5.2, 5.0, and 6.5 mm) can also achieve the same inner diopter of D=-10 correction. However, the second method will require a deeper center ablation than that of the first method. The first method may be more complex in software design.

The Corneal Power After LASIK may be calculated by:

$$DC=378/r1-41/r2 \quad (4)$$

which requires a measurement of keratometry power k = 337/r1 (postoperative) and the posterior surface radius (r2) after the LASIK surgery. The conventional keratometry-based reading has been used to estimate the post-LASIK corneal power may suffer 5% to 10% error since it assumes an average r2 at about 6.5 mm. A personalized r2 is required for true accurate corneal power which has major impact on the required IOL power for eyes post-LASIK or postcataract.

High-Order Formulas in LASIK

The center ablation depth in LASIK (myopia) including high-order term is given by:

a. single zone case

$$h1 = (DW^2/3)(1 + C2) \quad (5.a)$$

$$C2 = 0.19 (W/r1)^2 \quad (5.b)$$

where C2 is the high-order term, W is the ablation zone diameter (in mm), h1 is ablation depth (in micron) and D is the "absolute value" of the correction power (in diopters) for myopic or hyperopic LASIK. For hyperopic correction, h1 stands for the maximal depth of the ablated outer ring

b. Multi-zone case

$$h2 = (RF)\, h1 \quad (6)$$

RF = (0.6 – 0.8) is a reduction factor depending on system software designs and in general is given by the square of the ratio of (W1/W3), W1 and W3 being the inner and outer zone diameter as shown earlier.

For a typical ablation diameter of W = W3 = 6.0 mm, and corneal radius r1 = 7.8 mm, we found single zone depth (per diopter correction) h1/D = 12 (1 + 0.114) = 13.36 (micron/D), reduced to 10.56 in a 3-zone design, which ablates 52.8 micron for a D= -5.0 myopic LASIK. We note that the ablation depth is very sensitive to optical zone (W), it goes by the square of W.

For high myopic case, say D = –10 and higher, one shall reduce W (or W3) to about (5.0 – 5.5) mm to keep enough stroma margin (about 250 micron bed) after a 160-micron flap. Furthermore, as shown by the correction term of C2 (about 12%), keratometry power (k) shall also be included, particularly for subjects with r1 deviating to its mean value 7.8 mm.

The typical hyperopic ablation zone is about (5.5 – 6.0) mm plus additional 2 mm transition zone is recommended. Given the ablation depth, the remaining stroma bed thickness at various W may be easily calculated by T(remain) = T_0 – h, where T_0 is the preoperative corneal thickness (about 500 to 600 um) and h is the maximal ablation depth. A safety stroma bed margin about 250 um is recommended. The above formulas are based on spherical corneal surface which typically is a prolate (aspherical) surface. LASIK procedures not only change the corneal surface power, but also its shape (or asphericity) to be discussed as follows.

Aspherical Profile

It was known that corneal surface aberration (or its asphericity) increases after myopic-LASIK. Therefore the conventional Munnerlyn formula (even the exact formula is used) can not describe the aspherical profile of the cornea initially or post-LASIK.

For an aspherical corneal surface, the ablation profile may be expressed as follows (up to the 4th-order power of d) for a myopia correction.

$$H(y) = Z2 + Z4, \quad (7.a)$$

$$Z2 = -(4D/3)(d^2 - y^2), \quad (7.b)$$

$$Z4 = 1000[(d^4 - y^4)/8R^3]\,(p1 - Bp2) \quad (7.c)$$

where p1 and p2 are the preoperative and postoperative corneal shape-factor related to its asphericity by pj = Qj + 1 (j = 1, 2); B = $(R/R')^3$ defined by the ratio of the corneal anterior surface radius R (preoperative) and R′ (postoperative); y is the distance away from the optical axis and d is the ablation radius. In the above expression, H in micron, D in diopter and R, d, y in mm.

The measured increasing asphericity after LASIK may be easily analyzed by Z4 which is proportional to the Zernike coefficient of Z(4, 0) defined by Lee and associates for spherical aberration and shows the role of refractive power correction (D) on the magnitude of spherical aberration by the B-factor in Eq.(1) which is further related to D by B = $(1 + 0.0204\,D)^3$ for a typical preoperative corneal radius of R = 7.7 mm. For examples: For a -5.0 D myopia correction of a cornea having p1=0.8 (a prolate cornea with Q1 = – 0.2), Z4 (at y = 0) = 0.8% of H_o (for p2 = 1.0); and Z4 (at y = d) = 7.8% of H_o for a +5.0 D hyperopia correction for P2 = 0.6 and d = 3.0 mm where a revised profile for hyperopia is needed to calculate Z4.

Therefore, the impact of Z4 on the ablation depth and the shape of the cornea is sensitive to the correlation ratio defined by $P1/P2 = B^N$, where N=(0.66 – 1.0) depending on the approximation used for the conical surface function expansion. In the parabolic (second-order) approximation N = 1.0 (Jimenez et al), and the infinity-order or asymptotic value of N is 2/3 (Lin, to be published). Greater detail of asphericity control may be found in another chapter of Lin in this book.

MICROKERATOME TECHNOLOGY

Microkeratome is a device to make the corneal flap, the step prior to LASIK. It was developed in 1963 by Bauaquer based on the Castroviejo Electrome. Krumeich developed a microkeratome without the need to freeze the corneal in 1985. In the 1990's, the mechanical design increased the predictability of flap diameter, thickness, hinge size and location, and edge characteristic.

Manual microkeratome offers the surgeon to choose parameters based on corneal thickness, diameter and surface curvature, whereas automated design offers the advantages of shortened learning curve and more consistent results. The currently available commercial systems include the following:

a. Manual model made by: SCMD, Eye Technology, Moria
b. Automated model made by: Schwind, Phoenix, Universal Keratome, Draeger Flap Maker where a rotating rather than oscillating blades was first introduced by Draeger and offers a "superior" hinge flap.

   Two nonmechanical microkeratome (for bladeless LASIK) designs have been developed as the alternatives:

c. Ultrashort (picosecond or femtosecond) pulsed Nd:YLF laser made by: Escalon Medical Corp. and IntraLase, Inc.
d. Waterjet device (or hydrokeratome) made by: VisiJet and MediJet.

Typical flap thickness includes 130, 160, 180 and 200 microns and the hinge diameter of 8.5 to 10 mm. These two factors depend on patient's preoperative corneal thickness (about 0.45 to 0.6 mm) and the correction power. For example, high refractive error and thin cornea would require a thinner flap (130 um) in order to keep the safety margin (about 250 um) of the remaining stroma bed. Surgeons also have the alternative to choose nasal or superior hinge.

The bladeless devices of (c) and (d) have the advantages of minimal blade-related complications (cutting chatter, irregular astigmatism, epithelial ingrowth, etc.) in addition to less tissue trauma, smoother surface and more consistent. The hydrokeratome is also much faster than mechanical microkeratome, less than one second vs. few minutes.

Disposable microkeratomes are also developed and offered by LaserSight, Refractive Technologies and Moria. The disposable units have the following pros:

- Minimal errors caused by disk assembly, cleaning and handling.
- Require no maintenance.
- Economical for low volume surgeons.

New microkeratome is completely automotive and does not use gears. It is propelled by flexible cable with high pressure (300 psec). The gearless device has the advantages of minimal problems of lashes and other debris which may accumulate in the gear, and minimal torgue during its translation.

The short pulsed laser currently offers a ALL laser LASIK procedure. The ultimate technology would be a LASIK procedure to ablate the corneal stroma without creating a flap, where a focused, scanning laser may be computer controlled to create the desired intrastroma profile for a given refractive error.

LASIK SYSTEM

Several beam delivery devices have been used in refractive surgery laser (RSL) systems by both excimer and nonexcimer lasers. They include: circle/linear scanning, slit scanning, expanding diaphragm, rotating disk, combined device of slit scanning and expanding diaphragm, erodible mask, absorbing cell, and fiber coupling.

Joysticks are used by some of the manufacturers, where the surgeon is able to steer the laser beam for centration and also for following slow eye motion. This feature is an advantage over conventional foot-switch control systems in which the laser beam cannot be steered and the surgeon has to control the patient chair for centration.

The expected post-LASIK surface quality, or smoothness of the ablated corneal surface, has usually been checked by ablation of PMMA sheets. Only those systems using a scanning device achieve very smooth PMMA surfaces (which also provide readable diopters by lensometer). The conventional broad-beam laser using diaphragm devices have generated step-like rings that cause rough PMMA surface ablations, which are hard to read in a lensometer checking. Eye fixation light was used in earlier systems which are now integrated with an eye tracking to avoid problems of decentration.

The Advantages of Scanning Laser

The first generation LASIK systems using a large beam size of 5 to 6 mm (such as systems made by Summit and VISX), or a slit beam of 1x7 mm (such as Meditec and Nidek systems), require a perfectly uniform beam for uniform surface ablation. Beam profiles of these systems are critical, since any "hot" or "cold" spots could cause serious safety problems. A typical laser energy per pulse of 200 to 400 mJ is also required in order required to obtain a uniform beam energy of 30 to 40 mJ on the corneal surface. Complicated optics usually employed for beam homogeneity in these systems cause an overall energy delivery efficiency of less than 20 %.

In contrast to the first-generation "broad-beam" technology, which uses industrial-type, high-power and low repetition rate (about 20 Hz) excimer lasers, the newest generation scanning laser system uses the recent technology of compact, high-repetition-rate (up to 250 Hz) excimer laser operated at a smaller beam spot size of 0.5 to 1.5 mm. It only requires a beam energy per pulse of only 0.8 to 2.5 mJ on the corneal surface to achieve the same range of fluence (or energy density) (160 to 200 mJ/cm^2) as that of the high-power excimers.

The advantages of scanning laser for LASIK include:

Efficient Beam Delivery

Only few optics (5 to 8) are required in the scanning system, more than 60% of the initial beam energy exiting from the laser cavity can be delivered onto the corneal surface, where beam reshaping and/or uniformity is not critical. For comparison, 15 to 25 optics were used in the high-power excimers using nonscanning modes which have an overall efficiency less than 30%.

Compact, Low Cost, and Reliable

Due to the high efficiency of beam delivery, only 2 to 3 mJ of energy/pulse is needed on the corneal surface. The problems suffered by high-power lasers (200 to 400 mJ) such as optics/coating damage and sensitivity to moisture and dust can be largely reduced in the low-energy scanning laser, which also has a lower maintenance cost.

Smooth Surface Ablation

The common problems of step-like rings and/or transition zones found in the diaphragm method (such as Summit and VISX earlier systems) were not found with scanning laser. The scanning mode produces a smoother surface, where a large number of pulses (2000 to 5000) are overlapped and delivered onto the corneal surface.

Customized Ablation Patterns

The software-driven scanning device (with eye-tracking) allows flexible ablation patterns suitable for customized ablate on including: The treatment of irregular , off-centered surface, local correction for astigmatism and customized ablation combined with the digitalized corneal topography or elevation map such as Orbscan, so-called topography-guided LASIK.

Minimal Surface Aberration (SA)

SA may be minimized by eliminating the high-order aberration for supervision.

Other Clinical Advantages

Smooth ablation boundary transitions should reduce the regression particularly in high diopter corrections, where epithelium filling of the ablated area may be triggered by a "deep" transition edge on the ablated zone. A "shallow" transition can be easily achieved in the scanning mode. In addition, a final "polishing" of the ablated area can also be easily conducted to further reduce the Haze effect. Shock-wave-induced tissue damage and central islands occurred in the high-power excimers have not been found in the scanning mode.

Optimal Scanning Parameters

Smooth PMMA profiles of myopic correction may be generated and used as the calibration at various overlap parameters (L) defined by $L = 1 - d/r$, with d being the displacement between each scanning spot and r being the diameter (or spot size) of the beam. For a spot size of 1.0 mm and d = 0.2 mm, L = 0.8 or 80% overlap. It should be noted that given a spot size, smaller beam displacement d (or larger beam overlap) always gives a smoother ablation surface in which, however, the thermal effect may also increases accordingly.

Therefore, the key issue for LASIK procedure is to optimize the parameters of d, L and the procedure time (T). It should be noted that laser average power (P) rather than the energy (E) is the determining parameter of the procedure time (T), assuming the laser fluence is above the ablation threshold.

Furthermore a smaller energy per pulse (E) and/or lower fluence (F) will achieve a smoother ablation surface. However, the procedure time (T) is inverse proportional to the ablation rate A and the laser repetition rate R. Therefore, the second optimization is to adjust the parameters of E (or F), A and R in addition to d and L. Regarding this aspect, the following relations are useful:

T proportional to $W^2/(E/r^2)R$, were W is the outer ablation zone diameter, $(E/r^2) = F$ (fluence) or the energy per unit area of each scanning spot.

Another important issue is beam uniformity. A compact scanning laser system did not include complicated optics for beam uniformity. Instead, the beam overlap technique is used to minimize the need of beam uniformity. A smooth overall ablation surface was achieved by enough beam overlap (typically, L= 60% to 80%), which is, however, limited by the minimal procedure speed required. Typical LASIK preferred procedure should be completed within 15 to 20 seconds for a -5 diopter correction at an ablation zone of 6.5 mm. In addition to the beam overlap, a uniform profile may also be achieved by beam "spinning" (or rotation by a so-called K-mirror) or by beam orientation when it is linearly scanned such as in Nidek system.

Yet another important issue is the ablation profile, which must match the theoretical curve in order to achieve the desired diopter correction. In the scanning mode approach, unlike the diaphragm mode, the profile is software-driven with profile accuracy limited by the beam spot size, that is, a small spot size of 0.5 to 0.8 mm is preferred. A smaller spot size takes a longer time to scan over the entire ablation zone, although it is easier to achieve an accurate profile. Therefore, the third optimization rule is the spot size and procedure speed at a given average power P. Given an optimized spot size, higher average power will always speed up the procedure without losing the accuracy of ablation profile.

Yet another issue of scanning laser is the increase of thermal effects in high repetition rate laser, say 200 Hz. This accumulated thermal effect from the spatially overlapped pulse may be minimized by a so called "random scanning" such that pulse to pulse or scanning layer to layer may be separated for minimal thermal effects although the UV laser is considered to be a "cold" laser.

Irregular or customized correction is another challenging task that may be performed by the scanning laser described here. Topographic analysis would be required for focal treatment of asymmetric astigmatism. Using software-driven ablation patterns, scanning would be an ideal method for these localized selective, ablations that require adjustable zone sizes, shape, and orientation. Greater details about customized corneal ablation will be shown later.

To summarize, the advantages of scanning laser over the high-power broad-beam systems include: Low-energy (less optical damage), low-cost, flexible ablation patterns, smooth surface and transition boundary (for less haze and regression), unlimited ablation zone size (for hyperopia and high myopia), and simplicity (without the need of complicated beam uniformity optics). The scanning device integrated in the system is computer-controlled to meet the optimization criteria, which are characterized by several parameters such as laser beam spot size, energy, fluence, average power, laser repetition rate, tissue ablation rate, scanning speed, and overlap function.

Positive Cylinder Correction

Most corneas have a prolate shape (flatter at the periphery) and an oblate (or more prolate) shape will be created after a myopia (or hyperopia) correction. For astigmatism correction, a cylinder (positive or negative) ablation pattern is needed. Typical excimer laser generated patterns on a zip thermal paper are shown in Fig. 4.7, the negative and positive cylinders are rotated by 90°. The most interesting correction strategy is to convert the negative cylinders to a positive cylinder for less corneal tissue removed and maintaining the same spherical equivalent (SE) and cylinder. Examples are shown as follows.

Compound (Toric) Error

Astigmatism causes a distorted image on the retina and is usually combined with a myopia or hyperopia to form a compound error (or toric) given the prescription of [a, b × angle] which has a spherical equivalent (SE) of a + 0.5b. Therefore, the following compound astigmatisms have the same SE but expressed in different formats (noting that the angles are rotated by 90°):

Negative cylinder	*Positive cylinder*
[+5.0, -3.0 × 180]	[+2.0, +3.0 × 90];
[+2.0, -2.0 × 180]	[plano, +2.0 × 90]

Above conversions are based on the general formula:

$$[a, b \times \text{Angle}] = [(a+b), -b \times (\text{Angle} - 90^\circ)]$$

For compound error correction, one may use the simultaneous elliptical method (SEM) for both the spherical and cylinder error. However, a hyperopic-shift is normally induced if the treated eye has no positive spherical preoperatively. To avoid the above problems, a consecutive or sequential method which uses a positive cylinder ablation to steepen the flat meridian and followed by central spherical (either myopic or hyperopic) ablation has been used.

WAVEFRONT TECHNOLOGY

Wavefront devices for the detection or reconstruction of optical aberration (OA) become increasingly important resulted from the induced OA after refractive surgeries of RK, PRK, LASIK, LASEK and others. The OAs are important particularly for low light levels and large pupil apertures, say larger than 3.0 mm where the Gaussian optics or paraxial-ray approximation fails and the ray tracking for peripheral area is required. There are four different principles by which wavefront OA may be measured and the related devices are commercially available: The Shack-Hartmann using the outgoing reflection, the Tscherning and ray tracing using retinal imaging, the spatially-resolved refractometry and the slit light bundle double pass aberrometry.

Shack-Hartmann aberrometry (SHA) is the most promising device today which was first tested by Liang and Williams in 1994, although the method was introduced by Hartman in 1900 and later by Shack in 1971. SHA uses the outgoing array of spot image to determine the wavefront shape. The array of spot images formed by the microlenslet array was

Table 2.5: Summary of optical aberration defined by Zernike coefficients

A. Monochromatic	
Defocus (second-order)	Coma (third-order)
Spherical (fourth-order)	Field curvature (second-order)
Astigmatism (second-order)	Distortion (first-order)
B. Chromatic	
Longtitudinal, Transverse]	
1. Seidel Aberration (surface contribution, relaxed eye) Cornea (+80%, – 10.4%), cornea-lens separation (– 5.6%) Lens (+13.1%, +22.9%), total power 60.29 diopter. For (r1, r2) = (7.8, 6.5), (R1, R2) = (10.5, 6) and S = 6(all in mm)	
2. Typical aspherical data (Q-value) for (front, back) surface Cornea (– 0.3, – 0.66), ideal surface Q = – 0.527 Lens (– 0.94, +0.96), for relaxed eye (Louis and Brennar)	

captured by a CCD sensor and analyzed by a computer to estimate the eye's aberration map. The OA is expressed as Zernike polynomical derivatives and the fitted coefficients and used to reconstruct the shape of the wavefront which is aberrated by the surfaces of the cornea and the lens and their coupling effects.

Table 2.5 summarizes the Zernike polynomial and the related OA including spherical surface aberration, cornea and other high-order terms.

Zernike Analysis for Different Devices

Six major wavefront devices made by Alcon, Nidek, Bausch & Lomb, Topcon, Tracey and Wavefront Sciences have been evaluated and compared by system repeatability and their performance with raw Zernike data and wavefront mapping by Durrie and Stalk (2004).

This study concluded that:

- Different wavefront devices cannot be easily studied interchangeably, where raw Zernike data from different devices can only be fed to specific therapeutic system.
- Devices with a higher data point (85 to 200 points in a 6 mm pupil) only slightly performs better than that of lower data points (< 70).

SHAPE FACTOR ANALYSIS

Optimization of retina image quality in customized LASIK via Zernike polynomials has been largely emphasized on the change of the conic surface of the cornea. The initially prolate cornea front surface having a negative Q-value (typically about – 0.2 to 0.3) may become positive or negative post-LASIK. However, changing cornea's Q-value via laser ablation alone could not completely eliminate system optical aberration which, 92% is due to defocus and astigmatism, and 8% due to third-order (coma-like), fourth-order (spherical aberration) and other higher-order aberrations. Much work has been done on the correction of surface aberration (SA) of cornea which contributes about 70% of the total SA, whereas less work is reported regarding the roles of the posterior cornea surface (about 10% of total SA), the lens surfaces (about 37%) and the coupling between cornea and lens (about 7% reduction of the total positive SA).

The Zernike analysis is useful for measuring corneal SA and total SA to obtain their difference for the SA due to internal optics. However, it provides little information regarding the compensation between corneal negative SA and lens positive SA. Lin presented a comprehensive theory, without using Zernike polynomials, based on three "shape factors

(SF)": S1 (for the cornea), S2 (for the lens) and S3 (for the whole system) to demonstrate how the asymmetric shapes of the corneal and lenticular surface can be compensated with each other for minimal spherical aberration and coma, which improves the overall retina image quality characterized by primary aberrations, namely defocus, astigmatism, coma, spherical aberration, field curvature and image distortion. Furthermore, system SF is a nonlinear function of S1 and S2, and minimal SA or spherical aberration is governed the ratio of between the effective focal length of the cornea and the lens, rather than their individual values, where anterior chamber depth also plays certain role.

Retina image quality (RIQ) is determined by refractive errors, ocular aberration, diffraction and scattering, where the first three factors depend upon wavelength (or color), pupil size and the shape of the cornea and lens. As shown by Table 2.5 , the Zernike second-order (defocus and astigmatism) contributes about 92% of the total optical aberration. The spherical aberration (SA) is proportional to surface power, therefore, it is contributed about 70% from cornea surface (+80% from front and -10% from back surface).

For young eye (before age 6) the negative SA gradually increases to a positive SA and considerable increased for age older than 35 due to the increase of negative asphericity of the lens. For young eye, lens accommodation may eliminate or minimize the SA caused by the imperfect compensation between the "prolate" cornea (with positive SA) and lens (with negative SA).

It was reported that post-LASIK has increased high-order Zernike aberration which may be reduced by customized ablation. Advanced IOL for aged eye with negative SA may also improve image quality. The RIQ may be analyzed by Zernike polynomials or alternatively by a simple method using the shape factor of the cornea and lens as shown above.

We note that Q-value of cornea (about – 0.2 to – 0.3) is not "prolate' enough for an ideal surface of Q = – 0.527, therefore, it contributes positive SA, which is partially compensated by the negative SA from the lens (mainly its posterior surface). It was reported that negative SPA predominated before age 6, but considerably increased to positive SPA after 35 years. However, mean aberration becomes zero by (2 to 3) diopter of accommodation in young eyes. Wavefront device has been used to analyze the surface aberration (SA) of cornea and the system and their difference gives the SA due to lens. Corneal reshaping by LASIK, therefore, is limited to the change of cornea SF (S1). Theory goes one step further to analyze the role of lens and its separation to the cornea (or ACD) on the whole system SA would be required.

To summarize the natural shapes (at relaxed state) of corneal and lens surfaces are constructed such that their optical aberrations are largely balanced, whereas the small remaining positive spherical aberration further reduced by lens accommodation for optimal retinal quality. Individual ocular information including the shape function of the lens and whole system is required for customized laser ablation, in addition to the power and shape of the cornea.

CUSTOMIZED CORRECTION

Two major technologies have been developed in the past two decades from cornea reshaping: The "broad beam" laser patented by L'Esperance in 1986 (US Pat. 4,580,559) and the "flying spot" scanning laser patented by the present author in 1996 (US Pat. 5,520,679). The scanning system using a smaller laser spot about 0.5 to 1.5 mm and integrated with an eye tracking make it possible to correct irregular or customized corneal surface. Advanced corneal mapping device provides the localized elevation map (EM) of the corneal surface, whereas the conventional topography measures the "averaged curvature" to define an overall diopter of the corneal surface. For irregular corneal surface or off-centered cornea after refractive surgery, corneal surface diopter is no longer well defined, and therefore, localized (or customized) information based on an EM is required in vision correction. Recent wavefront technologies further provide the optical aberration (OA) measurement, preoperatively and postoperatively, such that so called "super vision" becomes possible by minimizing or eliminating the OA.

Wavefront devices and topography may be used to correct higher-order surface aberration (SA) and surface irregularity. Empirical correction factors introduced by laser manufacturers to compensate the increase of SA after LASIK based on the averaged population patient data are, strictly speaking, not a true customized correction which requires individual specific needs including the following considerations:

- Age and occupation needs
- Corneal thickness and pupil size
- Anterior and vitreous depth
- Anterior and posterior surface of the cornea (r1, r2)
- Anterior and posterior surface of the lens (R1, R2)
- Axial length
- Keratometry power
- Ablation zone size
- Microkeratome flap thickness
- Alternative procedure of LASIK, LASEK, phakic IOL, or combined procedures.
- Monovision or bifocal
- Center or peripheral myopia.

  For example, the LASIK central ablation depth depends on r1 or keratometry; for a given lens power, the effective anterior chamber depth (ACD) depends on the thickness and shape of the lens (or the ratio of R1 and R2); the total SA is affected by the combined and coupling of the SA of cornea and lens. Furthermore, keratometry power alone cannot determine the actual corneal power which also requires accurate measurement of r2 LASIK flap (120 to 180 um thick) and corneal thickness are correlated to the ablation zone size (W) in order to keep a minimal 250 um bed after LASIK.

  Customized correction would require one or more than one of the following:

- Corneal topography
- Wavefront measurements based on the commercially available devices including:
  - Shack-Hartmann sensor
  - Crosscylinder aberrometer
  - Tscherning aberrometer
  - Tracey device (Ray tracking)
  - Slit-light bundle
  - Spatially resolved refractomer

Wavefront-guided ablation (WGA) is designed to reduce the high-order optical aberration of the whole eye to increase retinal image resolution and contrast, whereas topography-guided ablation (TGA) is designed to correct mainly corneal wavefront. Therefore, the ideal design would be a combined WGA and TGA to separate the wavefront of the whole eye and the cornea for a true customized treatment.

In addition, the aged-reduced positive SA must also be included as one of the factors to be considered. It was known that the natural crystalline lens has a SA of – 25 um, 0 and +25 um at age 20, 40 and 60, although cornea SA remains constant throughout the whole like. When the positive SA increases in the eye, the presence of glare and night halos also increase. It was proposed that aging causes a gradient refractive index in the lens and causes a change from negative SA of the lens over time. Therefore, as the eye ages, the combined positive SA of cornea and lens increases. The idea of customized IOL is to cause a perfect compensation of the positive SA of a prolate-cornea (with $Q < 0$) by the implanted aspherical IOL having a negative SA, or a oblate structure (with $Q > 0$) for most of the cataract patients. However, an opposite strategy will be needed for the 10% abnormal patients having negative SA after cataracts.

Topography-Guided LASIK

The recent developed corneal topography provides the elevation maps for corneal surface which also provides more information than the regular Placido maps or axial maps. Systems made by Orbscan and others having the elevation maps open the possibility of customized corneal reshaping based on the preoperative data. Lin and Hwang presented the first irregular corneal reshaping based on preoperative computer simulation in 1997 at ISRS meeting including off-center astigmatism, undercorrection enhancement and zone enlargement and some irregular shape ablation. These simulation data are based on the semielevation map provided in a system made by Opticon-2000. Although the true elevation is not provided, these simulation data demonstrated that customized corneal reshaping is possible, when detailed elevation maps are integrated into a scanning laser.

A true topography-linked corneal reshaping (TOPCOR) at this time is limited by factors of : (1) Real-time-fast process of the topographic measurement is not ready when integrated with a scanning refractive system, where the ablated corneal surface, either in LASEK or LASIK, may not be measured in real time, (2) physical integration of a topography to the delivery unit of the laser has not been developed, (3) scanning software based on the localized "mean-point" of a corneal surface is not yet developed.

In a paper presented by Lin and Hwang (in World Refractive Surgery Symposium, Miami, July, 1999), these authors proposed a mesh-point method for preoperative simulation for certain selected cases and under some assumption for certain selected cases and under some assumptions of the corneal shape. However, a true TOPCOR for an irregular cornea operated in real time or intraoperatively is still under development. Furthermore a new "concept" based on "localized" corneal elevation rather than the "averaged-curvature" or diopter must be redefined in order to customize the laser reshaping procedure. The preoperative irregular corneal shape, radius and line-of-sight and other factors affecting a patient's vision must be considered all together so that improved vision better than 20/20 may be possible even in a irregular cornea. Summary of the paper of Lin and Hwang is as follows.

To demonstrate a true topography-linked software for the corrections of regular and irregular cornea and define a new mesh-point method (MPM) different from any of the existing methods which the authors believe are not a true mapping.

Based on elevation map and the converted coordinate "relative heights" of each local point of the corneal preoperative surface with respect to the "desired" correction surface, either regular or irregular, we define a mapping with mesh points of each 0.25 × 0.25 mm area. A scanning laser (made by PDI), under the control of the predetermined software, is then used to fix each local mesh point of the mapping and achieve the desired final corneal map. The results using this MPM can be confirmed by various methods. PMMA flat sheets measured by a micron-sensor, curved PMMA button measured by a topography, or computer simulation on selected maps.

Using the MPM, the authors were able to demonstrate the corrections of the following cases (confirmed by simulation and PMMA data): (i) Regular myopic and hyperopic correction in consistent with the nonmapping method, (ii) off-centered astigmatism, (iii) off-centered and undercorrected myopic followed by a enlargement in ablation zone, and (iv) irregular cornea profile corrected by a customized mapping.

The mesh-point method (MPM) is a unique method which provides the true topography-linked corneal mapping for particularly irregular correction and other postoperative enhancement. The existing methods based on the "averaged corneal curvature" are limited only to almost regular corneas and cannot achieve the localized or customized results as that of the MPM. A real-time, true mapping, scanning laser system integrated to a topography may become possible, if MPM can be processed fast, within few miniseconds per map.

Figure 2.5 shows the computer-simulated topography for pure cylinder correction, in which (A) and (B) are the preoperative map in axial mode and in elevation mode, (C) is the laser ablation for a negative cylinder along the follow-the-rule direction for a negative cylinder along the follow-the-rule direction, and (D) is the 90-degree rotated, positive cylinder ablation. Figure 2.6 shows the ablation profiles for a pure negative and positive cylinder corresponding to (C) and (D), respectively.

Figure 2.7 shows the computer-simulated topography for an off-centered cylinder correction, in which (A) and (B) are the preoperative maps in

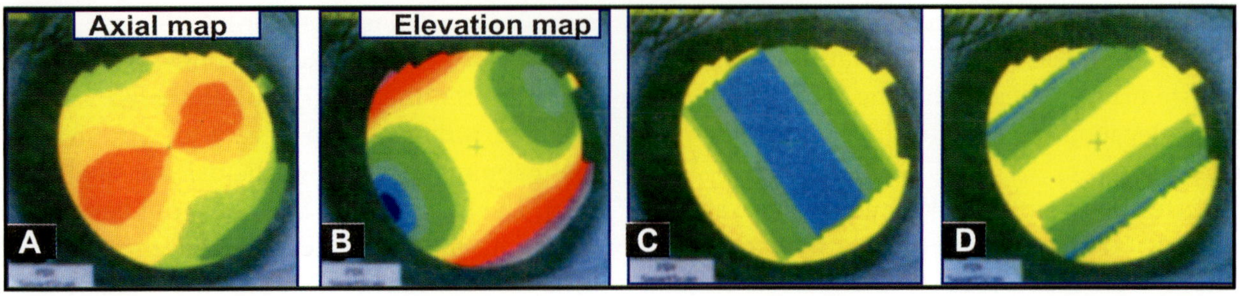

Figs 2.5A to D: Computer-simulated topography for pure cylinder correction, in which (A) and (B) are the preoperative maps in axial mode and in elevation mode, (C) is the laser ablation for a negative cylinder along the follow-the-rule direction, and (D) is the 90° rotated, positive cylinder ablation

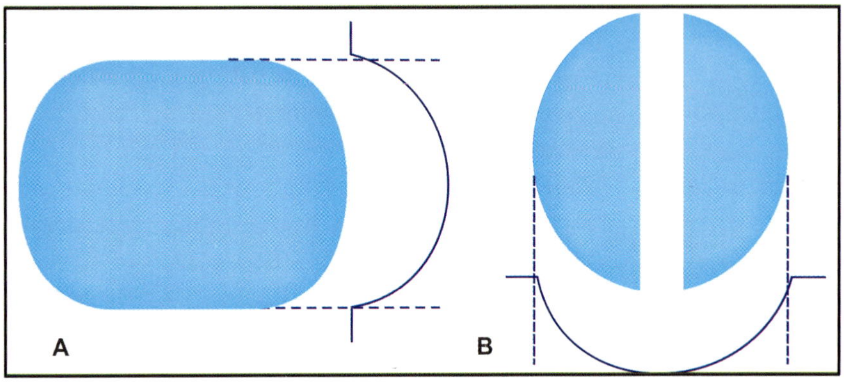

Fig. 2.6: Shows the ablation profiles for a pure negative and positive cylinder corresponding to (C) and (D) in Figure 2.3 to 2.6, respectively

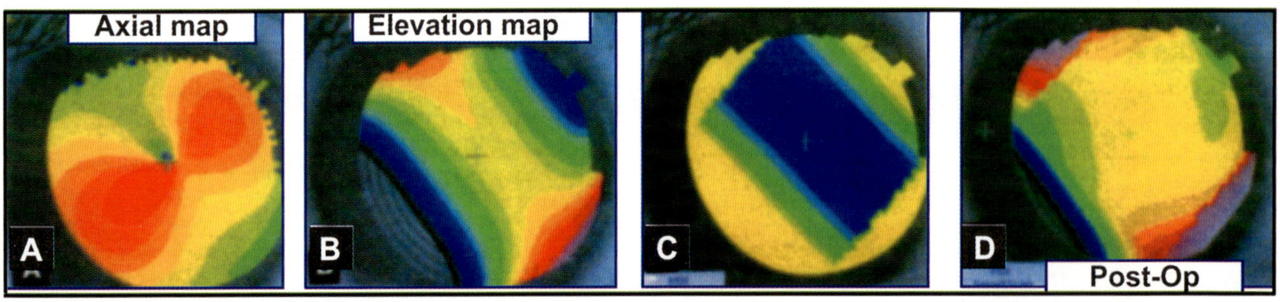

Figs 2.7A to D: Computer-simulated topography for an off-centered cylinder correction, in which (A) and (B) are the preoperative map in axial mode and in elevation mode, (C) is the laser ablation patent which is off-centered accordingly and (D) is the postoperative result

axial mode and in elevation mode, (C) is the laser ablation profile which is off-centered accordingly, and (D) is the postoperative map.

The third example for results generated from PDI's SmartScan is shown in Figure 2.8. The preoperative topography (A) shows an off-centered and undercorrected case (conducted by a PRK procedure) which is corrected (B) by a two-step procedure: Step 1 is to treat the undercorrection and step 2 is to enlarge and center the corrected area.

Limitations of CCR

Laser manufacturers have claimed the use of customized corneal reshaping (CCR), however, they did not address the technical difficulties which have not yet been overcome for a true, real-time CCR.

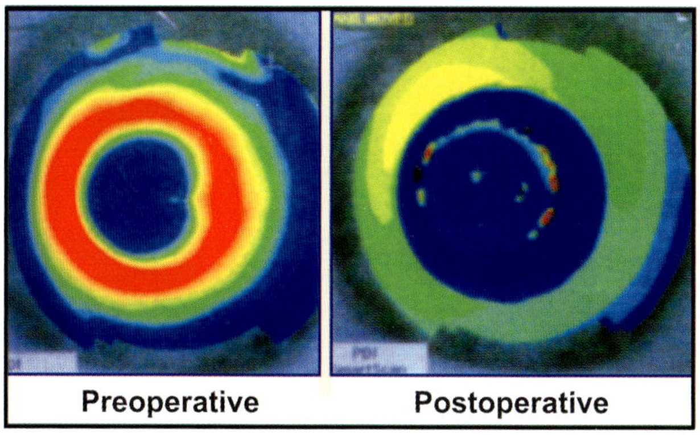

Fig. 2.8: The preoperative topography (A) shows an off-centered and undercorrected case (conducted by a PRK procedure) which is corrected by a two-step procedure: First treat the undercorrection and then enlarge the ablation zone and center the corrected area, shown in (B)

The scanning lasers currently used for LASIK were designed with the intent for customized surface ablation. However, they are all based on average corneal surface data for "approximate" large area correction. A localized, small area correction for CCR based on the EM has not yet been developed since the concept was first presented by Lin in 1999 (Fall World Refractive Surgery Symposium, Oct. 1999, Orlando, FL).

Most of the systems on the market (made by Nidek, LaserSight, Alcon, Bausch and Lomb and others claiming the capability of customized reshaping are simply misleading without mentioning the limitations. For example, in correcting a post-PRK off-centered eye, a portion of the off-centered corneal surface was ablated and followed by another correction on the resultant refractive error, where "symmetry" ablation profiles were typically used and the correction power is defined by an averaged surface diopter. This procedure, most of the time, will ablate too much corneal tissue with the high risk of corneal weakening and is limited only to symmetric-type corrections. Therefore, the existing systems having input parameters based on the surface diopter cannot correct localized irregularity of the surface which requires the EM data as well as the calculated profile difference between the desired regular profile and the initial irregular profile.

In addition, all the existing LASIK systems using a fixed laser beam spot size limit the accuracy of corrected profile, particularly when the localized irregularity is smaller than the laser spot size, typically about 0.8 to 1.5 mm. It should be noted that smaller beam spot provides more accurate ablation profile but slower procedure, whereas larger spot gives faster procedure with poor accuracy. Current excimer laser technologies can only offer up to about 250 Hz repetition rate which also limits the procedures speed to be about 3.0 seconds per diopter. Therefore, the ultimate solution for accurate and fast procedure would require a system having an adjustable beam spot size. For example, one may use 0.3 mm laser spot to correct smaller or irregular profile, whereas a 2.0 mm spot for large area and smoother profile. A two-step CCR with adjustable spot size has been recently proposed accordingly. (Lin, JT. US pending patent, 2005).

Theoretically, one may always achieve a desired corneal surface profile (F) given by $F(x,y,z) = G(x,y,z) + C(x,y,z)$, where C is the ablating (correcting) profile and G is the initial (regular or irregular) profile. However, before a CCR becomes clinically practical, several technical difficulties need to be overcome.

First, both C and G are 3-D functions, or (x,y,z) dependent. The commonly used correcting profile assuming symmetric in x and y is not an acceptable solution, when G (measured by EM) has asymmetric depth in (x, y) plane.

Second, patient's refractive error based on large area averaged curvature is not well-defined in an irregular profile G and cannot be used as an input parameter for the profile C.

Third, a true CCR shall be based on the EM data for the initial profile G which is then used to calculate the correcting profile given by the difference of G and F, $C = F - G$.

The most difficult part of removing the irregularity of G is the surface roughness after the ablation. The desired profile F normally is a well-defined, regular surface which can be generated by a software program, where a typical "single" spatial overlap parameter of 50% to 70% (in both x and y direction) is used in a Gaussian profile laser in order to minimize the surface roughness. For irregular profile G, the overlap parameters in x and y directions, in general, are different and require irregular "multiple" overlap parameters which is almost "mission impossible" for a software design. It would be possible only by using a "flat-top" laser profile and without any overlap which, however, has another problems of roughness resulting from the edges of each spot, unless each of the scanning spots are perfectly displaced. Fig. 2.9 summarizes the procedures involved in CCR and their difficulties, where step one is to remove the irregularity of G (without changing the refractive power), and step two is to correct the refractive error.

To conclude, the current technologies combining scanning beam, eye-tracking, elevation map and wavefront device may offer a customized corneal reshaping (CCR), but is only limited to large area averaged correction, such as off-center correction. A true, real-time CCR, particularly for high-degree, preoperative small-scale irregularity, will remain technically impossible, until the surface smoothness and irregular beam overlap issue addressed above can be resolved.

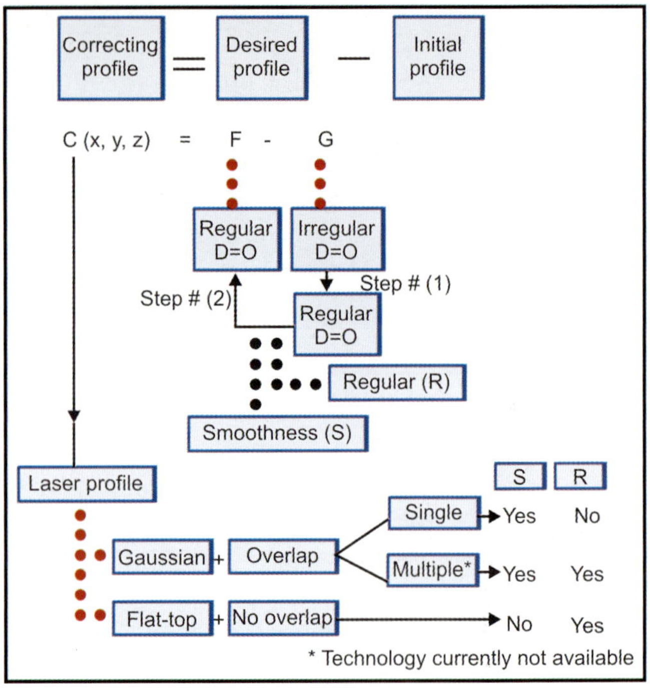

Fig. 2.9: Flowchart for customized Lasik

BIBLIOGRAPHY

1. Anera R, Jimenez JR, Barco LJ. Equation for corneal asphericity after corneal refractive surgery. J Refract Surg. 2003;19:65-69.
2. Anera RG, Jimenez JR, Barco LJ, Hitta E. Change in corneal asphericity after laser refractive surgery, including reflection loss and nonnormal incidence upon the anterior cornea. Opt Lett. 2003;15:417-19.
3. Avalos G, Silva A. Presbyopia LASIK-the PMMA technique. In: Agarwal A. ed. Presbyopia, a surgical textbook. Thorofare NJ: SLACK 2004;139-46.
4. Cantu R, Rosales MA, Tepichin E, et al. Objective quality of vision in presbyopic and nonpresbyopic patients after pseudoaccommodative advanced surface ablation. J Refract Surg. 2005(Suppl.);21:S603-05.
5. El-Danasoury A, Baines HS. Optimized prolate corneal ablation: Case report for the first treated eye. J Refract Surg. 2005;21:S595-602.
6. Gatinel D, T Hoang-Xuan, Azar D. Determination of corneal asphericity after myopia surgery with the excimer laser: a mathematical model. Invest Ophthalmol Vis Sci 2001;42:1736-1742.
7. Gills J, et al. Corneal topography: The state of the art. SLACK Inc: Thorofare 1995.
8. Gordon M et al. Photorefractive keratectomy (PRK) at 193 nm using an erodible mask. Proc SPIE. 1992;1644:11-19.
9. Jenkins TCA. Aberration of the eye and their effects on vision. Br J Physiol Opt 1963;20:59-91.
10. Jimenez JR, Anera RG, Diaz J, Diaz A, Perez-ocon F. Corneal asphericity after refractive surgery when the Munnerlyn formula is applied. J Opt Soc Am (A) 2004;21:98-103.
11. Jimenez JR, Anera RG, Barco LJ. Refractive changes due to ablation parameters after photorefraqctive surgery. J Refract Surg. 2004;20:182-182.
12. Lee H, Oh JR, Reintein DZ, et al. Conservation of corneal tissue with wavefront guided laser in situ keratomileuse. J Cataract Refract Surg. 2005; 31:1153-58.
13. Lin JT: In Program and Abstract, ISRK, pre-AAO, 1994-99.
14. Lin JT. Multiwavelength solid state laser for ophthalmic applications. Proc SPIE 1992;1644:266-75.
15. Lin JT. Mini-excimer laser corneal reshaping using a scanning device. Proc SPIE 1994;2131:228-236.
16. Lin JT. Scanning laser technology for refractive surgery. In: Garg et al. Mastering the techniques of corneal refractive surgery. New Delhi, India, Jaypee Brothers 2005;20-36.

17. Lin JT. Critical review on refractive surgical lasers. Opt. Engineer. 1995;34:668-75.
18. Lin JT. A new formula for ablation depth in 3-zone LASIK. J Refract Surg 2005;21:413-14.
19. Lin JT. Prediction and control of corneal asphericity after refractive surgery. J Refract Surg 2006;22:(in press)
20. Machat JJ. Excimer laser refractive surgery: Practice and principles. SLACK Inc: Thorofare, 1995.
21. Mackee SM, Krueger RR, Applegate RA. In: Customized corneal ablation. Ed. Mackee SM, Krueger RR, Applegate RA. (SLACK, Thorofare, NJ, 2001),3-9.
22. Manns F, Ho A, Parel JM, Culbertson W. Ablation profile for wavefront-guided correction of myopia and primary spherical aberration. J Cataract Refract Surg 2002;28:766-74g.
23. Marcos S, Cano D, Barbero S. Increase in corneal asphericity after standard laser in situ keratomileusis for myopia is not inherent to the Munnerlyn algorithm. J Refract Surg 2003;19:S592-96.
24. Mrochen M, Seiler T. Influence of corneal curvature on calculation of ablation patterns used in photorefractive laser surgery. J Refract Surg 2001;17:S584-87.
25. Niemz MH, et al. Intrastromal ablation for refractive corneal surgery using picosecond infrared laser pulses. Laser Light Ophthalmol 1993;5:149-55.
26. Puliafito CA, et al. Excimer laser ablation of the cornea and lens. Ophthalmology. 1985;92:741 48.thermokeratoplasty by means of a pulsed holmium:YAG laser for hyperopic correction. Refract Corneal Surg 1990:6:335-39.
27. Ren Q, Lin JT, et al. Ultraviolet solid-state laser (213 nm) photorefractive keratectomy. Ophthalmology 1993;100:1828-34.
28. Rozakis G. Refractive Lamellar keratoplasty. SLACK Inc: Thorofare 1995.
29. Seiler T, et al. Laser thermokeratoplasty by means of a pulsed holmium:YAG laser for hyperopic correction. Refract Corneal Surg 1990;6:335-39.
30. Sher NA. Surgery for hyperopia and presbyopia. Williams and Wilkins, 1997.
31. Srinivasan R. Ablation of polymers and biological tissue by ultraviolet lasers. Science 1986;234:559-65.
32. Tabaoda J, et al. Response of the corneal epithelium to ArF excimer laser pulses. Health Phys 1981;352.
33. Telando A. Pseudo-accommodative cornea: a new concept for correction of presbyopia. J Refract Surg 2004;20(Suppl.):S714-17.
34. Trokel SL, et al. Excimer laser surgery of the cornea. Am J Ophthalmol 1983;92:741-48.

Orbscan Corneal Mapping in Refractive Surgery

3

FRANCISCO SÁNCHEZ LEÓN (MEXICO)

INTRODUCTION

Today corneal topography plays several critical roles in different refractive surgery decisions. Conventional axial and tangential topography maps are not enough to demonstrate a healthy cornea and we can not decide either if Lasik surgery, any type of surface laser refractive procedure or intracorneal rings for early keratoconus are suitable procedures indicated for any case based only on surface topographic evaluation.

Maw 1, mentioned that he served as consultant of six cases of postoperative LASIK ectasia ocurred in low to moderate myopia, unfortunately none of the eyes he examined had undergone a preoperative evaluation with Orbscan, so he was unable to analize the posterior elevation or the displacement of either the posterior float or corneal thinning. This is unfare for a LASIK patient, in the times when technologies are capable of such analysis.

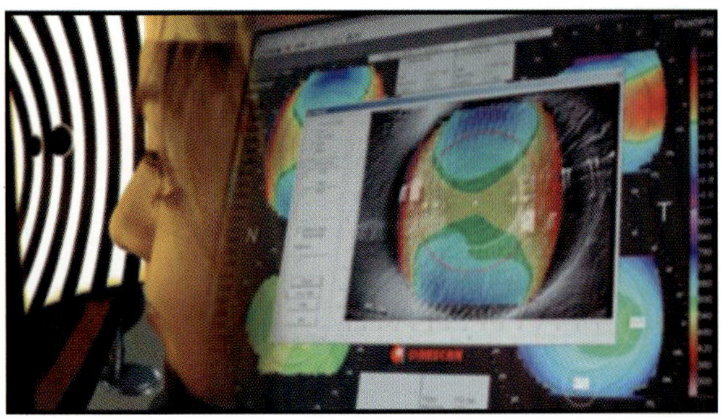

Fig. 3.1

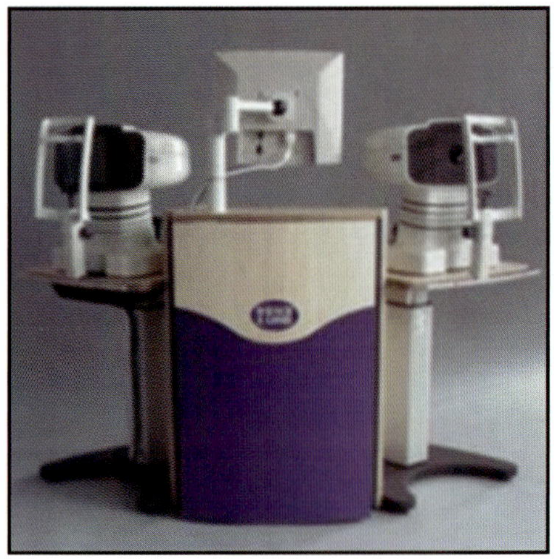

Fig. 3.2: Zyoptix dual work station. Integrates OrbscanZII and Zywave Aberrometer

Bausch and Lomb's Orbscan® IIz is a fully integrated multidimensional diagnostic system that elevates diagnostics beyond mere topography. Unlike current topography systems which scan the surface of the eye at standard points, the Orbscan II acquires over 9000 data points in 1.5 seconds to meticulously map the entire corneal surface (11 mm), and analyze elevation and curvature measurements on both the anterior and posterior surfaces of the cornea.

The Orbscan® system (Bausch and Lomb, Rochester, NY) uses the principle of projection. Forty scanning slit beams (20 from the left and 20 from the right with up to 240 data points per slit) are used to scan the cornea from limbus to limbus and to measure independently the x, y, and z locations of several thousand points on each surface . The images captured are then used to construct the anterior corneal surface, posterior corneal surface, and anterior iris and anterior lens surfaces. Data regarding the corneal pachymetry and anterior chamber depth are also displayed. In the newer version of the Orbscan® system, a placido disk has been mounted to this device in order to improve the accuracy of the curvature measurements.

An advantage of this device is that it measures all surfaces of the anterior segment. Scanning time (1.2-1.5 seconds) is required, this device use a tracking system to track the eye movements in order to minimize the influence of involuntary eye movement.

By providing more comprehensive preoperative diagnostics and planning, exclusionary criteria such as keratoconus, prekeratoconus, and corneal thinning can be identified to optimize outcomes in both primary treatments and enhancements. The Orbscan II may help explain decreased visual acuity postoperative, and is designed to allow the surgeon to more accurately prescribe retreatments, if necessary. This technology is capable of detecting and analyzing posterior corneal abnormalities where corneal anomalies first appear.

Orbscan Corneal Mapping for Refractive Surgery Diagnostics

The Orbscan II, together with other diagnostic tools such as aberrometry , pupillometry and pachymetry, provides us with an unprecedented opportunity to select patients for an appropriate technique (LASIK, LASEK, PRK, Phakik IOL, Intracorneal Rings), minimising complications such as long-term corneal posterior ectasia.

Posterior ectasia has been identified after refractive surgery techniques such as Lasik, where insufficient corneal tissue has been left behind postoperatively.[2] It has manifested itself as a forward 'bulging' of corneal tissue (Fig. 3.3), developing from the posterior corneal surface. Indeed, several researchers indicates that up to 90 percent of kerataconus developing in the untreated eye appear first from the posterior surface. This is thought to be related to leaving the cornea with too little tissue postoperatively; and indeed although this is established, there are other indicators which could also put a patient at risk. *The Orbscan II provide us additional information to predict these risk.*

It has become a universally accepted the standard to leave at least 250 µm residual stromal bed as a safety measure in Lasik, and the Orbscan II has played its part to make it happend. However, the true validity of this limit is in some doubt.[4] The average cornea can range in thickness from 490 to 600 µm, so it is not logical to leave a standard 250 µm in all cases.

A number of surgeons support the view that a percentage thickness of the cornea should remain instead, and/or that a minimum of at least 260 µm to 280 µm is a more realistic standard. To facilitate this, intraoperative pachymetry (corneal thickness measurement) can be performed to provide a more accurate idea of how much tissue will remain after a

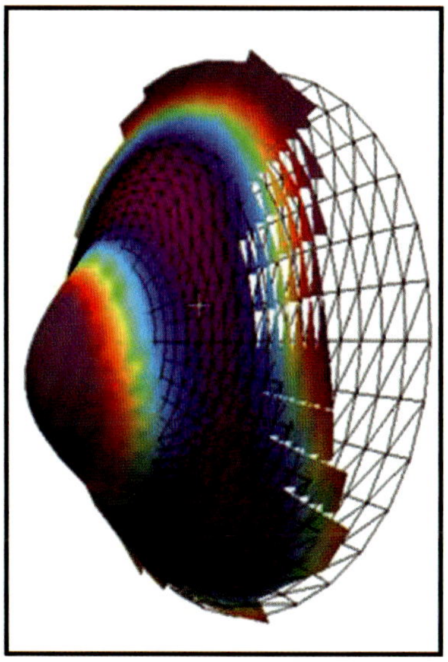

Fig. 3.3: Three dimensional representation of 'bulging' from posterior corneal tissue in a ectasia case after LASIK by Orbscan II

procedure.[5] This in itself has limitations, but gives an additional safety criterion, rather than merely relying on manufacturers' estimations of flap thickness.

In summary, the residual stromal bed is by far from our clinical perspectives the only indicator for safe preoperative screening. So how does the Orbscan II influence decisions on whether or not to treat? It is important to understand that selection criteria for refractive surgery never stands alone, and it is the clinician's responsibility to bring together all the information gathered in the screening process, before deciding whether it is safe to proceed. The Orbscan influences this decision in a number of ways.

Unlike other modern topography systems, the Orbscan is based on slitscanning technology in addition to traditional placido-based techniques (Fig. 3.4).

The placido image gives us information on axial keratometric readings, by converting distortion of the rings into topographical data. A series of illuminated annular rings are projected onto the cornea. Using the corneal tear film as a mirror, the reflected image of the rings is captured by a digital video camera. The captured image is then subjected to an algorithm to detect and identify the position of the rings in relation to the video keratographic axis. Once these borders are detected, the digital image is 'reconstructed' to show anterior corneal curvature.

Orbscan goes much further than this; slit-beam scanners and triangulation are used to derive the actual spatial location of thousands of points on the surface. Each beam sweep across the cornea gives information on corneal elevation, or height, from the anterior corneal surface, posterior surface and iris. To represent the corneal surface data in a way that is easily understood, the computer calculates a hypothetical sphere that matches as close as possible to the actual corneal shape being measured. This is called the best fit sphere (BFS). It then compares the real surface to the hypothetical sphere, showing areas 'above' the surface of the sphere in warm colors, and areas 'below' the surface in cool colours.

This has many uses, but for the purposes of refractive surgery selection, 'bulges' in both the posterior and anterior surface can indicate patients who may be at risk of ectasia development. This enables the surgeon to screen them out early in the selection process.

A 'quad map' can be produced, which gives four different maps each portraying different information about the cornea (Fig. 3.5). The bottom left hand map is the axial keratometry map, based on placido technology. This is similar to maps produced from the majority of commercially available topography systems, and provides detailed keratometric information across the diameter of the cornea.

For LASIK selection, this information is important for a number of reasons. The 'K' readings it is important, because limits of K readings are between

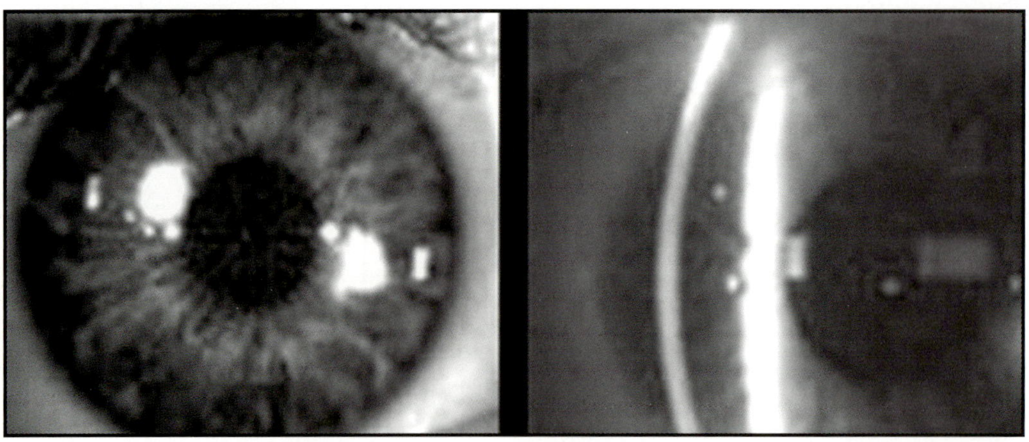

Fig. 3.4: Orbscan is based on slit-scanning technology, in addition to placido-based techniques

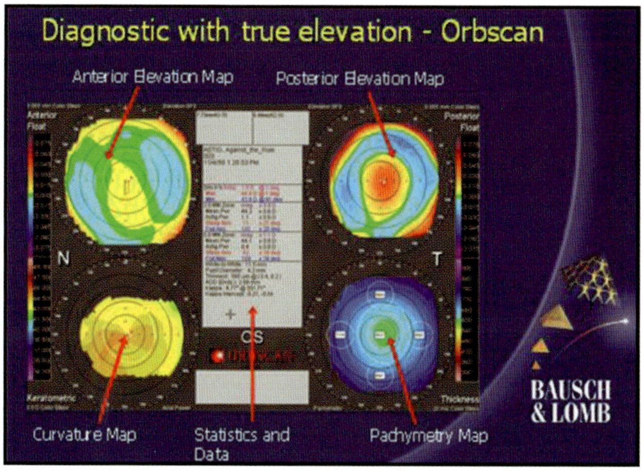

Fig. 3.5: A 'Quad map' gives four different maps, each portraying different information about the cornea

certain values; the cornea must be neither too steep nor too flat. It is difficult for the microkeratome (blade designed for flap cutting), to create a good quality corneal flap in LASIK if either of these extremes is the case, as this can lead to surgical flap complications.

In addition, K readings of more than 48D are an indication of potential kerataconus, particularly where this is decentered inferonasally. Details of the K readings can be found in the stats and data information in the centre of the quad map.

The top left hand map of Figure 3.6 is the anterior elevation map, and as with the top right hand posterior elevation map, slit scanning provides the means of creating the information. As mentioned before, slit scanning provides elevation data, and this also can create a 3D interpretation of the cornea. Looking at both elevation maps, if it is imagined that the green tissue is at sea level, then the warmer colors are above sea level, or towards the viewer, and the cooler colors are below, or further away from the viewer.

A 3D interpretation of both elevation maps can be seen in Figures 3.6A and B. The meshwork affect indicates how the cornea would appear if it were entirely spherical and is referred to as the reference sphere.

This elevation data can be interpreted usefully in a number of ways. First the difference between the highest and lowest points is a potential kerataconus indicator, if over 100 µm; Rousch criteria 6 (Fig. 3.7).

In addition, on the posterior map, the highest elevation value can again be interpreted as a kerataconus indicator, or at least as a screen for those patients who may be at risk of developing kerectasia postoperatively. This provides safety criteria to avoid treating patients at risk. From the work of Vukich 7 and Potgeiter 8, 55D elevation has been recommended as an absolute cut off. As can be seen from Figures 3.6 and 3.7, the elevation on the right hand side (posterior elevation) is more advanced than that on the left (anterior elevation), indicating that 'bulges' develop from the posterior surface of the cornea in the first instance.

From studying the relationship between the two elevation maps, further information can be gleaned. A ratio can be calculated between the posterior and anterior surfaces, which gives an indication of the relative difference in curvature between the two maps 9. Figure 3.8 shows two corneal cross-sections.

This very simplistic diagram shows us that the same elevation data for the posterior surface can have a different impact on the stability of the cornea. In diagram B where the ratio is high at 1.27, it can be seen that a weak area (indicated by the arrow) develops which is not apparent in A, even though posterior elevation data is the same for both. This information on elevation and ratio would rarely be used as exclusion criteria alone, but by considering these together, more conclusive information can be obtained. For example, a high ratio of say 1.26 would be far more concerning if the posterior elevation was

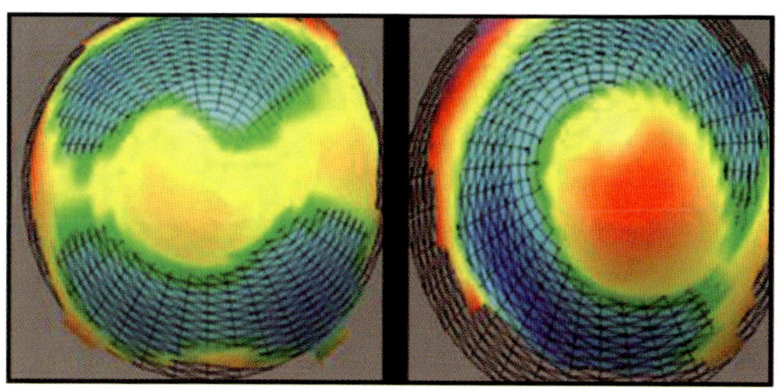

Figs 3.6A and B: Anterior elevation posterior elevation map – 3D view map – 3D view

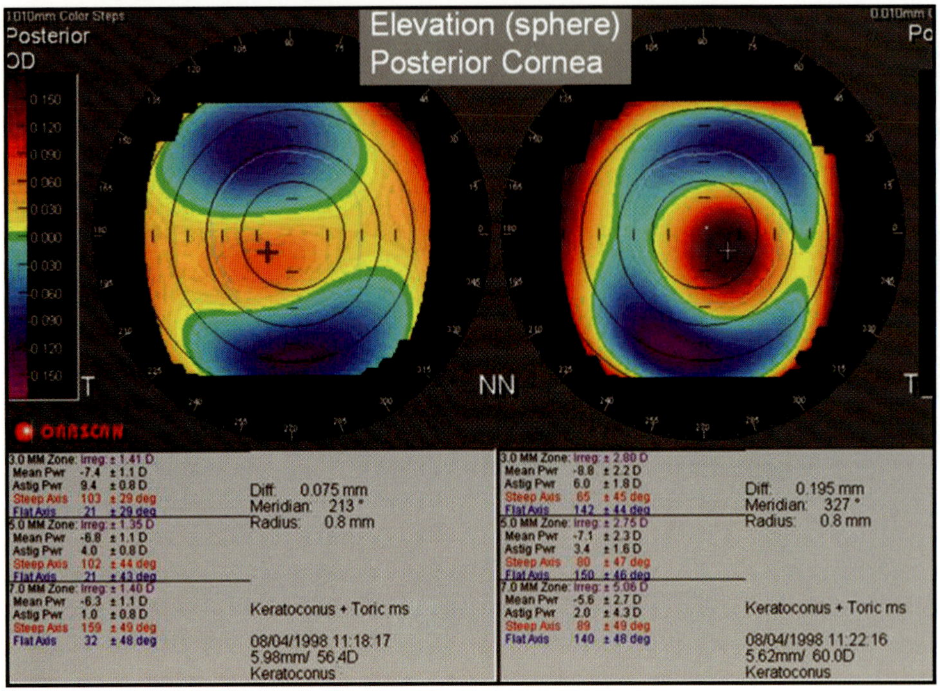

Fig. 3.7: The elevation on the right hand side (posterior elevation) is more advanced than that on the left (anterior elevation)

high at 55D, the cornea was of borderline thickness, and the preoperative prescription high.

The final map to study is the pachymetry map. This is map four of our quad map in Figure 3.5. Traditionally, pachymetry has been measured using ultrasound, which provides a reading of corneal thickness from Bowman's membrane to Descemet's membrane. Through slitscanning technology, Orbscan provides us with a pachymetry reading from the precorneal tear film to the endothelium, therefore slightly thicker readings can be expected.[10] The Orbscan can, however, be calibrated to take this into consideration when comparing readings. The true advantage of the pachymetry map is that it provides us with thickness information across the cornea from limbus to limbus, not just in single points as with ultrasound. This once again gives the opportunity to detect areas of weakness, thinning or scarring. Auffarth et al[11] state that the relationship between the highest point on anterior and posterior elevation maps, and the thinnest point (shown by a yellow dot) is an indicator of kerataconus.

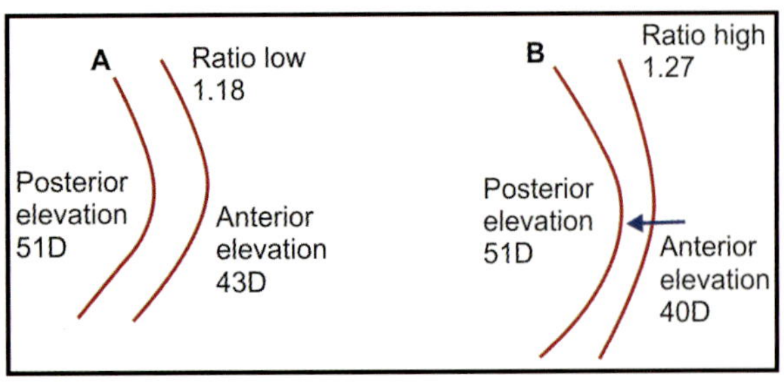

Fig. 3.8: Two corneal crosssections

The relationship between pachymetry readings can be looked at, and it has been suggested that 100 μm should be a cut-off criteria between thickness regions on the map. Figure 3.9 shows the relationship between the central reading in the white circle, and the four peripheral readings, indicated by the arrows. Once again these criteria would be used alongside other information, but alone would not exclude a patient. The readings within the circles are averages of measurements within the area, but the Orbscan also flags the thinnest point, indicated by a yellow dot.

In conclusion, it can be seen that much information can be obtained from analysis of Orbscan

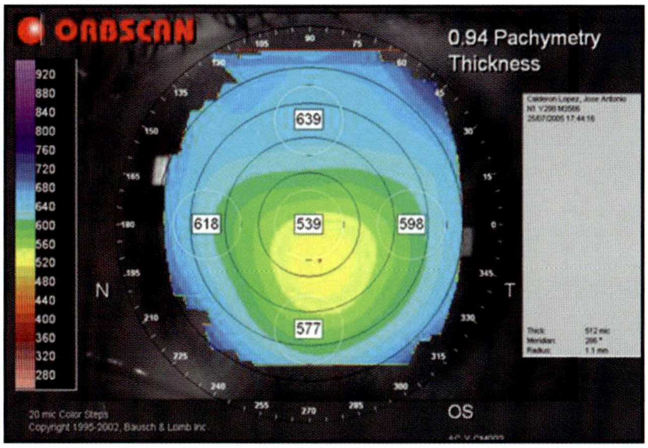

Fig. 3.9: The relationship between the central reading in the white circle, and the four peripheral readings

maps, and this information does not have the scope to cover it all. The most important message is that the criteria does not stand alone, and by looking at all the maps together along with other information, an informed decision can be made as to whether it is safe to proceed to surgery.

Selection Criteria

The diagnosis of keratoconus proper, seldom proves to be problematic, and represents the undisputed black end of the spectrum, as would be the case for the patient with simple with the rule astigmatism who would be on the white end of the spectrum. However, in between a large grey area exists, consisting of aginst-the rule astigmatism, asymmetric astigmatism, non-orthogonal astigmatism, irregular astigmatism and forme fruste keratoconus.

Over the past number of years since true elevation corneal topography became available, a set of criteria (Tables 3.1, 3.2)[6,8,9] were developed to distinguish to distinguish among these entities. Altough corneal topography provides us with the most clues for the diagnosis of early keratoconus, other clinical criteria also need to be considered.

These would include the patient's age, a family history of keratoconus, history of systemic or local pathology, asociated with keratoconus, refractive stability, as well as wheter a good and crisp endpoint could be achieved on refractive testing of the subject.

No single cornea topographic sign is in its own right diagnostic of fruste keratoconus, but rather a combination of a set of criteria. One might look at each of these criteria as a "alarm sign" noted, with the probability for early keratoconus proportionate to the number of alarms present.

These criteria can be divide into the following categories:

a. Power map changes
b. Posterior elevation maps
c. Pachymetry
d. Composite/integrated topography information

Power Maps

Mean corneal curvature >45 diopters. Mean corneal curvature measuring in excess of 45 diopters is a well established feature of keratoconus.

Bow –tie/broken-tie pattern. In addition to steep corneal curvatures, the bow-tie or broken bow-tie appereance of astigmatic pattern might be indicative

Table 3.1: Rousch's Orbscan criteria for subclinical keratoconus detection

1. Elevation difference superior of 100 mm at the central optical zone of 7 mm.
2. Clinical difference superior of 100 mm at the central optical zone of 7 mm.
3. Anterior elevation superior of 40 mm at the central optical zone of 7 mm from BFS.
4. Posterior elevation superior of 50 mm at the central optical zone of 7 mm from BFS.
5. Posterior BFS reference > 55D.

Table 3.2: Efkarpides's Orbscan criteria for subclinical keratoconus detection

1. Anterior/Posterior BFS of reference difference in mm superior to 1.25 to 1.27.
2. Morphological difference between anterior and posterior face (warpage).
3. Remarkable convergence of points (highest point on anterior elevation, highest point on posterior elevation, thinnest point in pachymetry, steepest curvature on the power map).
4. Infero-temporal displacement of these remarkable points
5. Color code statistical analysis (Normal Band Scale). Elevation values, curvature, pachymetry of more than 2 standard deviations from controls.

of early keratoconus, and also a well known criteria. Central corneal asymetry. A change within the central 3 mm optical zone of the cornea of more than 3 diopters from superior or inferior can be correlatedwith the presence of vertical coma. However, this may be merely a sign of asymetrical astigmatism, and is not necesarily an indicative of pathology.

Posterior Elevation

The elevation map displays corneal height or elevation relative to a reference plane, which may be a spherical or aspherical surface depending on the topographer. It is important to note that the elevation display depends on reference surface size, shape, alignment, and fitting zone. This map shows the three-dimensional shape of the cornea and is useful in measuring the amount of tissue removed by a procedure, assessing postoperative visual problems, or planning/monitoring surgical procedures

Many surgeons think the first sign of keratectasia appers on the posterior surface of the cornea, not on the anterior topography map . Considering this, the importance of recognizing a change in the posterior surface deserves special emphasis.[1-3] While one would not perform corneal laser surgery on eyes with keratoconus, keratoconus suspects or posterior ectasia defined by technologies with the capability of posterior corneal float analysis, it might prove useful to look at the criteria for early form of keratoconus in order to define those cases, and distinguish them from eyes that would be suited to laser refractive surgery.

Laser clinics had shown that 5 to 8% of patients screened for refractive procedure are not good candidates because keratoconus detection by simple axial topography, however, a mexican study demonstrated that 3.13% of population screened for laser eye surgery had posterior ectasia criteria by Orbscan, despite having axial topography clasified as normal (unpublished data).[3]

We have found four different posterior float patterns in patients screened for laser eye surgery: Complete positive band 71.87%, incomplete postitive band 18.75%, butterfly wings common in patients with high astigmatism 6.25%, and central island 3.13% (Fig. 3.10). In other words, if we don´t know posterior float features from every case, we have at least 3% risk of unstable LASIK result or iatrogenic ectasia in the worst case.[3]

Best fit sphere > 55 diopters. The most common reference surface for viewing elevation maps is the "best fit sphere". This geometric surface is constructed by fitting a spherical spline with the least square of difference values though the three dimensional elevation data from the cornea, whether it be the anterior or posterior profile. The sphere can thus be employed to judge the average profile of the surface in question. A best fit sphere (BFS) with the power of 55 diopters or more on the posterior profile, could be indicative of posterior ectasia. This criterium is not diagnostic as a sign of early keratoconus per sé, as this sign may also be seen in small diameter corneas.

Posterior high point >50 micron above BFS. Early keratoconus is often seen first on the posterior corneal profile. *Whenever a localized elevation above BFS on the posterior surface measures more than 50 micron in elevation, this might be indicative of an early posterior ectasia.*

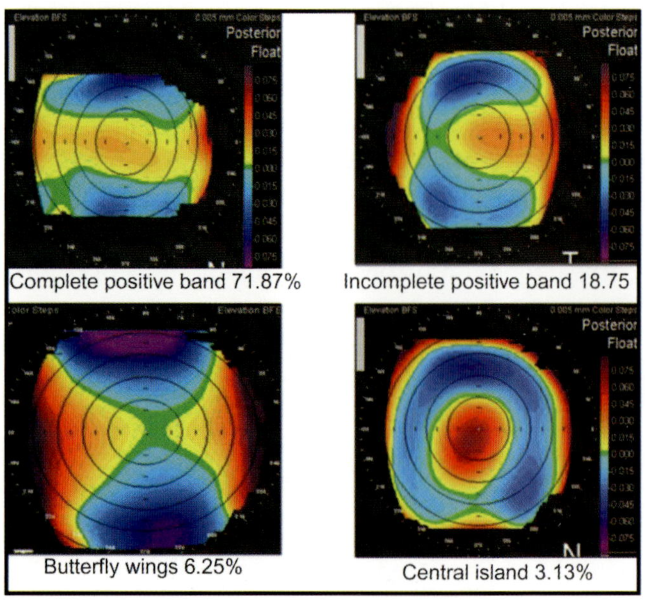

Fig. 3.10: Orbscan posterior float, 4 different types in patients screened for Laser eye surgery

Many authors have review the posterior surface's response to LASIK, and Orbscan is an unique technology to evaluate this changes.[12-15] Increased forward shift of the posterior corneal surface is common after myopic LASIK and correlates with the residual corneal thickness and ablation percentage per total corneal thikness.[12]

An excessively thin residual cornea bed or a large ablation percentage may increase the risk of iatrogenic complications, such ectasia. Others have considered that even if a residual corneal bed of 300 mm or thicker is preserved, anterior bulging of the cornea after LASIK can ocurr. Eye with thin corneas and high myopia requiring greater laser ablation are more predisposed to an anterior shift of the posterior central cornea.[13,14]

Roberts 15 with the help of Orbscan proposes a new theory to explain the increased posterior elevation postLASIK, she suggests that the mild ectasia appereance may be due to a backward sweling of the peripheral redistributed cornea rather than a pathological forward bulging of the central cornea.

Pachymetry

Thinnest point < 470 micron.This constitutes an absolute contraindication to corneal refractive surgery. In pathological corneas, this thinnest point is often displaced inferotemporal.

Difference of > 100 microns at 7 mm optical zone. A difference of more than 100 microns from the thinnest point to the values at the 7 mm optical zone implies a steep gradient of thinning from the midperiphery towards the thinnest point. These, in conjuntion with other signs, can be indicative of early pathology.[9]

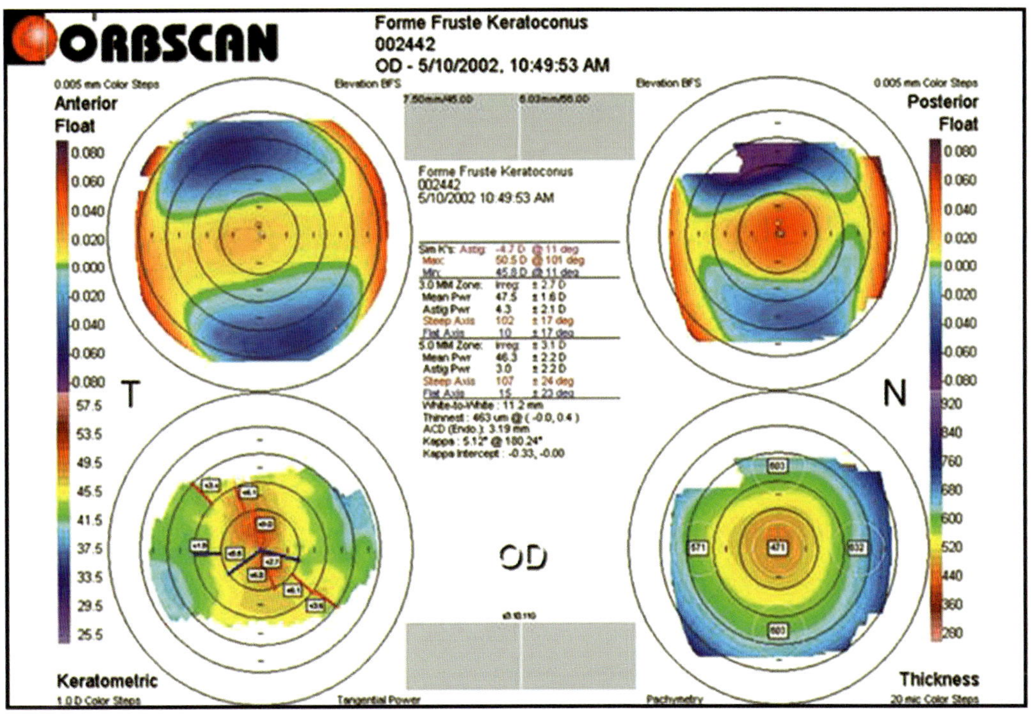

Fig. 3.11: Similarity between the anterior and posterior elevation profiles might indicate early kerato-conus,especially if bending of the profile is in relation to the point of thinnest pachymetry on the cornea. However, one has to consider all the information available. An example is present, a pathologically thin cornea in lieu of a posterior best fit sphere exceeding 55 diopter, as well as anterior curvature values of more than 45 diopters, which raises the suspicion of early of early keratoconus

Composite/Integrated Information

As a default, four corneal maps are routinely presented by the Orbscan II (Bausch and Lomb, Orbtek, Salt Lake City, Utha). Elevation topography System. These include the anterior elevation profile, posterior elevation profile, power map, and a total pachymetry map. Through integration of the information provide on these maps, one is able to detect subtle, but powerful signs not present on any individual map. These signs include the following:

Bent/warped cornea. Similarly between anterior and posterior profiles implies a forward bending of those areas shown above the BFS. If these bending is in association with the thinnest point on the cornea. It could related to structural weakness in the cornea, irrespective of wheter the thinnest point still shows and adequated pachymetry. These sign has to be evaluated within the context other signs above.

Inferotemporal displacement of the highest point. Infero-temporal displacement of the highest point on the anterior as well as the posterior elevation profile can be indicative of early keratoconus, but must also be seen in context (Fig. 3.11).

Correlation of signs of the highst point on the posterior elevation. This is probably the strongest topographic sign indicative of early keratoconus. If the highst point on the posterior elevation coincides with the highst point of anterior elevation, the thinnest point on pachymetry, and the point of steepest curvature on the power map, one has to very carefull regarding your decision to operate. This signs implies that the thinnest point represents an structural weakness, wich cause a forward bending of the cornea (as is noted on the posterior and anterior elevation maps), further supported by the curvature change on the power map (Fig. 3.12).

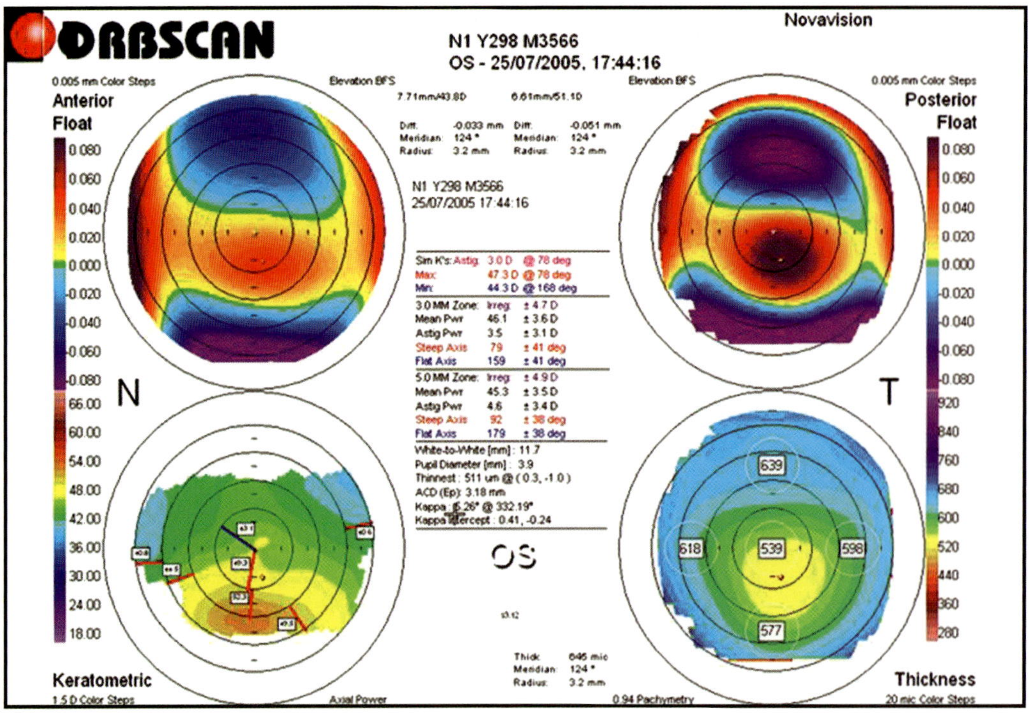

Fig. 3.12: Correlation of signs with the highest point on the posterior elevation is the surest indication of keratoconus . If the highest point on the posterior elevation coincides with the highest point on the anterior elevation,the thinnest point on pachymetry,and the point of steepest curvature on the power map, the diagnosis is indicative of keratoconus. This sign implies that the thinnest point represents a structural weakness,which causes forward bending of the cornea (as is noted on the posterior and anterior elevation maps) further supported by the curvature change on the power map

Recognizing keratoconus an the other forms of corneal pathology like pellucid marginal degeneration that contraindicate corneal laser refractive surgery is central to safe clinical practice. As profesionals is our own responsibility to keep the prestige of refractive surgery, and LASIK safe desicion must be our mision.

Finally, if some criteria of unhealthy cornea or posterior ectasia have been found, other refractive surgical techniques can be attepted such as phakic IOL in the case of fruste keratoconus or thin cornea for a of high myopia patient (Fig. 3.13); or in the scenario of a keratoconus, intracorneal rings can be attempted, orbscan offers us the posibility in helping to take this decision and follow up.

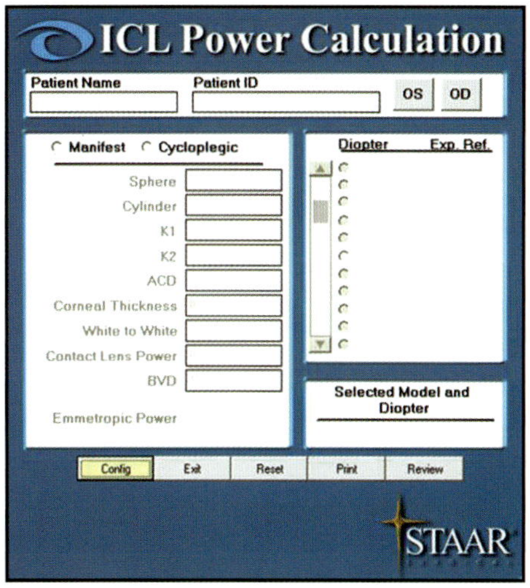

Fig. 3.13: ICL Power Calculator, OrbscanII can also help to obtain the data requiered to calculate ICL

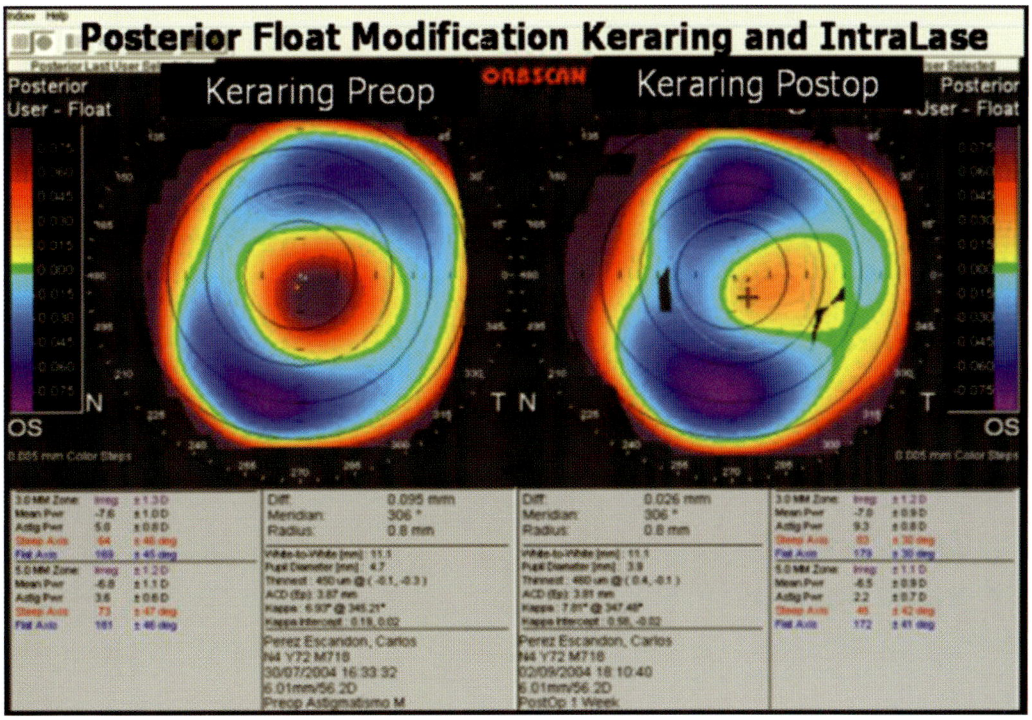

Fig. 3.14: Ferrara/Keraring case implanted with IntraLase, a dual posterior float map demostrates an improvement of the preop posterior elevation of 92 microns (pathological) to postoperative posterior elevation of 26 microns (pseudo-normal)

REFERENCES

1. Maw R. Avoiding Postoperative LASIK Ectasia. Cataract and Refractive Surgery Today. Nov-Dec 2003.
2. Seiler T, Koufala K, Richter G. Iatrogenic keratectasia after laser in situ keratomileuisis. J Cataract Refrac Surg 1998;14:312-17.
3. Vaca, Oscar. Posterior Float Features in Population Screened for Laser Eye Surgery. Mexican Cornea and Refractive Surgery Society, 1999.

4. Ambrosio R, Klyce SD, Wilson SE. Corneal topogrphic and pachymetric screening of keratorefractive patients. J Refractive Surg 2003;19:24-29.
5. Ou RJ, Shaw EL, Glasgow BJ. Keratectasia after laser in situ keratomileusis (LASIK): evaluation of the calculated residual stromal bed thickness. Am J Ophthalmol 2002 Nov; 134(5):771-73.
6. Roush C. Orbscan II Manual (Salt Lake City, Utha. Orbtek).
7. Vukich J, et al. Early spatial changes in the posterior corneal surface after laser in situ keratomileusis. J Cataract Refract Surg 2003;29:778-84.
8. Potgeiter F. Custome Lasik Surgical Techniques and Complications. Buranto L, Brint S. Slack 2004;435-37.
9. Assouline M. Chirugie Ceil–Le Kératocone. De nouveaux critéres de detection de kératocone infra-clinique. www.inclo.com/le-keratocone.php
10. Fakhry M, Artola A, Belda J, Alio J. Comparison of corneal pachymetry using ultrasound and Orbscan II . J Cataract Refract Surg 2002;28:248-52.
11. Auffarth GU, Tetz MR, Biazid Y, Volcker HE. Keratoconus evaluation using the Orbscan Topography System. J Cataract Refract Surg 2002;26:222-28.
12. Lee DH, Seo S, Jeong KW, et al. Early spatial changes in the posterior corneal surface after laser in situ keratomileusis. J Cataracy Refract Surg 2003;29;778-84.
13. Twa MD, Roberts C, Mahmound AM, Chang JS Jr. Response of the posterior corneal surface to laser in situ Keratomileusis for myopia. J Cataract Refract Surg 2003;31:61-71.
14. Miyata K,Tokunaga T, Nakahara M, et al. Residual bed thickness and corneal foward shifth after laser in situ Keratomileusis. J Cataract Refract Surg 2004;30: 1067-72.
15. Grzybowski DM, Roberts CJ, Mahmound AM, Chang JS Jr. Model for nonectatic in posterior corneal elevation after ablative procedures. J Cataract Refract Surg 2005;31:72-81.
16. Cairns G McGhee NJ, Collins MJ,et al. Accuracy of Orbscan II slit scanning elevation topography. J Cataract Refract Surg 2002;28:2181-87.

Advances in Microkeratomes

4

KUMAR J DOCTOR, DIPTI N SHAH (INDIA)

INTRODUCTION

Microkeratomes have come a long way since they first appeared in the early 1980's. This still is an evolving technology and has significant improvements in both, the safety and predictability of procedures. The very limited role of Microkeratomes for almost two decades was followed by widespread use over the last half decade as their predictability and safety has increased.

All refractive procedures that were performed during the last two decades modified optical properties only by indirectly altering corneal power and curvature. Microkeratomes were introduced to improve two procedures, Ketatomileusis and Keratophakia. Laser ablation and corneal lamellar procedures have evolved over time. Designs of Microkeratomes continue to evolve to meet the same demands and its role and importance in LASIK continues to grow.

Fortunately improvements in the last 1990's in mechanical microkeratome design increased the predictability of flap diameter, thickness, hinge size and edge characteristics and this led to decreased flap complications. These improvements have provided safety and finally enabled microkeratomes and LASIK to gain wide spread acceptance.

Manual microkeratome designs offers the surgeons the ability to vary microkeratome parameters based on corneal diameter and curvature to decrease complications but the surgeon requires to be ambidextrous to achieve consistent flaps.

The newer Automated Microkeratomes have definitely helped to decrease the LASIK learning curve as a result of newer automated machines.

It still remains to be demonstrated whether laser and waterjet microkeratome will be more convenient, safe and predictable than the latest generation mechanical microkeratomes. Will they offer advantages for wave front guided ablations? It will be interesting to see the future of microkeratomes.

EVOLUTION

The microkeratome utilized to make the corneal flap was developed and refined by Jose Barraquer, MD of Bogota, Columbia. The development of this instrumentation began in 1950's and continues today. Although there are many microkeratomes in the market today, all follow the basic design principles developed by this father of refractive surgery. Roles and designs of microkeratomes continue to evolve as laser ablation procedures improve. Manual dissection of the recipient bed was used until 1962, however as the dissection plane was not smooth enough, Barraquer developed the Microkeratome based on Dr Castroviejo's electro keratome and this new instrument was capable of performing consistently smooth lamellar sections.

Microkeratomes work like a carpenter's plane. All current designs have a suction ring which attaches to the eye and raises the intraocular pressure so that the cornea is firm. The microkeratomes then have an applanation plate which flattens the Cornea while an oscillating blade is advanced through the tissue with an offset of 130, 160, 180 or 200 Microns. The corneal section is made by advancing the microkeratome across the applanated surface of the cornea while the oscillating blade creates a smooth incision. A successful hinge of the flap is created by stopping the advancing blade at a predetermined spot.

There have been several attempts to improve the design of the original microkeratome to improve the quality of lamellar cutting and reduce the incidence of microkeratome related complications Viz those related to suction and increased IOP include Vascular occlusion, subretinal neovascular hemorrhage, thin, thick and irregular flaps; and intraoperative discomfort and anxiety. The high-speed oscillating blades also may contribute to cutting chatter within the bed and along its edge, which may contribute to irregular astigmatism and epithelial ingrowth. Finally, the adjacent gears can result in jamming of the unit by eye lashes or the obstructive elements, which would result in an irregular cut and a need to abort the procedure. Today surgeons have many choices nasal or superior hinge, disposables or reusables, automatic or manual, mechanical or non mechanical, etc. Among the newer mechanical microkeratomes, several offer automated advancement without using gears (Schwind, Phoenix, Universal Keratome, Draeger and Refractive technologies flap maker), while others offer only manual advancement [Eye Technology MLK, SCMD, and Moria]. Modifications in the blade angle approach (range: 0° to 25°), the oscillating frequency of the steel blade (range: 8000 to 16000) and the material of the blade (Schwind: Sapphire blade, Mastel: diamond blade) have been attempted to improve flap cutting and reduce chatter and irregular astigmatism. Rotating rather than oscillating blade has been introduced by Draeger.

Consequently efforts have been made to consider an alternate method of—sectioning that does not require the use of mechanical microkeratomes. Two such alternative technologies include that of the ISL neodymium: YLF [yttrium lithium fluoride] picosecond laser (Escalon Medical Corp, Skillman, NJ) and the water-Jet technology (Hydro Blade Keratome medjet Inc. Edison, NJ). The former is a laser microkeratome that deposits laser Pulse energy intrastromally to create a corneal flap without a mechanical blade or significant suction. The latter is a water Jet microkeratome that uses a thin high-pressure beam of water in place of a mechanical blade to cleave a lamellar flap without section or tissue hydration.

A perfect lasik procedure has 3 components.

1. A perfect corneal flap.
2. A perfect laser ablation profile.
3. A perfect post-operative course.

Imperfection in any of these 3 stages leads to sub-optimal optimal results.

The corneal flap is crucial for visual outcome because if the corneal flap is imperfect or if the alignment is not accurate, the resulting optical quality will be poor even with a perfect laser ablation.

Thus the microkeratome design, mechanism and accuracy with consistency plays a very important role for a successful lasik procedure

Ideal Microkeratome

- Can fit all ocular dimensions
- Consistent suction
- Control over flap diameter, flap thickness, hinge width and hinge orientation.
- Normal effects on cap
- Economical
- Easy to use
- Safe

BARRAQUER APPLANATION TONOMETER (FIG. 4.1)

Basic Mechanism of Microkeratome

A suction plate-ring assembly stabilizes and pressurizes the eye, admitting the corneal dome for cutting, and a moving assembly with applanation

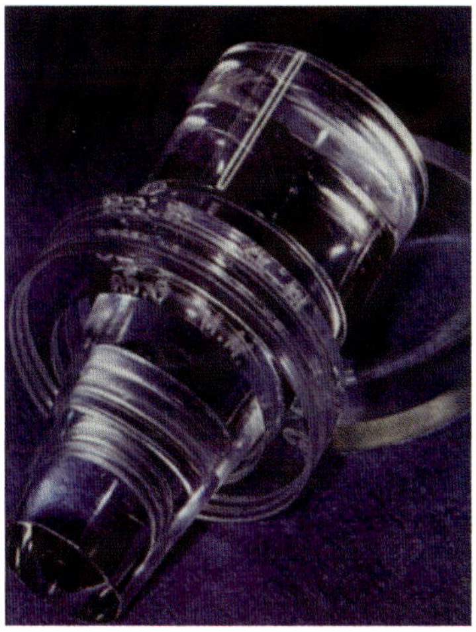

Fig. 4.1: Barraquer applanation tonometer

plate and blade is used to cut the corneal dome and create a flap.

Microkeratomes are held to the eye by the combined forces of air pressure and vacuum pump suction. The eye and cornea become hard and exhibit an equal and opposite force. The microkeratome head progressively flattens the cornea as it powers across, generating a resultant upward force. Passage of the cutting head over the pressurized eye produces resistance and upward force on the microkeratome as it encounters and flattens the corneal hill.

As the applanation plate of the microkeratome approaches the steepest point of the cornea, the plate is pushed upward and away from the cornea. corneal volume is related to lift. Suction plate aperture and corneal curvature are variables that relate to lift. As either factor increases more corneal volume is admitted to encounter the keratome head as it crosses the cornea. At a certain critical point corneal volume reaches a high enough level to force the microkeratome upward. The size of the aperture in the suction plate controls the volume of cornea presented for flattening and cutting.

Steep corneas and/or large aperture openings increase the presented corneal volume and the upward forces on the microkeratome. Smaller aperture sizes are used for steeper corneas to decrease the presented corneal volume. If a way could be found to match the suction plate aperture prospectively to the corneal curvature optimal flaps could be created on every eye.

If K is 1.35 or less, flaps have optimal thickness and regularity because keratome lift does not occur, on the other hand if K is greater then 1.36, flaps can be thin, irregular or perforated, because keratome lift may occur. Using this relationship (K) it is now possible to create custom microkeratomes with aperture sizes specially designed to limit exposed cornea properly for differing corneal curvatures.

MECHANICAL MICROKERATOMES

SKBM-Summit-Krumeich-Barraquer-Microkeratome (Fig. 4.2)

SKBM is a microkeratome that produces consistently size and quality flaps with a very low incidence of any complications. The automated SKBM is easy to use and safe. Its handpiece features *dual motors* which regulate blade oscillation and translation speed independently and a drive band controls the blades traverse across the cornea.

Another key feature of the SKBM is its *preview window* a calibrated transparent applanation plate that provides surgeons complete visualization of the cornea and the diameter available for the flap.

This window can optimize ring selection and make last minute console adjustments that will ensure the best possible flap.

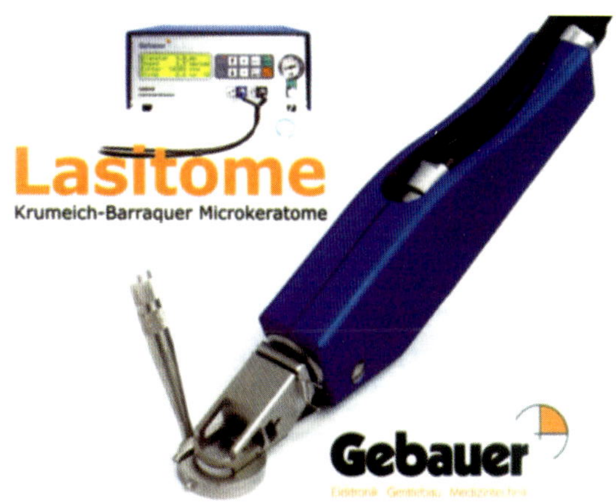

Fig. 4.2: Krumeich-Barraquer-microkeratome

The SKBM has five vacuum rings defined by their diameters and the height of the vertical side wall along with the standard head and an alternative H head that features a lower window and exerts more pressure on the cornea. As a result the SKBM is adaptable to eyes varying in orbit configuration or corneal steepness.

Moria M2

The new automated version of the manual Carriazo-Barraquer microkeratome.It has dual motor system. You can place the hinge either superiorly or nasally by simply rotating the ring position. You can chose from between 110 and 130 micron plates and can alter flap dimensions with the availability of the 4 ring sizes ranging in 0.5 mm and various choices of stops for the hinge size ie.You can tailor the flap characteristics. Also the M2 offers a small diameter ring allowing for placement on deep set eyes and those with tight lids.

M2 should not be used where there is >then 3D difference between the K in the two meridians or with a pachymetry value of less then 500 microns. Flap thickness varied by pre-operative pachymetry and K values. Thicker flaps were achieved in corneas which were flatter while flaps were relatively thinner than average in flatter corneas.

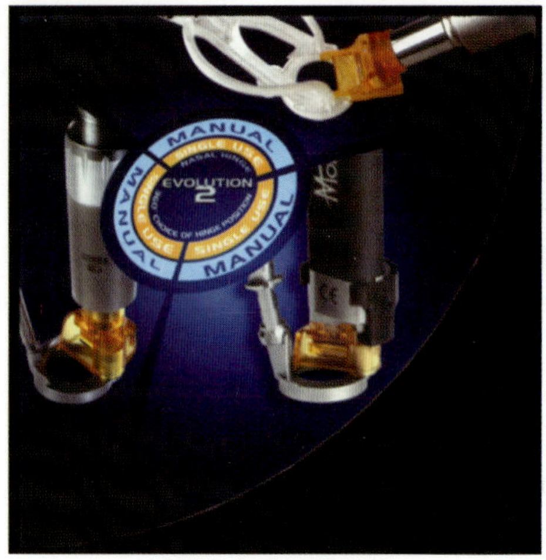

Fig. 4.3: Moria M2

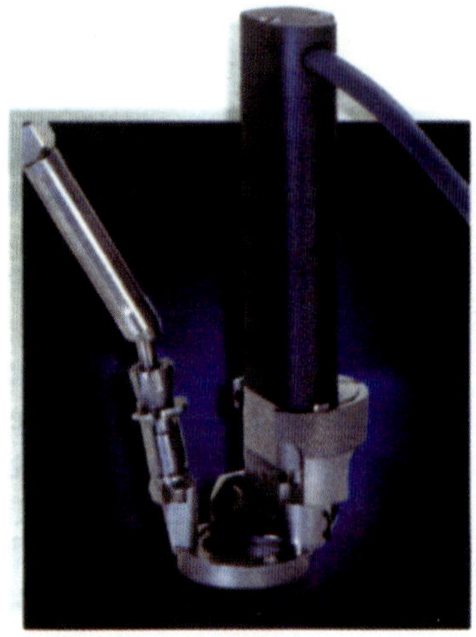

Moria M2

Fig. 4.4

STEPS FOR ASSURING ACCURATE APPLANATION AND PROPER SUCTION

- Initial drying of central cornea before the suction ring is applied
- Pressing down on the suction ring using both the handle and a finger on the port before suction is engaged
- Verifying the suction with tonometry,pupil dilatation when possible and visual blackout.

AMADEUS (ALLERGAN)

Constructed to maintain the surgical field as a protected space clear of lids and lashes, the AMADEUS design also affords the surgeon added safety with full visualization of the flap during the cutting procedure and software that performs ongoing checks of numerous operation parameters. Furthermore, the Amadeus offers versatility with its high walls, it can be used without a speculum in eyes with tight orbits. Users can vary hinge width as well as the translation speed and oscillation rates of the motors and a number of choices are available for ring and plate sizes. Currently there are two rings – 8.5 mm and 9.5 mm.Plates are available in 140, 160and 180 micron depths, 220 and 300 micron plates will be added to the line up. Pre assembled and featuring only 3 pieces the Amadeus microkeratome is easy to use and to clean. Suction time is minimized using the Amadeus because it is easy to put on and take off the eye.

MK–2000

The MK–2000 (Nidek) is an easy- to- use automated microkeratome it is FDA approved. This system has a single hand piece design.

Nidek, the Japanese manufacture of the MK2000, designed this device for use in oriental eyes and it fits well into any small eye. With its small foot print, this microkeratome also allows the surgeon to do any type of tonometry to confirm the adequacy of suction before cutting is begun.

The suction ring also features dual suction so that IOP rises immediately and is sustained at over 100 mm Hg.

The construction of the MK-2000 prevents obstruction from lids and lashes Jamming during cutting is not an issue because there are no gears, guides or external stoppers.

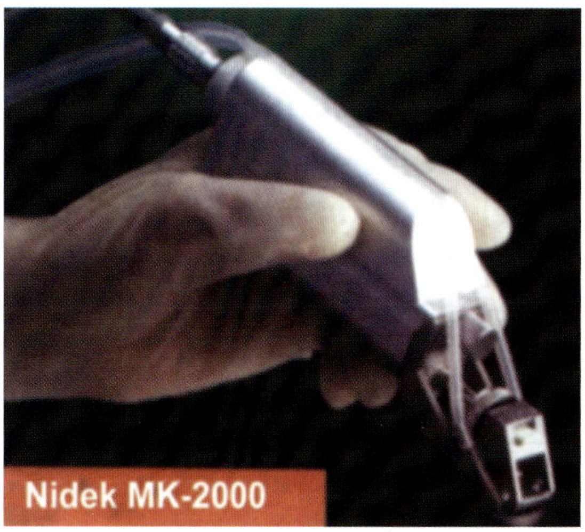

Fig. 4.5: Nidek MK-2000

Independent motors control blade oscillation and advancement. There is no oscillation in reverse mode, so the risk of epithelial defects is minimised. The design also allows surgeon to visualise flap creation while it is occurring.

The MK2000 only creates nasally hinged flaps.

Three ring sizes available are 8.5 mm, 9.0 mm and 9.5 mm.

Salient Features of MK-2000

- Single hand piece design
- One hand operation possible
- No assembly
- No external gears
- Dual suction lines
- Fits into all eyes
- No oscillation in reverse pass
- Nasally hinged flaps

Hansatome Microkeratome (Bausch and Lomb)

The creator of this device is a German engineer in Miami. It was designed to replace the ACS which is now no longer available. The Hansatome Microkeratome is engineered for high volume surgical efficiencies. This corneal resection instrument features an automated pivoting Motion that provides smooth, resistance-free travel with a superior-positioned hinge.

Key Features

- Ergonomic Pivot post allows simple loading.
- Simple 3-step assembly.
- 8.5 mm and 9.5 mm diameter resection.
- Elevated gear rack features a nasal location, away from the lid and speculum (Preventing impeded forward progress).
- Single rolling gear for smooth translation.
- Disposable blade with fixed holder for convenient insertion and smooth oscillation.
- 160, 180, 200 head.
- 4 suction ring handles.
- 2 left / right eye adaptor.
- Motor cord and motor.
- Single foot switch.

Power Supply

- Internal diagnostics feature ensures system integrity prior to each procedure
- Cutting motion will not start until appropriate vacuum level is reached.

- Cutting stops if vaccum drops below threshold.
- Electronic compensation delivers constant motor speed.
- New quiet, high out put vacuum with backup power system.

Salient Features

- Availability of both a microsuction ring which is designed for use in deep-set eyes or those with very small fissures and a series of *Zero Compression Heads* [160 180 and 200 microns] which essentially eliminate flap compression and thus the risk of epithelial defects.
- The microsuction ring has a 19 mm foot print and can create 8.5 mm or 9.5 mm flaps.
- The rate of suction build is quite rapid with the micro ring and the level of suction achieved is excellent, so there is no tendency for the ring to move on the eye. Furthermore with this relatively smaller ring, patients who are Squeezers and those with small fissures no longer pose a challenge to the successful completion of the case.

CENTURION SES MICROKERATOME–PLANAR MICROKERATOME

The device is manufactured by BioVision AG Bern, Switzerland and distributed by CIBA vision corp.

The centurion SES Microkeratome approved by the FDA has features that differentiate it from conventional micro keratomes used for standard LASIK procedures: *a combination blade/cartridge component, a bar applanator, and a resultant gutterless flap.*

The microkeratome is able to flatten the cornea directly in front of the blade by means of a bar applanator.

Bar applanator applies lens force to the Cornea during the microkeratome pass, *Epi-Edge Technology*, allows the safe, reliable use of the suction ring with 50% less suction compared with other microkeratomes currently in use. This results in a safer, more comfortable procedure for the patient.

Also provides a feathered cut with smoother-edged corneal flaps, which may account for the gutterless edge that heals more quickly than conventional flaps. The smoother edge on the flap also has decreased the incidence of diffuse lamellar keratitis (DLK) that results from inflammation.

SET UP

The blade cartridge system is sterile and ready to use.

The microkeratome is set up in four steps:

1. The suction ring is inserted into place.
2. The appropriate blade cartridge system is selected.
3. The lid on the system is pulled back.
4. The blade cartridge system is snapped on.

Advantages of This Planar Microkeratome

- The oscillating blade/cartridge system provides smooth consistent cuts.
- The simple design allows for single-handed use without "on-the-eye" assembly.
- The device is fully automated has programmable surgeon settings. And uses 50% less pressure than a conventional microkeratome.
- It is able to produce flaps that are consistent.
- Can be used in eyes with prominent brows, and small palpebral fissures.
- Facilitates faster patient recovery, less epithelial ingrowth, less-flap slippage and less DLK.

An attachment that will become available soon to surgeons using the—SES Microkeratome is the subepithelial separator handpice, which creates an epithelial flap for subepithelial LASEK or epi LASIK. This device eliminates the need for alcohol, which is used in some laser procedures and is toxic to epithelial cells in separating epithelium from the basement membrane. The hope is that by eliminating the toxicity, the surgical site will heal faster than is now possible and with less pain.

When using the subepithelial separator, there are no sharp blades, knives or chemicals needed. Surgeons can reposition an intact epithelium with the worst complication being a corneal abrasion. As the epithelium is intact, there is no risk of haze. Also with no flap, there are no striae or flap debris, and the subepithelial debris is eliminated. In addition, unlike many other laser procedures, the epi LASEK procedure is wave front compatible Epi-LASIK is perfectly suited for surface ablation.

The surgeon does not have to manipulate the epithelial layer during the procedure, making SES a "*non-touch*" surgical approach.

CARRIAZO PENDULAR

Invented by Cesar Carriazo, MD Barranquilla, Columbia.

Introduction

Microkeratomes of the 1st generation rely on a linear cutting action, the 2nd generation evolved to a pivoted rotational cutting action and now the 3rd generation features a pendulum like cutting action.

The carriazo-pendular microkeratome is based on the principle of convex applanation of the cornea during the cut. This results in the cornea being applanated evenly from the beginning of the cut to the end. This ensures that the intraocular pressure does not vary to the extent it does with conventional flat plate applanation.

Ergonomically designed, the carriazo pendular microkeratome makes placing the head into the suction ring extremely simple and takes just two steps due to its *drop-and-go* mechanism.

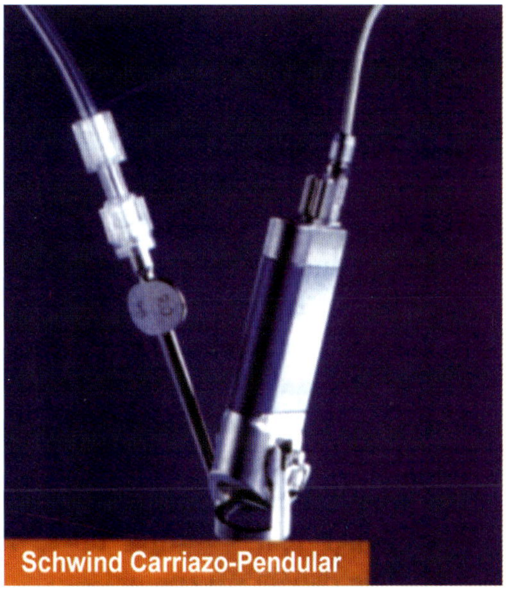

Fig. 4.6: Schwind Carriazo-Pendular

The spherically molded system with carriazo pendular blade oscillation can produce high quality flaps in any quadrant of the cornea.

Salient Features

- Unique pendular movement.
- Ball shaped cutting head protects the corneal centre.
- Vertically centered coupling of ring and head in front of the eye.
- 360 degree free choice of hinge position.
- Also well suited for very small and deep set eyes due to minimum dimension of suction rings (19 mm).
- Multiple built in safety features.
- The drive unit with its two separately driven micro-motors.
- New revolutionary design of the suction ring (the suction ring has a very small footprint and suction is obtained fast and efficiently).
- The calibrated OP vacuum and the intelligent electronics of the user console.
- No additional step of latching in the head with the suction ring with the carriazo pendular it is simply a matter of "drop and go".

The Bdk –3000 /Bection –Deckinson K-300 (Insight Technologies)

This microkeratome is a precision cutting device uniquely designed on added comfort speed and accuracy.

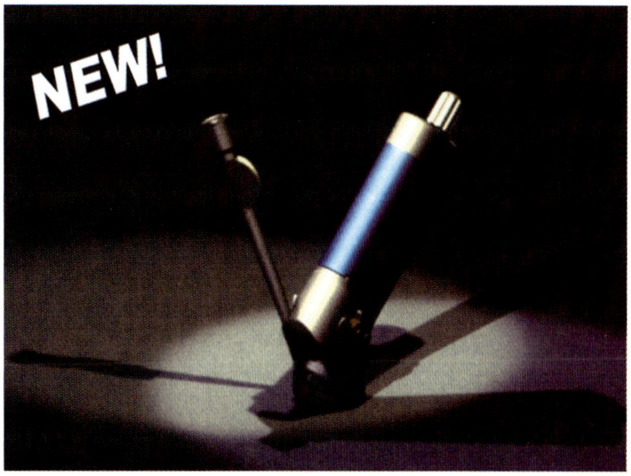

Fig. 4.7

Salient Features

- One piece allowing completing assembly prior to positioning on the eye.
- Ergonomically designed to increase surgeon's comfort.
- All components fully interchangeable for flexibility.
- The blade and the blade holder come pre-assembled and are disposable.
- Applanator assures accuracy.
- Applanator prior to the actual cut prevent smaller than desired caps with 9 mm are three applanator sizes 8.5 mm 9.0mm and 9.5 mm with in 10.0 mm are 9.5 mm, 10.0 mm and 10.5 mm sizes.
- Sizes include 8.5 mm,8.8 mm ,9.0 mm,9.5 mm and 10.0 mm

Keratome Head

The single piece stainless steel keratome which houses a precision bearing delivers constant drive alignment. A horizontal groove mount provides stable oscillation of the blade, essential in super smooth stromal beds. The keratome allows viewing of the flap as it being dissected.

Suction Ring

360 suction port combined with special vacuum system assures fixation of eye. It can be used for very small and deep set eyes.

Blade

- Medical grade stainless steel Blade, 25 angle
- Honed trifaceted cutting edge
- Nonmetallic blade holder, Preassembled, sterile.

Hand Piece

- Titanium construction, Ergonomically designed and light
- Dual Swiss motors control Translation.

Power Unit and Vacuum

- Independent power source for added safety
- Dual vacuum pumps; low vacuum option for greater control
- Automatic stop and rest if suction lost.

Golden Tips

- Avoid hurting the lid Speculum; this can create an irregular bed.
- Use good technique.
- Examine carefully and discard any defective blades.
- Discard blades that do not go easily into the keratome.
- Test to make sure the blade and the motor are engaged to avoid partial and incomplete cuts.
- Follow the manufacturer's guidelines for testing the microkeratome and blades.
- Use only the manufacturer's blade for each micro-keratome.

NON-MECHANICAL MICROKERATOMES

The So Called Bladeless Lasik

Introduction

Majority of microkeratomes in use today are dependent on one common denominator - *BLADE*. It is this component that will "Make or break the keratectomy".

Blades are vulnerable to damage and thus microkeratome safety will increase considerably if the blade is eliminated.

This has led to the entry of two new entities. (I) *Water-Jet based microkeratomes and (II) Femtosecond laser ablated flaps.* The major advantages are that the blade related complications are eliminated. Also the flaps are smoother and more consistent.

Water-Jet Microkeratomes/Mechanical Microkeratomes

- Interlamellar vs. intralamellar cuts.
- Less tissue trauma vs greater tissue trauma.
- Smooth surface vs thermally and physically damaged.
- Miniscule distorting forces < 2g vs 10's g Wt.
- Ultra fast < 1 sec Vs minutes.
- Slight 10 P increase < 60 mm Vs > 60 mm Hg.
- Debris free water jet microkeratomes.

The Water Jet Microkeratome: Bladeless Microkeratome

Water Jet technology is already being used in the industry as a very effective cutting tool for even the hardest materials and is under consideration for surgical procedures in a variety of different medical fields.

The water jet based microkeratome is a non mechanical device which is capable of making clean reproducible flaps with a smooth interface. The refractive cut is created by a high speed stream of saline propelled under ultra high pressure of about 15000 Psi. The rectilinear liquid stream has a diameter of 30 Microns and is forced through a small nozzle to make the corneal lamellar dissection.

The Water-Jet device cuts are cleaner and smoother because they make inter-lamellar cuts.

Electron Micrographs indicate that the water-jet cuts by separating the corneal surface and that there is little collateral damage and the vast majority of collagen in the stroma remains undisturbed.

This new microkeratomes allows a full and easy view of the cornea while the procedure is being carried out through the applanation window and it can be easily halted or altered if it becomes necessary. Another advantage of the water jet is the observation that the energy level used cuts the cornea so easily that the intraocular pressure is almost unchanged. It may be temporarily elevated by the suction ring, but is negligible when performing the incision.

Types

The *lipshitz Bass knife water-jet keratome* is among the first of the new device to be discussed in the medical literature (Journal of Refractive Surgery January-February 1996, PS. 181-186) it consists of three parts; a pressure generator, a robotics subunit that directs the cutting head along an X-Y-Z axis and the instrument head itself. It has a multiple size suction ring to immobilise the eye, which allows deformation of the anterior corneal curvature at the time of incision to a predetermined curvature. That is achieved by changing the size of the ring and the intraocular pressure or by using different templates over the eye, so as to precisely cut the desired amount of tissue.

Once the cut is made the ring or template is removed and the newly created surface becomes curved again into the desired shape by the eye's normal intraocular pressure. The system operates by using a very thin (50 mm), high pressure stream of water applied coronally to remove a narrow disc of the anterior cornea; this is done by means of a computer controlled program to ensure precise refractive correction.

After the water crosses the eye, it is collected by a small suction cup. The surgeon can monitor the procedure accurately and control it. The operation can be stopped at any time with the foot-pedal. Another safety device is a He-Ne laser beam that is attached to the cutting head exactly parallel to the water-jet. Further more numerical limitations can be entered into the computer or the mechanical robot to stop the procedure when desired.

MEDIJET

The waterjet device (Hydro Blade) developed at Medijet, Inc. in New Jersey, USA, consists of a plastic hand-piece, connected by a small diameter, flexible plastic tubing capable of sustaining high pressure to a flexible bottle of saline. The bottle is inserted in pressurizing cylinders controlled by a foot-pedal. The activating force for the high hydrostatic pressure (15,000 Psi) created within the bottle to power the water jet is derived from a light weight disposable cartridge containing carbon dioxide.

VISIJET

Another water-based device now under investigation is called the Hydrokeratome and has been developed by Visijet, Inc, a subsidiary of Surgijet, Inc, in Irvine, California.

The components of the Visijet Hydrokeratome system include a titanium hand-piece, the applanation suction ring, the console, and an activating foot switch. The hand piece measures about 14.0 × 1.0 × 2.2 cm, weighs approximately 20 gm and contains the beam orifice through which the water beam is emitted. It connects to the console via a high pressure hose and to an inter changeable applanation suction ring. The suction rings are available in sizes ranging from 140 to 200 microns, and they feature a clean plate to provide the surgeon good visibility of the cornea during the entire procedure.

The console contains both primary and back-up vacuum pumps thus assuring vacuum function of the eye is maintained even if the primary pump fails, as well as a hydraulic pump, which creates high levels of hydraulic pressure using nitrogen gas and sterile water for injection. The sterile water for injection that ultimately exits the hand-piece is twice-filtered, first through a 0.2 micron, stainless steel fitter and again through a 20-Micron stainless steel filter.

After set-up is completed, operation of the Hydrokeratome is begun with depression of a foot switch. A motor carriage assembly into which beam orifice is mounted is then driven by a 12 V DC Motor, laterally across the cornea from a home to a re-programmed stop position. Flaps of up to 10 mm in diameter can be treated – it takes 1.2 seconds for the water to reach full velocity, to assure cut initiation begins only once full velocity level is achieved the system features a built-in delay between the carriage assembly and food switch activation with that mechanism assembly movement does not begin until 1.5 seconds after the foot switch is depressed.

Then the carriage assembly reaches it pre-programmed stop position, the high hydraulic pressure is vented to the atmosphere via a valve with in the console and the flow of high pressure water through the orifice ceases in about 30 milliseconds. Overall, the resection is completed in about 2 seconds and with less than 1 ml of sterile water.

Differences in Design

The Visijet device is some what simpler than the Medijet Hydrokeratome. The latter has an eye fixation device and uses custom-designed templates to create each cut. On the other hand, the Visijet instrument uses eye holders in several sizes. There are also subtle differences in the size and speeds of the two devices. International clinical trials involving both in instruments were initiated in late 1997.

FEMTOSECOND LASER

The new Pulsion (femtosecond) technology the only ***ALL LASER*** solution for the correction of the corneal flaps. The Pulsion FS laser marks the first significant advancement in flap creation technology in nearly 50 years.

With its computer controlled software, the femtosecond laser brings a level of accuracy and precision to flap creation procedures that is not attainable with mechanical blade technology. This all laser approach, with its patented femtosecond technology, provides patients with a safe blade less alternative to the microkeratome and offers the surgeon a computer controlled, minimal invasive technique that reliably creates precise corneal flaps. The Pulsion FS femtosecond technology brings a new level of accuracy, precision and safety to flap creation for lasik surgery. This laser uses infra red light to precisely cut tissue by a process called photo disruption. The laser beam is focused via optics into a tiny three micron spot that passes harmlessly through the outer layers of the cornea until it reaches its exact focal point within the stroma (central layer of the cornea).When it reaches this focal point, the beam forms a microscopic cavitation bubble of carbon dioxide and water vapour by making an inter connecting series of these bubbles in a tightly wound, inside the spiral, a dissection plane is created at a precisely controlled depth within the corneal stroma. The laser beam then stacks a pattern of bubbles along the periphery of the dissection plane, leaving uncut section of tissue to act as a hinge .This final dissection to the surface is beveled, meaning the outer diameter of the flap is slightly wider than the inner diameter. This unique shape assists in re alignment and seating of the flap upon completion of the treatment. Because the low energy pulse from the laser is in the femtosecond range a mere quadrillionth of a second there is no heat damage to the surrounding tissue thus it is less invasive then the mechanical microkeratome and is well suited for delicate corneal surgery. Since the laser eliminates the need for mechanical microkeratome no abrasions of the corneal membrane can occur. Also as the laser makes a near vertical beveled incision at the flaps margin as opposed to a more horizontal incision with the microkeratome, the flap reseats better and provides a better seal at the margins of the flap. This greatly reduces the possibility of flap slippage post operatively. This tighter seal also reduces the probability of epithelial in growth into the incision.

The Pulsion laser eliminates much of the uncertainty in a flap creation because it is computer controlled with a point and click function for easy selection of surgical parameters. As a result flaps can be made that are both accurate and consistent in thickness amd diameter.

Another important safety aspect using a laser lies in the method of stabilizing the eye during the flap creation.

Two different approaches are being investigated for using the femtosecond laser microkeratome. One involves fixation of a contact glass to the laser system using a suction holder applanated to the cornea and focusing of the laser beam to a fixed reference depth. The second is a contact free technique that establishes the intra stromal reference plane through very precise eye tracking.

The contact and non contact methods each have advantage and draw backs. Achieving a cut of predictable and constant depth may be facilitated with the contact glass method that establishes a reference frame and keeps the eye from moving.

To assure accuracy in the depth of the cut a good Z reference is critical, very careful control is needed because the beating heart causes the eye to move in this plane .Since the applanation glass with applied suction flattens the cornea at its distal surface, creating a flap of consistent thickness requires only that the laser focus be scanned at a single, specified distance from the laser surface of the glass.

In contrast the contact free method requires additional technology to track the X,Y and Z movements with the necessary high precision .The eye movements have to be controlled by optical means and the position of the laser focus has to be actively controlled in order to generate a contiguous treatment pattern when placing the laser shots.

Because the cornea maintains its normal curved shape, as the laser spot scans circumferentially within the stroma, the depth of focus has to be varied to achieve constant flap thickness.

The contact free technique may have a cost advantage since a new applanation glass and holder have to be used for each eye due to etching of the glass when the anterior –posterior flap cut is made.

Salient Features of the Femtosecond Laser

- Only a very minimal increase in IOP (30 MM) is required during creation of the flap.
- Very precise corneal depths can be achieved.
- Corneal thickness will be very consistent throughout the flap.
- Management of flap complication due to loss of suction is better as a new flap can be made within 45-60 minutes.
- No tendency to create epithelial sloughing or recurrent erosions due to it's relatively a traumatic mechanism of action.
- Lasik without blade.

NEW DISPOSABLE MICROKERATOMES

Three Disposable units -The Laser Sight Automated Disposable Keratome (ADK), The flap maker, from Refractive Technologies, Moria Be One up Disposable Keratome.

The Laser Sight Automated Disposable Keratome (ADK) uses a disposable head, eye cup and vacuum assembly. It's propelled by a dual gear track mechanism, with one gear on each side. The Maker says this may pose less of a risk of jamming than a single gear device which can torque. The gear drives are covered to minimize entrapment of the lids and eyelashes. All of the on eye components are transparent to make visualization easy.

The flap maker from Refractive technologies is a completely transparent disposable unit that uses a cable rather than gears for propulsion. This reduces the risk of chatter as the cut is being made.

Disposable Microkeratome removes some of the major problems associated with the care and setting up of conventional microkeratome. There is no need for a dedicated microkeratome technicians and all that is required is to remove the unit from its sterile pack, attach some cables and suction tubing and take place it on the eye.

Because the unit is disposable, there is no cleaning required. The microkeratome is similar in design to modern Barraquer style microkeratomes but it is fabricated from transparent, injection-molded polycarbonate plastic. Because it is transparent it allows better cent ration and it makes it easier for the surgeon to visualize the cornea while creating the flap. It also has a fixed suction ring diameter and a fixed blade gap depth.

That feature is of critical importance because it eliminates the possibilities of the surgeon incising into the globe, as may occur with the presently available microkeratome if the plate is not set properly. The initial unit of the disposable microkeratome will have gap depth of 160 microns, but later models may be thinner or the thicker, depending on the needs of the surgery.

Additionally, there is feedback mechanism so that if suction is lost during the LASIK procedure, the blade will stop oscillating. Further more the blade will oscillate only while it is moving forward and stops oscillating during reverse translation. To ensure the quality of the blade, each unit will come with a photomicrograph of the blade edge. Because the blade is already set in the microkeratome, it doesn't have to be assembled.

New microkeratome is completely automated, does not have any gears. It is a propelled by a flexible cable which produces more than 300 psi of force, the lack of gears eliminates problems of lashes and other debris which may accumulate in the gear and interfere with the passage of microkeratome. Gear system can also cause the microkeratome to torque during its translation, but because the cable of this new disposable device pushes the microkeratome away from the center, the torque possibilities eliminated.

The Pros of Disposable Microkeratomes

- They minimize the possibility of an error during disk assembly, cleaning and reassembling.
- They require no maintenance.
- They are relatively economical particularly for low volume surgeons.
- They are good for beginners.

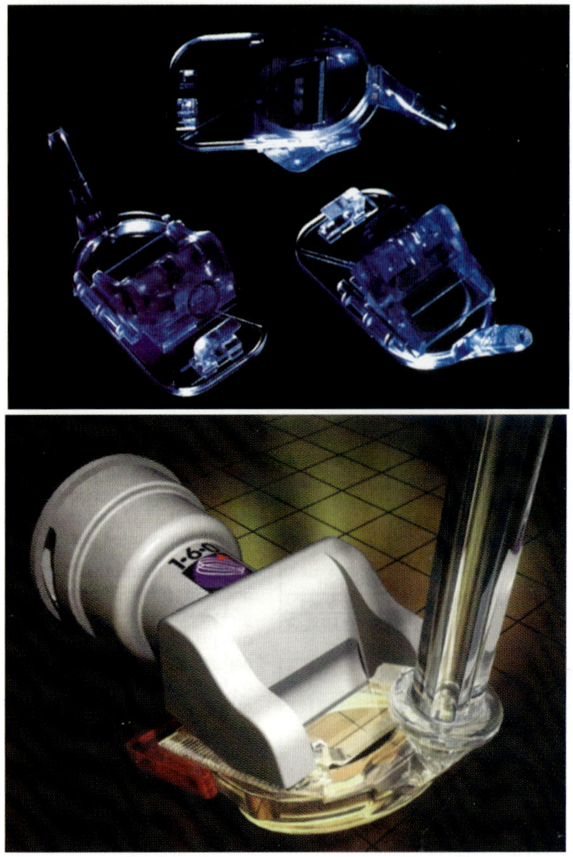

Figs 4.8 and 4.9: Flap maker

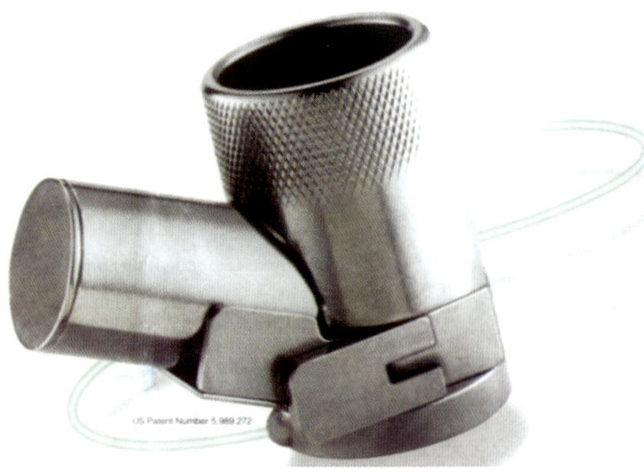

Fig. 4.10: Katena all stainless steel microkeratome

Conventional | *Disposable*

Product name	***Amadeus***	***Moria M2***	***NIDEK MK-2000***	***Schwind Carrazio Pendular***	CB single use
Manual/automatic	Automatic	Automatic	Automatic, no exposed gears	Both, no external gears and two seperately driven motors	Manual
Advanced rate	Customizable	Two advance speeds available	2 mm/sec	Blade translation standard speed 5 mm/sec	Can be varied by surgeon
Cutting mechanism	Surgical steel blade	Blade	Blade	Ball shaped cutting head protects the central cornea	Blade/ disposable head
Oscillation/min	Cutomizable	15000 rpm	9,000 rpm	15,000 rpm	15,000 rpm
Flap diameter	8.5/9/9.5/10 mm All in standard size, narrow size and Asian	Upto 10.5 mm	8.5/9.5/9 mm (Optional)	8, 9, 10 mm (6 Suction rings right and left for 8,9, 10 mm diameter each available)	Up to 10.5 mm
Blade angle eye fixation	25 degrees yes	Proprietary suction rings (sizes- –1,0,+1,+2,+3)	25 degrees suction ring	39 degrees Suction ring	Proprietary suction rings (sizes-1,0,+1,+2)
Depth	140/160/ 180 microns	130 and 160 microns	130+,160+ and optional 180 microns	3 cutting head available for different flap thickness, choice of hinge position	130 and 160 microns
Variable flap Orientation	Yes	Yes	Yes	Yes, 360 degrees free choice of hinge orientation	Yes
Power source	115-250 V, 50-60 Hertz,AC with battery	Battery	115 V, 230 V	115 V/230 V	Battery
Handpiece composition	Swiss made surgical titanium	N/A	Hand piece, suction ring, blade holder with wedge tip	Single piece cutting head (surgical stainless steel)	N/A
Regulatory status	510(k) approved	CE marked and 510 K approved	FDA approved	FDA in process	CE marked and 510 K approved

CONCLUSION

Technology is racing to develop the perfect procedure for refractive surgery. It is essential that the eye care practitioner maintains an awareness of current technological developments, ongoing research and future designs so as to best advise the patients.

Finally, research is on going to develop a successful procedure which directs the ablation to the stroma without any flap being created at all!

Femtosecond Laser for Corneal Flaps

5

BOJAN PAJIC (SWITZERLAND)

INTRODUCTION

The mechanism of femtosecond laser flap has been described extensively.[1-5] The system produces short-duration (600 to 800 femtosecond) light pulses at 1053 nm infrared wave-length. Multiple pulses are focused to an approximately 3 µm spot diameter at a preset depth, leading to photodisruption and creation of a corneal resection plane. Once the bed of the flap has been created, the device creates a side cut from the level of the resection plane, moving anteriorly through the epithelium. Cavitation bubbles created during photodisruption generally remain in the resection plane; however, they may migrate anteriorly, posteriorly, or peripherally in the cornea.

Initial experience in the United States with the IntraLase FS laser began in May 2000 and showed excellent results with no postoperative complications.[3, 4] To date, several studies have documented improved flap predictability and refractive outcomes compared with that of the mechanical microkeratome.[6-8] Use of technology has been reported to reduce or eliminate many of the minor and severe complications associated with flap creation.[4-9]

Methods and Patients

In a prospective study femtosecond laser (Intralase) with 15 KHz is compared with a mechanical keratome (SIS Amadeus) regarding the LASIK flap creation. 651 myop cases were carried out for LASIK surgery, in 310 patients in the femtosecond laser group 1 and 341 patients in the mechanical keratome (SIS Amadeus) group 2 between November 2004 and April 2006. Mean age of patients was in group 1 35 ± 8.5 years (range: 20-60 years) and group 2 35 ± 8.6 years (range: 21-62 years). In group 1 148 patients (47.7%) were female, 162 patients (52.3%) male and in group 2 154 patients (45.2%) were female, 187 patients (54.8%) male. In group 1 156 cases (50.3%) the right eye in 154 cases (49.7%) the left eye and in group 2 174 cases (51.0%) the right eye in 167 cases (49.0%) the left eye were treated. The preoperative mean refractive spherical equivalent was –3.71 ± 2.68 in the femtosecond laser group (range –9.75 to 4.50 D) and –3.40 ± 2.56 in the mechanical keratome group (range –9.88 to 4.25 D). The mean cylinder was –0.99 D in the IntraLase group (range –5.00 to 0.00 D) and –1.07 D in the Amadeus SIS group (range –6.00 to –0.50 D). There is no significant difference between the groups regarding the mean preoperative spheroequivalent and cylinder ($p>0.05$). All soft contact lens use was discontinued for at least 1 week.

In all patients, preoperative evaluations included uncorrected visual acuity (UCVA), manifest refraction, best-spectacle-corrected visual acuity (BSCVA), cycloplegic refraction, intraocular pressure (IOP), topography, pachymetry, wavefront aberrometry and slitlamp examination. With online OCT the pachymetry was acquired before surgery and immediately after the flap was cut and lifted of the unmoistened stromal bed. With a confocal laser microscopy the cornea was analyzed after the femtosecond laser surgery and pachymetry was controlled. Patients were evaluated preoperatively and 1 day, 1 week and 1, 3 and 6 months after surgery.

Femtosecond laser flaps were programed to deliver equivalent geometric dimensions with following settings. 120 µm tickness, 8.5 mm diameter, 45-degree superior hinge angle to achieve equivalent corneal stromal surface exposure, 70-degree side-cut angle, laser raster pattern spot/line separation 10/10 µm with a 15 KHz repetitionsrate, and stromal energy of 3.0 µJ with a side-cut energy of 4.0 µJ. Mechanical flaps were created using a 140 µm head and 8.5 or 9.5 mm ring depending of the corneal radius.

Confocal Corneal Laser-Microscopy

The development of in vivo confocal laser-scanning microscopy permitted precise three-dimensional (3-D) visualization of microstructures of the ocular fundus in particular with its optic nerve head and the peripapillary retina. Modern digital image processing technology enables quantitative data to be collected non-invasively, rapidly and with a low level of illumination. The precision of laser-scanning ophthalmoscopy in this context is based on the principle of the confocality of the examined object with the light source and the detector plane. A laser light source is focused through a pinhole diaphragm to one point on the object. The reflected laser light is separated by a beam splitter from the incident laser beam path and deflected through a second confocal diaphragm to reach a photosensitive detector. Because of the confocal design, light originating from outside of the focal plane is highly suppressed, and only the object layer located at the focal plane contributes to the image. In order to build up a two-dimensional image perpendicular to the optical axis of the device, the laser beam has to scan the sample point by point. This is achieved by introducing two oscillating mirrors into the beam path. By moving the focal plane optically, an image can be acquired from a deeper layer of the examined object, thus enabling a data cube to be built up in a successive series. By contrast, in slit-lamp biomicroscopy examination of the cornea, an optical section that is essentially perpendicular to the corneal surface is seen in up to X50 magnification or, with an additional lens for endothelial viewing (specular microscopy), in up to X200 magnification. Nowadays, documentation is generally performed using digital photography. All other cellular structures, e.g. the epithelium, cannot be imaged with this technique because of the high proportion of scattered light.[10]

Optical tomography perpendicular to incident light path has only become possible with adaptation of confocal microscopy, as described above, for the examination of the living eye.[11-17]

Slit-Scanning Techniques

Techniques based on principles of rotating NIPKOW disk or tandem slit-scanning were used initially for confocal microscopy of anterior segment of eye. For the purposes of corneal assessment these microscopes can be used to image confocal sections, with an optical layer thickness of approx. 5-10 µm. Synchronization of slit-scanning[16,18,19] with video rate of a residual light camera yields sharp and motion-independent image sequences at 25 frames/s.[20,21] Three-dimensional image distortion due to eye movements with this noncontact microscopy technique can only be minimized by faster image acquisition. However, more rapid movement of the confocal plane along the optical axis (z-scan) is accompanied by a loss of resolution. Loose optical coupling to the cornea using a gel limits the precision of depth information relating to the optical section in the cornea, and hence the 3-D reconstruction of cell structures.[22-24] Systematic errors such as inhomogeneous image illumination and image distortion also arise as a result of the electromechanical slit-scanning technique used. Linear movement along the z-axis during individual image acquisition also produces distortion along the z-axis. These fundamental sources of error can only be prevented by a rapid laser scanning system unhampered by mass inertia and incorporating a serial dot raster technique, with stepwise advance of confocal plane during the z-scan.[10]

Laser-Scanning Microscopy and Pachymetry

As an alternative to confocal slit-scanning microscopes, a confocal laser-scanning microscope for the anterior segment of the eye was developed at the Rostock Eye Clinic on the basis of an already commercially available laser-scanning system. Not least because of its compact construction, the Heidelberg Retina Tomograph II (HRT II. Heidelberg Engineering GmbH, Germany) was selected as the basic device for a digital confocal corneal laser-scanning microscope. In laser-scanning ophthalmoscopy of the posterior segment, the optically refractive media of the eye forms part of the optical imaging system. For anterior segment applications, a high-quality microscope lens is positioned between the eye and the device, providing a laser focus less than 1 μm in diameter. The result is a high-resolution, high-speed, digital confocal laser-scanning microscope permitting in vivo investigation of cornea. Movement of the confocal image plane inside the cornea can be achieved manually at the microscope lens or by using the automatic internal z-scan function of the HRT II. Laser-scanning tomography is consequently possible in anterior segment of the eye.[10]

This technique permits rapid and reliable visualization and evaluation of all the microstructures in the cornea, including the epithelium, nerves, and keratocytes, as well as the endothelium and bulbar conjunctiva. For the first time, the dendritic (or Langerhans') cells can now also be visualized in vivo with an image quality that permits quantification.[25]

Results

The mean acuities in both groups improved significant from baseline to 1 day after surgery and remains stable in the further follow-up. The mean acuities were not significantly between the groups at each interval ($p > 0.05$). The mean UCVA and standard deviations were not significantly between the groups ($p > 0.05$). In the Intralase group 1 were within ± 0.5D of the intended manifest refractive spheroequivalent at 1 month 94%, at 3 months 95% and at 6 months 97% (Fig. 5.1) respectively in the mechanical SIS Amadeus Keratome at 1 month 96%, at 3 months 97% and at 6 months 95% (Fig. 5.2). There is no significant difference between the groups ($p > 0.05$). Regarding the predictability, there was in the femtosecond laser group 1, a slightly over correction

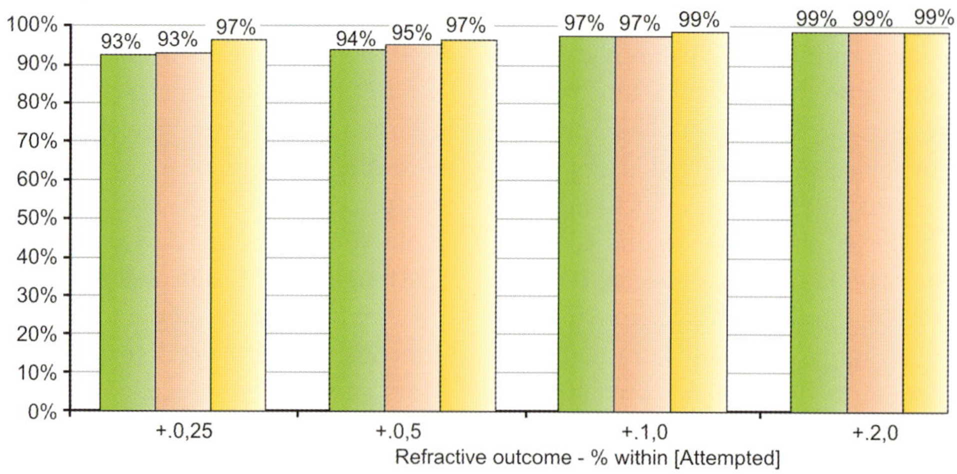

Fig. 5.1: Femtosecond laser: Refractive outcome - % within attempted

of 0.25 D (Fig. 5.3). In group 2 as higher the preoperative refraction is, the higher is the undercorrection over a surgery refraction of 5 dpt (Fig. 5.4). After the procedure the mean flap thickness was in the IntraLase group 1 119 ± 4.6 µm (range 111 to 129 µm) and in the SIS Amadeus group 2 148 ± 38 µm (range 124 to 196 µm). The femtosecondlaser was significant more accurate than the mechanical keratome ($p < 0.01$). In the group 1 and 2 no significant endothelial cell loss was found at 6 months postop.

In group 1 the best visual acuity was unchanged at 1 month in 55%, at 3 months in 34% and at 6 months in 56%, improved by one line at 1 month in 30%, at 3 months in 43% and at 6 months in 33% and improved by two lines at 1 month in 15%, at 3 months in 14% and at 6 months in 10%. No patient lost lines of visual acuity (Fig. 5.5). In group 2 the best visual acuity was unchanged at 1 month in 50%, at 3 months in 57% and at 6 months in 32%, improved by one line at 1 month in 6%, at 3 months in 22% and at 6 months in 34% and improved by two or more lines at 1 month in 6%, at 3 months in 4% and at 6 months in 8%. Best visual acuity was lost by one line at 1 month in 33%, at 3 months in 13% and at 6 months in 8% and by two

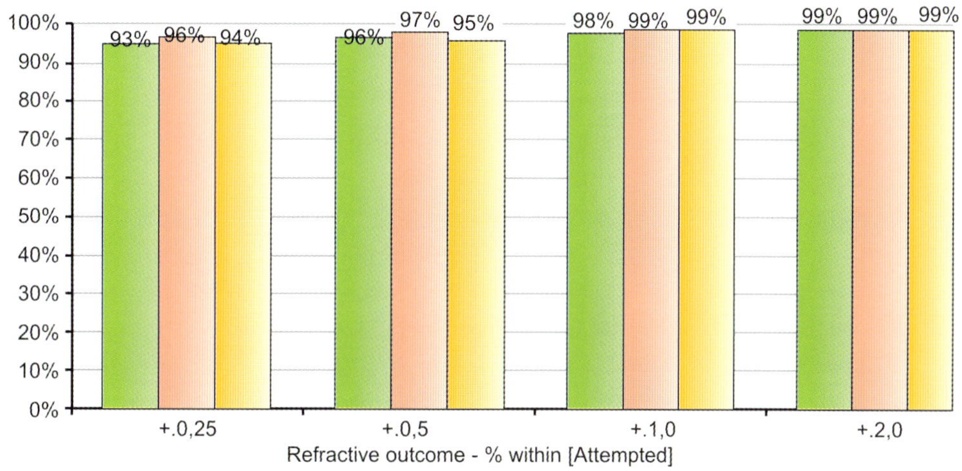

Fig. 5.2: Mechanical keratome: Refractive outcome - % within attempted

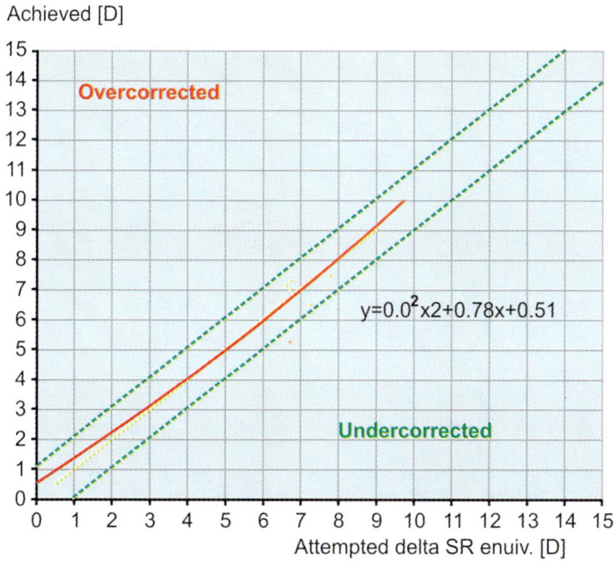

Fig. 5.3: Femtosecond laser: Predictability

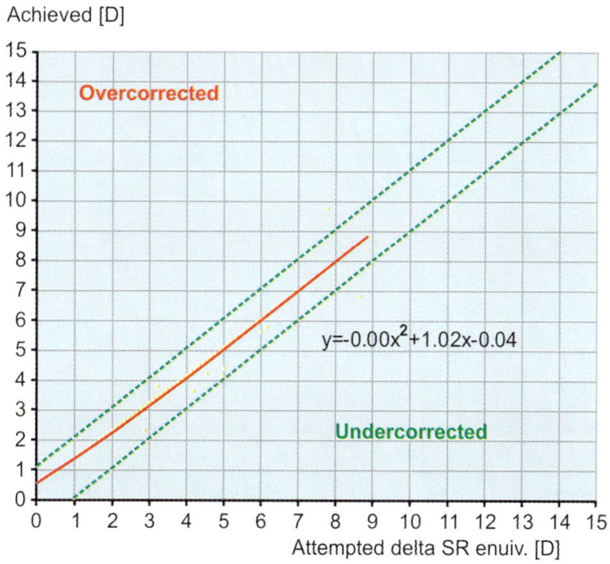

Fig. 5.4: Mechanical keratome: Predictability

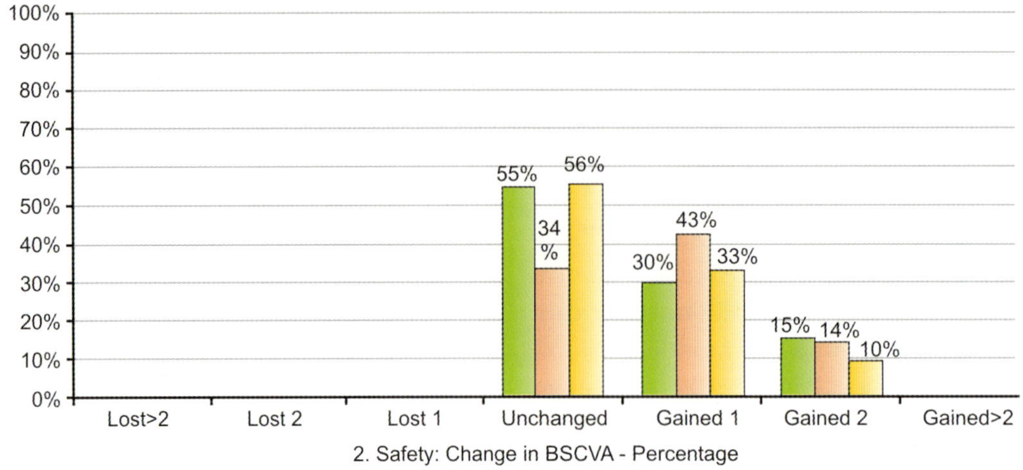

Fig. 5.5: Femtosecond laser: Safety

lines at 1 month in 6%, at 3 months in 4% and at 6 months in 8% (Fig. 5.6). Regarding the safety there was a significant difference between both groups, it's said the femtosecond laser group has a better outcome ($p < 0.01$).

Complications were seen in group 1 overall in 5 cases, 2 striae and 3 diffuse lamellar keratitis and in group 2 overall in 19 cases, 9 striae, 5 diffuse lamellar keratitis, 2 epithelial ingrowth, 1 flap dislocation and 2 incomplete flaps.

The external temperature has an impact on the delivery of femtosecond laser energy to the tissue. The hotspot of the laser was investigated at 17°C and at 24°C. Experimental we could show, that with the raise in temperature, the spot loses homogeneity (Fig. 5.7 and 5.8).

Discussion

This prospective study compared LASIK outcomes obtained using 2 devices for flap creation: The IntraLase femtosecond laser and the standard compression head Amadeus SIS mechanical Keratome. Flap creation with IntraLase femtosecond laser has high predictability, safety and low complication rate, comparing with a mechanical keratome. Femtosecond laser flap cutting is a highly reproducible technique with a high rate of predictability. Comparing with a mechanical

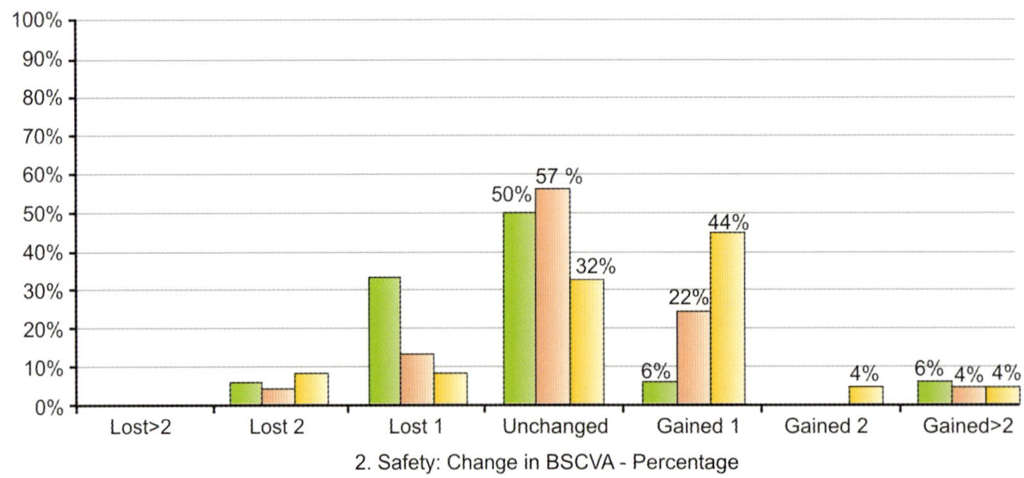

Fig. 5.6: Mechanical keratome: Safety

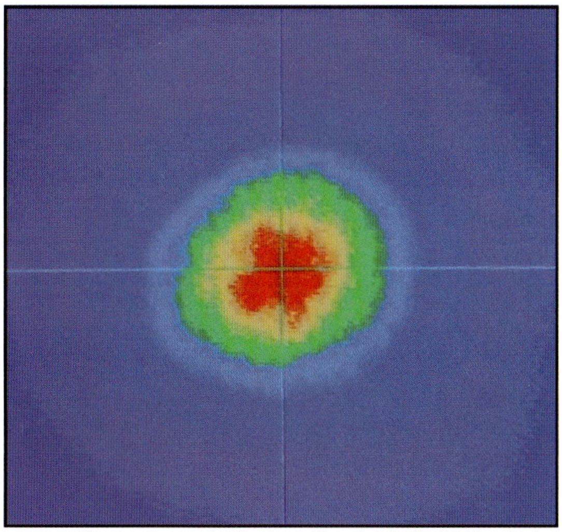

Fig. 5.7: Hotspot of femtosecond laser at room temperature of 17°C

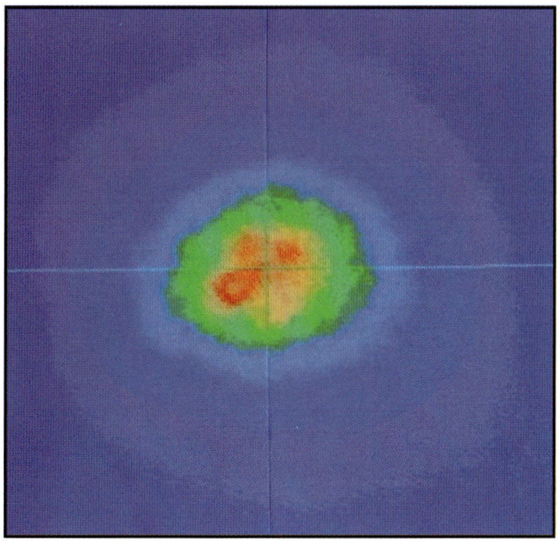

Fig. 5.8: Hotspot of femtosecond laser at room temperature of 24°C. The spot is less homogenous

keratome there is possible to rely on the flap thickness, performed by a femtosecond laser, with low range of less than 10 µm. A further advantage of a femtosecond laser comparing with a mechanical keratome is the precision and safety of cut is independent of preoperative corneal curvature. The predictability was high in both patients groups. In the femtosecond laser group 1 a slightly over correction of 0.25 D was seen. It could be explained, that the overall treatment time with the femtosecond laser, is longer as with the mechanical keratome, thus the interface is more dry with a consecutive overcorrection. Cutting a LASIK flap with a femtosecond laser is a very safe treatment. No patient lost lines of visual acuity with a very low rate of complications. An interesting correlation was found between interface edema and room temperature. Confocal microscopy observation of cornea after surgery showed, that eyes which were exposed to a warmer environment tended to develop proportionally more edema than eyes operated on at a slightly lower temperature (Fig. 5.9 and 5.10). The external temperature has an impact on delivery of femtosecond laser energy to the tissue. Experimental we could show, that with the raise in temperature, the spot loses homogeneity (Fig. 5.8). We suggest that the ideal surgery room temperature should be between 17° and 22°C. In conus of IntraLase, the laser beam is outside of the device where the temperature could have an influence on the hotspot.

In future new femtosecond laser systems will be developed with a higher pulsfrequency, a lower energy application per effect and a shorter treatment time. So the bubble formation caused by photodisruption will be much smaller and the cutting

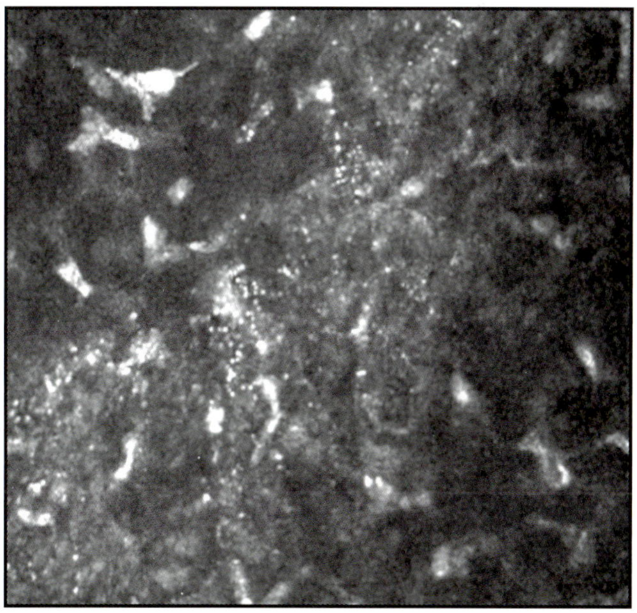

Fig. 5.9: Confocal microscopy. Corneal edema postoperative is less pronounced in the cornea, exposed at a room temperature of 19°C

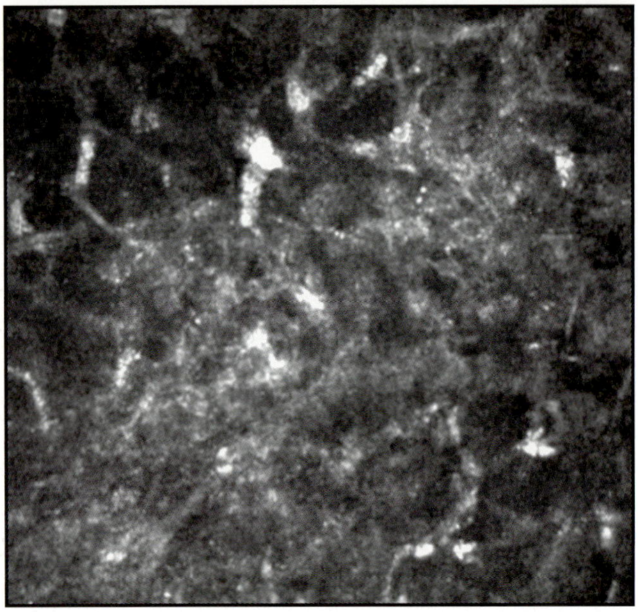

Fig. 5.10: Confocal microscopy. Corneal edema postoperative is more pronounced in the cornea, exposed at a room temperature of 22°C

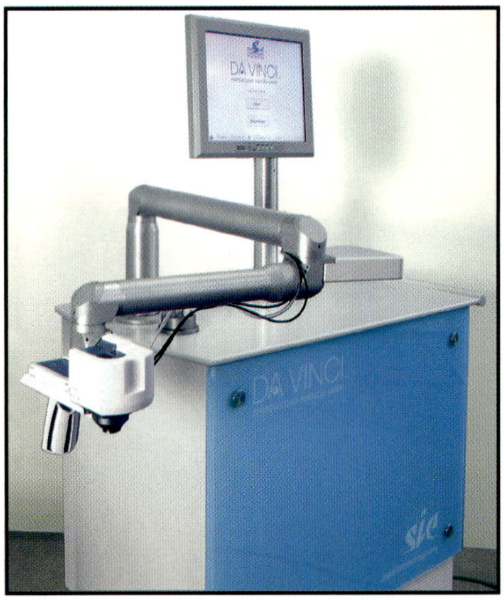

Fig. 5.11: New femtosecond laser system DaVinci

surface smoother. The next developing steps are already done by IntraLase with a pulsfreqeuncy of 30 KHz and 60 KHz. The treatment time reduces with the 60 KHz below 30 seconds. Up to now, advantage of IntraLase femtosecond laser is comparing with other systems, that there is customize treatment possible, not only in the refractive but also in cornea surgery, e.g. for cornea grafting.

Soon we perform a pilot study of new DaVinci femtosecond laser with a pulsfrequency in a MHz range (Fig. 5.11). The first outcomes shows nearly no bubbles with very smooth surface in the interface. The results will be reported.

REFERENCES

1. Kurtz RM, Liu X, Elner VM, et al. Photodisruption in the human cornea as a function of laser pulse width. J Refract Surg 1997; 13:653-58.
2. Sugar A. Ultrafast (femtosecond) laser refractive surgery. Curr Opin Ophthalmol 2002; 13:246-49.
3. Ratkay-Traub I, Juhasz T. Horvath C, et al. Ultra-short pulse (femtosecond) laser surgery; initial use in LASIK flap creation. Ophthalmol Clin North Am 2001; 14(2)347-55.
4. Nordan LT, Slade SG, Baker RN, et al. Femtosecond laser flap creation for laser in situ keratomileusis: six-month follow-up of initial US clinical series. J Refract Surg 2003; 19:8-14.
5. Ratkay-Traub 1, Ferincz IE, Juhasz T, et al. First dinical results with the femtosecond neodynium-glass laser in refractive surgery. J Refract Surg 2003;19: 94-103.
6. Kezirian GM, Stonecipher KG. Comparison of the IntraLase femtosecond laser and mechanical keratomes for laser in situ keratomileusis. J Cataract Refract Surg 2004; 30:804-11.
7. Binder PS. Flap dimensions created with the IntraLase FS laser. J Cataract Refract Surg 2004; 3026-32.
8. Iran DB, Sarayba MA. Bor Z, et al. Randomized prospective clinical study comparing induced aberrations to IntraLase and Hansatome flap creation in fellow eyes: potential impact on wavefront-guided laser in situ keratomileusis. J Cataract Refract Surg 2005;31:97-105.
9. Anderson NJ, Edelhauser HF, Sharara N, et al. Histotogic and ultrastructural findings in human corneas after successful laser in situ keratomileusis. Arch Ophthalmol 2002;120:288-93.
10. Guthoff RF, Stave J. Essentials in Ophthalmology Cornea AND External Eye Disease; In Vivo Micromorphology of the Cornea: Confocal Microscopy Principles and Clinical Applications, Hrsg. Reinhard Th., Larkin F.; Springer-Verlag Berlin Heidelberg 2006;173-208.
11. Bohnke M, Thaer AA. Untersuchung der Kornea mit einem neuen konfokalen Mikroskop. In: Lund OE, Waubke TN (eds) Bildgebende Verfahren in der

Augenheilkunde. Methoden und Indikationen. Enke, Stuttgart, 1994;47-53.
12. Cavanagh HD, Jester JV, Essepian J, Shields W, Lemp MA. Confocal microscopy of the living eye. CLAO J 1990;16:65-73.
13. Cavanagh DH, Petroll WM, Alizadeh H, He YG, McCulley JP, Jester JV. Clinical and diagnostic use of in vivo confocal microscopy in patients with corneal disease. Ophthalmology 1993;100:1444-54.
14. Koester CJ, Roberts CW, Donn A, Hoefle FB. Wide field specular microscopy. Clinical and research applications. Ophthalmology 1980;7:849-60.
15. Maurice DM. A scanning slit optical microscope. Invest Ophthalmol 1974;13:1033-37.
16. Thaer A, Geyer OC. Die Anwendung der konfokalen Spaltscanning-Mikroskopie auf die In-vivo-Untersuchunge der Kornea-Mikrostruktur im Zusammenhang mit dem Tragen von Kontaktiinsen. Contactologia 1997;19:157-77.
17. Tomii S, Kinoshita S. Observations of human corneal epithelium by tandem scanning confocal microscope. Scanning 1994;16:305-06
18. Masters BR, Thaer AA. In vivo human corneal confocal microscopy of identical fields of subepithelial nerve plexus, basal epithelial, and wing cells at different times. Microsc Res Tech 1994;29:350-56
19. Wiegand W, Thaer AA, Kroll P, Geyer OC, Garcia AL. Optical sectioning of the cornea with a new confocal in vivo slit-scanning videomicroscope. Ophthalmology 1995;102:568-75
20. Masters BR, Thaer AA.Real-time scanning-slit confocal microscopy of the in-vivo human cornea. Appi Optics 1974;33:695-701.
21. Masters BR, Bohnke M. Three-dimensional confocal microscopy of the human cornea in vivo. Ophthalmic Res 2001;33:125-35.
22. Moller-Pedersen T, Ehlers N. A three-dimensional study of the human corneal keratocyte density. Curr Eye Res 1995;14:459-64
23. Patel SV, McLaren JW, Camp JJ, Nelson LR, Bourne WM. Automated quantification of keratocyte density by using confocal microscopy in vivo. Invest Ophthalmol Vis Sci 1999;40:320-26.
24. Stave J, Slowik C, Somodi S, Hahnel C, Grummer G, Guthoff R. Keratozytendichte der In-vivo-Kornea. Automatische Messung mit einem modifizierten konfokalen Mikroskop Microphthal®. Klin Monatsbl Augenheilkd 1998;213:38-44.
25. Suzuki T, Sano Y, Kinoshita S. Conjunctival inflammation induces Langerhans cell migration into the cornea. Curr Eye Res 2000;21:530-33.

Rotational Eyetracker System, Its Importance and Clinical Outcomes

6

BOJAN PAJIC, HERMANN ANHALM JÖRG MÜLLER (SWITZERLAND)

INTRODUCTION

In the last years several improvements on the diagnostic side of refractive corneal surgery have been introduced which contributed to higher precision and the availability of new sets of information such as Wavefront aberration maps and 3 dimensional corneal maps with high precision elevation data.

On the indication and algorithm side parallel developments have been started by expanding the treatment ranges to high levels of astigmatism, aspheric ablation profiles and the correction of high order aberrations.

As a result of these developments the therapeutic side of the refractive platform needs to be equipped with new technologies to enable the therapeutic laser system to deliver the appropriate and needed level of precision to be able to utilize the new level of available information.

One of the essential components to achieve this goal is an appropriate eye tracking technology. Basically there is no refractive leaser system in the field which does not utilize an eye tracking feature in one of the possible implementations.

B and L's H.EYE.TECH eye tracking system is a video based system operating in the infrared. Using infrared radiation to illuminate and to capture the image combines the advantages of being independent of surrounding and iris color conditions and the illumination level of the surgical field. In this implementation the position of the eye is captured by a camera and the eye tracker module determines the position and size of the pupil. This information is transferred to the laser software and the corrective parameters related to the positional change are used to redirect the laser pulses.

The relevance of cyclotorsion and its negative effects on the effectiveness of the ablation process are well known and several companies started to include compensating technologies into their platforms.

As the observed rotational misalignment during the ablation can not be neglected, the next logical step was to expand the applicability of this technology to also include the ablation phase itself. The importance of the intraoperative rotational tracking is especially in the treatment of high order aberrations and mild to high astigmatisms given.

DESCRIPTION OF THE IMPLEMENTED IRIS RECOGNITION TECHNOLOGY

By introducing the rotational eye tracker the already approved X/Y tracker which compensates actively for transversal movements of the eye will be upgraded to compensate misalignments in rotation. While the uses the acquired pupil images only, additional objectively acquired information is needed to provide a rotational tracking capability.

B and L's H.EYE.TECH rotational tracker module is based on the iris pattern recognition technology. It is well known that Iris patterns are similar to finger prints unique biometric properties of an individium.

By using the appropriate technology not only the individual eye can be recognized (which is a safety feature for itself), but also specific match parameters such as rotational misalignment between two images of the same iris can be obtained.

Clinical Evidence for the Need of Rotational Tracking

Almost all diagnostic examinations such as objective measures like wavefront and topography as well as subjective refraction are measured while the patients are seated. However the LASIK treatment is performed on the supine patients. During the surgery the cyclotorsion is a dynamic phenomena, it is said that the angle can change up to 15 degrees within the treatment.

Therefore there are two main reasons for possible cyclotorsion of the eye. First the patient and especially the patient head might lay not properly and straightly onto the bed and secondly the tension within the ocular muscles may change while the patient lies down and the eye will rotate.

Finally loss or reduction of fixation for the time in which the flap is opened my be an additional reason for a torsional movement of the eye.

Published Literature

Different studies investigated the amount of cyclotorsion of eyes during LASIK treatments. Swami et al marked 240 eyes preoperatively while the patients were seated. Immediately before beginning the treatment they measured the rotational misalignment of the eyes on the supine patients. They found a mean cyclotorsion of 4.1° (± 3.7°) while 8% of the eyes showed a deviation greater than 10°. *[Swami et al, Rotational malposition during laser in situ keratomileusis, Am J Ophthalmol. 2002 Apr;133(4):561-2]*

Ciccio et al repeated the measurements. They marked the horizontal axis of 1019 eyes prior to wavefront measurements and detected the mark on the supine patient under the laser. The angle of mismatch were measured and analysed. They reported a mean rotational angle of the eyes from seated to supine patient of 4.05° (± 2.9°). Moreover they found a difference between left eyes and right eyes in the predominant trend of the rotation. 46% of the patients showed bilateral excyclotorsion and only 1.7% displayed bilateral incyclotorsion. *[Ciccio AE et al, Ocular cyclotorsion during customized laser ablation, J Refract Surg., 2005 Nov-Dec;21(6):S772-4]*

Own Datas of Cyclotorsional Measurements with B and L's Rotational Tracker

We measured and adjusted the eyetrackersystem in LASIK treatments on overall 1242 eyes, 654 eyes with B and L's H.EYE.TECH rotational tracker in group 1 and 588 eyes with only X/Y tracker system. The cyclotorsion from upright to supine position were measured using iris image comparison and it was not necessary to mark the cornea.

Mean age of patients was in group 1 36 ± 7.9 years (range: 23-61 years) and group 2 36 ± 8.2 years (range: 21-62 years). The preoperative mean refractive spherical equivalent was -3.43 D ± 2.61 D in group 1 (range –10.5 to –1.5 D) and -3.69 D ± 2.55 D in group 2 (range –8.75 to –1.75 D). The mean cylinder was -1.14 D ± 1.00 D (range -5.75 to –0.75) in group 1 and -1.08 D ± -0.75 D (range -6.00 to –0.75) in group 2. There is no significant difference between the groups regarding the mean pre-operative spheroequivalent and cylinder ($p > 0.05$). All soft contact lens use was discontinued for at least 1 week.

The postoperative mean refractive spherical equivalent was -0.08 D ± 0.36 D D in group 1 (range –2.5 to –0.0 D) and -3.69 D ± 2.55 D in group 2 (range –8.75 to –1.75 D). The mean cylinder was -0.02 D ± 0.13 D (range -0.5 to –0.0) in group 1 and -1.08 D ± -0.75 D (range -6.00 to –0.75) in group 2. There is no significant difference between the groups regarding the mean preoperative spheroequivalent ($p > 0.05$) but there is highly significant regarding the cylinder ($p < 0.01$). The mean cyclotorsion can be calculated to 3.75° with a standard deviation of 3.1°. The total range of torsion was from –14.9° to +12.6.

The frequency rate of the integrated iris based rotational eyetracker was 25 Hz. After successful detection of the cyclotorsion angle the position of the Excimer laser beam was adjusted actively with 25 Hz to apply the intended ablation profile on the desired position on the cornea.

Technical Background of B and L's HEYE TECH Iris Pattern Recognition

As already mentioned, it is well known that iris patterns are unique properties of an individium (such as finger prints) and the probability to find two objects with the same iris pattern is extremely low.

The challenge is to utilize this fact in a way that the realization provides an accurate determination of the special alignment of the mentioned unique pattern if compared to a reference image of the same eye.

Therefore the following three factors have been considered to provide the rotational tracking capability:

- Reliability to distinguish between different iris patterns with a high confidence level.
- Accuracy to determine the rotation with sufficient resolution.
- Speed of processing to provide ease of use and real time intraoperative tracking.

The basic strategy to fulfill these criteria is given by a sophisticated strategy to analyze the complex iris structures and to transform this information into a digital code of the iris which is sufficiently unique but still compact enough to provide a realistic processing time according to the desired application.

A central iris recognition and comparison module is used in all these mentioned applications. This module is the main tool in the identification of the iris patterns as well as the determination of the rotational misalignment between two specific images.

The initial point for an iris recognition process is always the availability of two iris images which will be compared to each other according to the questions whether they belong to the same eye or not and if yes is there a measurable rotational angle between the two images.

Design of the Iris Pattern Recognition Tool

The basic data which are used to analyze iris patterns are the infrared images of acquired iris images. The important fact here is the special normalization and implementation of the technology in a way that iris images can be processed which are acquired at different illumination conditions (large and small pupils) or even at different systems (such as Zywave wavefront sensor and laser system) (Tables 6.1 and 6.2).

IMPLEMENTATION INTO THE PLATFORM

In the following section the implementation of the rotational eye tracking technology into B and L's H.EYE.TECH refractive platform will be described. As already mentioned, both the diagnostic module as well as the therapeutic module need to be modified to provide the required information for the rotational eye tracking.

While the diagnostic tool will be upgraded by modified software to collect and analyze the iris pattern and the derived information, the laser system will be equipped with a second camera to capture the iris image. The algorithm to detected the rotational error resides on an upgraded eye tracker board. Finally the communication between the eye tracker board and the controlling PC of the laser will be extended to include iris data and rotational information.

The acquired rotational information will be then finally applied to the successive pulses to be applied to the cornea.

The following graph gives an overview over the implementation of the iris recognition module in the B and L H.EYE.TECH platform.

Table 6.1: Digital code creation

Step	*Description*	*Example*
1.	Create digital code of the image: Determine pupil boundary and limbus boundary of the reference image. Certain sanity checks are applied to ensure that the identified pupil and limbus geometries are within reasonable measures.	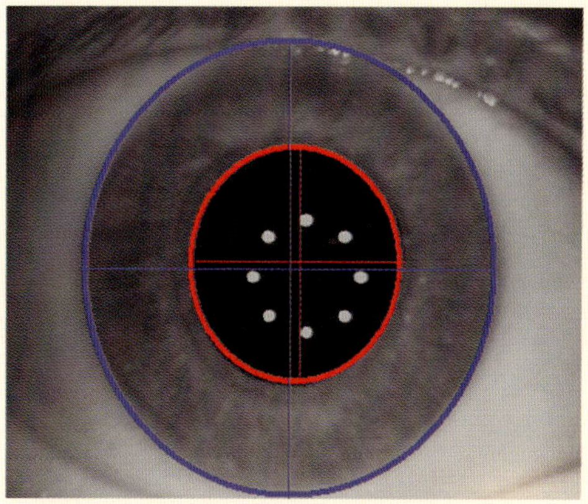
2.	The visible iris pattern defined as the structures between the pupil boundary and the limbus edge will be used. All operations which lead to the final digital iris code are performed within this normalized band	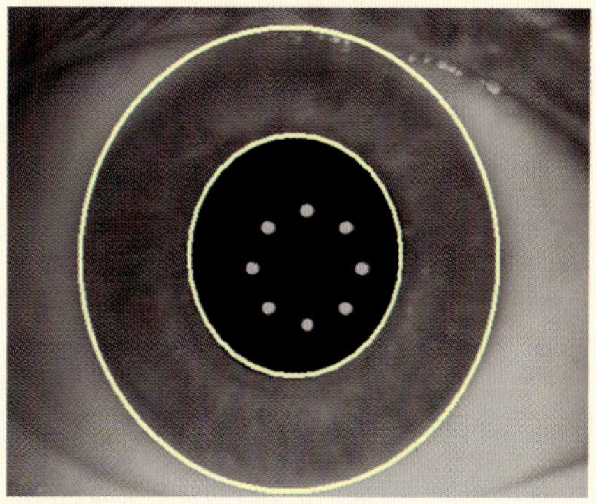
2.1.	Within this band a digital code is generated. Mathematical operators are used to generate a digital code. These operators are aligned in a specific predefined pattern.	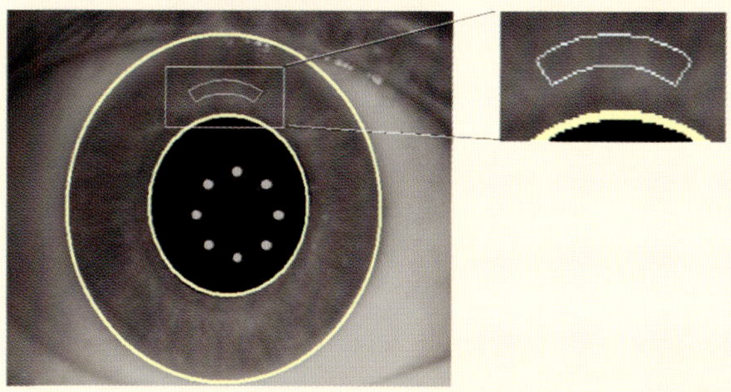
2.2.	The basic data stream of the digital code consists of information of 3920 irisdata at 980 different irislocations	Digital Code = [01001111011.....10111011111]

Table 6.2: Output parameter of the rotation eye tracker system

Output parameter	*Specification*
Images belong to same eye OR not	Logical parameter having possible values: Yes or No. Confidence level: 6σ
Pupil radius	Resolution: less than 30 μm
Pupil center	Resolution: less than 30 μm
Limbus radius	Resolution: less than 30 μm
Limbus center	Resolution: less than 30 μm
Rotation angle between images	Resolution 0.7° (= 360°/512), range ± 14.8°
Quality factor of recognition:	Percentage value. If > 62% then confidence level higher than 6 s.
Response time	40 msec (25 Hz)

The iris data are generated from one acquisition and can be directly exported without performing an additional iris recognition a the diagnositic instrument. This option is available for different treatment modes (Wavefront and Tissue Saving) (Fig. 6.1).

Therapeutic Module (H.EYE.TECH)

In the following section an overview about the eye tracking module in the H.EYE.TECH refractive laser system is given:

Starting shortly with the already existing lateral system the discussion will be extended to include the

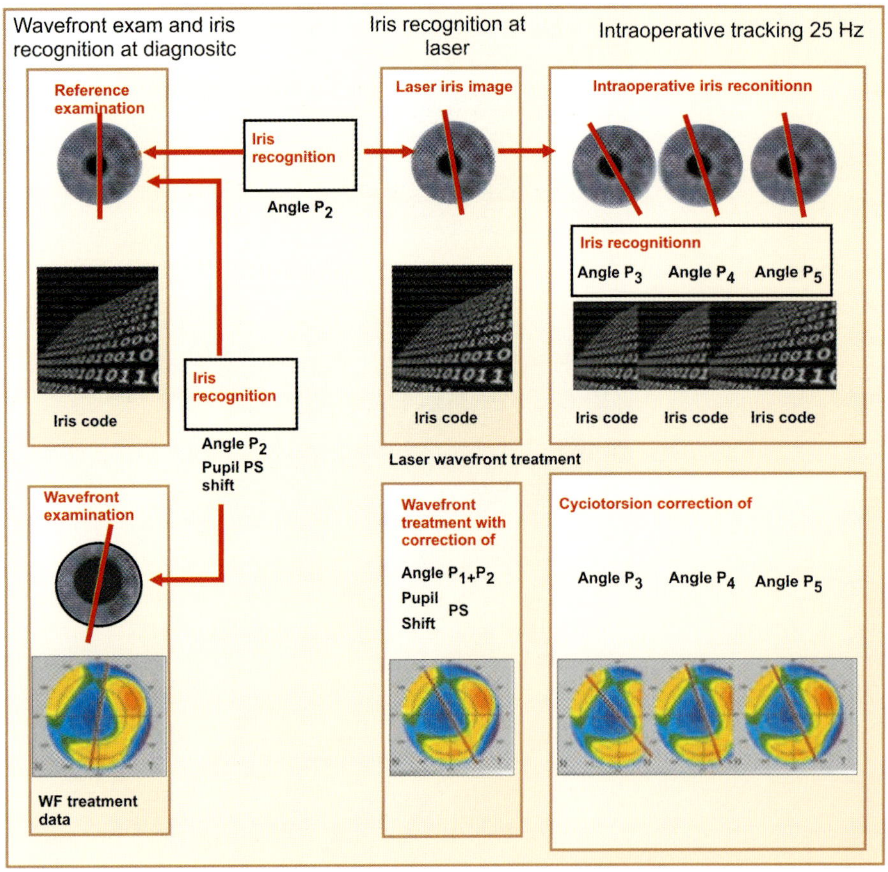

Fig. 6.1: Function of the rotational eye tracking technology

implementation and the functionality of the rotational eye tracking system.

General Functionality of the Eyetracker System

To observe and to track the eye movements of a patient during surgery, the laser is equipped with two different cameras for the eye tracking system. One camera detects eye movements in the x/y direction. It is optimized for the area of the pupil and works with a frequency of 240 Hz. The other eyetracker camera detects the rotational movements of the eye and has a wider display window, so that the iris and limbal region can be observed. This camera works with a frequency of 25 Hz. The slower frequency of the rotational eyetracker camera is justified in the slow speed of cyclotoric movements of eyes, while the x/y tracker must handle also with very fast saccadic movements in the x/y direction (Fig. 6.2).

Due to the different observation angles of the two camera systems it is possible to detect also movements in the height of an eye. So the eye tracker system is able to detect movements in the z direction by observation of the pupil centers of both cameras.

The lateral eye tracker systems works independently. Both cameras can block a laser pulse if the position is not accurate. The surgeon is able to deactivate the rotational eyetracker system (including z-tracking) at any time of surgery, while the x/y tracker will still be activated. A possible manually deactivation of the x/y tracker will switch off both eyetracker systems.

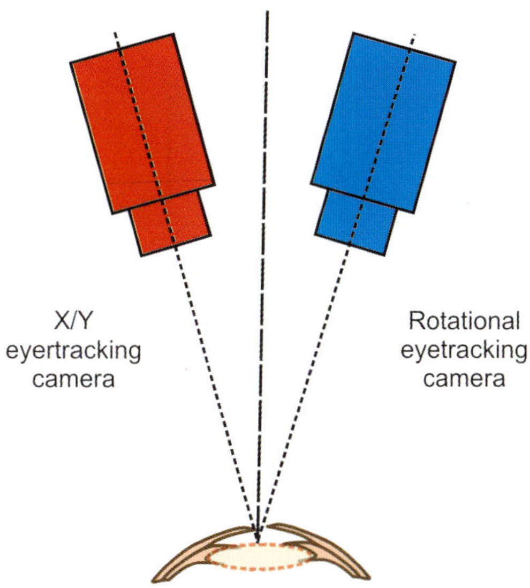

Fig. 6.2: Eye tracker camera system

Lateral Eye Tracker System

With the additional rotational eyetracking feature, the performance of the lateral eyetracker system will not change to the currently available system of the B and L H.EYE.TECH platform.

The current Bausch and Lomb H.EYE.TECH lateral eye tracker consists of an infrared imaging camera system capturing the geometric center of the undilated pupil plus a scanning system to respond and compensate for any pupil movement.

The active x-, y- tracking range is ±1.5 mm from original fixation. Within this active range the eyetracker adjusts the Excimer laser pulses to the intended location according to the pupil position, outside this range it will pause the laser pulsing until the eye is repositioned.

Additionally an active scanner feedback mechanism ensures correct scanner mirror position prior to activating a laser pulse.

For the ease of using the eye tracker system the surgeon defines the treatment center according to pupil reference always having full visual control throughout the entire treatment. The surgeon can also modify the treatment center at any time.

Both eyetracker systems (lateral and rotational) are active and passive systems. So both systems will compensated the pulse position, if eye movements occur as long they are in the defined range. If an eye movement exceed the trackable ranges, the eyetracker systems will block the pulse as long as the correct pulse position is not ensured.

Rotational Eye Tracker System

The following steps are performed in the course of a rotational eye tracking procedure.

Initial recognition procedure To determine the rotation angle of an eye between the upright position of a person at the diagnostic and the supine position under the laser, the software requires the alignment information collected during the diagnostic procedure. These information are delivered within the *.TLS file, which is uploaded to the laser software. This file contains the ablation pattern for the zero degree axis of the iris and the digital iris code of the corresponding eye.

Before starting the laser surgery, when the patient is positioned under the laser the iris recognition procedure is started. During this step the software compares the digital reference iris code (delivered from the diagnostic step) with the digital code of the current images of the rotational eyetracker camera from the laser (Fig. 6.3).

After a successful recognition process, the treatment pattern is rotated to the calculated angle of the last image of the three valid images (φ_3) and shifted by the calculated pupil shift if available.

So the treatment for the correct eye is identified and the accurate orientation of the treatment is ensured.

Surgeons, using the current available version of this rotational eyetracker system reported a successes rate for the initial iris recognition of more than 90% of the patients eyes.

If no recognition is possible within 15 seconds, the process is aborted and an info message is displayed. In this info box the surgeon is asked to check possible reasons for unsuccessful recognition as correct patient, correct eye, misaligned head, dehydration of epithelium, etc.

So the surgeon is able to decide to start a new recognition procedure with improved conditions or to start the laser treatment without compensation of cyclotorsion between diagnostic and laser. Bausch and Lomb H.EYE.TECH application recommendation describes up to three recognition tries, before starting the laser surgery without rotation information.

Continuous recognition procedure during laser ablation The rotational eyetracker system has the ability, not only to correct the rotation of an eye due to a change of the body position. It also capable to correct cyclotoric movements intraoperativly. This intraoperative cyclotorsion can occur, for example due to loss of fixation of the patient, excitement or small head rotations.

To ensure the accurate pulse position also during treatment, the recognition process is continuously applied during the laser ablation.

These images are compared continuously to the reference image, which is the last image of the initial recognition process. For each image the quality factor and rotation angle is calculated and the remaining pulse list is rotated to the actual valid rotation angle (Fig. 6.4).

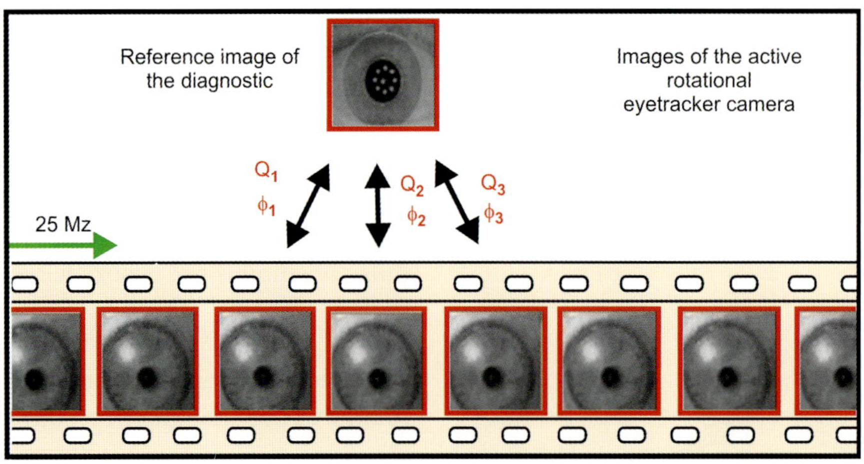

Fig. 6.3: Scheme of initial iris recognition process under the laser

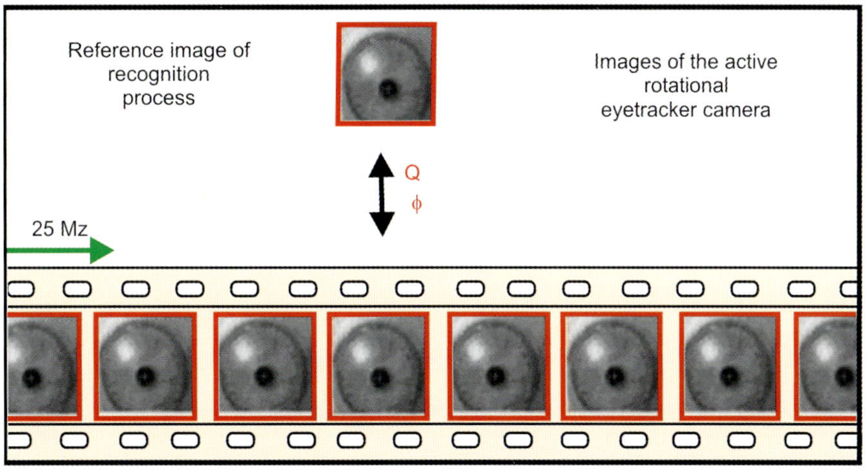

Fig. 6.4: Scheme of online iris recognition process during laser treatment

So even if intraoperatively cyclotorsions occur, the dynamic application of the iris recognition process and the following correction ensures the accurate pulse positioning during the treatment.

During laser treatment the images of the eye can loose contrast, for example due to dehydrating of the corneal surface, so that the difference between the reference image and the actual real time images is increased. In this case the software is capable to record a new reference image with the last valid rotation angle and continue to track the rotation angle using the new reference image.

The rotational eyetracker module will block the application of the next pulse, if the rotation of the eye exceeds a range of ± 14.8 ° (absolute and relative to the initial angle), or the quality factor is not sufficiently high for longer than 0,8 seconds.

Is the patient's eye repositioned or the patient fixates again, the rotational eyetracker will enable the system to continue the treatment when an image and angle is valid.

It is also important to mention that in the case, that the initial patient recognition fails, or no iris picture of the diagnostic is available, the surgeon is not forced to abandon the advantages of intra-operative rotational eye tracking.

In this case the software will automatically generate a reference image when the x/y tracker is logged to the treatment center and the system starts the rotational eye tracking using this reference image.

ACKNOWLEDGEMENTS

The authors thank for distinct support of Dr. Gerhard Youssefi and Anton Hilger (Technolas) for personal and technical advice.

Posterior Corneal Changes in Refractive Surgery

7

Amar Agarwal, Soosan Jacob, Sunita Agarwal,
Athiya Agarwal, Nilesh Kanjiani, Ashok Garg (India)

INTRODUCTION

The development of corneal ectasia is a well-recognized complication of LASIK and amongst other contributory factors, unrecognized preoperative forme fruste keratoconus is also an important one. Patients with this disorder are poor candidates for refractive surgery because of the possibility of exacerbating keratectasia. It is known that posterior corneal elevation is an early presenting sign in keratoconus and hence *it is imperative to evaluate posterior corneal curvature (PCC) in every LASIK candidate.*

TOPOGRAPHY

Topography is valuable for preoperative ophthalmic examination of LASIK candidates. Three-dimensional imaging allows surgeons to look at corneal thickness, as well as the corneal anterior and posterior surface and it can also predict the shape of the cornea after LASIK surgery. Topographic analysis using three dimensional slit scan system allows us to predict which candidates would do well with LASIK and also confers the ability to screen for subtle configurations which may be a contraindication to LASIK.

ORBSCAN

The ORBSCAN (BAUSCH and LOMB) corneal topography system uses a scanning optical slit scan which makes it fundamentally different from the corneal topography that analyses the reflected images from the anterior corneal surface. The high-resolution video camera captures 40 light slits at 45 degrees angle projected through the cornea similarly as seen during slit lamp examination. The slits are projected on to the anterior segment of the eye: the anterior cornea, the posterior cornea, the anterior iris and anterior lens. The data collected from these four surfaces are used to create a topographic map. Each surface point from the diffusely reflected slit beams that over-lap in the central 5-mm zone is independently triangulated to x, y, and z coordinates, providing three-dimensional data.

This technique provides more information about the anterior segment of the eye, such as anterior and posterior corneal curvature, elevation maps of the anterior and posterior corneal surface and corneal thickness. It has an acquisition time of 4 seconds.[1] This improves the diagnostic accuracy. It also has passive eye-tracker from frame to frame and 43 frames are taken to ensure accuracy. It is easy to interpret and has good repeatability.

PRIMARY POSTERIOR CORNEAL ELEVATION

The diagnosis of frank keratoconus is a clinical one. Early diagnosis of forme fruste can be difficult on clinical examination alone. ORBSCAN has become a useful tool for evaluating the disease, and with its advent, abnormalities in posterior corneal surface topography have been identified in keratoconus. Posterior corneal surface data is problematic because it is not a direct measure and there is little published information on normal values for each age group. In the patient with increased posterior corneal elevation in the absence of other changes, it is unknown whether this finding represents a manifestation of early keratoconus. The decision to proceed with refractive surgery is therefore more difficult.

Posterior Corneal Topography

One should always use the ORBSCAN system to evaluate potential LASIK candidates preoperatively to rule out primary posterior corneal elevations. Eyes are screened using quad maps with the normal band (NB) filter turned on. Four maps include (a) anterior corneal elevation: NB = ± 25 μ of best-fit sphere. (b) posterior corneal elvevation: NB = ± 25 μ of best fit sphere. (c) Keratometric mean curvature: NB = 40 to 48 D (d) Corneal thickness (pachymetry): NB = 500 to 600 μ. Map features within normal band are colored green. This effectively filters out variations falling within the normal band. When abnormalities are seen on normal band quad map screening, a standard scale quad map should be examined. For those cases with posterior corneal elevation, three-dimensional views of posterior corneal elevation can also be generated. In all eyes with posterior corneal elevation, the following parameters are generated (a) radii of anterior and posterior curvature of the cornea, (b) posterior best fit sphere, (c) difference between the corneal pachymetry value in 7 mm zone and thinnest pachymetry value of the cornea.

Preexisting Posterior Corneal Abnormalities

Figures 7.1 to 7.6 show the various topographic features of an eye with primary posterior corneal elevation detected during pre-LASIK assessment. In Figure 7.1 (general quad map) upper left corner map is the anterior float, upper right corner map is posterior float, lower left corner is keratometric map while the lower right is the pachymetry map showing a difference of 100 μm between the thickest pachymetry value in 7 mm zone of cornea and thinnest pachymetry value. In Figure 7.2, normal band scale map of anterior surface shows "with the rule astigmatism" in an otherwise normal anterior surface (shown in green), the posterior float shows significant elevation inferotemporally. In Figure 7.2 only the abnormal areas are shown in red for ease in detection. Figure 7.3 is three-dimensional representation of the maps in Figure 7.2. Figure 7.4 shows three-dimensional representation of anterior corneal surface with reference sphere. Figure 7.5 shows three-dimensional representation of posterior corneal surface showing a significant posterior corneal elevation. Figure 7.6 shows amount of elevation (color coded) of the posterior corneal surface in microns (50 μm).

In the light of the fact that keratoconus may have posterior corneal elevation as the earliest manifestation, preoperative analysis of posterior corneal curvature to detect a posterior corneal bulge is important to avoid post LASIK keratectasia. The rate of progression of posterior corneal elevation to frank keratoconus is unknown. It is also difficult to specify that exact amount of posterior corneal elevation beyond which it may be unsafe to carry out LASIK. Atypical elevation in the posterior corneal map more than 45 μm should alert us against a post LASIK surprise. ORBSCAN provides reliable, reproducible data of the posterior corneal surface and all LASIK candidates must be evaluated by this method preoperatively to detect an " early keratoconus".

Elevation is not measured directly by Placido based topographers, but certain assumptions allow the construction of elevation maps. Elevation of a point on the corneal surface displays the height of the point on the corneal surface relative to a spherical reference surface. Reference surface is chosen to be a sphere. Best mathematical approximation of the actual corneal surface called best-fit sphere is calculated. One of the criteria for defining forme fruste keratoconus is a posterior best fit sphere of >55.0 D.

Ratio of radii of anterior to posterior curvature of cornea ≥ 1.21 and £ 1.27 has been considered as a keratoconus suspect. Average pachymetry difference between thickest and the thinnest point on the cornea in the 7 mm zone should normally be less than 100 μm.

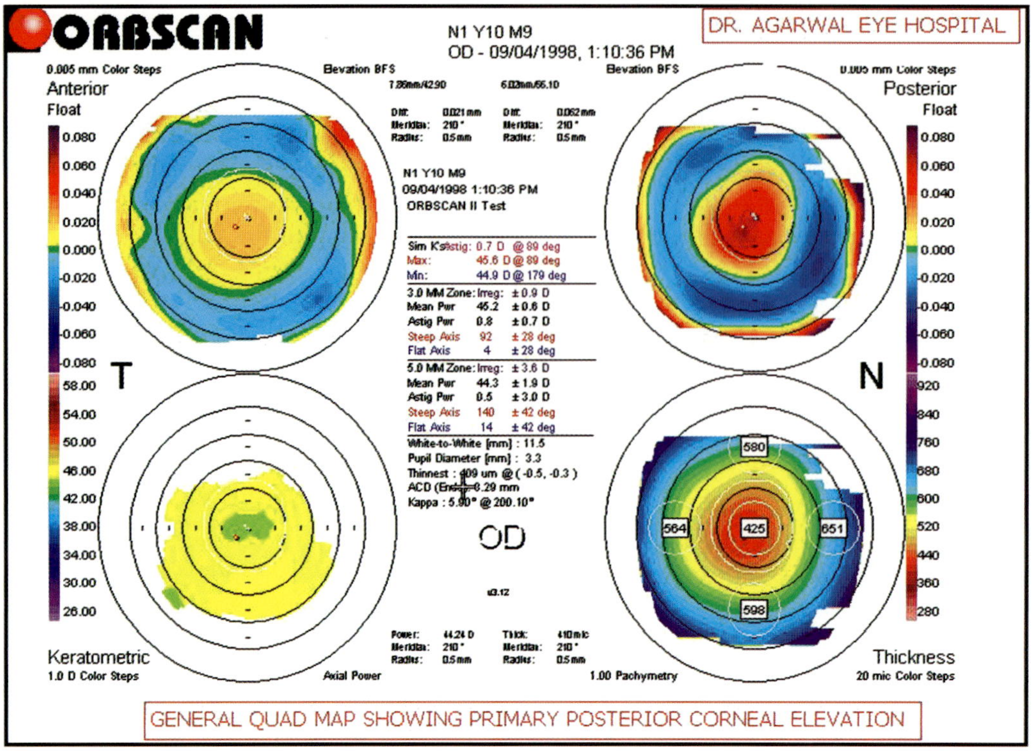

Fig. 7.1: Showing general quad map of an eye with primary posterior corneal elevation. Notice the red areas seen in the top right picture showing the primary posterior corneal elevation

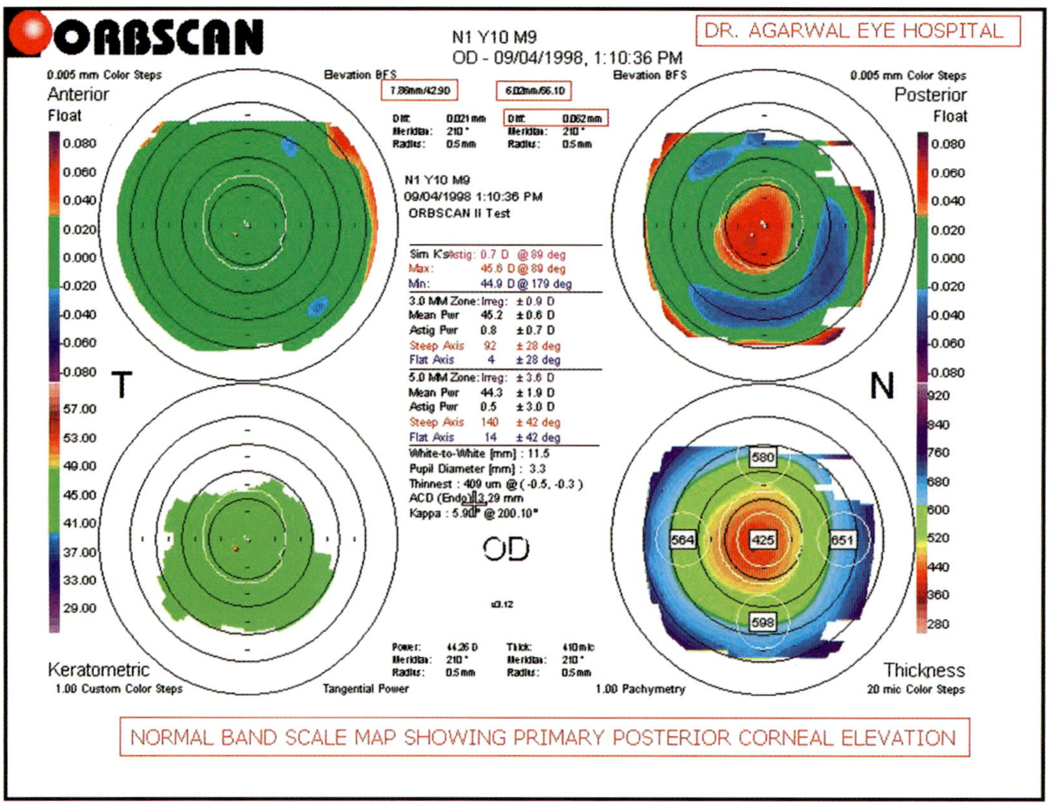

Fig. 7.2: Showing quad map with normal band scale filter on in the same eye as in Figure 7.1

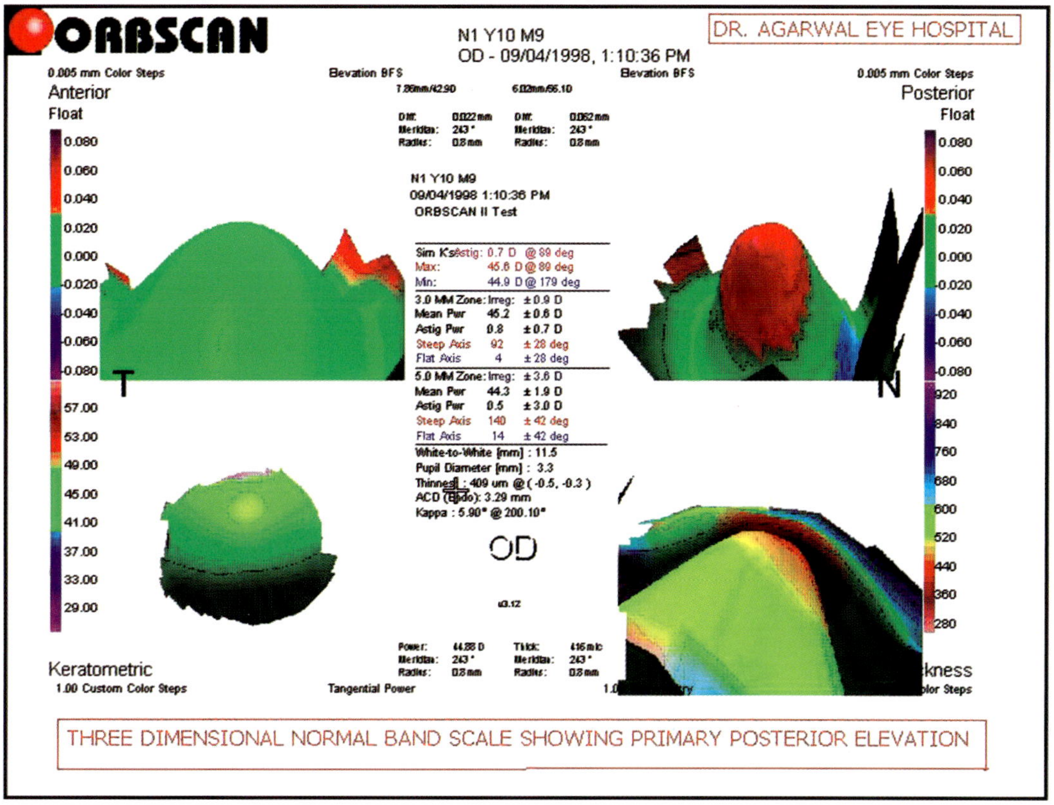

Fig. 7.3: Showing three-dimensional normal band scale map. In the top right note the red areas which shows the elevation on the posterior cornea. The anterior cornea is normal

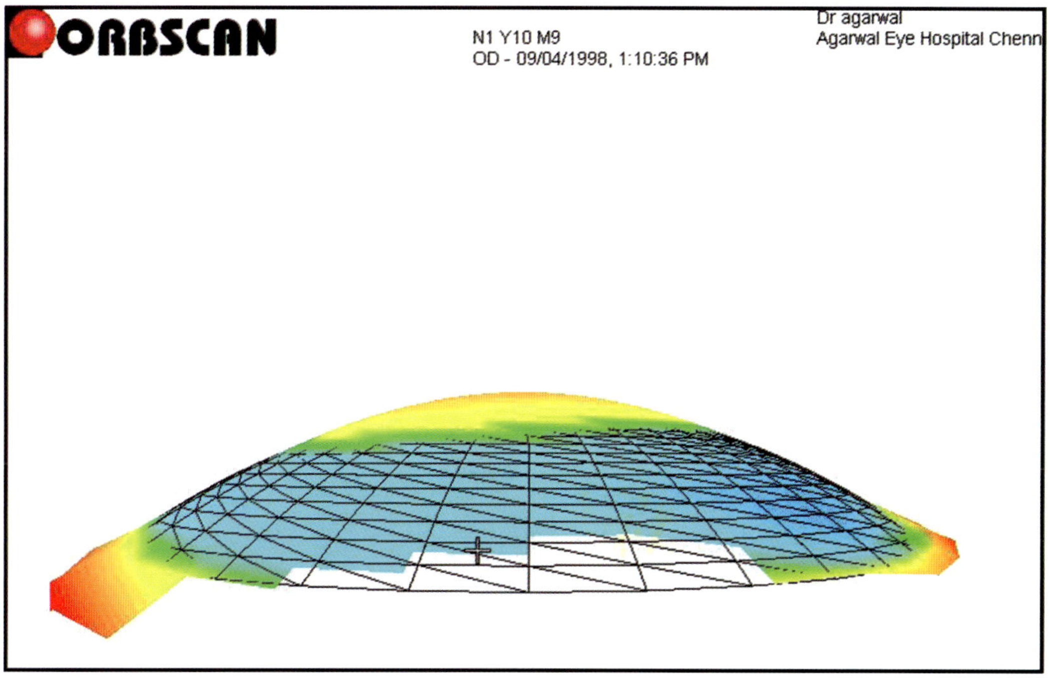

Fig. 7.4: Showing three-dimensional anterior float. Notice it is normal

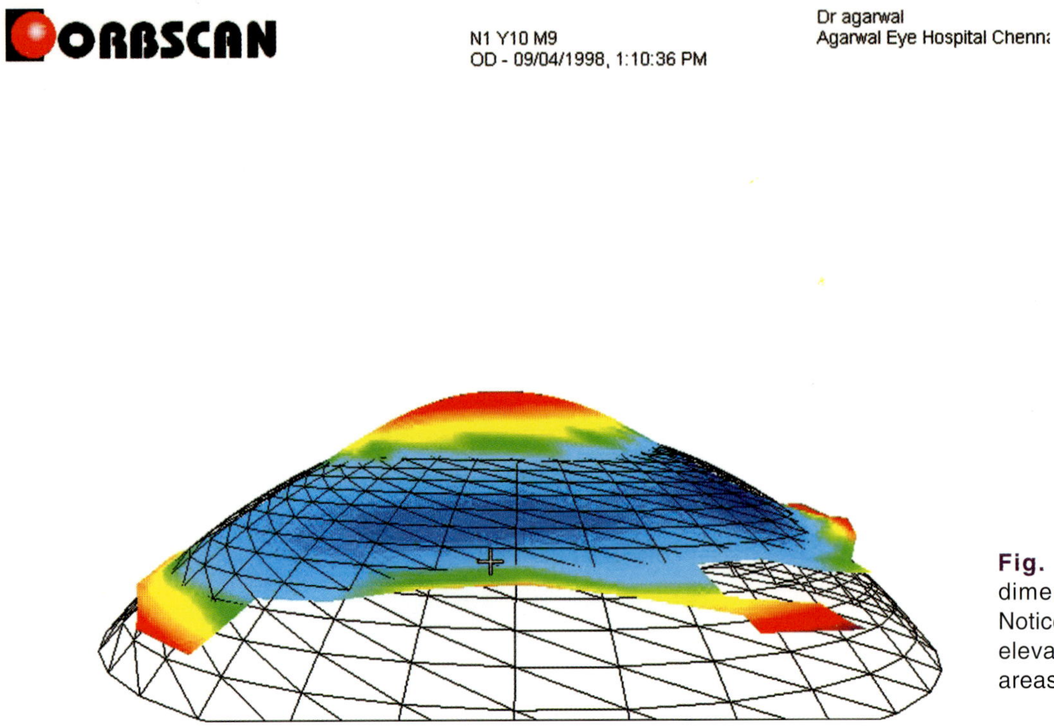

Fig. 7.5: Showing three-dimensional posterior float. Notice in this there is marked elevation as seen in the red areas

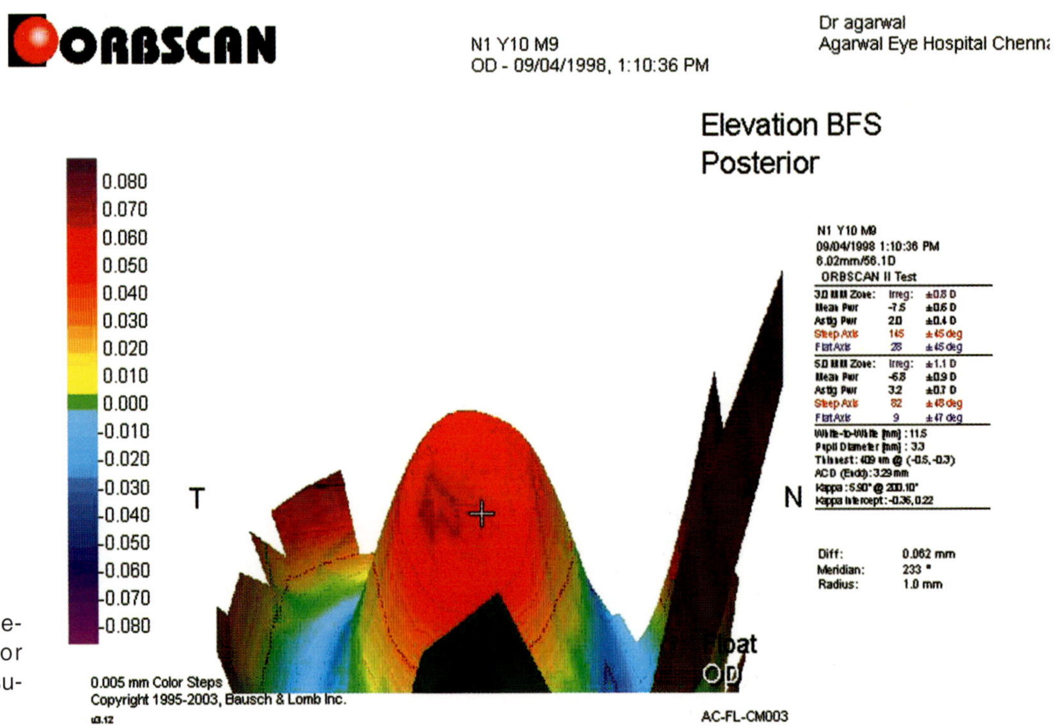

Fig. 7.6: Showing three-dimensional posterior corneal elevation measured in microns

Agarwal Criteria to Diagnose Primary Posterior Corneal Elevation

1. Ratio of the Radii of anterior and posterior curvature of the cornea should be more than 1.2. In Figure 7.2 note the radii of the anterior curvature is 7.86 mm and the radii of the posterior curvature is 6.02 mm. The ratio is 1.3.
2. Posterior best fit sphere should be more than 52 D. In figure 7.2 note the posterior best fit sphere is 56.1 D.
3. Difference between the thickest and thinnest corneal pachymetry value in the 7 mm zone should be more than 100 microns. The thickest pachymetry value as seen in figure 7.2 is 651 microns and the thinnest value is 409 microns. The difference is 242 microns
4. The thinnest point on the cornea should correspond with the highest point of elevation of the posterior corneal surface. The thinnest point as seen in figure 7.2 bottom right picture is seen as a cross. This point or cursor corresponds to the same cross or cursor in Figure 7.2 top right picture which indicates the highest point of elevation on the posterior cornea.
5. Elevation of the posterior corneal surface should be more than 45 microns above the posterior best fit sphere. In Figure 7.2 you will notice it is 0.062 mm or 62 microns.

IATROGENIC KERATECTASIA

Iatrogenic keratectasia may be seen in some patients following ablative refractive surgery (Figs 7.7 and 7.8). The anterior cornea is composed of alternating collagen fibrils and has a more complicated interwoven structure than the deeper stroma and it acts as the major stress-bearing layer. The flap used for LASIK is made in this layer and thus results in a weakening of that strongest layer of the cornea which contributes maximum to the biomechanical stability of the cornea.

The residual bed thickness (RBT) of the cornea is the crucial factor contributing to the biomechanical stability of the cornea after LASIK. The flap as such does not contribute much after its repositioning to the stromal bed. This is easily seen by the fact that the flap can be easily lifted up even up to 1 year after treatment. The decreased RBT as well as the lamellar cut in the cornea both contribute to the decreased biomechanical stability of the cornea. A reduction in the RBT results in a long term increase in the surface parallel stress on the cornea. The intraocular pressure (IOP) can cause further forward bowing and thinning of a structurally compromised cornea. Inadvertent excessive eye rubbing, prone position sleeping, and the normal wear and tear of the cornea may also play a role. The RBT should not be less than 250 mm to avoid subsequent iatrogenic keratectasias.[2-4] Reoperations should be undertaken very carefully in corneae with RBT less than 300 mm. Increasing myopia after every operation is known as "dandelion keratectasia".

The ablation diameter also plays a very important role in LASIK. Postoperative optical distortions are more common with diameters less than 5.5 mm. Use of larger ablation diameters implies a lesser RBT post-operatively. Considering the formula: Ablation depth [mm] = 1/3. (diameter [mm])^2 × (intended correction diopters [D])),[4,5] it becomes clear that to preserve a sufficient bed thickness, the range of myopic correction is limited and the upper limit of possible myopic correction may be around 12 D.[6]

Detection of a mild keratectasia requires knowledge about the posterior curvature of the cornea. Posterior corneal surface topographic changes after LASIK are known. Increased negative keratometric diopters and oblate asphericity of the PCC, which correlate significantly with the intended correction are common after LASIK leading to mild keratectasia.[6,7] This change in posterior power and the risk of keratectasia was more significant with a RBT of 250 µm or less.[8] The difference in the refractive indices results in a 0.2 D difference at the back surface of the cornea becoming equivalent to a 2.0 D change in the front surface of the cornea.[6] Increase in posterior power and asphericity also correlates with the difference between the intended and achieved

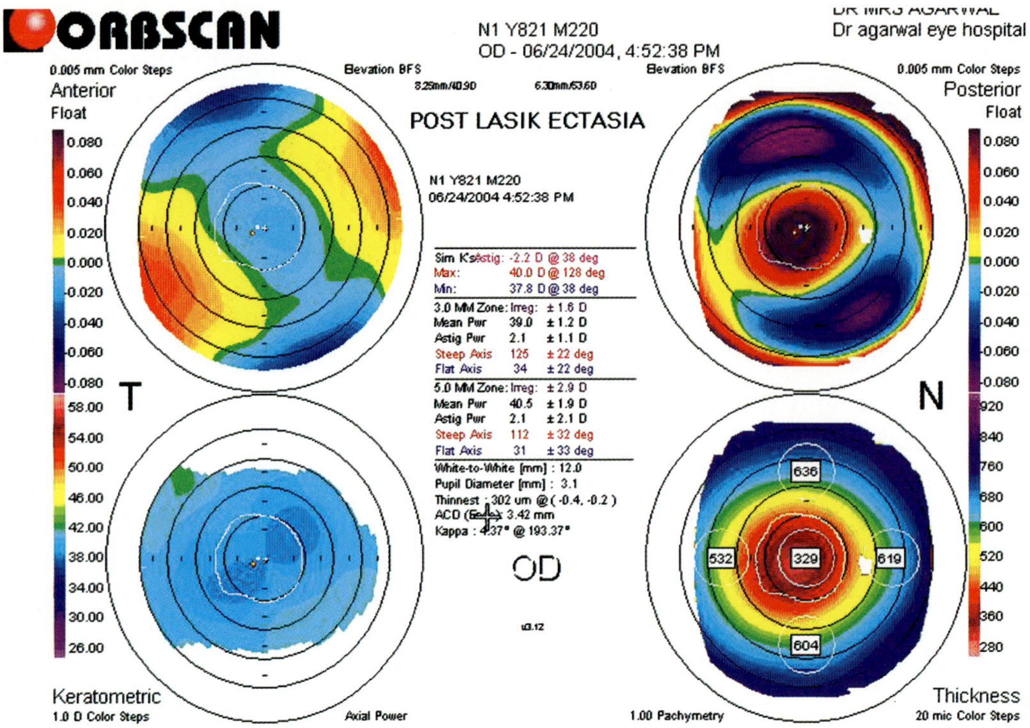

Fig. 7.7: Shows a patient with iatrogenic keratectasia after lasik. Note the upper right hand corner pictures showing the posterior float has thinning and this is also seen in the bottom right picture in which pachymetry reading is 329

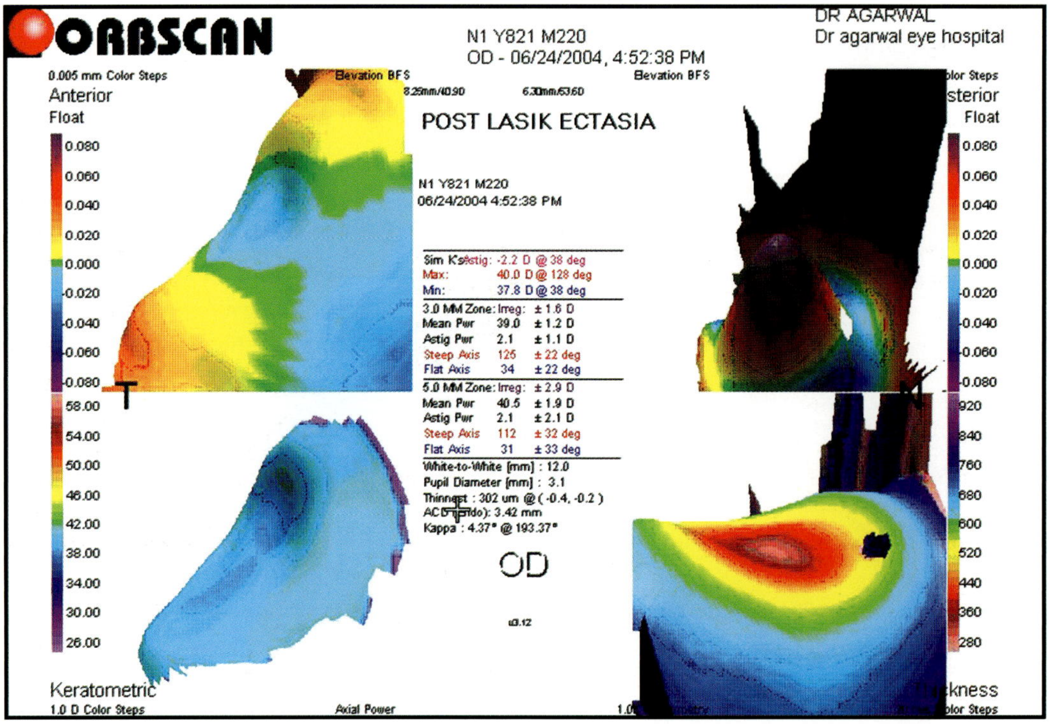

Fig. 7.8: Shows the same patient with iatrogenic keratectasia after lasik in a 3D pattern. Notice the ectasia seen clearly in the bottom right picture

correction 3 months after LASIK. This is because factors like drying of the stromal bed may result in an ablation depth more than that intended.[6] Reinstein et al predict that the standard deviation of uncertainty in predicting the RBT preoperatively is around 30 μm. [Invest Ophthalmol Vis Sci 40 (Suppl):S403, 1999]. Age, attempted correction, the optical zone diameter and the flap thickness are other parameters that have to be considered to avoid post LASIK ectasia.[9,10]

The flap thickness may not be uniform throughout its length. In studies by Seitz et al, it has been shown that the Moris Model One microkeratome and the Supratome cut deeper towards the hinge, whereas the Automated Corneal Shaper and the Hansatome create flaps that are thinner towards the hinge. Thus, accordingly, the area of corneal ectasia may not be in the centre but paracentral, especially if it is also associated with decentered ablation. Flap thickness has also been found to vary considerably, even upto 40 μm, under similar conditions and this may also result in a lesser RBT than intended.[11-17]

It is known that corneal ectasias and keratoconus have posterior corneal elevation as the earliest manifestation.[18] The precise course of progression of posterior corneal elevation to frank keratoconus is not known. Hence, it is necessary to study the posterior corneal surface preoperatively in all LASIK candidates.

EFFECT OF POSTERIOR CORNEAL CHANGE ON IOL CALCULATION

IOL power calculation in post-LASIK eyes is different because of the inaccuracy of keratometry, change in anterior and posterior corneal curvatures, altered relation between the two and change in the standardized index of refraction of the cornea. Irregular astigmatism induced by the procedure, decentered ablations and central islands also add to the problem.

Routine keratometry is not accurate in these patients. Corneal refractive surgery changes the asphericity of the cornea and also produces a wide range of powers in the central 5 μm zone of the cornea. *LASIK makes the cornea of a myope more oblate so that keratometry values may be taken from the more peripheral steeper area of the cornea, which results in calculation of a lower than required IOL power resulting in a hyperopic "surprise". Hyperopic LASIK makes the cornea more prolate, thus resulting in a myopic "surprise" post cataract surgery.*

Post PRK or LASIK, the relation between the anterior and posterior corneal surface changes. The relative thickness of the various corneal layers, each having a different refractive index also changes and there is a change in the curvature of the posterior corneal surface. All these result in the standardized refractive index of 1.3375 no longer being accurate in these eyes.

At present there is no keratometry, which can accurately measure the anterior and posterior curvatures of the cornea. The Orbscan also makes mathematical assumptions of the posterior surface rather than direct measurements. This is important in the LASIK patient because the procedure alters the relation between the anterior and posterior surfaces of the cornea as well as changes the curvature of the posterior cornea.

Thus direct measurements such as manual and automated keratometry and topography are inherently inaccurate in these patients. The corneal power is therefore calculated by the calculation method, the contact lens overrefraction method and by the CVK method. The flattest K reading obtained by any method is taken for IOL power calculation (the steepest K is taken for hyperopes who had undergone LASIK). One can still aim for -1.00 D of myopia rather than emmetropia to allow for any error, which is almost always in the hyperopic direction in case of pre LASIK myopes. Also, a third or fourth generation IOL calculating formula should be used for such patients.

REFERENCES

1. Fedor P, Kaufman S. Corneal topography and imaging. Medicine Journal 2001;2(6).
2. Seiler T, Koufala K, Richter G. Iatrogenic keratectasia after laser in situ keratomileusis. J Refract Surg 1998;14(3):312-7.

3. Seiler T, Quurke A W. Iatrogenic keratectasia after laser in situ keratomileusis in a case of Forme Fruste keratoconus. J Refract Surg 1998;24(7):1007-9.
4. Probost LE, Machat JJ. Mathematics of laser in situ keratomileusis for high myopia. J Cataract refract Surg 1998;24.
5. Mc Donnell PJ. Excimer laser corneal surgery: New strategies and old enemies {review}. Invest Ophthalmol Vis Sci 1995;36:4-8.
6. Seitz B, Torres F, Langenbucher A, et al. Posterior corneal curvature changes after myopic laser in situ keratomileusis. Ophthalmology 2001;108 (4):666-72.
7. Geggel HS, Talley AR. Delayed onset keratectasia following laser in situ keratomileusis. J Cataract Refract Surg 1999;25(4):582-86.
8. Wang Z, Chen J, Yang B. Posterior corneal surface topographic changes after laser in situ keratomileusis are related to residual corneal bed thickness. Ophthalmology 1999;106(2):406-89.
9. Pallikaris IG, Kymionis GD. Astyrakakis NI. Corneal ectasia induced by laser in situ keratomileusis. J Cataract Refract Surg 2001;27(11):1796-802.
10. Argento C, Cosentino M J, Tytium A, et al. Corneal ectasia after laser in situ keratomileusis. J Cataract Refract Surg 2001;27(9):1440-48.
11. Binder PS, Moore M. Lambert RW, et al. Comparison of two microkeratome systems. J refract Surg 1997;13: 142-53.
12. Hofmann RF, Bechara SJ. An independent evaluation of second generation suction microkeratomes. Refract Corneal Surg 1992;8:348-54.
13. Schuler A, Jessen K, Hoffmann F. Accuracy of the microkeratome keratectomies in pig eyes. Invest Ophthalmol Vis Sci 1990;31:2022-30.
14. Behrens A, Seitz B, Langenbucher A, et al. Evaluation of corneal flap dimensions and cut quality using a manually guided microkeratome [Published erratum appears in J Refract Surg 1999;15:400]. J Refract Surg 1999;15:118-23.
15. Behrens A, Seitz B, Langenbucher A, et al. Evaluation of corneal flap dimensions and cut quality using the Automated Corneal Shaper Microkeratome. J Refract Surg 2000;16:83-89.
16. BehrensA, Langenbucher A, Kus MM, et al. Experimental evaluation of two current generation automated microkeratomes: the Hansatome® and the Supratome®. Am J Ophthalmol. 2000;129:59-67.
17. Jacobs BJ, Deutsch TA, Rubenstein JB. Reproducibility of corneal flap thickness in LASIK. Ophthalmic Surg Lasers 1999;30:350-53.
18. McDermott G K Topography's benefits for LASIK. Review of Ophthalmology. Editorial, Vol No 9:03 issue.

Pre-Lasik Retina Examination and Its Clinical Relevance

8

S Natarajan, Chaitra Jayadev, Hijab Mehta,
Hitendra Mehta (India)

The Eye Disease Case-Control Study Group in its study on the "Risk factors for idiopathic Rhegmatogenous retinal detachment"[1] has determined that an eye with a spherical equivalent refractive error of –1 to –3 diopters has a four-fold increased risk of retinal detachment compared with a nonmyopic eye. If the refractive error was greater than –3 diopters, the risk is increased 10-fold. The data suggest that almost 55% of nontraumatic detachments in eyes without previous surgery are attributable to myopia. LASIK has proven to be an effective procedure for correcting these very same low-to-high myopes. There are relatively few reports on vitreoretinal complications in comparison with anterior segment complications associated with LASIK.[2, 3] Considering the large number of LASIK being done today, even these cases can amount to a significant visual insult. Keeping that in view it, an evaluation of the posterior segment of the eye (vitreous and retina) via binocular indirect ophthalmoscope is a must to rule out possible retinal diseases prior scheduling a LASIK.

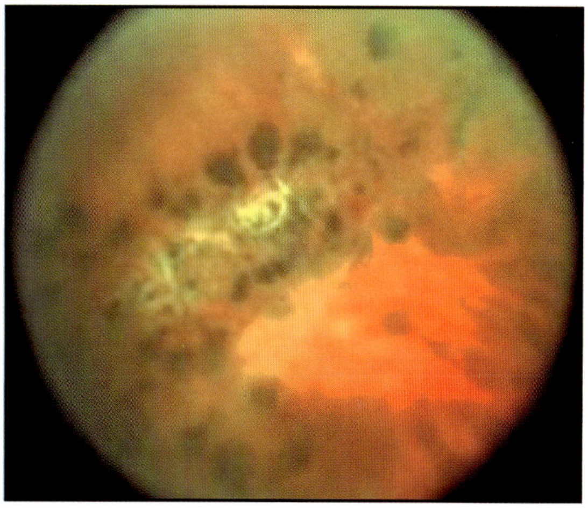

Fig. 8.1: Lattice lesion containing small atrophic holes

Methods of Retinal Evaluation

Include: indirect ophthalmoscopy with 360-degree scleral depression and/or 3-mirror contact lens examination. While performing scleral indentation maximum dilation is of utmost importance, this will greatly improve the ability to see the indented retina. As a rule scleral indentation is performed through the lids. However, there are times when one will have to use an anesthetic and place the depressor directly on the sclera to get a better view. A 3-mirror contact lens examination with a slit-lamp may accomplish adequate examination without scleral depression and serve to stabilize the eye in an uncooperative patient. Whatever the method used the clinician has to make sure that the entire 360-degree of the retinal periphery is well evaluated for any treatable lesions.

What is the Risk?

It has been known for long that myopia is associated with an increased incidence of retinal detachments.[1]

Lifetime risks were 0.2% in hyperopes, emmetropes, and myopes with refractive errors of as great as –1.00 D, but the risk increased to 7% for eyes with greater than –9.00 D of refractive error.[6] The incidence of these risks in eyes undergoing LASIK has been studied with one study[4] illustrating a 0.02% yearly incidence in patients who had an average refractive error of -6.00 D, a finding that indicates a lack of association between LASIK and retinal detachment while few other studies indicate a higher association. However, no large, long-term, case-controlled, prospective study has yet been undertaken to produce convincing associations.

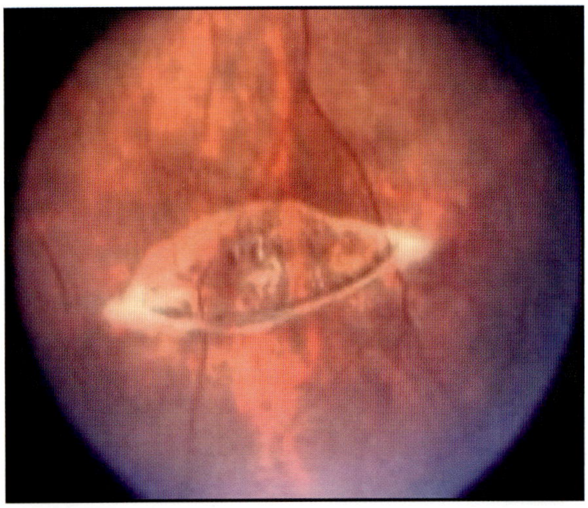

Fig. 8.2: A peripheral lattice lesion demonstrating the typical snail-track appearance, with overlying vitreal opacities (which may represent glial proliferations or regions of increased vitreoretinal condensation)

Mechanism of Retinal Changes during LASIK

Ozdamar in 1998 and Tsai in 2001[7, 8] published the case reports of two patients with RD due to giant tears, who have had their onset respectively 2 and 9 months after LASIK refractive correction. These patients had medium-high myopia. These authors ascribed an important role to the mechanic stress on the vitreous base caused by the microkeratome during the aspiration phase. In fact, during this surgical phase the ocular tone increases over 65 mm Hg. The fast change in the ocular tone during the aspiration alters the shape with a remarkable increase of the equatorial diameter and traction on the vitreous base with the eventual development of peripheral tears. This pathogenetic mechanism is very similar to that of contusive trauma. Other mechanisms of trauma during LASIK may include excimer laser-induced shock waves (pressure as high as 100 atm) caused by the high number of energy pulses required to achieve adequate surgical results in moderate and high myopes.[4, 5]

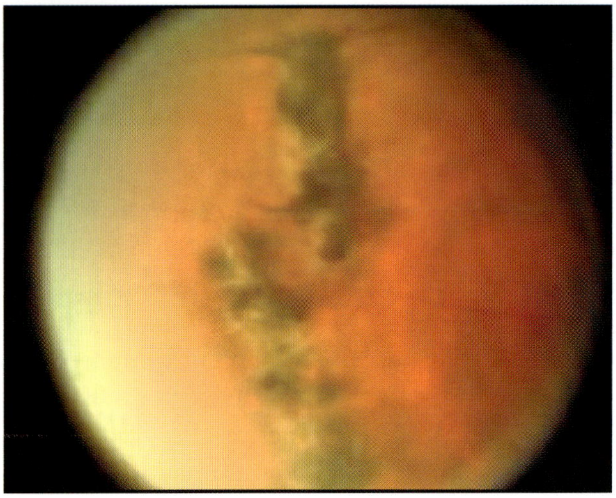

Fig. 8.3: An example of a heavily pigmented lattice lesion

Another study found that one (2%) of 50 patients with refractive errors of less than –4.00 D and five (10%) of 50 patients with refractive errors of greater than –7.00 D developed a PVD shortly after undergoing LASIK.[9] It has also been suggested that a delayed posterior vitreous detachment (PVD) from premature vitreous liquefaction associated with myopia can account for the time delay between the LASIK procedure and the development of an RRD.[5] In another study, 78% of the retinal breaks occurred in the temporal quadrant, a finding that could be attributed to the additional pressure that the microkeratome applied on the temporal side of the eyes.[4]

On the other hand, many ophthalmologists believe that the retinal detachments observed after LASIK are not related. They opine that these detachments are more due to the effects of myopia than LASIK. The time delay between the LASIK procedure and incidence of RRD goes against any direct causation, although a delayed PVD may be a contributing factor. Supporting this school of thought is a study, which has found that, for all cases in which retinal tears led to a detachment, the retinal detachment occurred within 6 weeks of the development of the retinal tears unlike in the case of post-LASIK detachments (average of 5 to14 months).[10]

Keeping in mind the large PVD frequency in high myopes of younger ages and the association of PVD with an increased risk of RRD, any PVD and subsequent RRD in a post-LASIK patient could simply be due to a spontaneous PVD that is unrelated to the prior LASIK surgery.

In addition, ocular pneumoplethysmography—the study of more than 69,000 tests of ocular blood flow using a device that applies suction to the globe to create IOPs in excess of 100 mm Hg—has never been shown to create a retinal detachment. Additional biomechanical studies on pneumoplethysmography patients have illustrated minimal eye-wall displacement and vitreous disturbance.[12]

Is Prophylactic Photocoagulation A Must?

Many ophthalmologists recommend prophylactic photocoagulation and routinely make their LASIK patients undergo a thorough retinal examination prior to the LASIK procedure.[4] Supporting this protocol is the study with the lowest incidence of RRD, in which every patient underwent a thorough retinal evaluation and prophylactic photocoagulation treatment if needed, prior to the LASIK procedure.[4]

Albeit this, there have been no prospective studies directly comparing prophylactic treatment versus no treatment or those showing any definite reduction in the incidence of Rhegmatogenous detachments in patients asymptomatic retinal lesions. On the other hand, there have been clinicians who have documented that the risk of retinal detachment in eyes with significant myopia or lattice degeneration is not altered by prophylactic treatment, and, therefore, the procedure is not indicated because its long-term complications are unknown.[13, 14]

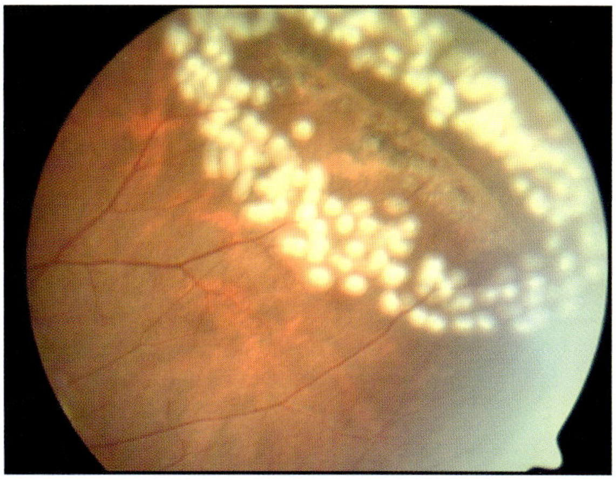

Fig. 8.4: Lasered lattice

Although it is assumed that LASIK induces some form of trauma and thereby causes detachments, it is known that eyes with lattice degeneration are not at an increased risk of detachment after a traumatic injury.[6]

Even if a patient has a treatable lesion and does undergo photocoagulation for the same, it does not ensure that the risk of retinal detachment is mitigated. In the eventuality of a post LASIK detachment, the surgeon is left with a dilemma of whether or not to use a scleral buckle to treat the condition. On one hand it is the most appropriate form of treatment and on the other hand it nullifies the effect of the LASIK procedure by inducing a myopic shift.

A patient requiring laser photocoagulation for a treatable retinal lesion, should be scheduled for LASIK at least 2 weeks after the laser treatment.

CONCLUSION

Until large-scale prospective studies are undertaken to prove than an association exists between LASIK and Retinal detachments, the use of prophylactic photocoagulation will remain physician-dependent. In the present senario, it seems most prudent to have patients undergo a dilated fundus examination prior to LASIK; symptomatic breaks and all horseshoe tears should receive treatment, but the value of treating asymptomatic operculated or atrophic holes is unknown.[11] Finally, even if a patient undergoes refractive correction using LASIK, the eye is inherently myopic and therefore required annual retinal check and reporting to a retinal surgeon on an emergency basis if symptoms occur.

REFERENCES

1. The Eye Disease Case-Control Study Group. Risk factors for idiopathic rhegmatogenous retinal detachment. Am J Epidemiol 1993;137:749-57.
2. Chan CK, Arevalo JF, Akbatur HH, et al. Characteristics of 60 myopic eyes with pre-laser in situ keratomileusis retinal examination and post-laser in situ keratomileusis retinal lesions. Retina 2004;24:706–13.
3. Arevalo JF, Ramirez E, Suarez E, et al. Incidence of vitreoretinal pathologic conditions within 24 months after laser in situ keratomileusis. Ophthalmology 2000;107:258–62.
4. Arevalo JF, Ramirez E, Suarez E, et al. Rhegmatogenous retinal detachment in myopic eyes after laser in situ keratomileusis. Frequency, characteristics, and mechanism. J Cataract Refract Surg 2001;27:674-80.
5. Aras C, Ozdamar A, Karacorlu M, et al. Retinal detachment following laser in situ keratomileusis. Ophthalmic Surg Lasers 2000;31:121-25.
6. Burton TC. The influence of refractive errors and lattice degeneration on the incidence of retinal detachment. Trans Am Ophthalmol Soc 1989;87:143-55.
7. Ozdamar A, Aras C, Sener B, Oncel M, Karacorlu M. Bilateral retinal detachment associated with giant retinal tear after laser-assisted in situ keratomileusis. Retina 1998;18(2):176-77.
8. Tsai YY, Lin JM, Tsai SC. Giant tear retinal detachment after laser in situ keratomileusis—a case report. Kaohsiung J Med Sci 2001;17(11):586-89.
9. Luna JD, Artal MN, Reviglio VE. Vitreoretinal alterations following laser in situ keratomileusis: clinical and experimental studies. Graefes Arch Clin Exp Ophthalmol 2001;239:416-23.
10. Davis MD. The natural history of retinal breaks without detachment. Trans Am Ophthalmol Soc 1973;71:343-72.
11. Comer G, Ciulla T. Is there a connection between LASIK and RRD? Cataract Refract Surg Today 2003;29-31.
12. Mazur Do, Hollifield R, Gee W. Retinal detachment in myopic eyes after laser in situ keratomileusis (comment). Am J Ophthalmol 2000;129:824-25.
13. Byer NE. Long-term natural history of lattice degeneration of the retina. Ophthalmology 1989;96:1396-1401.
14. Wilkinson CP. Evidence-based analysis of prophylactic treatment of asymptomatic retinal breaks and lattice degeneration. Ophthalmology 2000;107:12-15.

Pre-Laser Assisted Stromal In situ Keratomileusis [LASIK] Investigation of Dry Eye

9

Anand Shroff (India)

The popularity of LASIK has grown among the youth in recent years. So has the number of patients experiencing dry eye symptoms. According to the 2003 Refractive Surgery Survey, dry-eye symptoms are the most common problem encountered after LASIK and occur in 15-25% of patients.[1]

Several factors may influence these symptoms, of which decreased corneal sensation may play a significant role. Other potential factors include difficulty wetting the ocular surface due to mechanical and shape factors and a loss of neuroregulatory factors derived from the corneal nerves that promote epithelial health.[2]

Particularly since the advent of the computer, dry eye symptoms resulting from computer vision syndrome are so common, that the differentiation of tear film abnormalities is the concern of every clinician.

The definition of an abnormal tear film and its causes has been reviewed by many clinicians; they consider the following signs to be important when diagnosing the condition:

1. A scanty or uneven tear meniscus
2. The presence of excessive particulate matter
3. The rupture of the tear film prior to a subsequent blink
4. The production of hyperosmotic tears
5. The abnormality or absence of the superficial lipid layer
6. An abnormal or inadequate mucous layer
7. The presence of an epithelial surface disorder.

A large number of clinical, experimental and research techniques have been developed to study the tear film and its different components. The focus here is on relevant techniques that can be applied by the clinician to more accurately detect a dry eye.

Symptoms

They vary in type and severity and are dependent on the state of instability of the tear film and the resultant damage to the ocular surface. They include:

1. A sensation of burning in marginal cases, caused by a hypertonic shift in the tear film.
2. Tearing, as a reflex and protective mechanism, induced by external conditions of low relative humidity, smog or air-conditioning drafts, and associated with early break-up of the tear film.
3. Incomplete lid closure may result in difficulty in opening the eyes on awakening.
4. Mucous discharge may indicate instability of the mucous layer and its dehydration.
5. Foreign-body sensations may be caused by improper lubrication and should be a warning of the possibility of a more severe tear film condition.
6. Dryness itself, reported as dry, scratchy, gritty, or sandy.

7. Photophobia may occur with continuing irritation.
8. Blurred vision may occur from a non-wetting surface in Sjögren's disease and keratoconjunctivitis sicca.

Slit-lamp Examination

Assessment of Appearance of the Tear Film Meniscus

The observation of the lid meniscus height[3] and its irregularity[4] is a guide to the diagnosis of dry eye. The shape of the meniscus can be observed in the specular reflection zone of the slit-lamp as a bright central band bordered by dark, non-reflective areas. The lower meniscus is easier to examine for regularity, height, width and curvature. Its estimated width is 1 mm.[5] A scanty appearance or area of discontinuity is a sign of an aqueous tear deficiency or lipid abnormality.[5]

An uneven border line and a height < 0.1 mm, combined with a sharp definition of the 'black line' separating it from the tear film, are signs of abnormality.

[On the corneal side of the meniscus, it is separated from the pre-ocular tear film by a localized thinning known as the 'black line', which is only visible when the film is stained with fluorescein].

Observation of Superficial Particulate Movement

Excessive particulate matter in the pre-ocular tear film and meniscus is abnormal. It often consists of mucous strands mixed with the superficial lipid layer. In filamentary keratitis these strands will be strongly attached to the epithelial surface. Increased cellular debris indicates surface damage when associated with contact lens wear or in conjunction with the use of preservatives.[6]

Observation of Surface Interference Phenomena either by Simple Specular Reflection or with the Tearscope Plus™ [Keeler Instruments]

Ehlers described the presence of embedded particles and various color dispersion phenomena visible in the portion lying slightly outside the direct 'mirror zone' formed by the light reflected from the cornea.[7] Most of the reflections originate from the oily layer. When the eye is opened wide, if a petrol-like pattern appears on the precorneal tear film, the lipid layer is at least 134 nm thick.[8] If the specular reflection is colorless or presents grayish lines, the lipid layer is thinner.

Abnormality of the lipid layer is caused by:

- An abnormal blockage of the secretion ducts[8]
- Poor apposition of the lid margins
- Contamination by skin lipid and/or make-up and skin lotions
- Presence of blepharitis or facial skin disorders
- Contamination by excessive or denatured mucus discharge.

The Tearscope Plus™ illuminates the tear meniscus along its entire length and permits non-invasive observation of morphological changes during the blink sequence. In its central area of observation is a black central band bordered by bright bands on either side. Any irregularity of the meniscus shape caused by degenerative lid changes or meibomian gland blockage is seen as a distortion of the central black band.

Measurement of Break-up Time [TBUT]

The pre-ocular tear film does not remain stable for long periods of time.[9] When blinking is prevented, the tear film ruptures within 15 to 40 seconds. Dry patches appear over the cornea. Reduced tear film break-up time or limited ocular surface wetting measured with or without fluorescein staining is one of the main signs of an abnormal tear film.

Technique

A moistened fluorescein strip is applied to the bulbar conjunctiva. After 2 to 3 blinks to spread the fluorescein evenly, the tear film is viewed with the help of the blue filter of the slit-lamp. When a dark area appears in the uniform green coloration, it represents a break in the tear film and the time elapsed since the last blink is recorded as tear film break-up time [TBUT].

Factors decreasing TBUT:

- Use of local anesthetic
- Exposure to benzalkonium chloride as a preservative agent
- Presence of air convection during testing
- Forced blinking before measurement or forcing the eyelids open

Fluorescein dyes the aqueous phase of the tear film and has little effect on the lipid or mucus layers. In view of the limited size of the aqueous phase it seems that a minimal amount of unpreserved dye, in an adequate concentration instilled in a precise volume will improve repeatability of the test.

Measurement of Non-Invasive Break-up Time [NIBUT]

Mengher developed a non-invasive technique for the assessment of preocular tear film break-up time without the use of fluorescein.[10] The method is based on observing changes in the specular image of a grid pattern projected on the open eye. A distortion of the grid line represents local thinning and discontinuity represents a break in the tear film. The first discontinuity from the last blink is taken as NIBUT. Normal values are 35 to 45 seconds.

Use of Vital Dyes to Study the Health of the Ocular Surface – Fluorescein, Rose Bengal, Lissamine Green

Fluorescein sodium is a water-soluble yellow-green dye that can be excited by a cobalt blue filter. The thickness and integrity of the tear film can be assessed by the intensity of coloration on the ocular surface. Less intense fluorescence despite repeated instillation occurs when tear volume or tear film thickness is reduced.

Rose Bengal is a water-soluble dye which stains degenerated and dead cells and mucus fibrils. It produces a punctuate coloration along the lacrimal rivus or line of Marx, which is probably due to pronounced cell degeneration in this area. One percent concentration is preferred as irritation increases with higher concentrations.

Conjunctival Signs

The presence of lip-like folds of the inferior conjunctiva is a sign of tear film related ocular surface problems. Three grades of folds:[11]

1. The folds are barely visible in the temporal corner
2. Clearly visible in the temporal bulbar conjunctiva
3. Also visible in the conjunctiva corresponding to the inferior corneal limbus

The folds disturb the morphology of the meniscus and its relationship with the lid edge. The presence of folds creates abnormal reservoir morphology, limiting the uptake of tears during a blink, decreasing the resurfacing of the ocular surface.

Examination of the lid borders, the lashes and related glands/orifices for any signs of blockage, abnormality or pathology, such as blepharitis and age-related degenerative changes

Blepharitis may cause secondary changes in the conjunctiva and cornea with associated tear film instability due to the intimate relationship between the lids and ocular surface.

The most common symptoms are burning, a foreign-body sensation, photophobia and lid crusting.

Examination of the meibomian glands when the lower lid is pulled down [using transillumination through the palpebral conjunctiva]

The meibomian orifices should be evaluated for distension or pouting caused by internal secretion in the underlying duct, protruding filaments, foam or bubbles surrounding the orifices or epithelial overgrowth.

Assessment of localized conjunctival hyperemia, preferably using grading scales for repeatability

Observation of the Blink Movement

Particularly observe for squeezing of eyelids during blinking and incomplete blinks.

Tear Flow—The Schirmer Test

Tear flow is of prime importance in maintaining a normal, wet eye. The Schirmer test uses a strip of filter paper 35 mm long and 5 mm wide. One bent end is placed in the lower conjunctival sac about one-third of the palpebral width from the temporal canthus. If anesthetic is instilled prior to the test, only basal secretion is observed. Otherwise reflex tearing is also calculated. Reflex lacrimation may increase the tear volume by a factor of 100. Less than 5 mm of wetting is considered a pathological dry eye, 5-10 mm suggests borderline dry eye and > 10 mm suggests a normal state of lacrimal secretion.

Suggested Sequence of Testing

1. Comprehensive patient history and symptoms should be recorded, preferably using a dry eye questionnaire.
2. As the tear film is very fragile, non-invasive tests should be carried out first – first topography and aberrometry followed by NIBUT and observation of the superficial lipid layer.
3. Slit-lamp examination of the lids for conjunctival hyperemia.
4. Perform Schirmer's test.
5. Tests using stains should be performed last in view of their effect on tearing and tear film composition.
6. Contact tests such as pachymetry are performed after assessment of tear film.

Mechanism of Dry Eye after LASIK

Dry eye after LASIK is at least partly caused by the corneal denervation associated with LASIK. In the normal eye, a neuronal feedback loop between the lacrimal gland and the ocular surface begins at the corneal surface and travels via neuronal pathways that are mediated by the brainstem in a single functional unit that is responsible for maintaining ocular surface homeostasis. It is suggested that basal tear production does occur but ocular drying between blinks induces subclinical corneal irritation that creates the blink reflex and stimulates the lacrimal gland to produce tears.[12] Only when ocular surface drying becomes severe does the patient experience discomfort. In LASIK, the corneal nerves are severed by the microkeratome and the deep corneal nerves are photoablated at the time of laser surgery. Both processes damage corneal innervation. The reduction in corneal neuronal feedback to the brainstem reduces brainstem reflex mediation of the lacrimal glands, diminishing tear production and inducing a corneal anesthesia or hypoesthesia that lasts upto 6 months. Many patients may not have the traditional symptoms of post-LASIK dry eye because of the lack of corneal sensation; visual fluctuation due to damage to the ocular surface may be their only symptom.

In a subset of patients with corneal staining after LASIK, it is hypothesized that the corneal breakdown is secondary to neurotrophic epitheliopathy in addition to dry eye.[13,14] Patients with neurotrophic keratitis with corneal staining after LASIK have been shown to have Schirmer tests that are not significantly different from those of post-LASIK patients without staining. Most cases of neurotrophic epitheliopathy resolve by 6 months.

Laser in situ keratomileusis significantly decreases TBUT, Schirmer test values, and basal tear secretion.[15,16]

Importance of Hinge Location during the LASIK Procedure

An advantage of the hinge on the LASIK flap is that it provides a conduit for corneal innervation. The corneal nerves that enter through the hinge are preserved, maintaining corneal sensation in this area. Since the corneal nerves predominantly enter the cornea at 9 o'clock and 3 o'clock,[17,18] a vertical flap (superior hinge) will transect both major areas of corneal innervation, whereas a horizontal corneal flap (nasal hinge) will transect only 1 area. Hypothetically, greater the loss of corneal sensation, greater is the risk for post-LASIK dry-eye syndrome. A wide hinge will preserve a greater percentage of the corneal neural architecture than a narrow hinge. The current data support this hypothesis. Eyes with a narrow nasal hinge flap showed a significantly greater loss of corneal sensation, a greater incidence of corneal and conjunctival lissamine staining, and lower Schirmer scores than eyes with a wide nasal hinge flap at 1 or more time intervals. Different microkeratomes cut flaps with different thicknesses and standard deviations. Hinge width has not been shown to affect flap thickness. The effect of flap thickness on corneal sensation and dry eye does not appear to have been studied.

Over the past few years, there has been increased documentation of dry eye after LASIK. There are many possible contributing factors to this, including increased physician and patient awareness. Other factors include an increased prevalence of superior hinge flaps, the need for larger flaps with smaller hinges to accommodate the larger ablation zones required for hyperopic treatments, and the larger optical and blend zones common to newer software delivery systems. These larger ablation zones may decrease the risk for glare and halos associated with scotopic conditions but may also be responsible for the increased incidence of post-LASIK dry eye.[19] It is recommended to use the smallest flap necessary with the largest hinge possible to complete the photoablation in the stromal bed without ablating the corneal hinge. Myopic patients with mild dry eyes who have small pupils and against-the-rule astigmatism (ablation profile is vertical) are good candidates for flaps with as large a nasal flap as possible. Corneal sensation improves at all time intervals but does not return to preoperative levels even 6 months postoperatively. Associated with the corneal denervation is an immediate postoperative increase in dry-eye syndrome signs and symptoms that improves at subsequent visits.

Furthermore, loss of corneal sensation and dry-eye syndrome were less pronounced in corneas with a wide nasal-hinge flap. This can be explained anatomically by the finding that the wider hinge flap severs a smaller percentage of the corneal innervation than a narrow hinge flap. Surgeons operating on patients with preexisting neurotrophic corneas or dry-eye syndrome should consider performing LASIK with as wide a nasal hinge flap as possible.

Many LASIK patients complain of the quality of their vision despite optimal uncorrected binocular visual acuity in the early postoperative period, related to disturbances in the tear film as discussed above. Accuracy of treatment may be compromised in cases with pre-existing dry eye. The stroma may be less hydrated and result in overablation. This author[20] has encountered 2 cases of overcorrection in patients with pre-existing dry eye and has evenly spread a microdrop of BSS on the stromal bed before ablation, which resulted in an optimal result. Both the above cases of overcorrection were enhanced by a similar procedure.

Schirmer test scores were higher in the wide-hinge group than in the narrow hinge group at all times, although the difference was only statistically significant at 1 month and not at longer time intervals. There were no significant between-group differences in TBUT.

Risk Factors for Chronic Dry Eye after LASIK[21]

1. Patients developing chronic dry eye after LASIK were significantly more likely to be female and have more dry-eye symptoms before surgery. Longer use of contact lenses was borderline significant ($P < .05$).
2. Those that develop chronic dry eye also exhibit significantly greater presurgical ocular surface staining, lower TBUT values and reduced presurgical corneal sensation.

   They also have a significantly higher attempted refractive correction and a greater ablation depth.
3. Chronic dry eye is also associated with reduced central corneal sensation upto 12 months after surgery.

The following guidelines should be considered by LASIK surgeons and potential patients:[22]

1. Patients with dry eye before LASIK should be advised that they have a significantly increased risk for developing chronic post-LASIK dry eye despite comprehensive ocular surface management before, during, and after surgery. There is also an association between chronic dry eye and poorer refractive outcomes. Other refractive management strategies should be discussed.
2. Women and patients requiring higher refractive corrections have an increased risk for developing chronic dry eye and regression. Again, alternative refractive correction options should be discussed.

3. If LASIK surgery is performed, the ocular surface and tear film must be managed with the best available treatment options and for a sufficient period of time. Unfortunately, corneal sensory denervation hinders the ability to detect and treat symptoms. Therefore, routine postoperative review in the first year after LASIK is advocated, even in asymptomatic patients.
4. Ocular surface management strategies may accelerate the recovery of ocular surface/lacrimal gland dysfunction after LASIK and improve visual quality. Therefore, routine use of non-preserved artificial tears in the first 6 months after LASIK is recommended.
5. Failure to identify and treat early signs of ocular surface/lacrimal gland dysfunction may permit a vicious cycle to occur with reduced ocular surface sensation leading to ocular surface damage, reduced tear secretion, and sustained reduction in corneal sensation. Regression of the refractive result may also occur as a consequence of this chronic post-LASIK integrated ocular surface/lacrimal gland dysfunction.
6. Enhancement surgery may exacerbate chronic post-LASIK dry eye and, hence, may be contraindicated in patients with chronic ocular surface dysfunction.
7. LASIK should be approached cautiously in patients with preexisting dry eye, particularly as dry eye and associated contact lens intolerance are significant motivating factors for patients to consider refractive surgery.[23-25]
8. Patients with chronic dry-eye symptoms after surgery also have less satisfaction with surgery.
9. Postmenopausal women on hormone replacement therapy are reported to have significantly inferior refractive outcomes after PRK surgery compared to age-matched controls in one study.[23-25] A significant correlation between female sex and the occurrence of corneal punctate epitheliopathy after LASIK was reported (GL Mayo, MD, T Starck, MD, "LASIK-Induced Neurotrophic Keratopathy: Incidence and Associated Risk Factors," ARVO, Ft. Lauderdale, Florida, USA, May 2002). These results highlight the strong influence of hormone levels on the ocular surface/lacrimal gland function unit.

REFERENCES

1. Solomon KD, Ferna´ndez de Castro LE, Sandoval HP, et al. Refractive surgery survey 2003. J Cataract Refract Surg 2004;30:1556-69.
2. Effect of hinge location on corneal sensation and dry eye after laser in situ keratomileusis for myopia Vroman DT, Sandoval HP, Fernández de Castro LE, Kasper TJ, Holzer MP, Solomon KD. Journal of Cataract and Refractive Surgery - October 2005 (Vol. 31, Issue 10, Pages 1881-1887).
3. Baum JL. Systemic diseases associated with tear deficiencies. Int Ophthalmol Clin 1973;13:157-84.
4. Rolando M, et al. Conjunctival damage distribution in keratoconjunctivitis sicca. An impression cytology study. Ophthalmologica 1990;200:170-76.
5. Holly FJ, Lemp MA. Tear physiology and dry eyes. Surv Ophthalmol 1977;22:69-87.
6. Bron AJ. Prospects for the dry eye. Trans Ophthalmol Soc UK, 1985;104:801-26.
7. Ehlers N. The precorneal tear film. Biomicroscopical, histological and chemical investigations. Acta Ophthalmol, 1965;81[Suppl], 5-136.
8. Norn MS. Semi-quantitative interference study of fatty layer of precorneal film. Acta Ophthalmol 1979;57: 766-74.
9. Holly FJ. Tear film physiology and contact lens wear. I. Pertinent aspects of tear film physiology. Am J Optom Physiol Opt 1981;58[4]:324-30.
10. Mengher LS, et al. A non-invasive instrument for the clinical assessment of the pre-corneal tear film stability. Curr Eye Res 1985;4:1-8.
11. Hoh, et al. Lid-parallel conjunctival fold [LIPCOF] and dry eye: A diagnostic tool for the contactologist. Contactologia 1995;17E:104-17.
12. Stern ME, Beuerman RW, Fox RI, et al. The pathology of dry eye: the interaction between the ocular surface and the lacrimal glands. Cornea 1998;17:584-89.
13. Wilson SE, Ambro´sio R Jr. Laser in situ keratomileusis-induced neurotrophic epitheliopathy. Am J Ophthalmol 2001;132:405-06.
14. Wilson SE. Laser in situ keratomileusis-induced (presumed) neurotrophic epitheliopathy. Ophthalmology 2001;108:1082-87.
15. Yu EYW, Leung A, Rao S, Lam DSC. Effect of laser in situ keratomileusis on tear stability. Ophthalmology 2000;107:2131-35.

16. Toda I, Asano-Kato N, Komai-Hori Y, Tsubota K. Dry eye after laser in situ keratomileusis. Am J Ophthalmol 2001;132:1-7.
17. Müller LJ, Pels L, Vrensen GFJM. Ultrastructural organization of human corneal nerves. Invest Ophthalmol Vis Sci 1996;37:476-88.
18. Müller LJ, Vrensen GFJM, Pels L, et al. Architecture of human corneal nerves. Invest Ophthalmol Vis Sci 1997; 38:985-94.
19. Effect of hinge width on corneal sensation and dry eye after laser in situ keratomileusis. Donnenfeld ED, Ehrenhaus M, Solomon R, Mazurek J, Rozell JC, Perry HD. Journal of Cataract and Refractive Surgery - April 2004 (Vol. 30, Issue 4, Pages 790-797).
20. Shroff AA, unpublished data.
21. Chronic dry eye and regression after laser in situ keratomileusis for myopia. Albietz JM, Lenton LM, Franzco, McLennan SG. Journal of Cataract and Refractive Surgery 2004;30(3): 675-84.
22. Toda I, Asano-Kato N, Hori-Komai Y, Tsubota K. Laser-assisted in situ keratomileusis for patients with dry eye. Arch Ophthalmol 2002;120:1024-28.
23. Corbett MC, O'Brart DPS, Warbuton FG, Marshall J. Biologic and environmental risk factors for regression after photorefractive keratectomy. Ophthalmology 1996;103:1381-91.
24. Toda I, Yagi Y, Hata S, et al. Excimer laser photo-refractive keratectomy for patients with contact lens intolerance caused by dry eye. Br J Ophthalmol 1996; 80:604-09.
25. McCarty CA, Ng I, Waldron B, et al. Relation of hormone and menopausal status to outcomes following excimer laser photorefractive keratectomy in women. Aust NZ J Ophthalmol 1996;24:215-22.

Dry Eye as Informed Consent Prior to Refractive Surgery

10

Y Ralph Chu, Jessica Matsumoto, Dan Davis (USA)

INTRODUCTION

As the first refracting surface of the eye, the ocular tear film plays a vital role in patient satisfaction following refractive surgery. By carefully analyzing and managing the tear film, a surgeon can have a greater degree of selectivity with refractive candidates and ultimately success in patient satisfaction.

Several techniques are used in my office in an attempt to stabilize the tear film perioperatively and afford the patient the fastest visual recovery possible. I will briefly discuss our methods of evaluation and management, and highlight aspects of patient communication of our findings.

Evaluation

The integrity and health of the ocular surface is evaluated at the pre-operative refractive examination. Thorough attention is given to the patient's past history of dry eye, including contributing systemic disease, current oral and topical medications and history of contact lens wear. It has been found that over 20-30% of patients who wear contact lenses have dry eye symptoms,[1] usually related to decrease in blink frequency and increased tear evaporation from the surface.[2]

Evaluation of the patient's habitual working and living environment are also important, as low-moisture environments can contribute to evaporative dry eye conditions.[3]

In my examination of the patient, we use the Schirmer II test as an evaluation of baseline tear secretion. More specifically, the Schirmer II test assesses basal tear secretion.[4] A patient is noted to have normal tear secretion values if the Schirmer paper strip is moistened to 10 mm or greater at 5 minutes. Values less than 10 mm are cause for initiating dry eye management prior to considering corneal refractive surgery.

A careful examination of tear film stability is also performed at the pre-operative refractive exam. A recent study indicated a correlation between ocular surface discomfort and tear integrity in patients with dry eye disease.[5] We use the fluorescein tear break-up time test on our patients. In those with instable tear film, the time it takes the tear layer to thin is less than 10 seconds.

The anterior segment is also examined at the pre-operative visit. Careful attention is given to the lid margins, investigating underlying lid disease such as meibomian gland dysfunction, which excess or deficient lipid secretion may contribute to poor tear quality. Surface inspection of the corneal epithelial cells will reveal any signs of superficial punctuate keratitis in patients with dry eye. Dry eye patients will also have low tear meniscus at the lid margin. Staining of the bulbar conjunctival with Lissamine green will help to uncover devitalized cells associated with dry eye syndrome.

Management

Our refractive patients are started on a routine regimen of non-preservative artificial tears four times a day and topical cyclosporin-A (Restasis®, Allergan Inc., Irvine, CA) twice a day, at least 2 weeks prior to surgery. If initial tear testing values (for example, Schirmer II test) were low and indicated poor tear quantity, or slit-lamp examination revealed significant ocular surface dryness, dry eye therapy is initiated sooner and corneal surgery is deferred until improvement is seen in tear quantity and quality. Patients who use soft contact lenses are advised to discontinue wear at least two weeks prior to surgery, and those who habitually wear rigid gas-permeable lenses or soft toric contact lenses are advised to discontinue wear at least three weeks prior to surgery.

Post-surgically, careful examination of subjective comfort levels and objective findings guide post-operative dry eye management. Patients are advised to continue their regular regimen of artificial tears and topical cyclosporine at least 6 weeks after surgery. Maintenance of a regular tear layer is important for visual clarity in the postoperative period. In study, it was found that patients who were symptomatic and asymptomatic for dry eye demonstrated significant improvement in uncorrected visual acuity after the use of non-preserved caboxymethylcellulose (CMC).[6] Thicker gel formulations are recommended for patients with symptoms aggravated in the evening and/or waking hours. Lid hygiene is advised for patients with chronic lid conditions such as blepharitis or ocular rosacea. In patients who continue to have dry eye symptoms after surgery despite the use of artificial tears and topical cyclosporin-A, the use of punctual occlusion is introduced to the patient. For patients with tear-deficient dry eye, the use of punctal plugs improves patient comfort as well as objective signs.[7] An evaluation studying the effectiveness of topical cyclosporin-A and punctal plugs found that its collective use provides more protection from dry eye disease. More specifically, there was less incidence of conjunctival staining and less use of artificial tears when topical cyclosporin-A was used with punctal plugs.[8]

Communication and Informed Consent

Evaluating patient expectations prior to refractive surgery is perhaps the most critical aspect of our screening process. The benefit of spending a few extra minutes of communication with a patient prior to surgery may prevent significant postoperative confusion or misunderstanding.

The importance of the role the ocular surface plays after corneal refractive surgery must be emphasized to the patient. The patient must understand that a uniform tear layer provides optimal visual quality and its maintenance is critical to the healing of the eye. Patients also need to be aware that they may experience more dryness in the acute postoperative time frame and use of artificial tears more than the required minimum will provide benefit to visual outcome.

Patients who are symptomatic for dry eye in the postoperative period may experience a foreign-body sensation and visual fluctuations. These symptoms are a part of the healing process and typically resolve in the six months following surgery. Our patients are counseled on the use of topical cyclosporin-A pre-operatively. Most of our patients continue its use for 6 weeks after surgery. In some cases of symptomatic dry eye prior to refractive surgery, patients are counseled on remaining on artificial tears and topical cyclosporin-A for an extended time period until their vision is stable

Dry eye following refractive surgery can be easily managed with proper identification of dry eye disease prior to surgery, thorough informed consent and realistic patient expectations.

REFERENCES

1. Bron AJ. Non-Sjögren's dry eye: pathogenesis, diagnosis and animal models. In: Sullivan DA (ed): Lacrimal Gland, Tear Film and Dry Eye Syndromes. New York: Plenum Press, 1994:471-88.
2. Lemp MA. Surface abnormalities in the preocular tear film and dry eye syndromes. Int Ophthalmol Clin 1973;13:191-99.

3. McMonnies CW. Key questions in a dry eye history. J Am Optom Assoc 1986; 57:512-17.
4. Schirmer O. Studien zur physiologie der tranenabsonderung und tranenabfuhr. Graefe's Arch Clin Exp Ophthalmol 1903;56:197-291.
5. Nally L, Ousler III GW, Albelson MA. Ocular discomfort and tear film break up time in dry eye patients: a correlation. Invest Ophthalmol Vis Sci 2000(Suppl); 41: S274.
6. Nilforoushan MR, Latkany RA, Speaker MG. Effect of artificial tears on visual acuity. Am J Ophthalmol 2005;140:830-35.
7. Albietz JM. Dry eye: an update on clinical diagnosis, management and promising new treatments. Clin Exp Optom 2001;84:14-18.
8. Roberts C. Comparison of topical cyclosporin, punctal occlusion and a combination for the treatment of dry eye disease. ARVO, 2005.

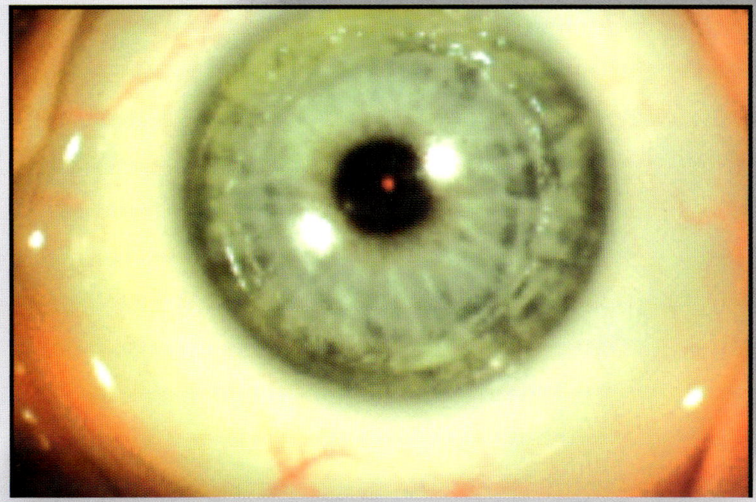

Lasik, Epilasik and Lasek Surgical Techniques

SECTION TWO

Aberropia: A New Refractive Entity

11

Amar Agarwal, Nilesh Kanjiani, Soosan Jacob, Athiya Agarwal, Sunita Agarwal, Tahira Agarwal, Ashok Garg

INTRODUCTION

The next evolution to come on to the visual science scene in refractive ocular imaging is the aberrometer, the Orbscan and wave front analysis. This technology is based on astrophysical principles, which astronomers use to perfect the images impinging on their telescopes. Dr Bille, the Director of the Institute of Applied Physics at the University of Heidelberg first began work in this field while developing this specific technology for astronomy applications in the mid-1970's. For perfect imaging, astrophysicists have to be able to measure and correct the imperfect higher-order aberrations or wavefront distortions that enter their telescopic lens system from the galaxy. To achieve this purpose, adaptive optics are used wherein deformable mirrors reform the distorted wavefront to allow clear visualization of celestial objects. Extrapolating these same principles to the human eye, it was thought that removal of the wavefront aberrations of the eye might finally yield the long awaited and much desired ultimate goal of "super vision".

So far, the only parameters that could be modified to obtain the optical correction for a given patients refractive error were the sphere, cylinder and axis even though this does not give the ideal optical correction many a times. This is because the current modes for correcting the optical aberrations of the eye do not reduce the higher order aberrations. The ideal optical system should be able to correct the optical aberrations in such a way that the spatial resolving ability of the eye is limited only by the limits imposed by the neural retina, i.e. receptor diameter and receptor packing.

Thus, there may be a large group of patients whose best corrected visual acuity (BCVA) may actually improve significantly on removal of the optical aberrations. These optical aberrations are contributed to by the eye's entire optical system, i.e. the cornea, the lens, the vitreous and the retina. This study was conducted to determine the existence of a hitherto unidentified entity which we label as *"aberropia"* wherein patients with best corrected visual acuity of less than 6/9 (0.63), corneal topography not accounting for the lack of improvement in BCVA and with no other known cause for decreased vision improved by more than two Snellen lines after refractive correction of their wavefront aberration.

Materials and Methods

16 eyes of 10 patients were included in this retrospective study carried out at the Dr Agarwal's Eye Institute, India between May and December 2002. Only patients who had visual acuity less than 6/9 (0.63) prior to the procedure and whose visual acuity improved by more than or equal to two lines after the procedure were included in the study. None of these patients had any other known cause for

decreased vision and their corneal topography did not account for the lack of improvement in BCVA. The routine patient evaluation including uncorrected (UCVA) and best corrected (BCVA), slit lamp examination, applanation tonometry, manifest and cycloplegic refractions, Orbscan, aberrometry, corneal pachymetry, corneal diameter, Schirmer test and indirect ophthalmoscopy had been performed for all the patients. Patients wearing contact lenses had been asked to discontinue soft lenses for a minimum of 1 week and rigid gas permeable lenses for a minimum of 2 weeks before the preoperative examination and surgery. Informed consent was obtained form all patients after a thorough explanation of the procedure and its potential benefits and risks.

The Zyoptix procedure was then performed using the Bausch and Lomb Technolas 217 Z machine. The parameters used were: wavelength 193 nm, fluence 130 mJ/cm^2 and ablation zone diameters between 4.8 and 6 mm. The Hansatome (Bausch and Lomb) was used in all the eyes. Either the 180 μm or the 160 μm plate was used in all the eyes. The aberrometer and the Orbscan, which checks the corneal topography, are linked and a zylink created. An appropriate software file is created which is then used to generate the laser treatment file.

Postoperatively, the patients underwent complete examination including UCVA, BCVA, slit lamp examination, Orbscan and aberrometry. The mean follow-up was 37.5 days.

For statistical analysis, the Snellen acuity was converted to the decimal notation. Continuous variables were described with mean, standard deviation, minimum and maximum values.

Results

Sixteen eyes of 10 patients satisfied the inclusion criteria. The mean age of the patients was 29.43 years (range 22 to 35 years). Six patients were females and 4 were males. The mean preoperative pupil diameter measured on aberrometer was 4.69 mm and mean postoperative pupil diameter measured on aberrometer was 4.53 mm.

The mean preoperative spherical equivalent was – 4.94 D (range –12.50 to –1.5 D). The mean spherical equivalent at 1 month postoperative period was – 0.16 ± 0.68 D (range –1.0 to 1.5) . Mean preoperative sphere was –4.95 D (range-12.50 to –0.75 D) and the mean postoperative sphere was –0.13 ± 0.68 D (range-1 to 1.5) at 1 month. The mean preoperative cylinder was –1.34 D (range 0 to –3.50). The mean postoperative cylinder was –0.08 ± 0.24 D (range 0 to –0.75 D) at one month. Postoperatively, at the end of first month, 70% of the patients were within ± 0.5D and 90% were within ± 1D of emmetropia (Fig. 11.1). Preoperatively mean RMS (Root Mean square) values (Fig. 11.2) were: Z 200 Defocus –9.22, Z 221 Astigmatism 0.12, Z 220 Astigmatism 1.02, Z 311 Coma –0.041, Z 310 Coma –0.04, Z 331 Trefoil 0.23, Z 330 Trefoil 0.016, Z 400 Spherical aberration –0.054, Z 420 Secondary astigmatism 0.103, Z 421 Secondary astigmatism 0.029, Z 440 Quadrafoil –0.103, Z 441 Quadrafoil –0.021, Z 510 Secondary coma 0.025, Z 511 Secondary coma –0.015, Z 530 Secondary trefoil 0.0049, Z 531 Secondary trefoil -0.00219, Z 550 Pentafoil 0.023, Z 551 Pentafoil 0.046. Postoperative mean RMS values were : Z 200 Defocus –0.429, Z 221 Astigmatism 0.07, Z 220 Astigmatism –0.07, Z 311 Coma 0.149, Z 310 Coma –0.079, Z 331 Trefoil –0.102, Z 330 Trefoil –0.004, Z 400 Spherical aberration -0.179, Z 420 Secondary astigmatism 0.015, Z 421 Secondary

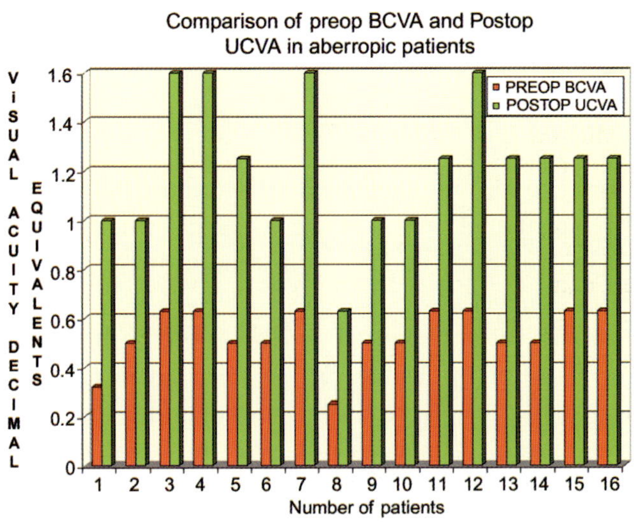

Fig. 11.1: Preoperative BCVA versus Post-op UCVA

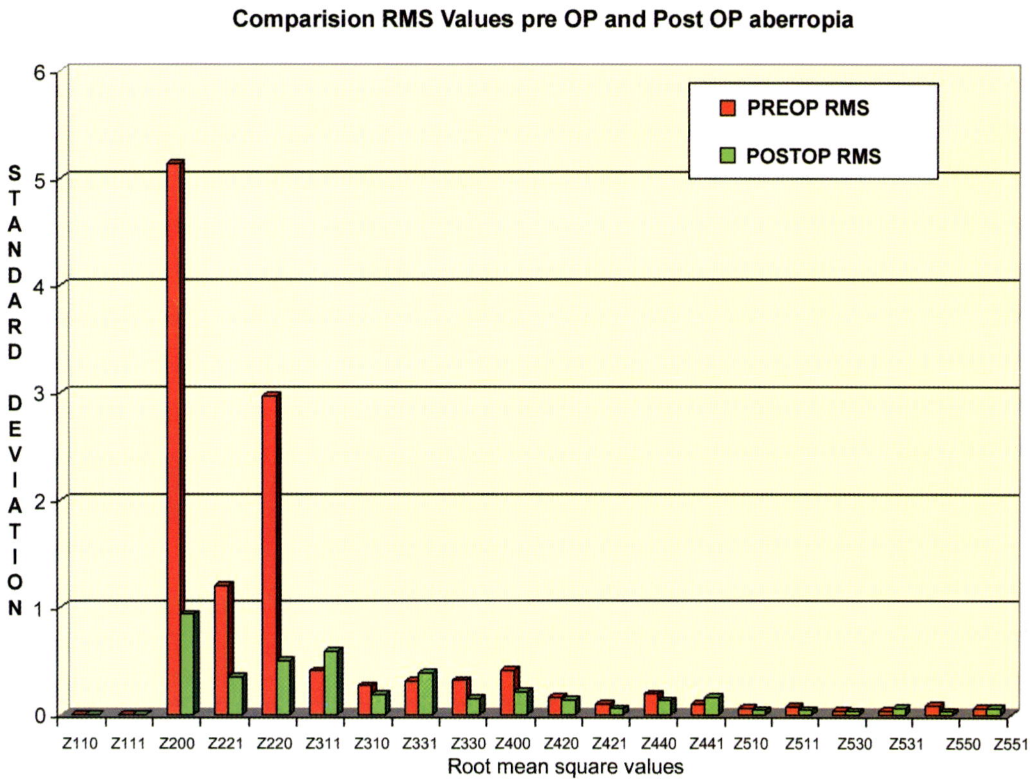

Fig. 11.2: RMS values pre-op and post-op

astigmatism 0.031, Z 440 Quadrafoil 0.019, Z 441 Quadrafoil –0.069, Z 510 Secondary coma –0.008, Z 511 Secondary coma 0.008, Z 530 Secondary Trefoil -0.002, Z 531 Secondary Trefoil –0.014, Z 550 Pentafoil 0.006, Z 551 Pentafoil 0.026.

RMS pre and post laser showed a reduction in the higher order aberrations (Tables 11.1 and 11.2). 6.25% patients achieved 6/9, 31.25% patients achieved ≥ 6/6 (1.00), 37.50% achieved a BCVA of 6/5 (1.25) and 25% achieved a BCVA of 6/4 (1.6) (Fig. 11.3). Figures 11.4 shows the pre-op Orbscan picture of a patient showing no abnormality. Figures 11.5 and 11.6 show the aberrometer maps of the right eye and left eye of a patient in which we can see the aberrations reduced post laser.

Discussion

Zyoptix is the new generation of excimer laser used for the treatment of refractive disorders. Until recently, refractive disorders were treated with standard techniques, which took into consideration only the subjective refraction. Zyoptix technique on the other hand, takes into account the patient's subjective refraction, ocular optical aberrations and corneal topography, with the latter not only for the

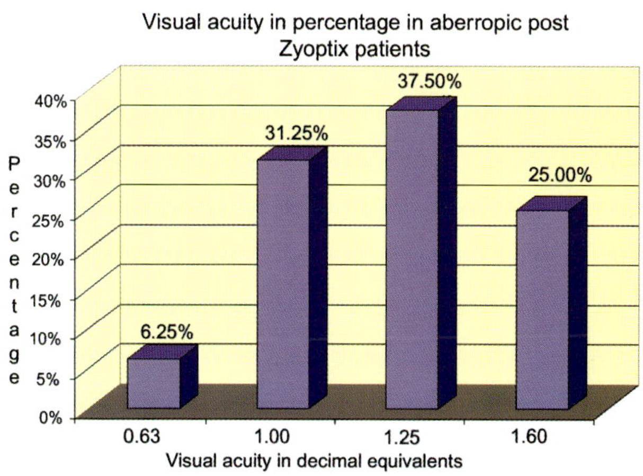

Fig. 11.3: Percentage values of visual acuity

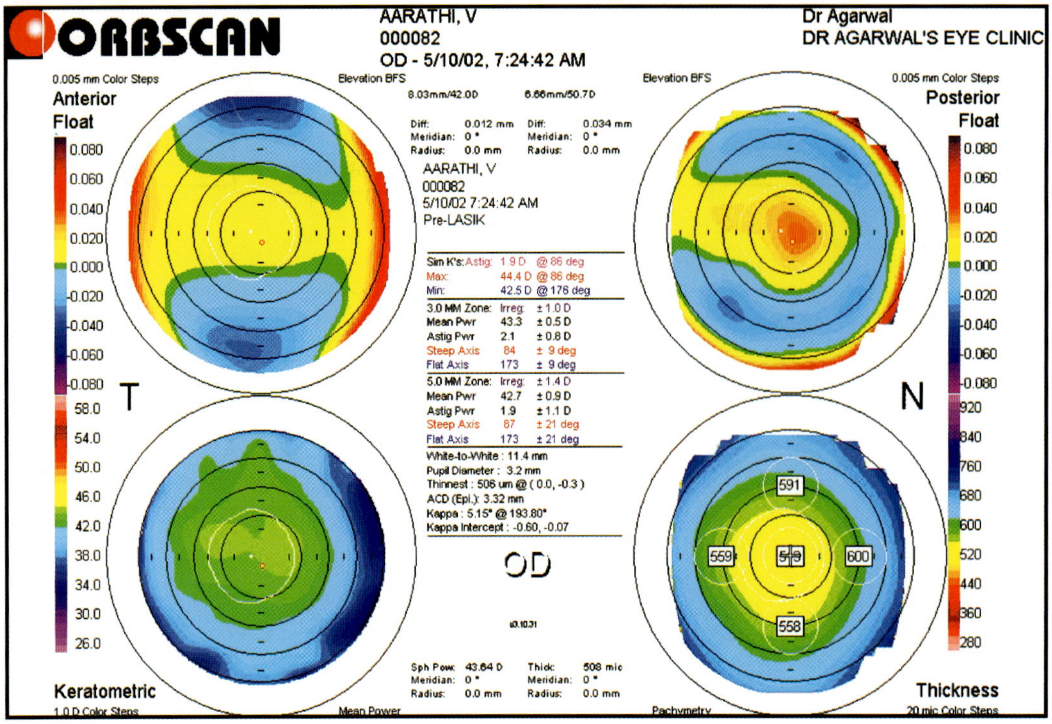

Fig. 11.4: Pre-operative orbscan

diagnosis, but also for the therapeutic treatment, in order to design a personalized treatment based on the total structure of the eye. The wavefront technology in Zyoptix uses the Hartmann Shack aberrometer based on the Hartmann-Shack principle[1] demonstrated by Liang et al[2] to measure the eye's wave aberration. This wavefront sensor has been improved by increasing the density of samples taken of the wave-front slope in the pupil.[3] All Hartmann-Shack devices are outgoing testing devices in that they evaluate the light being bounced back out through the optical system. A narrow laser beam is focused onto the retina to generate a point source. The out coming light rays which experience all the aberrations of the eye pass through an array of lenses which detects their deviation. The wavefront deformation is calculated by analyzing the direction of the light rays using this lenslet array. Parallel light beams indicate a good wavefront and non-parallel light beams indicate a wavefront with aberrations, which does not give equidistant focal points. This image is then captured onto a ccd camera and the wavefront is reconstructed. The data is explained mathematically in three dimensions with polynomial functions. Most investigators have chosen the Zernike method for this analysis although Taylor series can also be used for the same purpose[4]. Data from the wavefront map is presented as a sum of Zernike polynomials each describing a certain deformation. At any point in the pupil, the wavefront aberration is the optical path difference between the actual image wavefront and the ideal spherical wavefront centered at the image point[5].

Any refractive error which cannot be corrected by sphero-cylindrical lens combinations is referred to by physicists as higher order aberrations, i.e. comma, spherical aberration, chromatic aberration. The Zernike Polynomials, which describe ray points, are used to obtain a best fit toric to correct for the refractive error of the eye. The points are described in the x and y coordinates and the third dimension, height, is described in the z-axis. The local refractive correction of each area of the entrance pupil can be determined by calculating from the wavefront polynomial the corresponding local radii of curvature and hence the required spherocylindrical correction[6]. Thus each small region of the entrance pupil has its own three parameters that characterize the local

Table 11.1: RMS values prelaser

Patient No.	Z 110	Z 111	Z 200	Z 221	Z 220	Z 311	Z 310	Z 331	Z 330	Z 400	Z 420	Z 421	Z 440	Z 441	Z 510	Z 511	Z 530	Z 531	Z 550	Z 551	Z 6
1	0	0	-5.77	4.055.	-6.131	0.299	-0.113	0.725	-0.44	0.009	-0.03	0.102	-0.233	0.109	0.131	0.027	-0.048	-0.041	0.052	0.039	-9999
2	0	0	-4.323	-1.719	6.005	-0.273	0.022	-0.353	0.275	0.092	0.092	-0.145	0.199	-0.013	-0.006	0.011	0.034	-0.039	0.042	0.042	-9999
3	0	0	-11.8	-0.088	0.116	0.435	-0.658	-0.444	-0.567	-0.779	-0.089	0.043	-0.202	-0.053	-0.052	-0.057	-0.04	-0.001	0.13	0.111	-9999
4	0	0	-12.46	0.514	-0.155	0.29	-0.006	0.016	0.529	-0.91	0.124	0.124	-0.431	-0.222	0.074	-0.04	0.001	-0.063	-0.141	0.119	-9999
5	0	0	-6.535	-0.123	-0.886	0.156	-0.09	0.094	-0.128	-0.084	-0.072	0.035	-0.009	-0.044	0.001	-0.031	0.01	-0.005	0.001	-0.041	-9999
6	0	0	-7.867	0.185	1.704	-0.02	0.414	0.441	0.197	0.365	0.197	0.107	-0.155	-0.002	0.123	0.026	-0.001	0.049	0.048	0.032	-9999
7	0	0	-4.28	0.167	2.571	0.007	-0.089	0.356	0.125	0.585	0.101	-0.002	-0.17	-0.062	-0.077	0.198	0.001	-0.104	-0.022	0.029	-9999
8	0	0	-10.4	0.502	-0.587	-0.007	-0.331	0.165	-0.126	-0.054	-0.071	0.036	-0.118	-0.128	0.009	0.017	-0.007	-0.026	0.063	-0.052	-9999
9	0	0	-17.15	-0.414	-1.217	0.093	-0.106	0.343	-0.18	-0.254	0.009	0.002	0.001	-0.025	0.007	-0.022	-0.007	-0.042	0.037	0.04	-9999
10	0	0	-16.78	-0.162	-0.637	0.122	-0.159	0.279	0.2	-0.181	0.115	0.007	-0.002	0.042	-0.034	-0.028	0.021	-0.043	-0.006	-0.017	-9999
11	0	0	-4.513	2.916	4.661	-0.634	-0.205	0.477	0.44	0.094	0.377	0.058	-0.201	0.101	0.133	-0.147	0.009	0.011	-0.055	0.118	-9999
12	0	0	-5.736	-1.501	5.195	-1.126	0.32	0.665	-0.254	0.218	0.479	0.122	-0.253	-0.045	0.099	-0.025	0.012	-0.006	-0.05	0.11	-9999
13	0	0	-15.46	1.605	2.754	0.378	0.443	0.208	0.458	0.643	-0.083	0.09	0.407	-0.006	-0.021	0.09	0.033	0.032	0.239	0.149	-9999
14	0	0	-15.26	-0.557	2.865	-0.26	-0.059	0.107	0.122	0.168	0.025	-0.256	-0.003	0.257	0.007	0.051	0.136	-0.061	-0.114	0.124	-9999
15	0	0	-4.955	0.735	0.383	-0.401	0.003	0.62	-0.494	-0.676	0.391	0.163	-0.421	-0.264	0.039	-0.261	-0.079	0.241	0.103	-0.067	-9999
16	0	0	-4.367	-0.195	-0.238	0.28	-0.04	0.021	0.11	-0.112	0.084	-0.022	-0.061	0.013	-0.018	-0.063	0.004	0.063	0.044	0	-9999

Table 11.2: RMS values postlaser

Patient No	Z 110	Z 111	Z 200	Z 221	Z 220	Z 311	Z 310	Z 331	Z 330	Z 400	Z 420	Z 421	Z 440	Z 441	Z 510	Z 511	Z 530	Z 531	Z 550	Z 551	Z 6
1	0	0	-0.022	0.74	-1.294	0.117	-0.067	0.141	0.052	-0.063	-0.076	0.1	0.054	-0.037	-0.028	0.001	0.008	0.007	0.013	0.006	-9999
2	0	0	-0.508	0.12	0.194	-0.085	0.039	-0.12	-0.018	-9999	-9999	-9999	-9999	-9999	-9999	-9999	-9999	-9999	-9999	-9999	-9999
3	0	0	-1.398	-0.606	0.697	-0.558	-0.351	0.841	0.345	-0.39	0.392	0.038	-0.303	-0.038	-0.001	0.103	-0.066	-0.105	-0.021	0.137	-9999
4	0	0	-2.05	-0.499	-0.375	-0.027	-0.269	-0.534	-0.289	-0.58	0.114	0.058	0.236	-0.161	0.034	-0.083	0.004	0.039	0.01	-0.077	-9999
5	0	0	0.229	0.1	-0.123	-9999	-9999	-9999	-9999	-9999	-9999	-9999	-9999	-9999	-9999	-9999	-9999	-9999	-9999	-9999	-9999
6	0	0	-0.036	-0.17	0.425	-0.002	0.069	-0.045	-0.042	-0.342	-0.032	0.094	0.075	-0.05	0.068	0.03	0.064	-0.014	0.012	0.002	-9999
7	0	0	0.687	0.128	-0.028	-0.117	-0.043	0.062	0.088	-0.178	0.179	0.024	-0.045	0.055	0.013	0.016	-0.034	-0.013	-0.013	0.059	-9999
8	0	0	-2.164	0.279	-0.696	-0.25	-0.398	-0.147	-0.128	-0.581	-0.238	0.02	0.032	-0.088	-0.129	0.028	-0.029	0.007	0.089	0.059	-9999
9	0	0	-0.298	0.002	-0.311	0.158	-0.206	0.129	-0.116	-0.105	-0.045	-0.043	-0.1	-0.1	-9999	-9999	-9999	-9999	-9999	-9999	-9999
10	0	0	0.109	0.241	-0.503	0.233	-0.119	-0.16	-0.204	-9999	-9999	-9999	-9999	-9999	-9999	-9999	-9999	-9999	-9999	-9999	-9999
11	0	0	0.034	-0.092	0.076	0.013	-0.03	-0.067	0.003	-9999	-9999	-9999	-9999	-9999	-9999	-9999	-9999	-9999	-9999	-9999	-9999
12	0	0	0.187	0.061	0.004	-0.097	0.015	0.067	0.035	-9999	-9999	-9999	-9999	-9999	-9999	-9999	-9999	-9999	-9999	-9999	-9999
13	0	0	-0.701	0.291	0.598	2.161	0.349	-1.062	-0.201	-0.428	-0.013	0.204	0.258	-0.636	-0.082	0.113	0.069	-0.239	0.062	-9999	-9999
14	0	0	-0.638	0.094	0.391	0.517	-0.328	-0.336	0.188	-0.118	-0.077	0.003	0.157	0.034	-0.006	-0.025	0.004	0.018	-0.066	-9999	-9999
15	0	0	-0.148	0.493	0.017	0.261	0.017	-0.354	0.302	-0.111	0.053	0.07	-0.019	-0.084	-0.007	-0.051	-0.052	0.063	0.011	-9999	-9999
16	0	0	-0.161	-0.038	-0.331	0.072	0.049	-0.05	-0.086	0.025	-0.008	-0.059	-0.028	-9999	-9999	-9999	-9999	-9999	-9999	-9999	-9999

refractive correction: sphere, cylinder and axis[6]. The global aberrations of the entire optical system including the cornea, lens, vitreous and the retina are thus measured. The great advantage of wavefront analysis is that it can describe these other aberrations.

The first order polynomial describes the spherical error or power of the eye. The second order polynomial describes the regular astigmatic component and its orientation or axis. Third order aberrations are considered to be coma and fourth order aberrations are considered to be spherical aberration. Zernike polynomial descriptions for wavefront analysis typically go up to the tenth order of expression. The first and second orders describe the morphology of a normal straight curve. More local maximum and minimum points require higher orders of the polynomial series to describe the surface. Normal eyes exhibit spherical[7,8] and coma[9,10] aberrations in addition to exhibiting defocus and astigmatism.

Ideally, the difference in the magnitude of the local refractive correction of each area of the entrance pupil should not exceed 0.25 D. Lower spherocylindrical corrections are generally associated with lower wavefront aberrations[6]. These observations regarding variation in local ocular refraction along different meridians are also confirmed by Ivanoff[11] and Jenkins.[12] Van den Brink[13] also commented on the change in refraction across the pupil. Clinically significant changes of at least 0.25 D in one or both components of the spherocylindrical correction might normally be expected for decentrations of about 1 mm. Rayleigh's quarter wavelength rule states that if the wavefront aberration exceeds a quarter of a wavelength, the quality of the retinal image will be impaired significantly.[14] Thus the aberration in eyes starts to become significant when the pupil diameter exceeds 1-2 mm.[6] Thus it is not possible to correct the entire wavefront aberration with a single spherocylindrical lens. As conventional refractive procedures such as Lasik also reduce only the second order aberrations, the visual acuity will still be limited by aberrations of third and higher order aberrations. These patients are likely to undergo tremendous improvement in their BCVA after correction of their aberrations by Zyoptix.

In the Zyoptix system, the aberrometer and the orbscan, which checks the corneal topography, are linked and a zylink created. An appropriate software file is created which is then used to generate the laser treatment file. The truncated gaussian beam shape used in Zyoptix combines the advantages of the common beam shapes, i.e. flat top beam and the gaussian beam, creating a maximized smoothness and minimized thermal effect. Thus Zyoptix gives a smoother corneal surface, reducing glare and increasing visual acuity. The larger optical zones reduce haloes. Zyoptix also causes a reduction of the ablation depth by 15-20% and a reduced enhancement rate

In a patient with higher order aberrations, LASIK does not remove the higher order aberrations and the point-spread function is a large blur. Zyoptix on the other hand, performs customized ablation and removes the higher order aberrations thus minimizing the wavefront deformation. The point-spread function is therefore a small spot of light.

In our study, the mean preoperative spherical equivalent improved from –4.78 D to –0.16 D ± 0.68 and the mean preoperative cylinder improved from –1.34 D to –0.08 D ± 0.24. The aberrations were reduced drastically in all the eyes and the BCVA improved in all cases by [3] two lines. Reduction of the aberrations of the eye can thus result in an improved BCVA postoperatively.

Improving the optics of the eye by removing aberrations increases the contrast and spatial detail of the retinal image. Reduction of higher order aberrations may not improve high contrast acuity much more in eyes where spherocylindrical lenses alone improve the BCVA to 6/3 (2.00) or better. In contrast, in otherwise normal eyes where the BCVA is limited to 6/9 (0.50) or 6/6 (1.00) due to optical aberrations, reduction of higher order aberrations should improve visual acuity.

Realization of the best possible unaided visual acuity may be limited at the cortical, retinal and the spectacle, corneal, or implant level. All maculae may

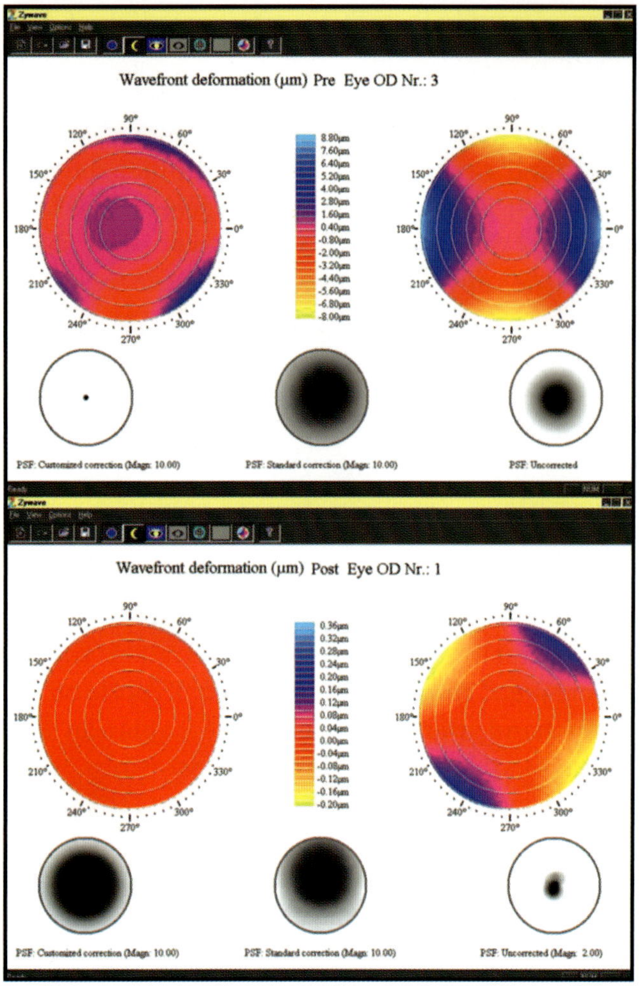

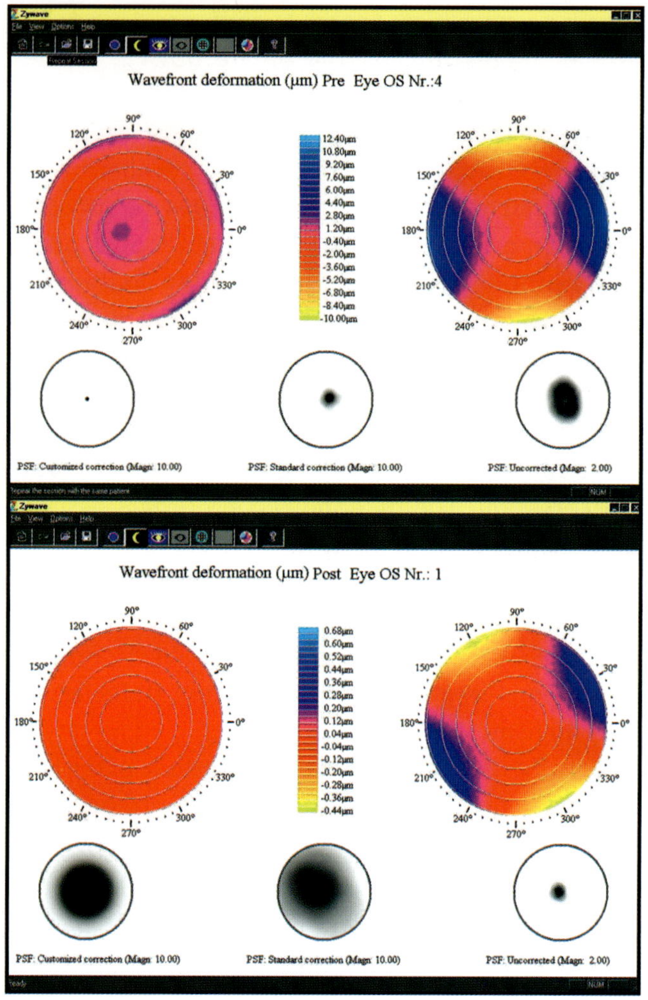

Figs 11.5 and 11.6: Pre and post-operative aberrometry of the right and left eye of the same patient showing removal of higher order aberrations

not be able to support 6/3 (2.00) vision. Insufficient cone density or sub-optimal orientation of cone receptors or a sub-optimal Stiles-Crawford profile of the macula may make 6/3 (2.00) vision impossible. Clinical or sub clinical amblyopia may make achievement of super vision impossible. But, in spite of this, there may be a certain patient population who have the potential for an improved BCVA on removal of their wavefront aberrations. The corneal topography does not account for the decreased preoperative visual acuity in these patients, neither do they have any other identifiable cause for the decrease in acuity except for an abnormal wavefront. It is important that this subgroup of patients are identified and their optical aberrations neutralized so that they are not deprived of the opportunity to gain in their BCVA.

Wavefront sensing technology, at present, does not in most cases define the exact locale of the pathology causing the aberration. Hence, clinical examination and other refractive tools, such as corneal topographic mapping, along with sound clinical judgment is required for proper understanding of the eye and its individual refractive status. Also, wavefront aberrations may not remain static. Numerous authors[15-18], have shown that ocular optical aberrations probably remain constant between 20 and 40 years of age but increase after that. Aberrations also change during accommodation.[19,20] and may be affected by mydriatics.[21] Thus, the patient should be informed about these possibilities while taking the consent for the procedure. Long-term studies are required to determine the stability of the post-operative refraction, residual aberrations and changes in BCVA if any.

The question of magnification factor improving visual acuity does not arise as these patients pre-operatively did not improve with contact lenses. Further the refractive error in some of these patients was not very large.

CONCLUSION

In conclusion, removal of the wavefront aberration may extend the benefit of an improved BCVA to patients with an abnormal wavefront. The subgroup of patients with higher order aberrations, normal corneal topography and no other known cause for decreased vision may thus benefit immensely with wavefront guided refractive surgery. Customized refractive surgery tailor-made for these individual patients, aimed at neutralizing the wavefront aberrations of the eye is safer, more predictable, provides better visual acuities and reduces the incidence of unsatisfactory outcomes. Further studies are required to assess the long-term outcomes.

Till now, when we discuss refractive errors we discuss about spherical and a cylindrical correction. But in todays world we have to think of a third parameter which is the aberrations present in the eye which can be anywhere in the optical media. These can be corrected in the corneal level by the laser treatment.

REFERENCES

1. B Platt, RV Shack." Lenticular Hartmann screen,"Opt Sci Center News (University of Arizona). 1971;5:15-16.
2. J Liang, B Grimm, S Goelz, J Bille. "Objective measurement of the wave aberrations of the human eye with the use of a Hartmann-Shack wavefront sensor" J Opt Soc Am 1994;11:1949-57.
3. J Liang, D R Williams, et al Aberrations and retinal image quality of the normal human eye. J Opt Soc Am A 1997;14(11):2873-83.
4. Oshika T, Klyce SD, Applegate RA, et al. Comparison of corneal wavefront aberrations after photorefractive keratectomy and laser in situ keratomileusis. Am J Ophthalmol 1999;127:01-07.
5. Fincham WHA, Freeman MH. Optics. 9th ed. London: Butterworths, 1980. Born M, Wolf E. Principles of Optics. 2nd ed. New York: Macmillan 1964;203-32.
6. WN Charman, G Walsh. Variations in the local refractive correction of the eye across its entrance pupil. Optometry and Vision Science 1989;66(1):34-40.
7. WM Rosenblum, JL Christensen. "Objective and subjective spherical aberration measurement of the human eye." In Progress in Optics, Wolf, ed. (North-Holland, Amsterdam 1976),13:pp 69-91.
8. MC Campbell, EM Harrison, P Simonet, "Psychophysical measurement of the blur on the retina due to optical aberrations of the eye,"Vision Res 1990;30: 1587-1602.
9. HC Howland, B Howland."A subjective method for the measurement of monochromatic aberrations of the eye. J Opt Soc Am 1977;67:1508-18.
10. G Walsh, WN Charman, HC Howland, "Objective technique for the determination of monochromatic aberrations of the human eye." J Opt Soc Am 1984;A1:987-92.
11. Ivanoff A. About the spherical aberration of the eye. J Opt Soc Am 1956;46:901-03.
12. Jenkins TCA. Aberrations of the eye and their effects on vision. Part 1. Br J Physiol Opt 1963;20: 59-91.
13. Van den Brink G. Measurements of the geometric aberrations of the eye. Vision Res 1962; 2:233-44.
14. Born M, Wolf E. Principles of Optics. 2nd ed New York: Macmillan 1964;203-32.
15. Kaemmerer M, Mrochen M, Mierdel p, et al. Optical aberrations of the human eye. Nature Medicine (in press)
16. Oshika T, Klyce SD, Applegate RA, et al. Changes in corneal wavefront aberration with aging. Invest Ophthalmol Vis Sci 1999;40:1351-55.
17. Calver RI, Cox MJ, Elliot DB. Effect of aging on the monochromatic aberrations of the human eye. J Opt Soc Am A 1999;16:2069-78.
18. Guirao A, Gonzalez C, Redondo M, et al. Average optical performance of the human eye as a function of age in a normal population. Invest Ophthalmol Vis Sci 199;40: 203-13.
19. Krueger R, Kaemerrer M, Mrochen M et al. Understanding refraction and accommodation through "ingoing optics" aberrometry: a case report. Ophthalmology (in press)
20. He JC, Burns SA, Marcos S. Monochromatic aberrations in the accommodated human eye. Vis Res 2000; 40:41-48
21. Fankhauser F, Kaemerrer M, Mrochen M, et al. The effect of accommodation, mydriasis, and cycloplegia on aberrometry. ARVO abstract 2248. Invest Ophthalmol Vis Sci 2000; 41:S461.

LASIK—Indications and Surgical Steps

12

Sanjay Chaudhary (India)

With LASIK, refractive surgery has finally come of age. With PRK, there was always an impending risk of corneal haze, more so when diopters of over 6 were corrected. Then there were also problems with post-operative pain, post op bandage, regression and a slow recovery. Lasik addressed all these problems as given below.

Advantages of Lasik over PRK

		PRK	Lasik
1.	Corneal haze resulting in blurring	possible in number over 6	Nil
2.	Bandage on eyes or BCL	3 days	Nil
3.	Pain	2 days	Negligible
4.	Stability in refraction	4-8 months	1 month
5.	Eye drops after procedure	4-8 months	2-3 weeks

However, Lasik has added a new set of complications as will be discussed later.

History

The history of Lasik goes back to 1989, when Buratto first used the Excimer laser to photo-ablate the corneal stroma in situ under a free cap. In 1991, Pallikaris used the hinge technique in the creation of a corneal flap.

The Micro-Keratome

This is the main instrument in performing Lasik. The main objective of a micro-keratome is to perform a uniform homogeneous planar cut on the corneal surface. The resulting corneal disc should have a precisely calculated thickness and diameter with a sufficient hinge to maintain its position and apposition during replacement.

A microkeratome has the following components:

A suction ring This allows the surgeon to fixate the globe, to maintain an IOP of 65 mm Hg., and allows the excursion of a microkeratome head on a given track. It also exposes the right diameter of corneal tissue to be resected.

The microkeratome head has an oscillating ***blade*** driven by a motor incorporated in the handle. The head also has a ***thickness plate***, which sets the exact depth of the cut. A ***stop*** mechanism ensures that the head stops at a pre set distance in the track on the

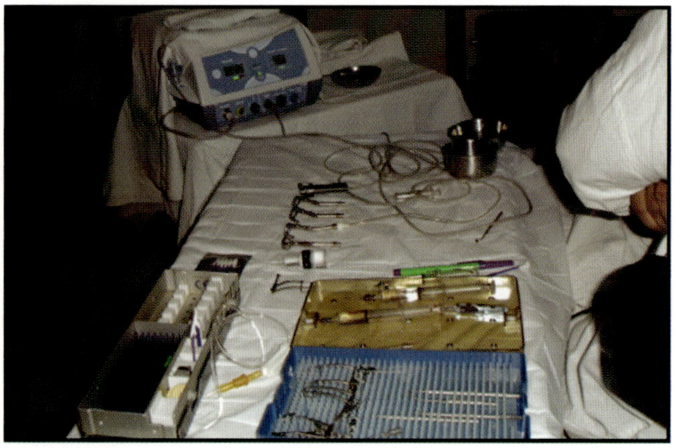

Fig. 12.1: The microkeratome layout (Moria M2)

suction ring during the cut to maintain a hinge of the flap. The movement of the head is either on a pivot or on gears and is driven either by a different motor or shared by the motor for blade oscillation.

How the Keratome Works

When the suction is activated, the cornea bulges out through the suction ring. The thickness plate decides the gap between the cutting edge of the blade and the edge of the thickness plate. During forward movement of the microkeratome, the plate flattens out the cornea while the blade cuts out a smooth flat flap.

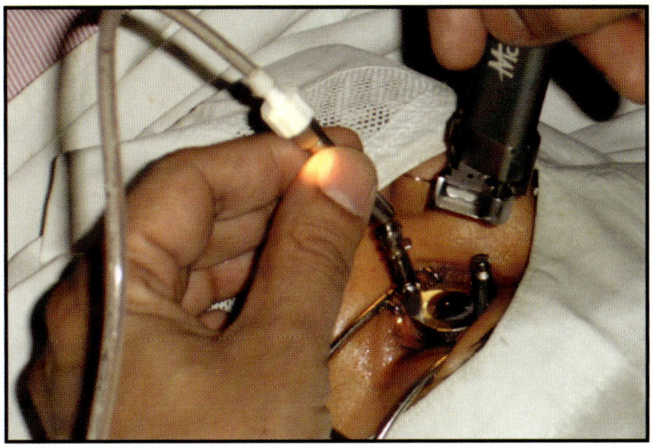

Fig. 12.2: Placing the keratome on the eye

Achieving a Good Quality Cut

A uniform smoothness and precision of a cut depends on a number of factors:

1. Speed of the pass. A rapid keratectomy will usually produce a thin cut while a slow pass will produce a thicker corneal resection. This is where an automated system scores over a manual system.
2. Oscillation of the blade. A slow oscillating speed tends to produce rougher surfaces, which may affect the quality of visual outcome. A higher oscillating speed produces greater friction of movement and hence greater heat production and dispersion. This may damage the tissue being cut. Greater oscillations may also damage the blade and its housing resulting in dispersion of metallic debris along the tract of the microkeratome. A good cut works at 10000 rpm.
3. The Blade edge should be sharp, smooth and uniform. Ideally one blade should be used per eye. The attack angle of the blade is 25 degrees in most of the machines.
4. IOP should be between 60 and 65 mm Hg during a cut.
5. The cornea should be doused with BSS to prevent friction with the thickness plate of the microkeratome.
6. A good eye exposure is a must.

The flap thickness is usually set to 160 microns. In a normal thickness cornea of 530 microns, and with a view to leave a stromal bed of 250 microns, this gives a flexibility to use 120 microns, which is good enough to correct myopia of 8 diopters. With interest in correcting higher diopters, the trend shifted too lasek and epilasik, but this replicated the corneal haze as seen in PRK. So lasik again gathered popularity but this time with a thinner flap enough to preserve the Bowman's membrane. The flap thickness now desired is 130 microns. The thinner flap gives another 30 microns of flexibility but the thinner flap is more liable to button holing and flap wrinkling.

Preoperative Counselling

In Lasik it is no different from other refractive surgeries.

1. The patient needs to understand that no refractive surgical procedure is 'perfect' and that possibility of over and under corrections exists as well as the possibility of enhancement especially with higher myopia. It is important to stress that enhancement may not always be possible nor advisable in all situations.
2. Patients with large pupil may be told of a possibility glare, halo's and night driving problems. Rare complication like the flap problems and infections should also be explained.
3. Explain that this procedure involves a series of steps and there is a possibility that the operation may be interrupted following any of these steps such as problems with the microkeratome, incomplete cut, poor flap or malfunction of the laser.

4. In patients nearing presbyopic age it is extremely important to explain presbyopia and the possibility of needing reading glasses in the near future. Some low to moderate myopes are used to reading without their spectacles, and when this is no longer possible following refractive surgery, they are unhappy with what the surgeon considers a perfect result.

Patient Selection

- Patient must be over 18 years of age (except for rare exceptions)
- Refraction must be stable for a year
- Patient should not be Pregnant or Lactating
- Range of correction should be
  - myopia – 1.0 to – 10.0 D
  - hyperopia + 1.0 to + 6.0 D
  - astigmatism 1.0 to 6.0 D
- Central corneal thickness in excess of 500 microns
- Corneas which are neither excessively flat (less than 40 D) or excessively steep (over 48 D).

Contraindications

- Keratoconus
- Current or previous history of eye inflammation such as herpes keratitis
- Pathology of Bowman's membrane or subepithelial layers
- Patients with unusually sunken eyes where it may be difficult to fix the suction ring
- Dry eye syndrome
- Marked pupillary decentration
- Patient with autoimmune disease
- Thin corneas (less than 450 microns).

Preoperative Examination

Orbital Anatomy

A good exposure is mandatory. One should have varying lid speculum especially the locking type to obtain maximal lid retraction and globe exposure. Unobstructed progression of the microkeratome during the pass on the suction ring is necessary. Patients with sunken eyes and small palpebral apertures may pose a problem.

Keratometry

K readings less than 42 D (flat corneas) result in greater possibility of free caps.

Topography

- Useful in evaluating postoperative results with preoperative findings
- Screening pre-op pathology such as keratoconus esp. in the sub clinical phase which may otherwise go undetected and may be considered a contraindication to surgery
- Monitor corneas following contact lens removal. It is recommended that soft contact lens be discontinued for two weeks and rigid or gas permeable contact lens four weeks prior to surgery. If corneal moulding is detected, continuous monitoring is required to allow stabilization.

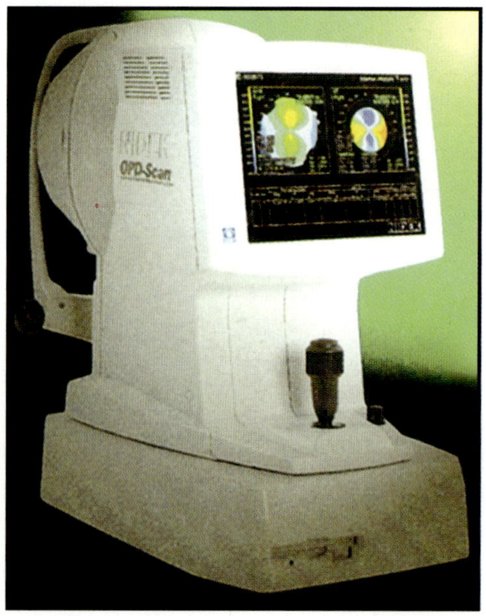

Fig. 12.3: Corneal topographer (OPD scan)

Pupil size

Large Optical Zones are required for people with large pupils. Young patients with large pupils must also be advised of potential glare, halo's, and night driving problems.

Refraction

Subjective, manifest and cycloplegic. Manifest refraction is the one selected and the manifest axis of the cylinder outweighs the topographic cylinder in case of a discrepancy. Use the least amount of minus correction for the best visual acuity. Vertex distance of 12 mm should be maintained as all lasers are fine tuned to this vertex distance.

Visual Acuity

With and without correction. Sometimes a vision of 6/9p in a high myope with spectacles results in 6/6p after Lasik. This improvement in the visual status is only due to the elimination of the minification effect of a high concave lens. A true comparison in such cases would be between visual acuity with a contact lens and that after Lasik.

Bio-microscopy

- For corneal clarity
- Tear film assessment
- Absence of conjunctival pathology which could cause difficulty in fixation of the suction ring
- Lens changes. An associated cataract could be better dealt with by an implant.

Tonometry

To establish pre op IOP level. Post op IOP levels are usually less than the pre-op levels due to reduction in tissue rigidity due to thinning of cornea.

Pachymetry

It is mandatory to do this at the center, 3, 5and 7 mm position to determine thickness of primary keratectomy and to determine the amount of available corneal tissue for ablation. Assuming that we use a 160 micron flap thickness, and we have to at least leave behind 250 microns of stromal base, so 410 microns have to be left behind. Thus a cornea with central thickness of less than 450 microns is a contraindication for the procedure. Minimal handling thickness should be 500 microns as this gives us 90 microns to work with

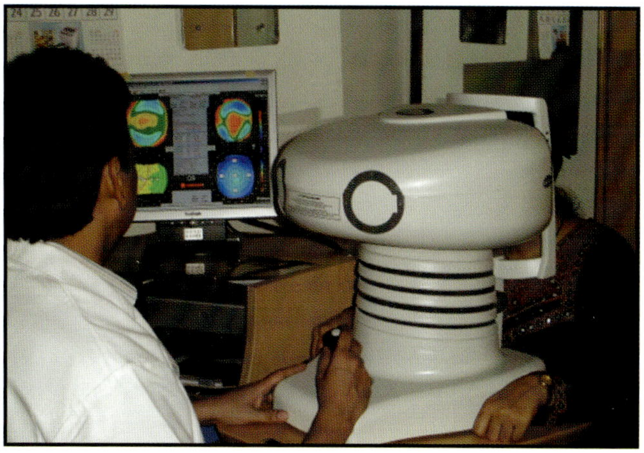

Fig. 12.4: Orbscan II for scanning corneal thickness, evaluating anterior and posterior elevation and corneal topography

Fundus

An Indirect Ophthalmoscopy and management of myopic peripheral degenerative changes cannot be over emphasized.

The Technique

Anesthesia

Topical anesthesia is the normal choice. We normally prefer proparacaine, however lignocaine may also be used. All anesthetics have a certain degree of epithelial toxicity so it is best to begin the instillation just prior to inserting the eye speculum.

Procedure

Eye lashes and eyelids are prepped with betadine outside the laser room. The patient is then made to lie on the table (or laser chair) under the laser. The eye is draped and a suitable speculum used which offers a good exposure. The cornea is marked with a gentian violet marker or pen. An ideal marker is one which has two radial and on para-radial marks. The para-radial mark is important in that it facilitates the correct orientation as well as alignment in the rare free flap situation. The suction ring is now fixed in place on the sclera and slightly decentered towards the side of the hinge. The suction is activated and as the IOP builds up over a few seconds to a level of 65 mm Hg., the pupil dialates and the patient remarks that he can no longer see. IOP is checked with a Barraquer tonometer. For a correct reading, the corneal surface and the tonometer should be dry. The surface of the cornea is then moistened with BSS to facilitate a smooth movement of the keratome. The microkeratome head is then fixed on the pivot of the suction ring. By depressing the forward foot pedal, the microkeratome makes a forward pass to cut a corneal disc/flap. By depressing the reverse foot pedal, it returns to its original position leaving behind a good corneal lamellar hinged disc/flap. At this point it is important to note whether an inadvertent free flap has not occurred. The suction is released. This period of raised IOP at 65 mm Hg should be as short as possible to prevent damage to the optic nerve head. The flap is retracted along the hinge. The stromal bed is ablated with Excimer laser to achieve the desired correction. Care should be taken that no fluid reaches the area where the ablation is in progress. Also protect the hinge during ablation. The flap is reposed. Irrigation is done under the flap to remove any debris and to allow the disc to smoothly float and settle on the stromal bed. The disc is then stroked with a moist Merocel sponge in a direction opposite to the hinge so that the flap is both aligned and distended properly. A drop of BSS is placed on the corneal dome to maintain hydration of the epithelium. The flap is allowed to dry naturally for 2 - 5 minutes to allow firm adhesion of the flap to the stromal bed. This is confirmed by the ***striae*** test whereby a dry Merocel sponge is used to depress the corneal periphery near the limbus producing striae, which can be seen radiating on to the flap. The speculum and drape are removed gently so as not to cause epithelial abrasion or a flap displacement. The patient is allowed to blink normally and this is observed through the operating microscope. The flap should appear well adhered and perfectly aligned. Antibiotic and anti-inflammatory drops are instilled.

The patient is reviewed after half an hour on the slit lamp to access the status of the flap.

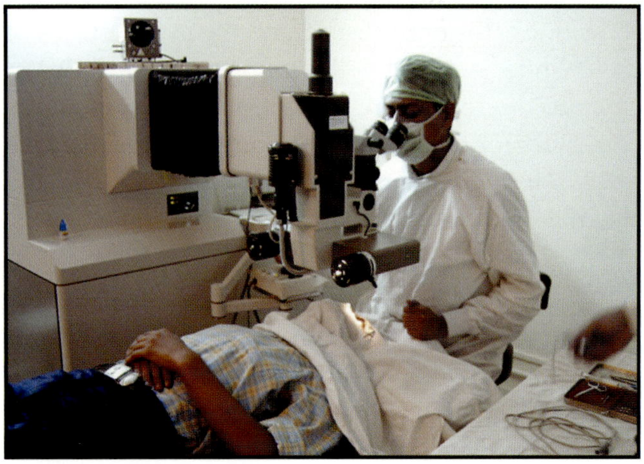

Fig. 12.5: The LASIK system comprising the excimer laser and the microkeratome

Postoperative Treatment

Local antibiotic and anti-inflammatory eye drops are used over a period of two to three weeks. My preference is Gatifloxacin and Fluorometholone eye drops. Lubricating drops like Artificial tears is also useful for the first few months. Lasik is relatively pain free post operatively as compared to PRK.

Follow-up

This is done on the first post op day and then after a month with instructions that in case of pain or sudden blurring of vision, the patient must immediately report to the doctor (could be a symptom of a dislocated flap)

Advice to Lasik Patients

- On returning home, rest or sleep for a few hours
- The patient can return to his/her routine activities the day after the operation
- No touching or rubbing the eye for two weeks
- No swimming for a month; light physical exercise is okay
- Avoid exposure to strong light or over use of the eyes for long periods

- Avoid activities which may cause trauma to the eyes
- The patient should be seen the next day for the first post op visit
- As Lasik is relatively painless, report pain or marked blurred vision to the doctor immediately (may be a symptom of a dislocated flap)

Complications

Intraoperative Related to the Keartome

- Incomplete primary cut
- Thin flaps and Button hole
- Free cap—360 degree flap resection and lack of hinge formation

Intraoperative Specific to the Use of Laser

- Incorrect ablation
- Decentration of the ablation
- Ablation of the hinge.

Postoperative

- Infective keratitis
- Diffuse Lamellar keratitis—Sands of Sahara
- Epithelia downgrowth
- Flap wrinkling—Traction folds on the flap
- Debris in the interface
- Corneal ectasia
- Dry eye
- Halo's and Glare
- Induced topographical alterations (central islands)
- Over and under corrections
- Irregular astigmatism
- Regressions
- Induced astigmatism (regular or irregular).

Corneal Wavefront Guided Lasik

13

Cyres K Mehta, Keiki R Mehta (India)

Lasik has gained in popularity worldwide. New flying spot lasers with Gaussian beam profiles and high speed infrared trackers provide precise, predictable and consistent ablation leading to exceptional accuracy.

The promise of "Supervision" is slowly becoming a reality with the availability of Hartmann Schack and Tscherning abberometry systems, with linkages to excimer laser platforms.

The Wavelight company, Germany, utilizes a Tscherning principle for its abberometer. Bausch and Lomb provide the Orbscan Corneal analysis system, a projection based videokeratograph system which relies on slits of light, with the 217 laser platform. Schwind Eye Tech Solutions a Refractive Solutions and Excimer laser manufacturer out of Germany provide an interesting variation on Abberometrically guided lasik.

Schwind provides the COAS abberometer as well as the ORK-W and ORK-CAM softwares which provide shot patterns based on the Optikon Keratron Scout Topographer, a placido principle-based videokeratoscope.

A Short Historical Account of Topography

- 1880-Placido invented a flat disk with alternating black and white rings
- 1889-Javal placed the discs into his ophthalmometer, behind the arc that carried the ophthalmometric mires.
- 1896-Alvar Gullstrand from the Uppsala University invented the Photokeratoscope and made very accurate arc-step calculations, with an 'algorithm' to plot the corneal meridian profiles. This won him the Nobel prize in 1911
- 1990's-Computerized corneal topography from EyeSys and a host of other companies basically all videokeratoscopes.
- 2001-Optikon 2000 an Italian company releases the Keratron Scout with a link to the Schwind ESIRIS flying spot laser.

TOPOGRAPHY AND WAVEFRONTS

A corneal topographer (CT) measures corneal shape while a Wavefront Analyser (WA) measures wavefront aberrations.

The Advent of the "Corneal Wavefront" ushers in a new era in refractive measurements.

The concept of the corneal wavefront The Corneal Wavefront is the part of the total aberrations of the eye, owed to the cornea.

So, Ocular Wavefront (OW) = Corneal Wavefront (CW) + Internal Wavefront (IW).

The Corneal Wavefront is easily calculated from the Corneal Topography by using an algorithm. An ***'algorithm'*** is the calculus procedure used to reconstruct corneal geometry from the calculation of the position of points on the corneal surface relative to axis or a reference sphere.

Ray tracing is used. Rays are traced from the fovea out of the eye.

Wavefront aberration is measured as the difference from a plane surface, at the entrance pupil, in object space. In ***Ray tracing*** we apply Snells law to the corneal surface to calculate (OPD) the Optical Path Difference. If a cornea is distorted (for example, has a bulge in the surface) the rays of light spend a longer time in the cornea (where the bulge is) so the rays that enter air first, from the flatter regions of the cornea, accelerate and create a deformed wavefront. In the time a ray travels 3 micron in the cornea, it travels 4 micron in air. So if the cornea is distorted from its ideal shape, we can follow the ***"rule of 3"***, i.e. Every 3 microns of distortion from the ideal shape of the cornea will produce a +1 micron difference in the OPD map and a -1 micron difference in the wavefront error map.

This Optical Path Difference, the basis of Corneal Wavefront theories, is the difference between the corneal wavefront and an Ideal wavefront. Its similar to the spherical offset which is the height difference between the cornea and a sphere.

Total aberration of the eye as measured by wavefront Analyzers depends on:

1. Size of the pupil-With the COAS analyzer, using a Hartmann Schack sensor, the abberometric map depends as with any analyzer on pupil size. If the pupil opens only 5 mm, then the map generated is only 5 mm, an unacceptably small ablation diameter.
2. Effect of Accommodation—Introduces another factor into the total wavefront, i.e. the effect of the Lens on the wavefront. As the lens changes shape to accommodate it itself induces aberrations.
3. Wavefront varies with age and from examination to examination and with epithelial factors.

In contrast. *Corneal Abberations* are:

1. Relatively stable over time and serial measurements.
2. Can be evaluated for different pupil Diameters.
3. Not affected by accommodation.
4. More than 80% of the total wavefront aberrations are attributed to the Corneal Wavefront and this measurement is stable!

ORK CORWAVE also called ORK-W "Corneal Wavefront" Software-Link is successfully being used for:

- Treatment of virgin eyes
- Individual improvement of visual acuity (in case of corneal aberrations)
- Re-treatment of decentered ablations, by increasing the ablation diameter
- Re-treatment to enlarged optical zones to combat glare and haloes
- Re-treatment of irregular ablations and smoothing effect for irregular corneas.

Methods

The combination of the future oriented ESIRIS Excimer laser system for Refractive Surgery (200 Hz pulse frequency, 330 Hz active high speed eyetracking and 0.8 mm scanning spot with gaussian beam profile) together with the high resolution topography systems Optikon Keratron Scout shows us new possibilities of measuring and interpreting the cornea. With this an indivdual and true "customized ablation" may be performed with the Schwind Excimer Laser ESIRIS. An intelligent software (Schwind ORK software for Optimized Refractive Keratectomy), which realizes the transformation of the cornea into an individual, customized ablation profile, is the most important link between the diagnostic unit (topography system) and the Excimer laser for the treatment. A Corneal wavefront generated by the software presents the cornea with its irregularities in form of a mathematic Zernike polynomial up to the 7th order. The projected "placido" rings and the information (data) resulting from it are the basis for the calculation. This is being described by the Optical Path Difference (OPD) with the help of ***Zernicke polynomials***. Corneal aberrations may now be calculated and compared with ocular aberrations.

ORK CORWAVE or "Corneal Wavefront Technology" delivers much more information about optical defects that may effect vision than just sphere and cylinder. It more or less describes the anterior corneal surface as a wavefront with its aberrations. Thus it is possible to qualify (describe) and quantify optical defects of the human eye. This information makes a real, individual ablation profile possible, which considerably increases and therefore improves postoperative visual quality of the patient.

Advantages of ORK CORWAVE (ORK-W)

- Pupil dilation of the patient, unlike abberometry is not necessary for measurement.
- Reliable measurement results, especially with irregular cornea, high astigmatism and "central islands".
- Selective simulation of corneal aberrations: Point Spread Function (PSF) - acuity chart or Modular Transfer Function (MTF - which relates to the contrast sensitivity).
- Individual treatment plan with decentrations and re-treatments.
- Extended diagnostic possibilities by comparing the complete aberrometry of the eye with the corneal aberrations.
- *Accommodation does not influence measuring results.*
- Treatment zone is *not limited by the pupil.*

The Keratron Scout—Manufactured by Optikon 2000S pA (Rome, Italy).

It uses a small cone with 28 edges for the projection of Placidos rings. This allows us to measure at least 85% of the corneal surface which is indispensable for peripheral treatments like hyperopia and also for retreatments by enlarging ablation diameter.

The software that connects the Laser to the Topographer is the Schwind ORK-W.

Steps in Performing a Corneal Wavefront Guided Ablation

1. Take a topographic picture from the Scout. Evaluate the picture for repeatability, artifacts, lashes, tear film abnormalities and adequate pupil recognition.
2. If the image meets the required criteria create a "Corneal Wavefront" map.
   The wavefront map can be broken down into and viewed as:
   a. Zernicke coefficients
   b. Point spread function
   c. Simulated Vision Chart
   d. Modulation Transfer Function (Like Contrast Sensitivity)
   e. A street scene where the patient can see a street scene simulated preoperatively and postoperatively. This is essential for patients undergoing treatment on highly abberated corneas to realize the meaning of wavefront and how it adds "sharpness" to vision.
3. Export the measurements to the ORK-W software which creates a shot file (an ablation pattern). ORK-W creates a Prolate cornea. The Optical Zone can include the entire topographic map and not just pupil diameter (like a Wavefront analyzer)
4. Perform the ablation
5. A week and a month after treatment, put the patient back on the topographer and analyse the difference map.

OUR EXPERIENCE

Over a 4 month period with the Schwind ESIRIS laser and the Keratron Scout with ORK-W software for 110 cases which included 9 cases of highly aberrated eyes.

1. On many cases of virgin eyes, we were able to reduce postoperative aberrations by one-third to half, of the RMS value
2. Patients perceived the vision as sharp. No patient lost lines and a few experienced a one line gain in BCVA (14 patients)
3. Minimum treatment diameter was 6.5 mm with a 0.5 mm transition zone. Thus with Indian pupils we did not get any case of Haloes or Glare
4. Nine highly aberrated eyes, Post Keratoplasty and Post-trabeculectomy and post ECCE were also treated with Corneal Wavefront.

Aberrations reduced by about a quarter in these complicated cases. Also in every case, the full cylinder was not eliminated. Postoperative BCVA, sometimes with spectacles (In cases where preoperative cylinder was as high as 10 D), improved about 1-2 lines in most cases (6 out of 9). No patient lost lines of BCVA!. So in our experience the system does work in the sense that it provides better postoperative best corrected visual acuity.

What matters is the ability of the operator to choose the appropriate topographic map from the 4 maps the topographer presents every sequence for analysis. Every map which is exported for wavefront correction must be screened thoroughly, *not by a technician* but by the Laser surgeon, for tear film, lash and position defects and for adequate pupil recognition.

CASE STUDY

Patient HM aged 70 presented to us with a BCVA of 6/24 (no improvement on pinhole) in his one functioning left eye.

This eye had been operated previously elsewhere for ECCE and trabeculectomy 10 years ago. The pupil was a 3 mm nondilating adherent pupil (to the PMMA IOL). Measured corneal thickness was 550 microns.

In the Figure 13.1—TOPO PREOP MATANI-Notice that the Keratron scout topographer has measured the pupil at 2.95 mm and the cornea looks grossly distorted, with a measured astigmatism of 8.98 diopters.

In Figures 13.2 and 13.2A—PREOP CORNEAL WAVEFRONT MAP. Notice that the software using an arc step algorithm has generated a wavefront map. In the Zernicke coefficients map we can see that third order aberrations are significant and the astigmatism is 9.59. The total RMS value of the aberrations in the cornea is more than 11 microns (top left part of the picture).

In Figure 13.2B—This is a shot file generated with ORK-W software. Notice that even though the patient accepts only +1-6D at 85 degrees, the topographer and software have decided the sphere

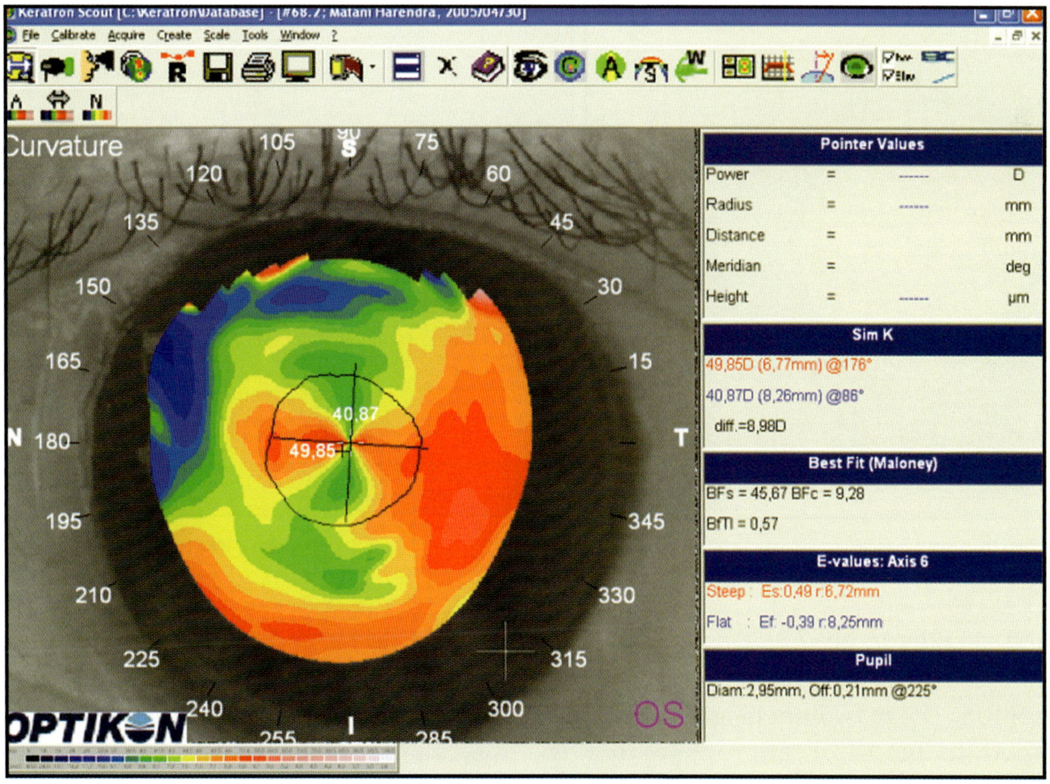

Fig. 13.1: Topo Preop

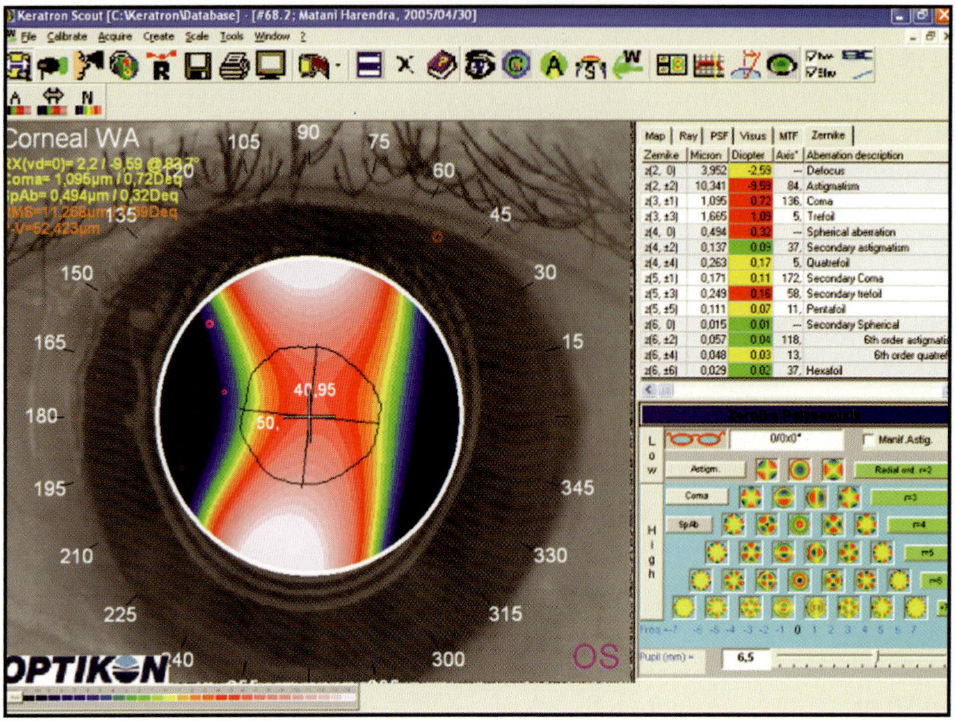

Fig. 13.2: Preoperative corneal wavefront map

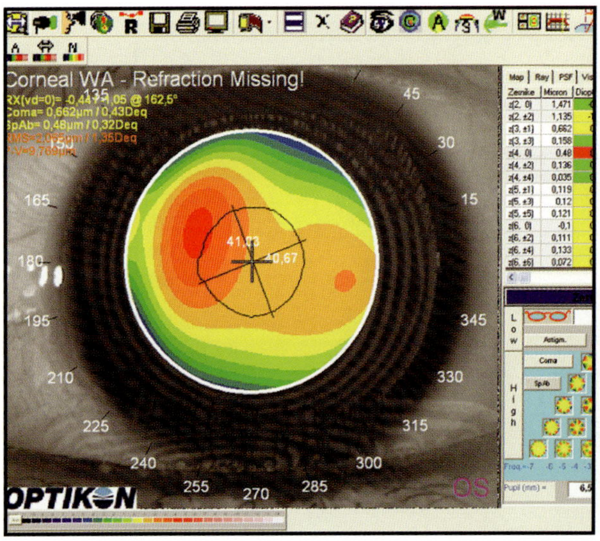

Fig. 13.2A: Preoperative corneal wavefront map

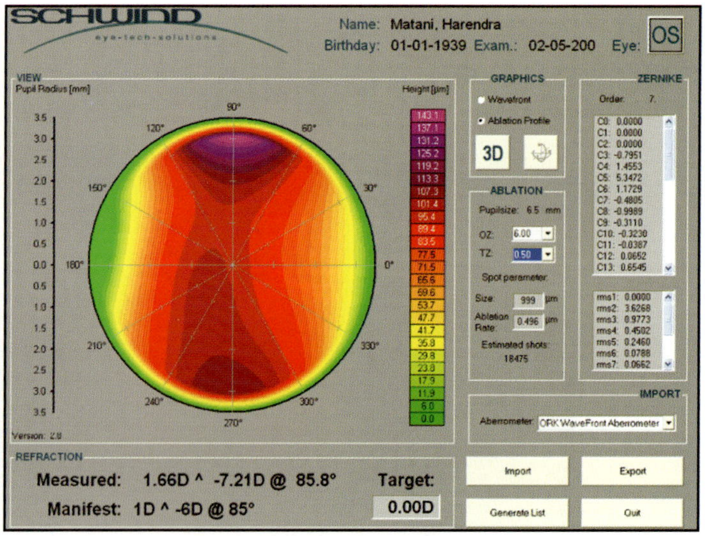

Fig. 13.2B: ORK-W shot file

to be 1.66 and cylinder to be -7.21.We have entered the ablation rate of 0.496 generated by the Fluence test on the ESIRIS. The maximum height of ablation is determined to be 143.1 microns which is acceptable. The ZIP is slotted into the laser and the ablation performed on the eye under a 110 micron flap.

Figure 13.3—POSTOP TOPO—at 1 week. Note the cylinder is greatly reduced to 4 D. The cornea looks much 'smoother' with less rapid transitions.

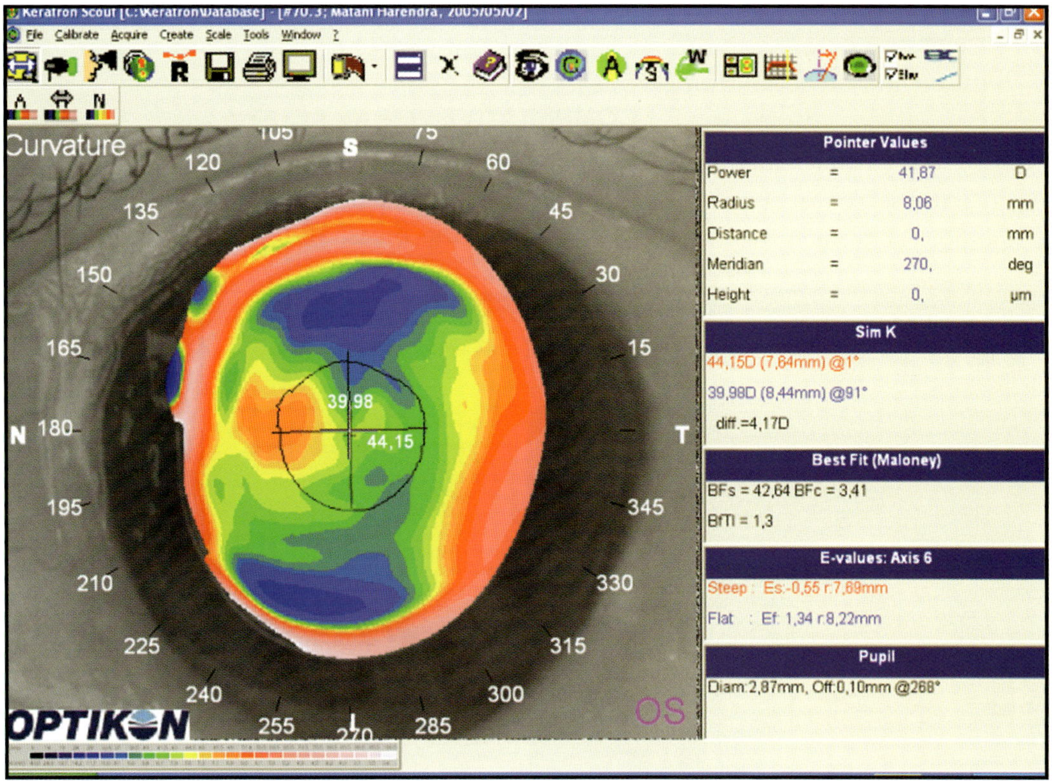

Fig. 13.3: Post-operative TOPO

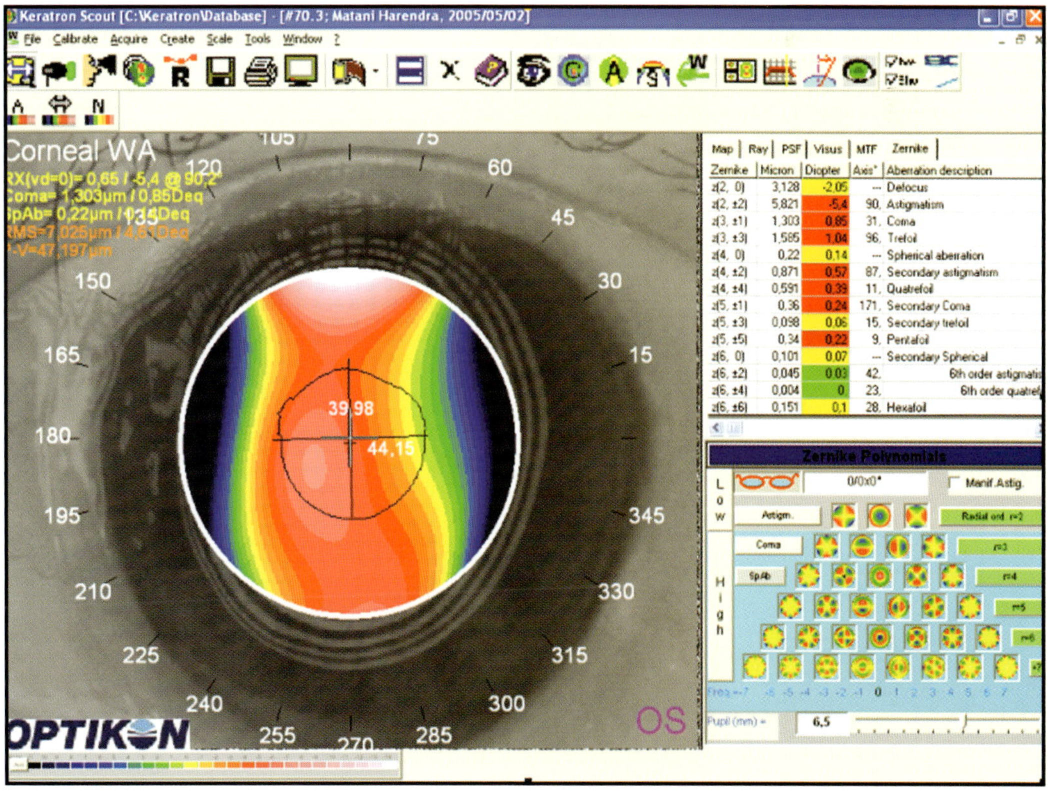

Fig. 13.4: Post-operative wavefront

POSTOPERATIVE WAVEFRONT (FIG. 13.4)

The RMS value is now reduced to 7 microns from 11, about a 30% drop

Astigmatism has dropped to 5 D from 9.4th order aberrations seem to have increased. We were baffled. Why? Reason. The flap had not yet perfectly settled.

A month after the case the patient was 6/12 with only 2.5 cylinder!!

COMPARATIVE VISUAL ACUITY SIMULATIONS (FIG. 13.5)

Here we can see that the simulated visual acuity is much better (the black and white picture) in the

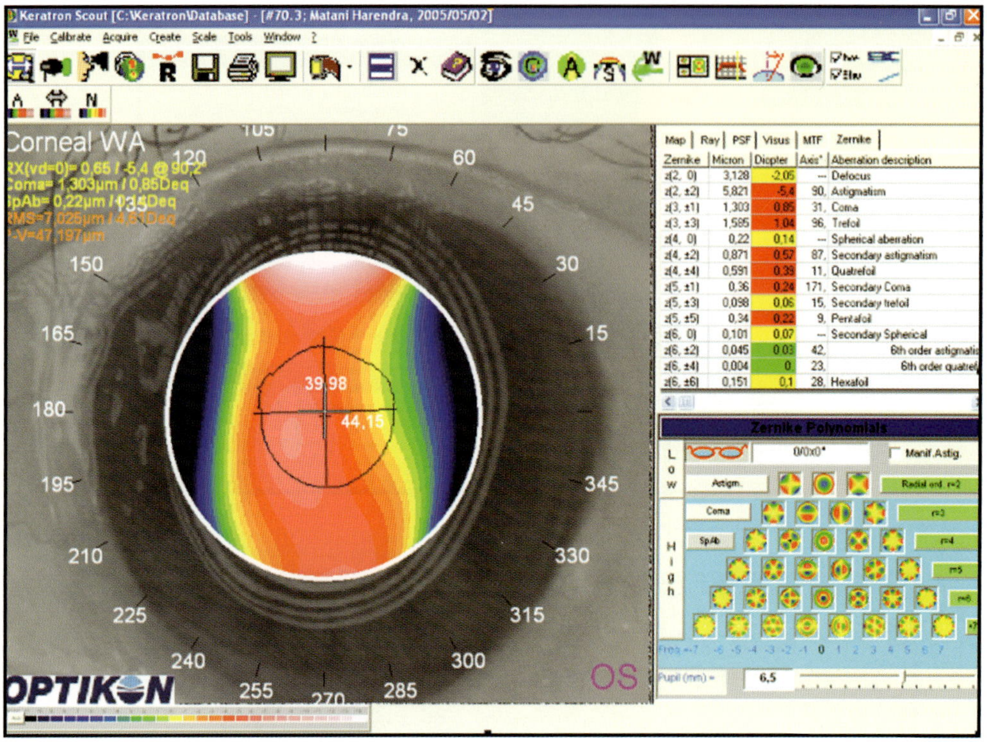

Fig. 13.5: Comparative visual acuity simulations

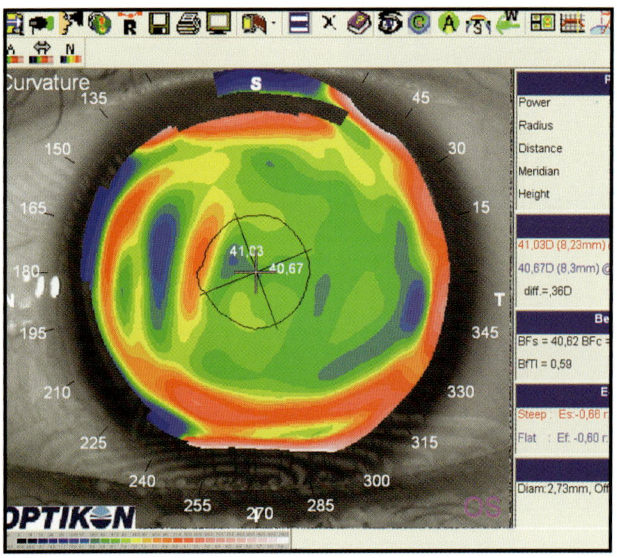

Fig. 13.5A: Comparative visual acuity simulations

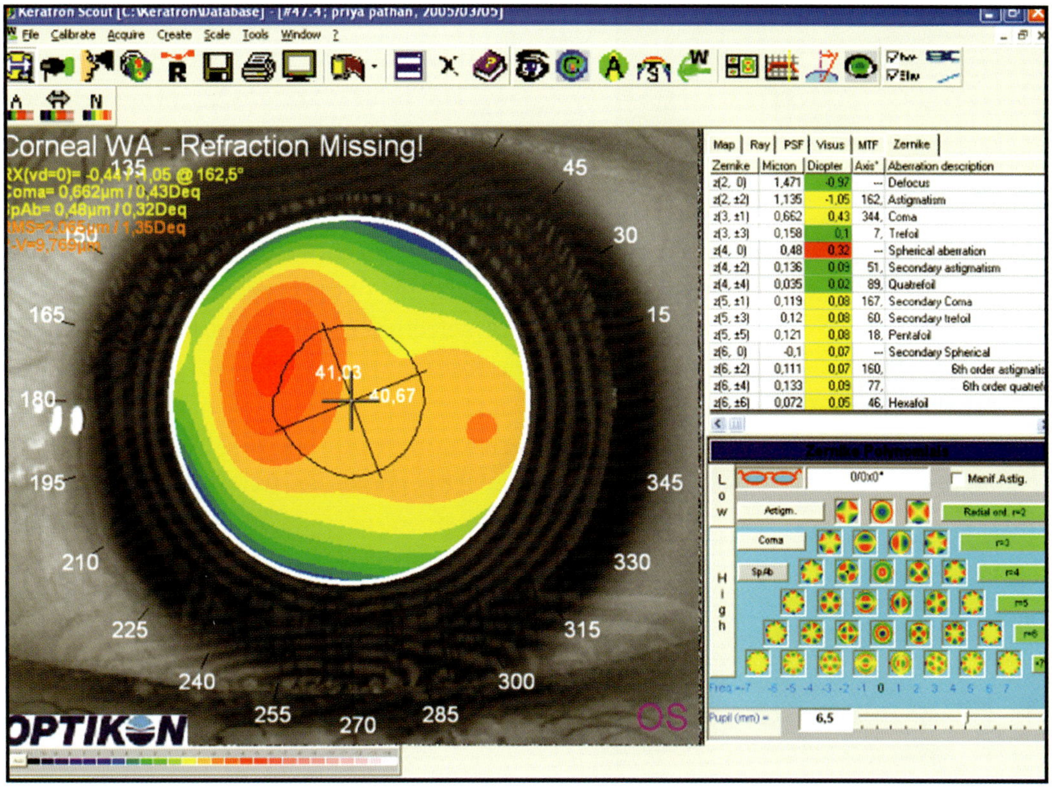

Fig. 13.5B: Comparative visual acuity simulations

postop case. Both UCVA and BCVA have both improved by 50% a month postoperative.

LET'S TAKE A LOOK AT ANOTHER CASE

This case underwent LASIK at another center that uses an ACS microkeratome that creates a nasal hinged flap. The flap was incomplete and part of the ablation fell on the hinge. Here even though the cylinder induced is barely 0.4 D (Fig. 13.5A) the patient complained of glare and ghosting and distortion of images. She was referred for an evaluation. On topographic evaluation we can see the blue and red areas where the flap was partial and laser energy fell on the upturned flap. Luckily for her pupil was only 3 mm in mesopic conditions.!

On corneal wavefront evaluation (Fig. 13.5B) we realized that a large amount of COMA and spherical aberration had been induced with total value of aberrations crossing 2 microns where more than 1 micron is significant. This explains her loss of BCVA. She has lost one line of BCVA(6/9) due to the aberrations. She would benefit from the ORCA wave procedure. Thus corneal wavefront guided procedures have a definite role to play in retreatments.

I would like to share one more case series from Germany which demonstrates the strength of the system in *Retreatments*

Experience, Results, and Cases Treated by Volker Rummelt, M.D., Oberstenfeld, Germany, with the Schwind 200 Hz. Excimer laser, ORK-Software, and Optikon Keratron Scout Topography System. This experience is based on corneal wavefront data, which had been obtained from the Optikon Keratron Scout Topography System and the Schwind ORK software, on 12 eyes which had undergone LASIK treatment 11 months earlier, and who had been *retreated* from May—December 2002. There was a decentered

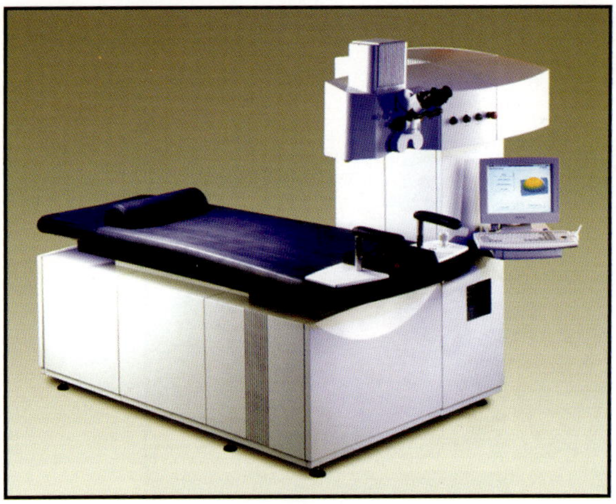

Fig. 13.6: Schwind Esiris laser platform

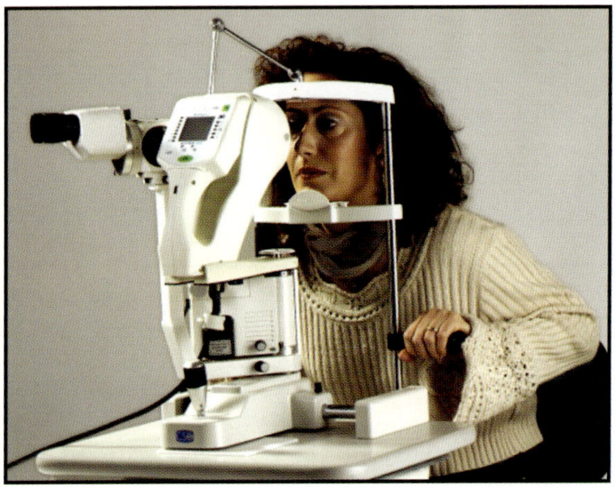

Fig. 13.7: Keratron scout

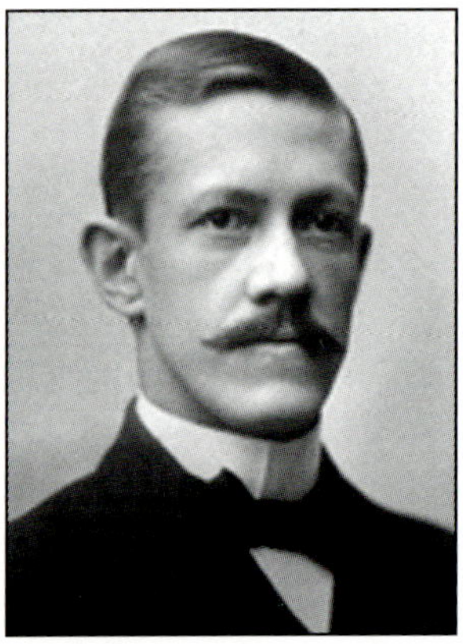

Fig. 13.8: Prof Alvar gullstrand—The father of corneal topography

ablation with a coma with 7/12 eyes pre-operatively, a relatively small optical zone (6.0 mm) with 6/12 eyes with large pupil diameter at mesopic conditions with subjectively increased Halos at night and with 3/12 eyes there was an irregular astigmatism with a partially lasered flap (hinge) after LASIK.

The optical zone (OZ) of all retreated eyes was enlarged (6.5 mm), and, if possible, completed *with a transition zone (1-1.5 mm).* Post-ORK showed a *clear visual improvement* (vision median (UCVA) pre-operative: 0.6; (UCVA) postoperative: >=1,0), a *'smoothing'* of the corneal ablation area and a decrease of selective corneal aberrations. From a subjective point of view, the visual acuity was considerably improved (increase of visual acuity and decreased perception of annoying Halos).

This shows us that Selective analysis of corneal wavefront permits an effective treatment of corneal ablation using the Schwind ORK-Software.

CONCLUSION

LASIK has entered its golden era where retreatments are possible to correct past errors, aberrated eyes can be effectively treated and the entire process has become to a great extent "pain-free for the Surgeon".With the new Topographic corneal wavefront, the possibilities for further precise correction is possible. A newer software is under trial, ORK-CAM which will allow greater translation of the corneal wavefront into excimer energy allowing us to treat a greater percentage of aberration.

Evolution and revolution are the markers of human history. *It is not the strongest of the species that survives, nor the most intelligent, but the one* ***most responsive to change.***"—Charles Darwin

FURTHER READING

1. Artal P, Berrio E, Guirao A, Piers P. Contribution of the cornea and internal surfaces to the change of ocular aberrations with age. J Opt Soc Am A 2002;19:137-43.
2. Roberts C. The cornea is not a piece of plastic. Editorial J Refract Surgery 2000;16:407-13.
3. Reinstein DZ, Srivannaboon S, Silverman RH, Sutton HFS, Coleman DJ. Limits of wavefront guided customized ablation: Biomechanical and epithelial factors. Inves Ophthalmol Vis Sci (Supple)2002;433942.

4. Reynolds A. Introduction: History of corneal measurement. In Schanzlin D, Robin J (Eds): Corneal topography measuring and modifying the cornea. New York: Springer Verlag, 1991:07-10.
5. Leven JR. The true inventors of the keratoscope and photokeratoscope. The British journal for the History of Science. 1965;2:8:324-42.
6. Gullstrand A. Photographic–Ophthalmometric and clinical Investigations of corneal refraction. Am J OptomArch Am Acad Optom 1966;43:143-214.
7. Koch DD, Foulks GN, Moran CT, Wakil JS. The corneal EyeSys system:accuracy analysis and reproducibility of first generation prototype. J Refract Corneal Surg 1989;6:423-29.
8. Mattioli R, Tripoli N. Corneal GeometryReconstruction with the Keratron videographer. Optom Vis Sci 1997; 74:881-94.
9. Guirao A, Artal P. Corneal wave aberration from videokeratography:accuracy and limitations of the procedure. J Opt Soc Am A 2000;17:955-65.

Zyoptix

14

Amar Agarwal, Ashish Doshi, Sonika Doshi, Nilesh Kanjiani,
Sunita Agarwal, Athiya Agarwal, Ashok Garg (India)

INTRODUCTION

Since as early as middle of 19th century it has been known that the optical quality of human eye suffers from ocular errors (aberrations) besides the commonly known image errors such as myopia, hyperopia and astigmatism.[1] In early 1970's Fyodorov introduced the anterior radial incisions to flatten the central cornea to correct myopia.[2] Astigmatic keratotomy,[3] Keratomileusis and Keratophakia, Epikeratophakia[4] and currently Excimer Laser[5] have been used to manage the various refractive errors. These refractive procedures correct lower order aberrations such as spherical and cylindrical refractive errors however higher order aberrations persist, which affect the quality of vision but may not significantly affect the Snellen visual acuity. Refractive corrective procedures are known to induce aberrations.[6] It is the subtle deviations from the ideal optical system, which can be corrected by wavefront and topography guided (customized ablation) LASIK procedures.[7]

ABERRATIONS

Optical aberration customization can be corneal topography guided which measures the ocular aberrations detected by corneal topography and treats the irregularities as an integrated part of the laser treatment plan. The second method of optical aberration customization measures the wavefront errors of the entire eye and treats based on these measurements.[7] Wavefront analysis can be done either using Howland's aberroscope[8] or a Hartmann Shack wavefront sensor.[9] These techniques measure all the eye's aberrations including second-order (sphere and cylindrical), third-order (coma–like), fourth-order (spherical), and higher order wavefront aberrations. Based on this information an ideal ablation plan can be formulated which treats lower order as well as higher order aberrations.

ZYOPTIX LASER

Zyoptix™ (Bausch and Lomb) is a system for Personalized Vision Solutions, which incorporates Zywave™ Hartmann Shack aberrometer coupled with Orbscan™ II z multi-dimensional device, which generates the individual ablation profiles to be used with the Technolas® 217 Excimer Laser system. Thus this system utilizes combination of wavefront analysis and corneal topography for optical aberration customization.

ORBSCAN

The Orbscan (BAUSCH and LOMB) corneal topography system (Fig. 14.1) uses a scanning optical slit scan that is fundamentally different than the corneal topography that analyses the reflected

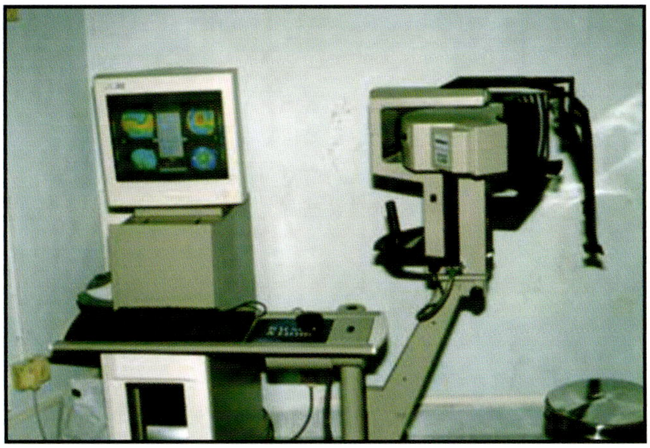

Fig.14.1: Orbscan

images from the anterior corneal surface. The high-resolution video camera captures 40 light slits at 45 degrees angle projected through the cornea similarly as seen during slit lamp examination. The slits are projected on to the anterior segment of the eye: the anterior cornea, the posterior cornea, the anterior iris and anterior lens. The data collected from these four surfaces are used to create a topographic map. This technique provides more information about anterior segment of the eye, such as anterior and posterior corneal curvature and corneal thickness.[10] It improves the diagnostic accuracy and it has passive eye-tracker from frame to frame, 43 frames are taken to ensure accuracy. It is easy to interpret and has good repeatability. Three different maps are taken, and the one featuring the least eye movements is used. The maximum movements considered acceptable are 200μ.

ABERROMETER

Zywave^{TM} is based on Hartmann –Shack aberrometry (Fig. 14.2) in which a laser diode (780 nm) generates a laser beam that is focused on the retina of the patient's eye (Fig. 14.3). An adjustable collimation system compensates for the spherical portion of the refractive error of the eye. Laser diode is turned on for approximately 100 milliseconds. The light reflected from the focal point on the retina (source of wavefront) is directed through an array of small lenses (lenslet) generating a grid like pattern (array) of focal points (Fig. 14.4). The position of the focal points are detected by Zywave^{TM} .Due to deviation of the points from their ideal position, the wavefront can be reconstructed. Wavefront display shows (a) higher order aberrations (b) predicted phoropter refraction (PPR) calculated for a back vertex correction of 15mm.(c) Simulated point spread function (PSF). Zywave^{TM} examinations are done with (a) single examination with undilated pupil (b) five examinations with dilated pupil (mydriasis) non-cycloplegic, using 5% Phenylephrine drops. One of these five measurements, which matched best with the manifest refraction of the undilated pupil, is chosen for the treatment.

ZYLINK

Information gathered from Orbscan and Zywave are then translated into treatment plan using Zylink^{TM}

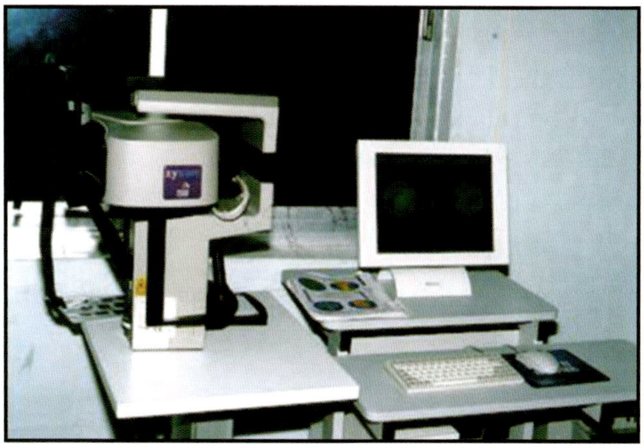

Fig.14.2: Hartmann Shack Aberrometer

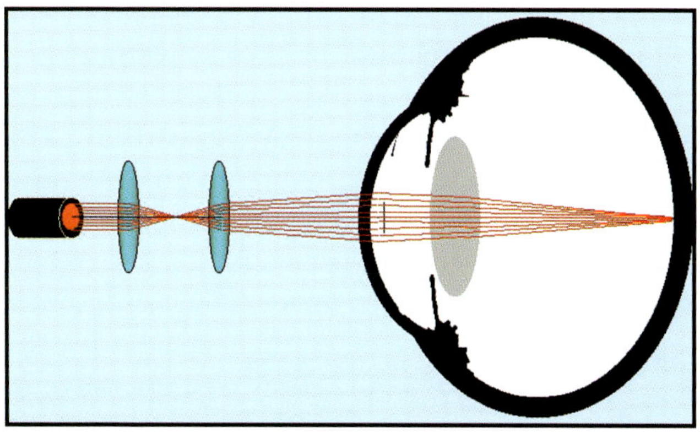

Fig.14.3: Zywave projects low-intensity HeNe infrared light into the eye and use the diffuse reflection from the retina

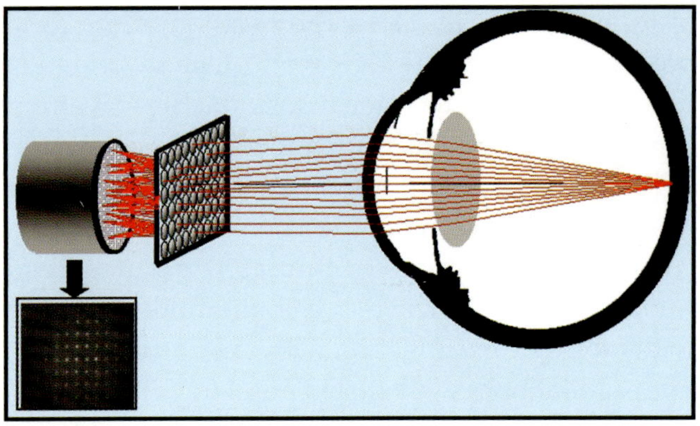

Fig.14.4: Schematic illustration of the Bausch and Lomb Zywave aberrometer. A low-intensity HeNe infrared light is shone into the eye; the reflected light is focused by a number of small lenses (lenslet-array), and pictured by a CCD camera. The capture image is shown on the bottom left

software and copied to a floppy disc. The floppy disc is then inserted into the Technolas 217 system (Fig. 14.5), fluence test carried out and a Zyopitx treatment card was inserted. A standard LASIK procedure is then performed with a superiorly hinged flap. A Hansatome^{TM} microkeratome is used to create a flap. Flap thickness varied from 160 μm to 200 μm. A residual stromal bed of 250 μm or more is left in all eyes. Optical zone varied from 6 to 7 mm depending upon the pupil size and ablation required. Eye tracker is kept on during laser ablation. Post–operatively all patients are followed up for at least 6 months.

Results

We did a study comprising 150 eyes with myopia and compound myopic astigmatism. Pre-operatively, the patients underwent corneal topography with Orbscan II z^{TM} and wavefront analysis with Zywave^{TM} in addition to the routine pre-LASIK work up. The results were assimilated using Zylink^{TM} and a customized treatment plan was formulated. LASIK was then performed with Technolas® 217 system. All the patients were followed up for at least six months.

Mean pre-operative BCVA (in decimal) was 0.83 ± 0.18 (Range 0.33- 1.00). Mean post-operative (6 months) BCVA was 1.00 ± 0.23 (Range 0.33 - 1.50). Difference was statistically significant (p = 0.0003). Out of 150 eyes that underwent customized ablation, 3 eyes (2%) lost two or more lines of best spectacle corrected visual acuity (BSCVA).

Safety Index = Mean post-operative BSCVA / Mean pre-operative BSCVA = 1.20 (Fig.14. 6). Mean pre-operative UCVA was 0.06 ± 0.02 (Range 0.01-0.50). Mean post-operative UCVA was 0.88 ± 0.36 (Range 0.08 – 1.50). Difference was statistically significant (p = 0.0001).

Efficacy index = Mean post-operative UCVA / Mean pre-operative UCVA = 14.66 (Fig.14.7). Pre-operatively, none of the eyes had UCVA of 6\6 or more and one eye (0.66%) had UCVA of 6/12 or more. At 6 months post-operatively, 105 eyes (69.93%) had UCVA of 6\6 or more and 126 eyes (83.91%) had UCVA of 6/12 or more.

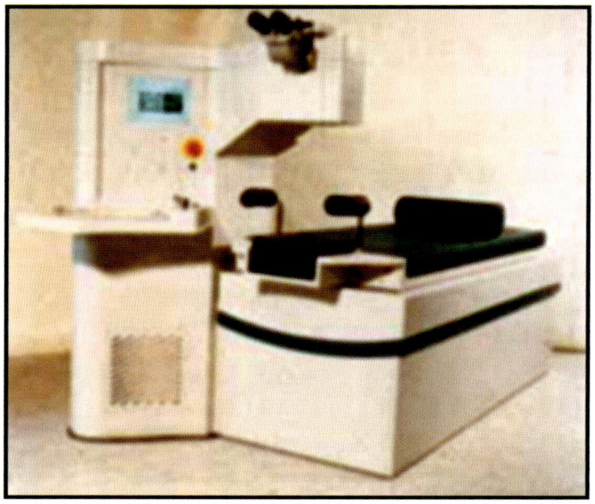

Fig.14.5: Technolas 217 z excimer laser system

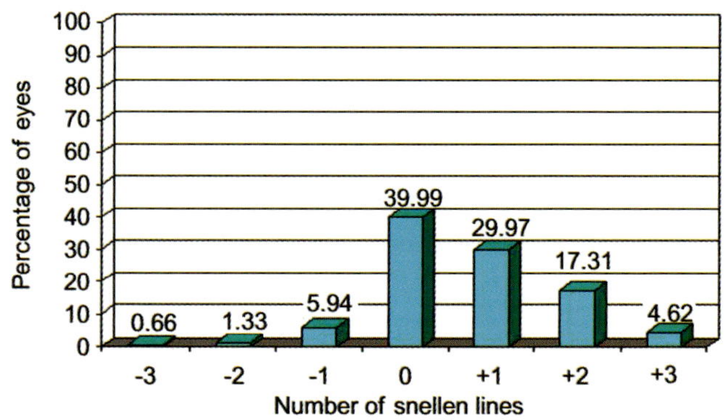

Fig.14.6: Shows changes in BSCVA 6 months post-operatively (Safety)

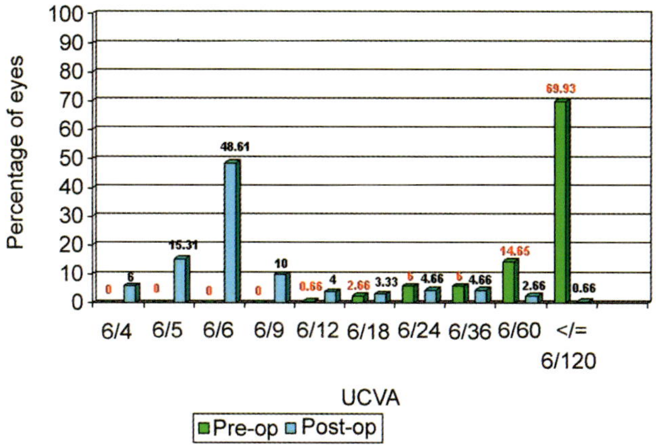

Fig.14.7: Compares pre-op and post-op UCVA (Efficacy)

Mean pre-operative spherical equivalent was -5.25 D ± 1.68 D (Range –0.87 D to –15 D). Mean post-operative spherical equivalent (6 months) was –0.36 D ± 0.931 D (Range –4.25 D to +1.25). Difference between the two was statistically significant ($p < 0.05$) (Fig. 14.8). 132 eyes (87.91%) were within ± 1.00 D of emmetropia while 120 eyes (79.92%) were within ± 0.05 D of emmetropia. 1 eye (0.66%) was overcorrected by > 0.5 D and 1 eye (0.66%) was overcorrected by >1D. The mean pupil diameter was 5.1mm ± 0.62mm. Preoperatively, 95 eyes (63.27%) had third order aberrations.42 eyes (28%) had second order aberration alone, while 13 eyes (8.65%) had fourth and fifth order aberrations. Post-operatively, 60 eyes (40%) had third order aberration 75 eyes (50%) had second order alone while 15 eyes (10%) had higher order aberrations.

DISCUSSION

Hartmann – Shack wavefront sensor was first used by Liang and colleagues to detect ocular aberrations.[11] They applied an adaptive optics deformable mirror to correct the lower and higher order aberrations of the eye. They reported a 6 times increase in contrast sensitivity to high spatial frequency when the pupil was large. This study demonstrated that correction of higher order aberrations could lead to supernormal vision in normal eyes.

In our series, using Zyoptix and Technolas 217 system, which is wavefront and corneal topography guided, we yielded results that are comparable to standard LASIK procedure.[12] In a series of 347 eyes, McDonald et al [12] reported a post-operative refraction of –0.29 ± 0.45 D (-0.36 ± 0.93 D in our series) with standard LASIK. 57% of the eyes in their series had post-operative UCVA of e"6/6. In our study, 70% of the eyes had UCVA of e"6/6, six months post-operatively.

Higher order aberrations were reduced post-operatively in our study. Third-order aberration (coma) was most common in our series, followed by second-order (defocus and astigmatism) and fourth-order (spherical aberration). Post-operatively, after

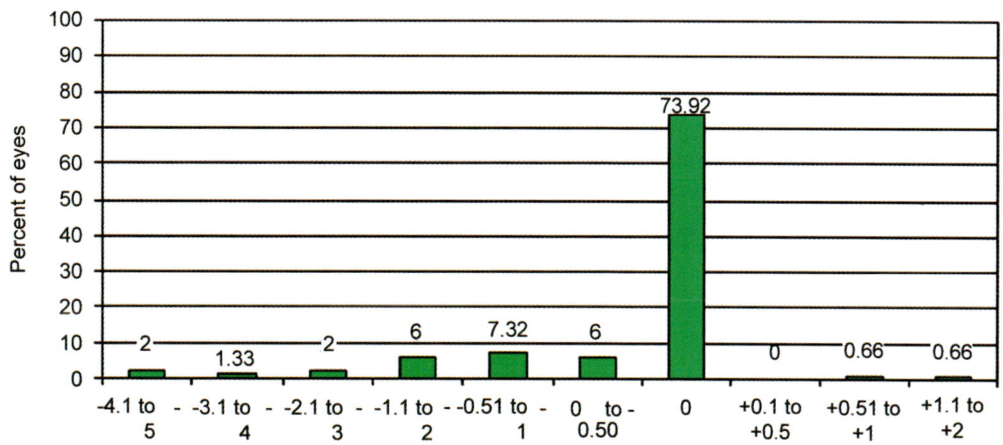

Fig.14.8: Shows the refractive results post-operatively after 6 months

6 months, there was considerable decrease in third-order and fourth-order aberrations. While most of the eyes had only defocus and astigmatism (i.e. second -order aberration). A slight increase in fourth-order aberration (spherical) was noted. Spherical aberration is known to increase after LASIK.[13-15] Roberts has reported that cornea changes its shape in response to ablation and this change, along with wound healing effects have to be taken into account before customized correction can nullify higher-order aberrations. Roberts and coworkers suggest that increase in spherical aberrations following LASIK may be caused by a biomechanically induced steepening and thickening that may occur in mid periphery of the cornea.[13] MacRae and coworkers have reported that simply creating a LASIK flap increases higher-order aberrations in unpredictable manner.[14] They suggest that improved results can be obtained using a surface ablation such as PRK or LASEK, or by doing a two-stage LASIK, with the second stage adjusting for the aberration created by the flap and initial ablation.

Scotopic visual complaints have been the bugbear of LASIK procedures, ranging from mild annoyance to server optical disability.[16, 17] Nighttime starbursts, reduced contrast sensitivity and haloes are the most common complaints.[16,17] Spherical aberration that is induced during LASIK may account for this scotopic complaints.[14] Pupil diameter is another factor that is important. When pupil diameter is large, as in young patients, dim light vision is improved after customized correction.[18, 19] In our series, 11% of the patients complained of haloes around light at night and difficult night driving. In dim light, the mean pupil diameter in these patients was 4.2 mm while it was 5.9 mm in other patients. Smaller pupil diameter and induced higher-order aberration may account for these scotopic visual complaints.

25% of the patients in our series reported improvement in bright light vision, while 40% showed improvement in dim light vision. A similar improvement was noted by Cox and co-workers (presentation by Cox IG at Zyoptix Alliance meeting, 2002 reported in *Ocular Surgery News*, July 2002 volume 13, number 7). In our series, treatment optical zone ranged from 6 to 7 mm. Treatment with larger optical zones and transition zones as compared to conventional LASIK may be possible since entire corneal topography and not just the central cornea overlying pupil along with wavefront ablation in dilated pupil are considered during treatment. This may induce lesser spherical aberration post-LASIK and account for improved scotopic vision.

Though we did not measure contrast sensitivity and glare acuity post-operatively, our results suggest improved quality of vision and fewer glare problems with Zyoptix treatment. A more temporal appraisal of the procedure has to be carried out with comparison to standard LASIK. Short-term results suggest wavefront and topography guided LASIK may be a safe and effective procedure which improves the visual performance.

CONCLUSION

Wavefront and topography guided LASIK procedure leads to better visual performance by decreasing higher order aberration. Scotopic visual complaints may be reduced with this method.

REFERENCES

1. Helmholtz H. Handbuch der physiologischen optik. Leipzig: Leopold Voss.1867;137-47.
2. Fyodorov SN, Durnev VV: Operation of dosaged dissection of corneal circular ligament.
3. Binder PS, Waring GO III: Keratotomy for astigmatism. In Waring GO III (Ed.): Refractive keratotomy for myopia and astigmatism. Mosby Year Book 1085–1198, 1992. in cases of myopia of mild degree. Ann Ophthalmol II: 1979;1885-90.
4. Kaufmann HE: Correction of aphakia Am J Ophthalmol 1980;89:1.
5. Mc Ghee CNJ, Taylor HR, Garty DS, et al: Excimer Lasers in Ophthalmology: Principles and Practice Martin Duntz: London, 1997.
6. MacRae S, Porter J, Cox IG, et al. Higher-order aberrations after conventional LASIK. ISRS: Dallas, Texas, 2000.
7. MacRae SM: Supernormal vision, hypervision, and customized corneal ablation. Guest Editorial J Cat Refract Surg 2000;26(2).

8. Howland HC and Howland B, A subjective method for the measurement of monochromatic aberrations of the eye, J Opt Soc Am 1977;67:1508-18.
9. Liang J, Williams DR, Miller DT. Supernormal vision and high-resolution retinal imaging through adaptive optics. J Opt Soc Am 1997;2884-92.
10. Fedor P, Kaufman S Corneal topography and imaging. Medicine Journal, 2001;2(6).
11. Liang J, Williams D. Aberrations and retinal image quality of the normal human eye. J Opt Soc AM A 1997;14: 2884-92.
12. McDonald MB, Carr JD, Frantz JM, et al. Laser in situ keratomilieusis for myopia up to –11 diopters with up to –5 diopters of astigmatism with summit autonomous LADAR Vision excimer laser system. Ophthalmology2001;108:309-16.
13. Roberts C. The cornea is not a piece of plastic. J Refract Surg 2000;16:407-13.
14. MacRae SM, Roberts C, Porter J, et al. The biomechanics of a LASIK flap. ISRS Mid-Summer Meeting: Orlando, Florida, 2001.
15. Applegate RA, Howland HC, Klyce SD. Corneal aberration and refractive surgery. In: MacRae S (Editor). Customized Corneal Ablation. Thorofare NJ: Slack, Inc., 2001.
16. Holladay JT, Dudeja DR, Chang J. Functional vision and corneal changes after laser in situ keratomileusis determined by contrast sensitivity, glare testing, and corneal topography. J Cataract Refract Surg 1999;25: 663-69.
17. Perez-Santonja JJ, Sakla HF, Alio JL. Contrast sensitivity after laser in situ keratomileusis. J Cataract Refract Surg 1998;24:183-89.
18. Applegate R, Howland H, Sharp R, et al. Corneal aberrations and visual performance after refractive keratectomy. J Refract Surg 1998;14:397-407.
19. Oshika T, Klyce S, Applegate R, et al. Comparison of corneal wavefront aberrations after photorefractive keratectomy and laser in situ keratomileusis. Am J Ophthal 1999;127:1-7.

Topography Assisted LASIK

15

Michael C Knorz (Germany),
Maria C Arbelaez (Sultanate of Oman)

INTRODUCTION

The invention of excimer lasers led to a tremendous improvement in the predictability of refractive surgical procedures. By moving the ablation inside the cornea, the introduction of laser-in-situ keratomileusis (LASIK) virtually eliminated scarring and regression, making it possible to treat high myopia as well as hyperopia. By adding LASIK to their spectrum, refractive surgeons were able to treat almost any refractive error.

Besides myopia, hyperopia, and astigmatism, we all know the rare cases with grossly irregular patterns following, e.g. penetrating corneal grafts, penetrating injuries, or peripheral corneal scars that cause irregularity. All these eyes could be treated rather unsuccessfully to date. In these eyes, we wished we had a software to custom-tailor the ablation and that is exactly what topography-assisted LASIK, (TA-LASIK) is about.

A custom-tailored ablation is also extremely useful and ultimately even more important in slight corneal asymmetries. Today, we use standardized and symmetrical ablation pattern, which is similar to buying a suit "off-the-rack". The individual corneas of our patients, however, show a lot of asymmetry. As many as 40 percent of eyes show some degree of asymmetry, and all these eyes would be far better off with a customised laser ablation. TA-LASIK is the ideal tool to create a perfect cornea as it allows us to reshape the cornea in any pattern we may decide. All that is required is corneal topography (Technomed C-Scan or EyeSys), the proprietary software, a Hansatome microkeratome (Bausch and Lomb Surgical), and a Keracor 117C or 217 excimer laser from Bausch and Lomb Surgical.

HOW DOES TA-LASIK WORK?

As in all refractive procedures, the first requirement to be met is stability of the cornea. It does not make sense to operate as long as the shape of the cornea is still changing. There should be a time interval of at least one year following penetrating grafts or large penetrating injuries. In small scars, of course, the interval could be shorter. Whenever uncertain, the surgeon should wait for three months and reexamine the patient. Now, as soon as the cornea is stable, a corneal topography is taken in the routine fashion. This topographic map should be of as high a quality as possible because it is used as the basis of the ablation. This means that the lids are wide open, that the tear film is regular, that there are no "dark spots" on the map, that the picture is well centered and well focused, and that the entrance pupil is visible on the map. All these requirements are easy to meet for experienced observers in normal corneas, but sometimes quite difficult in abnormal ones, which are the corneas we will treat with TA-LASIK. If it is not possible to obtain a good picture, the examination should be repeated at a later date. It is also a good idea to perform topography prior to any other examinations. In addition, we learned from mistakes in the beginning and now require a set of three topographic maps taken at the same day to calculate the ablation.

Assuming perfect maps were obtained, the respective data files are exported onto a disk which is either physically or electronically transferred to Bausch and Lomb Surgical Technolas, Munich, Germany. This procedure is state-of-the-art even today. Later on, the required software will definitely be available either on the laser or on the topography unit. The respective software then converts measurements of radii of curvature to true height values. Based on the height, the ablation is calculated by a proprietary algorithm. All we have to do is to tell the software which K-value it should target. This is another tricky issue in very irregular corneas, but only the correct K-value will create an emmetropic eye and therefore an extremely happy patient. Should the K-value not be accurate, however, this will result in some spherical deviations from emmetropia which is still much better than an irregular cornea. To establish the actual K-value of a specific cornea, we used topographic maps (normalized scale) and subjectively estimated the average refractive power of the part of the cornea overlying the entrance pupil. In irregular corneas, this requires some guessing.

In addition to the K-value, we must provide the diameter of the desired ablation zone and, of course, pachymetry of the central cornea. Pachymetry is especially important in repair procedures following previous refractive surgery, e.g. PRK (photorefractive keratectomy) or LASIK. The cornea is thinner after PRK or LASIK, which leaves less space for further ablations. Therefore, it is very important to measure corneal thickness in these cases.

After all parameters are set, the computer will calculate a treatment based on the corneal topography of the individual eye.

CASE REPORTS

Patient CW: Irregular Astigmatism after Penetrating Injury

This 6-year-old patient had suffered a penetrating injury in her left eye. A light bulb exploded, and glass fragments penetrated her eye, causing corneal lacerations extending from 10 to 12 O'clock peripherally. One year after the initial repair, scar formation caused significant irregular astigmatism. Uncorrected visual acuity (UCVA) was 20/200. With a correction of +0.5 sphere –5.0 cyl axis 170°, an acuity of 20/100 was achieved. Contact lenses were tried but not tolerated by the patient. Corneal topography showed marked irregular astigmatism. Therefore, the authors discussed treatment options with the parents of this child. As contact lenses were not tolerated, surgery seemed to be the only option to prevent amblyopia. We considered T-cuts, corneal grafts and TA-LASIK. LASIK was selected as the least invasive and most predictable option. Surgery was performed under general anesthesia. Figure 15.1 shows the topographic work place on which the ablation is planned. The preoperative topographic map (scale in diopters) is on the upper left, and the ablation profile suggested by the TA-LASIK software (scale in μm) is on the upper right. On the lower left, the surgeon can add individual fudge factors, and the expected result is displayed on the lower right hand side. Comparing maps, we can see that the flat area at the lower right (blue colors) of the preoperative topography map is steepened by the ablation (red color at the lower right of the ablation map). Superposing the two maps in the upper row, the resulting map, which is displayed at the lower right, should be a perfect sphere, at least theoretically.

Figure 15.2 shows the results of the calculated ablation we just described. The preoperative topographic map and the topographic map one day after surgery are shown in Figure 15.2. The color scale is the same in both maps, which can therefore directly be compared. As clearly visible, the steep area on the upper left is considerably flatter, and visual acuity

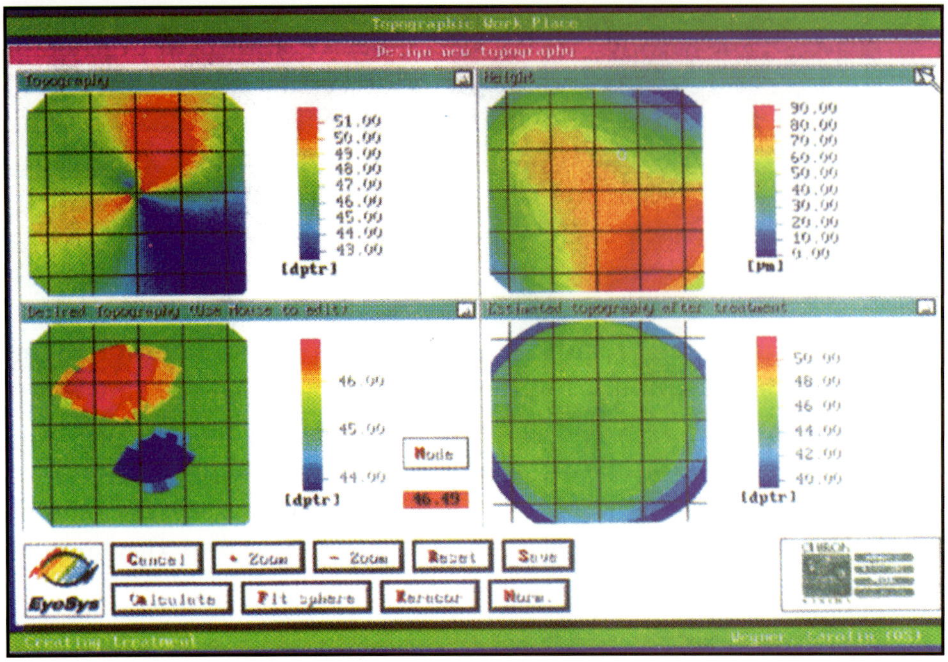

Fig. 15.1: Topographic workplace used to design the ablation of patient CW. The preoperative topographic map (scale in diopters) is on the upper left, and the ablation profile suggested by the TA-LASIK software (scale in µm) on the upper right. On the lower left, the surgeon can add individual fudge factors, and the expected result is displayed on the lower right hand side

without correction improved to 20/60 on day one. Figure 15.2 also shows the differential map. The change map, which visualizes the ablation that was performed, closely resembles the planned ablation (see Fig. 15.1, upper right, for comparison). One year after surgery, visual acuity without correction was 20/80, and with correction of –2 cyl axis 140° acuity was 20/60. To prevent amblyopia, the right eye was occluded 4 hours a day. Corneal topography at one year shows considerable regression of effect. The cornea was still more regular than preoperatively, but most of the effect had regressed. We considered a retreatment and calculated an ablation of 50 µ. Preoperatively, corneal thickness was 587 µ. Flap thickness was 160 µ, and ablation depth during the first TA-LASIK procedure was 86 µ. Central corneal thickness after the first procedure was 430 µ. We therefore decided against a retreatment to avoid possible late keratectasia due to corneal thinning.

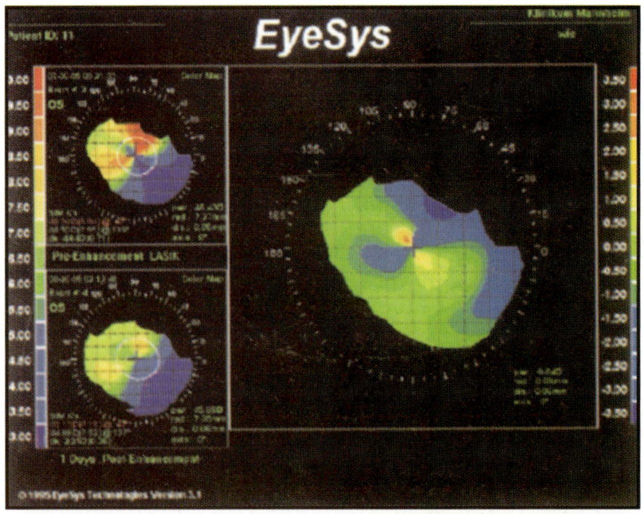

Fig. 15.2: Pre- and postoperative topographic maps and differential map of patient CW (penetrating injury with irregular astigmatism)

Patient AT: Decentered Ablation after PRK

Mr AT is a 40-year-old patient who had PRK in his right eye in July 1994 (Meditec MEL 60 excimer laser). His preoperative refraction was –8 D in his right eye. After PRK, he complained about halos and double vision, most pronounced in dim light and at night, and had refused PRK in his second eye because of these problems. He was referred to us for possible retreatment. Corneal topography revealed a small ablation zone which was also decentered superotemporally (Fig. 15.3, upper left). The average refractive power of the cornea overlaying the entrance pupil was estimated to be 41 D. UCVA was 20/30, spectacle-corrected visual acuity (SCVA) was 20/20 (–1.0 sphere –1.5 cyl axis 160°). Central corneal thickness was 469 μ. We decided to perform TA-LASIK. Considering a corneal refraction of, on average, 41 D and a manifest spherical equivalent (SE) of –1.75 D, we aimed for a target K-value (corneal refraction) of 39 D. Optical zone size was 6 mm, ablation depth 95 μ. As a flap thickness of 160 μ was used, this left a stromal bed of roughly 200 μ which we consider to be the minimum in order to avoid possible late ectasia. Corneal topography at day 1 shows a much larger ablation zone (Fig. 15.3, center). Visual acuity was 20/20 without correction on day one, and the halos had disappeared. Visual acuity and refraction remained stable throughout the postoperative follow-up which is now 6 months. Corneal topography is shown in Figure 15.3. The STARS display allows for evaluation of both the surgical change and the healing change, or regression. The differential map on the lower left (surgical change) shows that the ablation zone was enlarged and the central astigmatism was removed. The map on the lower right shows some regression of effect, indicated by the steepening (red colors) around the edge of the ablation zone.

Patient DK: Irregular Astigmatism after PKP and RK

The patient, a judge at a local court, had had a penetrating corneal graft because of recurrent stromal herpetic keratitis in 1992. He was first referred in 1993. Manifest refraction was +0.25 sphere –6 cyl axis 135°. Corneal astigmatism was –8 D axis 135° and slightly asymmetric. Initially, astigmatic keratotomy was performed in 1994. After AK, manifest refraction was –2.5 sphere –4 cyl axis 165°. UCVA was 20/400 and best-corrected visual acuity (BCVA) was 20/60. Corneal topography showed marked irregularity and axis shift (Fig. 15.4, upper left). We therefore decided to perform TA-LASIK. Average refractive power of the cornea overlaying the entrance pupil was estimated to be 45 D. Spherical equivalent of manifest refraction was –4.5 D. We therefore selected a target K-value of 40.5 D. A 5.4-mm optical zone was used, and ablation depth was 150 μ. Corneal thickness was 610 μ centrally, and both the internal and external margins of the graft were well aligned with the host cornea. It is very important to check alignment prior to the lamellar cut. In poor alignment or localized ectasia at the edge, corneal thickness might be reduced, and the keratome cut may cause further weakening of

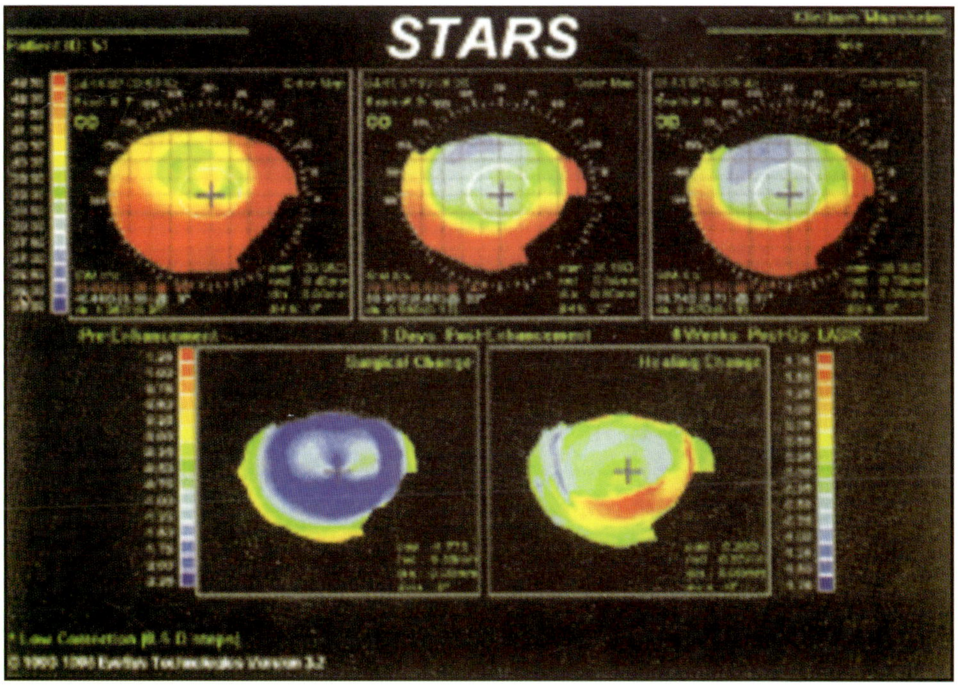

Fig. 15.3: STARS display of patient AT (decentered ablation after PRK). The preoperative map is shown on the upper left, the map on day 1 in the center, and the map at 1 month on the upper right. The differential map on the lower left (surgical change) shows that the ablation zone was enlarged and the central astigmatism was removed. The map on the lower right (healing change) shows some regression of effect, indicated by the steepening (red colors) around the edge of the ablation zone

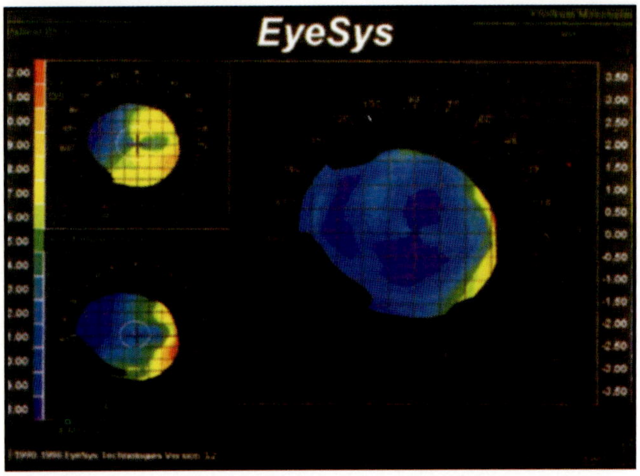

Fig. 15.4: Pre- and postoperative topographic maps and differential map of patient DK (irregular astigmatism after PKP and RK)

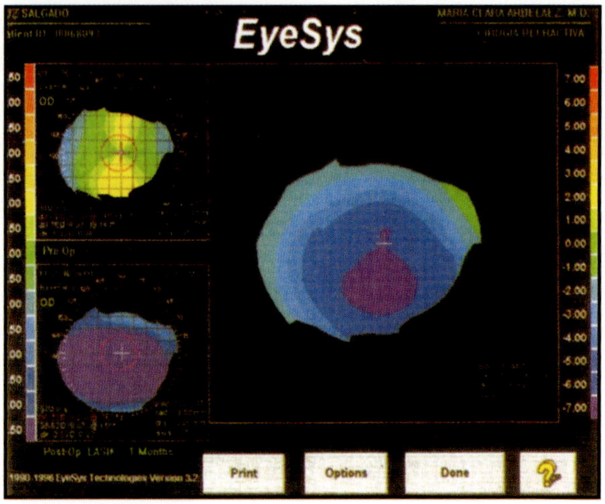

Fig. 15.5: Pre- and postoperative topographic maps and differential map of patient ASJ (asymmetric WTR-astigmatism)

the cornea, inducing more ectasia, or even a penetration of the anterior chamber. In this patient, alignment was perfect, and the LASIK procedure performed in July 1997 was uneventful. A 160 μ flap was used. One day after TA-LASIK, UCVA had improved to 20/30, and BCVA was 20/25 (correction: +0.75 sphere). After 4 months, UCVA was 20/30 and BCVA 20/25, but manifest refraction had changed slightly to +1 sphere –2.0 cyl axis 10°. Corneal topography 4 months after TA-LASIK showed marked improvement of the irregularity (Fig. 15.4). Some residual with-the-rule (WTR) astigmatism was still present, but the irregular astigmatism which was present preoperatively had virtually disappeared as shown by the differential map (Fig. 15.4).

Patient ASJ: Asymmetric WTR-Astigmatism

This patient is an excellent example for the use of TA-LASIK in a cornea with "just" some asymmetric astigmatism. Remember, as many as 40 percent of human corneas show some asymmetries like the one shown here ! This 29-year-old lady had a refraction of –7 sphere –1.25 cyl axis 170° in her right eye. SCVA was 20/20. Corneal topography showed asymmetric WTR-astigmatism, with the lower half-meridian being steeper than the upper half-meridian (Fig. 15.5, upper left). A symmetrical ablation pattern would have left part of the astigmatism in the lower half-meridian. We therefore decided to perform TA-LASIK in this patient. Preoperative pachymetry was 579 μ. An optical zone size of 5 mm was used. Flap thickness was 160 μ, and ablation depth was 109 μ.

On day 1, UCVA was 20/30 and BCVA (+1.25) was 20/20. At 1 month.

UCVA was 20/20, and results remained stable throughout the follow-up period of 6 months. Corneal topography showed a spherical surface after the ablation (Fig. 15.5, lower left). The differential maps nicely demonstrates the asymmetric ablation performed—flattening was greater in the lower half-meridian than in the upper half-meridian, as clearly visible by the asymmetric blue bow-tie pattern (Fig. 15.5).

PATIENTS AND RESULTS

In a prospective, noncomparative case series, we operated 29 consecutive eyes of 27 patients between July 1996 and July 1997. All eyes have one year follow-up, and the data were presented at the annual meeting of the American Academy of Ophthalmology in New Orleans in 1998. Results were evaluated in four groups:

Group 1 (post-keratoplasty group) consisted of six eyes (five patients) with irregular corneal astigmatism after penetrating keratoplasty. All grafts were performed more than 2 years ago.

Group 2 (post-trauma group) consisted of six eyes (six patients) with irregular corneal astigmatism after corneal trauma. The trauma dated back more than 2 years in all eyes.

Group 3 (decentered/small optical zones group) consisted of 11 eyes (10 patients) with irregular corneal astigmatism after PRK (one eye) or LASIK (10 eyes) due to decentered or small optical zones. All patients complained about halos and image distortion even during the day.

Group 4 (central islands group) consisted of six eyes (six patients) with irregular astigmatism after PRK (two eyes) or LASIK (four eyes) due to central islands or keyhole patterns. All patients complained about blurred vision or image distortion even during the day.

Corneal topography was performed using the corneal analysis system (EyeSys System 2000, Software Version 3.10 and 3.20, EyeSys Premier, Irvine, CA) and more recently the Technomed C-Scan (Technomed Co., Baesweiler, Germany). The topographic changes from the preoperative examination to the postoperative examination at 12 months were subjectively graded as follows—planned correction fully achieved (irregularity less than 1 D and optical zone size as predicted), attempted correction partially achieved (decrease of irregularity of more than 1 D on the differential map and/or increase of optical zone size by at least 1 mm), flattening or steepening of the corneal contour level only, no change of irregularity (change 1 D or less on differential map), no change at all. The term "topographic success rate" (Table 15.1) was introduced and defined to include eyes in which the planned correction was fully achieved and eyes in which the planned correction was partially achieved. In addition, a short questionnaire was completed 12 months after surgery by all patients. Patients were asked to rate their satisfaction with the result of the surgery (high, moderate, not satisfied).

The results of all groups are given in Table 15.1. In the postkeratoplasty group, corrective cylinder was significantly reduced as compared to the preoperative

Table 15.1: Refraction, visual acuity, corneal topography, and patient satisfaction 12 months after topographically-guided LASIK

	Group 1 postkeratoplasy	*Group 2 posttrauma*	*Group 3 decentered/small*	*Group 4 central islands*
No. of eyes	n = 6	n = 6	n = 11	n = 6
Cylinder preoperatively	5.83 +/− 1.25 D (4.00 to 8.00 D)	2.21 +/− 1.35 D (1.00 to 5.00 D)	0.73 +/− 0.71 D (0 to 2.00 D)	1.42 +/− 1.13 D (0 to 3.50 D)
Cylinder at 12 months	2.96 +/− 1.23 D* (1.50 to 4.50 D)	0.50 +/− 0.84 D** (0 to 2.5 D)	0.36 +/− 1.05 D (0 to 3.5 D)	0.50 +/− 0.84 D* (0 to 2.00 D)
UCVA improved 2 or more lines	83%	83%	55%	50%
UCVA +/−1 line	17%	17%	36%	17%
UCVA lost 2 or more lines	0%	0%	9%	33%
Topographic success rate	66% (n = 4)	83% (n = 5)	91% (n = 10)	50% (n = 3)
Patient response: "Very satisfied"	66% (n = 4)	66% (n = 4)	18% (n = 2)	34% (n = 2)
Patient response: "Moderately satisfied"	17% (n = 1)	0%	46% (n = 5)	0%
Patient response: "Not satisfied"	17% (n = 1)	34% (n = 2)	36% (n = 4)	66% (n = 4)
Reoperation rate	50% (n = 3)	50% (n = 3)	36% (n = 4)	50% (n = 3)

SE—spherical equivalent of manifest refraction, UCVA—uncorrected visual acuity, * p—0.01; ** p—0.001

value, and UCVA improved significantly. In the post-trauma group, corrective cylinder was also significantly reduced, and UCVA improved significantly. In the decentered/small optical zones group, both corrective cylinder and SE were reduced, and UCVA improved accordingly, but differences were not statistically significant.

In the central islands group, both corrective cylinder and SE were reduced, and UCVA improved accordingly, but the difference of corrective cylinders was statistically significant only.

Comparing the groups, UCVA improved most in the postkeratoplasty and the posttrauma groups. Results were worst in the central island group, with 33 percent loosing two or more lines of UCVA.

Results of corneal topography were best in the decentered/small optical zones group, with a success rate, defined as the percentage of eye with the planned result and the percentage of eyes that improved, of 91 percent, followed by the posttrauma group with a success rate of 83 percent. The lowest success rate was observed in the central island group, being 50 percent only (Table 15.1).

SUMMARY

We observed a significant improvement of UCVA, a significant reduction of corrective cylinder, and a more regular corneal topography in all but one of the treatment groups. However, results were poor in one group (central islands group). Our results confirm that topographically-guided LASIK works clinically, and that it is clearly indicated in decentered or small optical zones and useful in postkeratoplasty and posttrauma irregularities. Following refinement of targeting, ablation algorithms, and corneal topography systems, topographically-guided LASIK will in the near future be a tool to create hard-contact lens vision in patients with irregular or asymmetric corneas. Topography-assisted LASIK will take refractive surgery to new limits by ultimately providing a quality of vision which is better than ever before in those 40 percent of patients with corneal irregularities.

Bifocal Profiles and Strategies of Presbyopic-LASIK

16

JT Lin (USA)

INTRODUCTION

Bifocal corneal reshaping using laser in situ keratomileusis (LASIK) procedure to create either a central-myopia island or peripheral-myopia ring for near vision has been recently reported as an alternative for presbyopia treatment.[1-3] The intent of the presbyopic-LASIK procedure is to achieve a pseudo-accommodation[1,2] versus the true-accommodation achieved by the modification of sclera or ciliary body.[4] Combining with the conventional LASIK nomogram, bifocal reshaping may be used to treat presbyopic patients having myopia or hyperopia. The reported results presented the clinical strategies and the refractive outcomes without showing the actual algorithms behind and their limitations.

A multi-step procedure based on the linear superposition (LSP) (either subtraction or addition) of ablation profiles could simultaneously correct aged patents' far vision while creating a central or peripheral myopia for near vision. This Chapter will present formulas for the limitations of LSP, the change OF corneal asphericity and compare two treatment strategies for presbyopic-LASIK. As shown in Fig. 16.1(A) for center myopia (CM) to see near and with peripheral to see far; and Fig. 16.1(B) for peripheral myopia (PM) to see near whereas the center to see far.

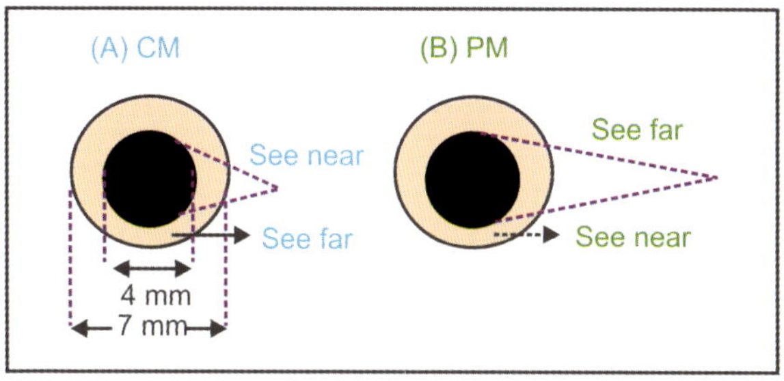

Fig. 16.1: Presbyopia-LASIK using bifocal corneal profile for (A) center-myopia (CM) and (B) peripheral myopia (PM)

TWO-STEP STRATEGY

The two-step strategy for correction myopic or hyperopic presbyopia (having a refractive error of D1 and D2, respectively) is based on the LSP of their ablation profiles f12 = f1 + f2 given by (derived in Appendix).

$$f12 = Z_0(1\text{-}aC_1d^2) + 1.33D12\,(1\text{-}aC_2y^2), \qquad (1)$$
$$C_1 = (p1\text{-}Bp2)/D1$$
$$C_2 = (p2\text{-}Ap3)/D12$$
$$a = 3/(32R1^3)$$

where $Z_0 = -DW^2/3$ being the first-order ablation depth of myopic correction [6] defined by the ablation diameter W. A and B are defined in the Appendix Eq.(A.1). D12 = D1 + D2 provides the additive (subtraction) power when D1 and D2 have the same (opposite) signs. The shape factors of p1, p2 and p3 stand for pre- and postoperative value of myopia and after hyperopia, respectively.

The above LSP will represent the resulting profile defined by D12 under two conditions: (a) the cornea surface is perfectly spherical (or p1 = p2 = p3 = 1.0, with asphericity Q = 0); and (b) the first-order approximation is valid (or when C1 = C2 = 0) such that the LSP profile f12 is independent to the preoperative corneal radius R1 and only characterized by D12.

For example, when D12 = 0 (or D1 = – D2), f12 stands for a profile parallel to the preoperative corneal surface, or equally shifted by Z_0 (the central ablation depth), and there is no refractive power change. This strategy of complete cancellation of refractive power (D1 = – D2) may be used to produce a wider transition zone, or larger effective zone, or for the treatment of off-centered eye followed by an enlargement of the treated area. Further discussions are shown in Appendix.

In general the LSP profile is affected by the corneal initial shape factor (p1) and the resulting values (p2 and p3) after the myopia-hyperopia combined procedures. These factors may contribute to only about 5% of the first-order central depth (Z_0). However, they are the key elements defining the change of corneal asphericity or its shape from prolate to oblate or vice versa.

COMPARISON OF ABLATION PROFILES

Case (a) initial cornea surface is spherical or p1 = p2 = p3 = 1.0; or asphericity Qj = 1-pj = 0. Eq.(1) becomes

$$f12 = Zo(1 - C'd^2) + (1.33D12)\, y^2 \quad (2.a)$$
$$C' = a\,(1 - B)/D1. \quad (2.b)$$

It shows that LSP profile f12 characterized by D12. For example, as discussed earlier, when D12 = 0 (or D1 = – D2), f12 stands for a profile parallel to the preoperative corneal surface.

Case (b) with the second-order correlation of Eq.(A.5) with N = N′ = 1, f12 becomes

$$f12 = Z_0 + (1.33D12)\, y^2 [1-(a/D12)(1-B^{-2})(p1)y^2] \quad (3)$$

which, when D1 = – D2, further reduces to

$$f12 = Z_0 - 1.33a\,(1-B^{-2})(p1)y^4, \quad (4)$$

which shows that the central ablation depth remains as Z_0, but corneal shape changes even when D12 = 0. This y-dependence feature is absent in the spherical case (a).

Case (c) with the nth-order approximation of Eq.(5) with N=N′=2/3, f12 becomes

$$f12 = Z_0 - [1-(a/D1)(1-B^{1/3})(p1)d^2] + (1.33D12)\, y^2[1-(a/D12)(1-B^{-4/3})(p1)y^2], \quad (5)$$

which further reduces to, when D12 = 0,

$$f12 = Z_0\, [1-(a/D1)(1-B^{1/3})(p1)d^2] - (1.33a)(1-B^{-4/3})(p1)y^4 \quad (6)$$

which has an extra term in Z_0 in comparing to Eq.(4), in addition to the difference in the correlation of y^4 term.

CENTRAL ABLATION DEPTHS

In the following, comparison of various approximation for the central ablation depth defined by f12 (y = 0) will be shown for a typical initial corneal anterior surface radius of d = 3.0 mm, R1 = 7.8 mm, a = 0.2 from Eq.(A.2.d) and B = (0.724, 0.882) for D1 = (-5.0, -2.0) diopter, B = (1.13, 1.34) for D2 = (+ 2.0, + 5.0) diopters calculated from Eq.(A.1.e) and Eq.(A.2).

For Case (a) with spherical surface, the central ablation depth from Eq.(2) f12(a) = 1.106 Z_0, for D1 = – 2.0 diopter. For Case (b), f12(b)= Z_0, and for Case (c), f12(c) = Z_0 ((1 + 0.036p1) which depends on the initial corneal shape factor.

For typical p1 value of 0.9 to 0.7 or asphericity Q1 = (p1-1) of -0.1 to -0.3 for a prolate cornea; and p1 = (1.1 to 1.2) for an oblate cornea, f12(c) equals 1.025 to 1.043 Z0 which are only 2 to 4.3% larger than the parabolic value Z0, or about 0.48 to 1.03 microns for Z0 = 24 micron (with D1 = – 2.0 diopter). These calculated values demonstrate that the shape-factor has very small impact on the ablation depth, whereas it plays a major role in the change of primary spherical aberration (PSA) calculated as follows.

BIFOCAL PROFILES (CM AND PM)

For simplicity the following strategies are based on the situation under conditions (a) and (b) described earlier. Table 16.1 compares the strategies based on a center-myopia (CM) with peripheral for distance and on a peripheral-myopia (PM) with center for distance vision. The PM strategies used in Nidek system offer the advantages of better contrast of sensitivity.[1, 2] However, CM would be preferred for a thin corneal and/or high diopter correction as shown in the following examples.

As shown in Table 16.1, case (c) as an example, the – 2.0 D myopic presbyopia (with a near addition of + 3.0 D) may be corrected by PM having two steps: first is to treat a larger zone of W = 7.0 mm at + 3.0D hyperopic correction and followed by a – 5.0 D myopic for the inner zone of 4.0 mm. The LSP provides the center area + 3.0 – 5.0 = – 2.0 D myopic treatment for far vision, whereas the outer zone (ring) has a +3.0 D overcorrection for the presbyopic eye to see near.

The PM method has a maximal ablation depth (MAD) about 3x7x7/3=49 um. In comparison, the CM method in case (c) consists of correcting a ring-shape area (defined between 4 and 7 mm circle) by – 2.0 D myopia which gives the outer ring (or peripheral) to see far. The second step of +1.0 D hyperopic treatment (with W = 4.0 mm) adding to the preoperative – 2.0 D myopia results a center-myopia of – 3.0 D which corrects the presbyopia having a +3.0 D near addition. The MAD in this CM case is about 2 × 7 × 7/3 = 37 um, or 25% less than PM (49 um).

Table 16.1: Strategies of presbyopia-LASIK using a center-myopia island (CM) or peripheral-myopia ring (PM)

Preoperative cases	*Correction diopter (zone size, in mm)* CM	PM
a. Plano	+ 2.0 (W = 7.0)	+ 2.0 (W = 4.0)
NA* = + 2.0 D	– 2.0 (W = 4.0)	No Wring needed
b. Hyperope + 1.0 D	+ 4.0	+ 1.0 (W_{ring})
NA = + 3.0 D	– 3.0	+ 4.0 (W =4.0)
c. Myope –2.0 D	+ 3.0	– 2.0
NA = + 3.0 D	– 5.0	+ 1.0
d. Myope –4.0 D	– 6.0	– 4.0
NA = +2.0 D	+ 2.0	– 2.0

* NA stands for the near addition power of a presbyopic eye.

** Each treatment consists of two steps: a large (7.0 mm) followed by a small (4.0 mm) zone correction in PM; and a ring-zone Wring(4/7 mm) followed by a central zone W = 4.0 in CM.

The advantage of CM over PM becomes even more significant in high-power correction cases. Case (d) shows the MAD of PM is about 6 × 7 × 7/3 = 98 um vs. that of CM 4 × 7 × 7/3 = 65 um (or 34% less); and case (b), MAD = 65 um (for PM) vs. 16 um (for CM).

DISCUSSION

The above calculated MAD values demonstrated that CM always removes less corneal tissue (in both depth and volume) resulted from the lower diopter correction required. Furthermore, the procedure of CM is faster than PM since less corneal tissue is removed, while it suffers worse contrast than that of PM.

The above discussed strategies based on LSP may be extended for non-linear profile or aspherical cornea, except that the ablation depth needs to be revised to include the nonlinear terms C1 and C2 in Eq.(1). For example, the LSP of + 4.0 D (with W = 7.0 mm) and -3.0 D (with W =4.0 mm) would result in +1.0 D hyperopic correction in the center 4.0 mm area using the first-order approximation which is about 0.12 D undervalued comparing to the second-order including C1 term.

The errors of LSP using first-order approximation in PM are significantly reduced in CM which treats the inner zone (4.0 mm) and outer ring-zone independently without using a linear superposition. In addition, the LSP in PM involves with two different ablation zones (4.0 and 7.0 mm) for aspherical surface which would be slightly distorted and f12 is no longer perfectly presenting a combined profile defined only by D12. It is also affected by the nonlinear terms C1 and C2 which are governed by the preoperative and postoperative corneal asphericities.

CONCLUSION

Ametropic presbyopia may be treated via CM or PM strategy which may be analyzed by LSP theory. An improved ablation algorithm shall include the nonlinear terms and asphericity of the cornea which have been ignored in most systems using the spherical Munnerlyn formula. Greater details of aspherical ablation will be presented in another Chapter of Lin in this book.

APPENDIX

The multi-step strategy for correction myopic or hyperopic presbyopia (having a refractive error of D1 and D2) is based on the LSP of their ablation profiles f1 (for myopia) and followed by f2 (for hyperopia) given by the Taylor expansion of conicoid surface, up to the 4th order, as follows:[7,8]

$$f1(y) = -(1.33D1)(d^2 - y^2) + (C1/8R1^3)(d^4 - y^4) \quad (A.1.a)$$

$$f2(y) = (1.33D2)y^2 - (C2/8R2^3)\, y^4 \quad (A.1.b)$$

$$C1 = p1\text{-}Bp2 \quad (A.1.c)$$

$$C2 = p2 - Ap3 \quad (A.1.d)$$

$$B = (R1/R2)^3,\ A = (R2/R3)^3 \quad (A.1.e)$$

where Rj (j = 1, 2, 3, 4) are related to D1 and D2 by using the paraxial formula for refractive error correction and corneal radius changes.[7,8]

$$1/R2 = 1/R1 + D1/0.377 \quad (A.2.a)$$

$$1/R3 = 1/R2 + D2/0.377 \quad (A.2.b)$$

where $Z_0 = -4Dd^2/3$ being the first-order ablation depth of myopic correction [6] defined by the ablation radius d; y is the distance from the optical axis; D12 = D1 + D2 provides the subtraction power because D1 and D2 have opposite signs in the myopia-hyperopia two-step procedure. The shape factors p1, p2 and p3 stand for value of pre- and postoperative myopia and the final state after hyperopia, respectively. Therefore the LSP profile of a myopia-hyperopia procedure is given by f12 = f1 + f2 and becomes Eq.(1) shown in the text.

Depending on the approximation of the Taylor expansion of the conicoid corneal surface, the initial and final shape factors, p1, p2, p3 may be correlated differently. The second-order approximation C1 = C2 = 0 in Eq.(1) which gives p1 = Bp2 and p2 = Ap3. This correlation was also reported by a least-square method.[8] In general, a power relationship may be used to correlate the final and the initial p-factor after a myopia and hyperopia treatment,

$$p2 = B^{-N}p1 \quad (A.3.a)$$

$$p3 = B^{-N'}p2 \quad (A.3.b)$$

where N = N′ = 1 corresponds to the second-order approximation. The n-th order approximation may be obtained by the n-th power Taylor expansion of the conicoid surface having the 2n-power term of y given by

$$(1 - B^{-k})\, p1y^{2n} \quad (A.4.a)$$

$$K = (2n - 1)/3 - (n - 1)N \quad (A.4.b)$$

which has an asymptotic value of N = 2/3 for n >> 1. Therefore, the final p-factor after hyperopia corrections correlated to the initial value (p1) by

$$p3 = B^{-M}p1 \quad (A.5)$$

where M = 2 for the second-order and M = 4/3 for the nth-order approximation, respectively.

In general the LSP profile is affected by the corneal initial shape factor (p1) and the resulting values (p2 and p3) after the myopia-hyperopia combined procedures. These factors may contribute to only about 5% of the first-order central depth (Z_0). However, they are the key elements defining the change of corneal asphericity or its shape change from prolate to oblate or vice versa.

REFERENCES

1. Cantu R, Rosales MA, Tepichin E, Curioca A, Montes V, Ramirez-Zavaleta G. Objective quality of vision in presbyopic and non-presbyopic patients after pseudo-accommodative advanced surface ablation. J Refract Surg 2005;21(Suppl): S603-605.
2. Telando A. Pseudo-accommodative cornea: a new concept for correction of presbyopia. J Refract Surg 2004;20(Suppl):S714-717.

3. Avalos G, Silva A. Presbyopia LASIK-the PMMA technique. In: Agarwal A. ed. Presbyopia, a surgical textbook. Thorofare NJ: SLACK 2004;139-46.
4. Lin JT, Mallo O. Treatment of presbyopia by infrared laser radial sclerotomy. J Refract Surg. 2003;19:465-67.
5. Lin JT. Scanning laser technology for refractive surgery. In: Garg et al. Mastering the techniques of corneal refractive surgery. New Delhi, India, Jaypee Brothers; 2005;20-36.
6. Lin JT. A new formula for ablation depth in 3-zone LASIK. J Refract Surg 2005;21:87-91.
7. Atchison DA, Smith G. Optics of the human eye. Woburn, MA: Butterworth-Heinemann 2000;14-16, 143-147, 160-62.
8. Jimenez JR, Anera RG, Barco LJ. Refractive changes due to ablation parameters after photorefractive surgery. J Refract Surg 2004;20:182.

Presbyopic Multifocal LASIK (PML): A New Approach in Corneal Refractive Surgery

17

Roberto Pinelli (Italy)

In all refractive surgery, our goal has been to surgically correct the visual defects, i.e. myopia, hyperopia, astigmatism, and presbyopia. Correction of these defects is possible through corneal surgical procedures or lenticular surgery.

Of all the visual defects, presbyopia has been the most challenging to correct, partly because the mechanisms of accommodation and the causes of presbyopia are complex and not fully understood. Thus far, it has largely been managed through the use of progressively stronger spectacles, which gradually take over the near focus work of the crystalline lens. Presbyopia is also unique in that it is the only refractive error that is considered to be progressive in nature. Although our management and most of our experience seems to point to the progressive nature of presbyopia, in truth, we don't know for sure that it truly progresses. It may be that in our "prosthetic culture" we have merely become unnecessarily dependent on our glasses and contacts.

In any case, a surgical alternative to the correction of presbyopia is appealing because of the enormous pool of presbyopic patients with a desire for good uncorrected vision. Mild hyperopes and emmetropes who have never worn glasses are particularly uncomfortable with presbyopia and its associated inconveniences.

APPROACHES TO THE SURGICAL CORRECTION OF PRESBYOPIA

The mission of presbyopic surgery-as with all other refractive surgeries-should be to eliminate the symptoms of the refractive error, rather than to correct the anatomical defect itself. For this reason, I think an approach that provides pseudo-accommodation is natural and appropriate. If we can provide patients with good functional vision at multiple distances, it is not necessary to restore true accommodative function in the form of a dynamically adjusting optical power of the eye.

There are several potential sites for correction of presbyopia. The cornea is probably the most common target, as it is the area refractive surgeons are most comfortable operating on. Theoretically, the anterior chamber provides another site for the correction of presbyopia, but this is as yet theoretical and would likely prove extremely difficult in reality. The human crystalline lens can be replaced with a multifocal or accommodative intraocular lens, of which many different styles are now under development and coming to market. Finally, a number of scleral implant or ciliary muscle surgical procedures have been developed. This approach, however, is complicated, largely untested, and seems "more surgical" than is necessary.

As a familiar corneal procedure, LASIK has been the most popular and easiest surgical approach. In addition to the surgeon comfort level with the procedure, patients in the presbyopic baby boomer generation are also familiar with and accepting of the procedure. In addition, LASIK can be performed bilaterally on the same day, is relatively quick and painless, and has proven to be quite safe.

Even with LASIK, we have several options for addressing presbyopia. Most conventionally, we have taken a monofocal approach with surgically-induced monovision, but bifocal and multifocal approaches are increasing. LASIK is ideal for presbyopia because of the absence of haze and its associated refractive complications, the absence of regression, and the presence of a regular and, hopefully, thin flap that can protect the multifocality created in the stroma.

In designing a multifocal LASIK procedure, we must take advantage of some of the lessons learned from current and past procedures. Some myopes treated with radial keratotomy have retained good near and distance vision well into the presbyopic age range. Why is that? Similarly, some hyperopic LASIK patients also have retained their pseudo-accommodative function well into their older years. Again, why would that be? The secret lies in the asphericity of the cornea. A prolate cornea seems to have the capability to focus both far and near better than an oblate cornea. We have seen that again recently with conductive keratoplasty, which I perform and have been involved in studying in Italy. CK is an excellent technique for correcting hyperopia and restoring near vision. It appears to provide some degree of multifocality because eyes corrected for near visual acuity with CK typically have much better distance visual acuity than would be expected. This may be due to the prolateness of the post-CK cornea. In any case, the "blended vision" of CK permits the presbyopic patient to read by treating just the non-dominant eye.

In the past three years, my purpose has been to create a truly multifocal corneal procedure that can be performed bilaterally if necessary, and that will work for any eye, regardless of preoperative refractive error. Intuitively, we know that many zones should do a better job of mimicking natural vision than just two zones, but obtaining a gradual but effective multifocality is nonetheless challenging. The ultimate presbyopic LASIK procedure must also be easy to perform, with standardized nomograms that any surgeon can use as a basis for successful surgery.

The PML™ Procedure

With the above goals in mind, I developed and have been investigating at ILMO a patented procedure which we call PML™ (Presbyopic Multifocal LASIK). This procedure can be performed on presbyopic myopes, hyperopes, astigmats, and emmetropes. Multifocality on the cornea is created using a multi-step treatment in which several independently calculated ablations are performed at various optical zones. Depending on the patient's refractive error, there may be anywhere from three to eight different concentric zones. In all cases, the goal is to treat the central cornea for distance vision, with a multifocal peripheral cornea that is able to provide functional near vision. Some other multifocal LASIK procedures take the opposite approach, with the near correction in the center. However, the central cornea provides an excellent site for distance vision because it is relatively aberration-free, while peripheral aberrations may actually be useful for near focusing.

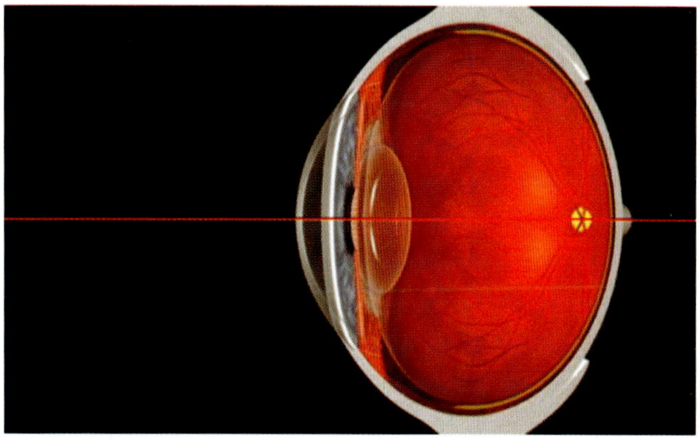

Fig. 17.1: Central area of the cornea: focus on the retina

In this multi-step process, we first treat astigmatism in the classic manner, as if we were doing a purely astigmatic laser correction. Next we treat the distance defect in a zone on the central cornea. Then, we treat the near defect in a larger optical zone. Finally, other zones may be created to ensure that the overall power of the cornea is emmetropic, even though there are varying powers in the different optical zones. It is a procedure that is highly customizable for each patient's optical needs.

I began doing this procedure in 2002, starting cautiously by treating 10 patients in only their non-dominant eyes. One year postoperatively, five of these patients were happy with their outcomes; the other five required retreatment. These unilateral patients experienced some of the benefits and problems of monovision. I became convinced that a bilateral approach would be more effective, and began to adjust and refine the nomograms towards this end.

For our first bilateral study cohort, we treated 100 eyes of 50 patients with. Our studies so far have been performed with the Technolas 217 Z (Bausch and Lomb) and the Lasitome microkeratome (Gebauer). However, the procedure is technology-independent and was designed to work with any keratome and laser combination.

Results

All 50 patients were seeing at least 20/25 for distance and at least J3 for near. Eighty percent had bilateral uncorrected vision of 20/20 or better for distance and

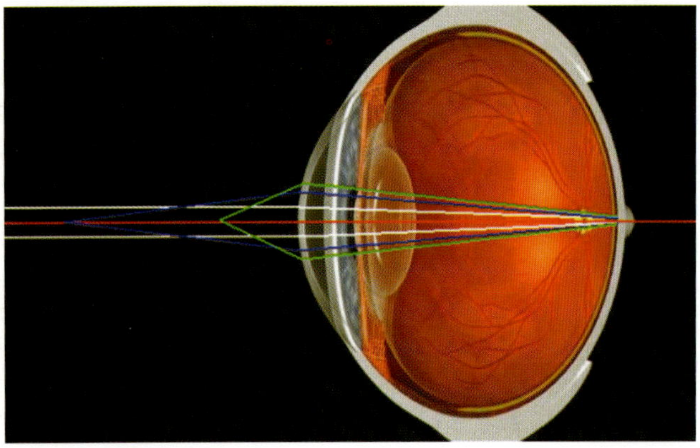

Fig. 17.2: Multifocality permits to focus both far and near objects on macula (pseudo-accommodation)

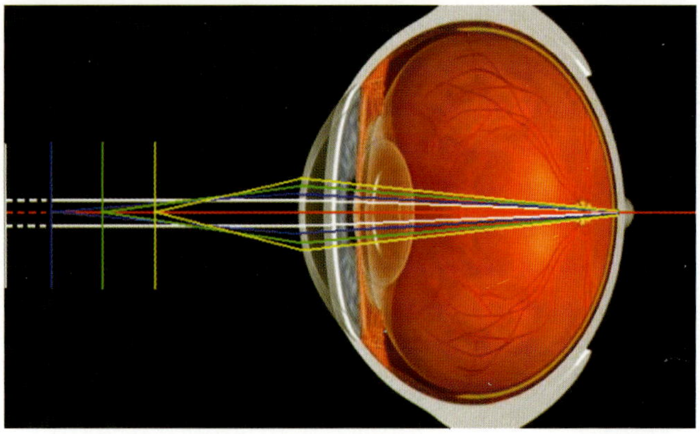

Fig. 17.3: Effects of a completely multifocal cornea

J2 or better for near. Another 10% were 20/25 and J2, while the remaining 10% were 20/25 and J3. Patient satisfaction levels have been very high, and there have been no retreatments thus far. Typically, patients experience a myopic shift during the first month postoperatively, then stabilize at plano.

A few cases illustrate well the potential of this procedure. The first example is a 50-year-old female

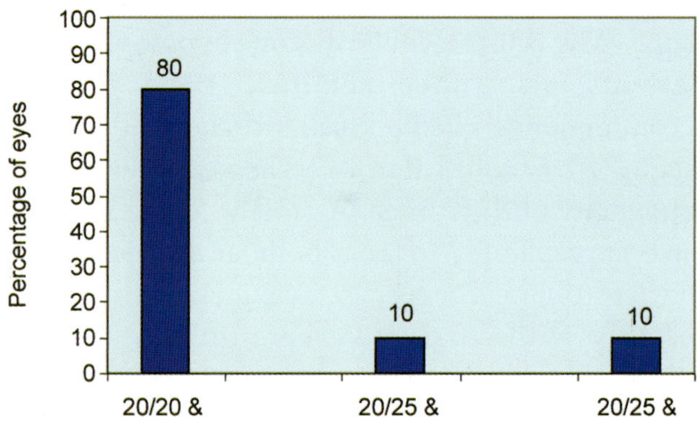

Fig. 17.4: 50 patients' eyes post-op results

who was a -6.0 D myope with a +1.5 D add for reading. We treated the cornea in six different zones: a -1.5 D correction in each of the following optical zones: 4.8, 5.2, 5.4, 5.6, and 6.0 mm; and a +2.00 D correction at the 6.5-mm optical zone. Six months postop, her uncorrected vision is 20/20 and J2 in both eyes.

The second case is a 54-year-old patient who was plano in both eyes preoperatively but using a +1.5 D add for near vision. We performed two treatment

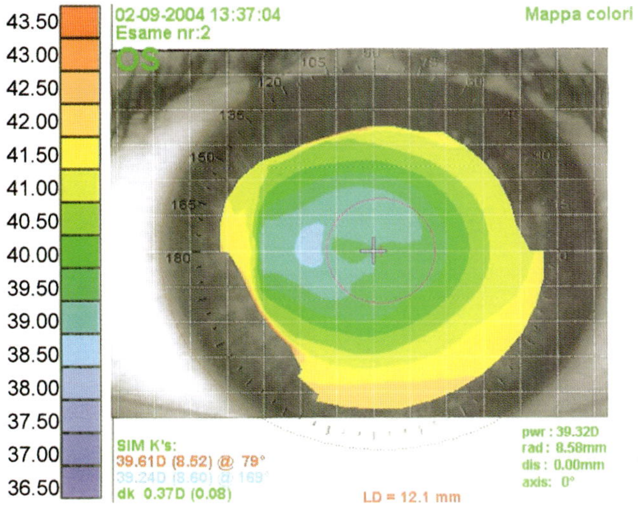

Fig. 17.5: A prolate cornea after PML™ case # 1

rings for near vision, each +0.75 D, at the 6.0 and 6.5-mm optical zones. In addition, I did three treatment rings for distance vision, ablating a –0.50 D spherical correction at the 5.0, 5.2, and 5.4-mm optical zones. After a myopic reaction initially, the eyes are now emmetropic, and six months postop, this patient's uncorrected visual acuity is 20/20 and J2 in both eyes. Ultimately, my goal is to be able to correct emmetropes like this as soon as they start experiencing presbyopic symptoms at age 45 or 50.

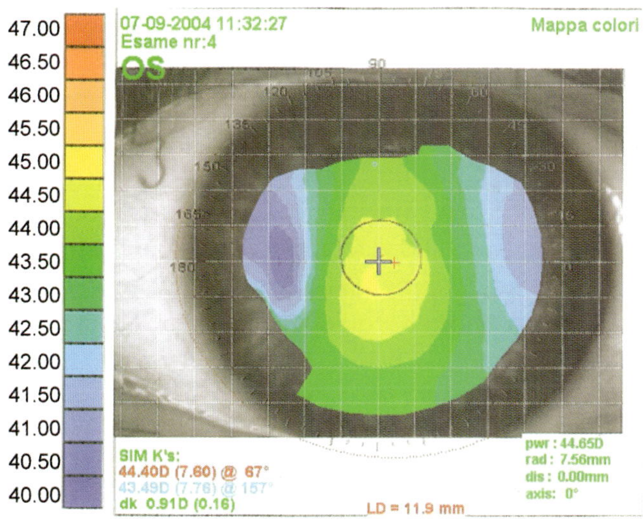

Fig. 17.6: An oblate cornea after PML™ case # 2

Pearls and Lessons Learned

We have found that it is better to overcorrect hyperopia and to undercorrect myopia, and that astigmatism must be fully corrected for a satisfactory outcome. In some cases (hyperopes and emmetropes), the cornea becomes more prolate; in other cases (primarily myopes) it actually becomes more oblate. Pupil size is not an important factor in determining outcomes from this procedure. We have not had to manage patients with especially large pupils any differently than we would with a monofocal LASIK procedure.

The PML™ technique uses the same or less tissue as other laser vision correction procedures, so although pachymetry is important, it is no more a factor than in monofocal LASIK. Keratometry is very important, as it is essential to keep the pre- and post-operative K values constant.

Patients must be willing to participate in training their eyes to learn how to see at near with the multifocal correction. Our patients are instructed not to use reading glasses after the procedure at all and to do visual exercises (for which we provide instruction) in order to maintain the eye's focusing power with age.

In our experience so far, is a very successful procedure that has been well-accepted by patients and is in high demand at our center. Currently, about 30% of our patients are PML™ candidates. The procedure and the excellent results experienced by patients have enhanced the reputation of our center and generated many referrals. Ongoing research is required to determine whether and when regression might occur.

Dr Pinelli is Scientific Director of the Istituto Laser Microchirurgia Oculare (ILMO) in Brescia, Italy. In 2004 he founded the Italian Society of Refractive Surgery (SICR) and was elected president of it. Dr Pinelli received his training in refractive surgery in the United States. He serves on the Publication Committee of the European Society of Cataract and Refractive Surgery (ESCRS) and the international editorial board of Cataract and Refractive Surgery Today. He's an invited member of the International Intra-Ocular Implant Club (IIIC).

Contact him at (+39) 030-24-28-248 or pinelli@ilmo.it.

Hormone Treatment and Refractive Surgery

18

Maeve O'Doherty (UK)

The theoretical concept that hormone status may be related to clinical and surgical outcome post refractive surgery is not new. There are several studies in the current literature that address this issue. McCarty et al has shown that post menopausal women have unfavourable results following photorefractive keratectomy (PRK) and those on hormone replacement therapy (HRT) have been found to have the poorest outcome.[1] O'Doherty, et al has further updated this information to show that females taking HRT have a poorer outcome post Laser in situ keratomileusis (LASIK) than younger females not taking HRT.[2] Furthermore there is evidence that there is a higher incidence of myopic regression in females who become pregnant at the time of refractive surgery.[3] However, it is generally accepted that the oral contraceptive pill has no effect on refractive outcome post laser surgery.[2,4]

The effect of hormone status on refractive outcome is most likely linked to the effect of these hormones on tear secretion. Control of the functional activity of human lacrimal and meibomium glands by sexual hormones is evidenced by the presence of estrogen receptors in the meibomium glands and androgen receptors in lacrimal and meibomium glands, cornea and conjunctiva.[5,6] Additionally, a strong role for androgens in maintaining an anti-inflammatory state at the normal ocular surface has been hypothesized.

Anecdotal evidence suggests an association between dry eye and systemic estrogens. Some women report symptomatic improvement of dry eye with systemic estrogen therapy for the treatment of estrogen deficiency. Akramian et al reported the treatment the dry eye in post menopausal women using estradiol ointment. They found only moderate improvement in Schirmer's test values and break up time, with modest benefits demonstrated by rose Bengal staining.[7]

The poorer outcome following LASIK surgery of the post menopausal group in this study when compared to controls or women taking the OCP may be attributable to the higher incidence of dry eye in these women.[8] Chronic dry eye has recently been shown to increase the risk of refractive regression post LASIK.[9] Post menopausal women are particularly likely to suffer from dry eye, a change most likely related to diminished concentrations of sex hormones.[8] Considering that hormone receptors (estrogenic and androgenic) have been identified in corneal and conjunctival tissues as well as in the meibomian glands it would seem rational that females taking HRT would benefit by improvements in tear production. However, a number of studies have shown that females taking HRT are even more vulnerable to dry eyes.[10,11] There is evidence that estrogen acts on lacrimal and meibomian glands inducing lacrimal gland regression and reducing tear output.[11] In premenopausal women, a negative correlation has been demonstrated between testosterone levels and tear production, whereas estrogen levels have been shown to increase tear production. In postmenopausal women, this correlation is reversed.[12] The relationship between hormone levels and tear production is obviously complex and as yet there is no definite answer to how fluctuations in levels affect tear secretion.

Furthermore changes in hormone levels can affect corneal thickness. Increased progesterone levels during pregnancy are associated with increased corneal thickness. In addition corneal topography and the level of corneal hydration alters with fluctuations in hormone levels.[13,14] Corneal hydration affects the rate and outcome of excimer laser.[15-17] The rate of dry component ablation determines refractive outcome following PRK, and there is an inverse linear relationship between corneal hydration and dry component ablation rate.[15] Because hormonal levels influence corneal hydration, it would follow that fluctuating hormonal levels associated with pregnancy, HRT and menopausal status could affect the outcome of refractive surgery.

Women taking the oral contraceptive pill are unaffected by this treatment.[2,4] It is most likely that the hormone dose in the oral contraceptive pill is insufficient to cause any negative effects on outcome. Also women taking the OCP in comparison to women taking HRT are much younger with healthier corneas and better tear secretion.

In conclusion, the role of hormones on refractive outcome is complex and difficult to identify with certainty because of the diversity of action of these hormones. Refractive outcome is dependent on multiple factors such as preoperative refraction, tear secretion, age and possibly hormone status. However, the latter three factors are intrinsically linked to such a degree that it is impossible to determine the individual effect.

REFERENCES

1. McCarty C, Ng I,Waldron B, Garrett S, Downie J, Aldred G, Wolfe R, Taylor H. Relation of hormone and menopausal status to outcomes following excimer laser photorefractive keratectomy in women. Aust and New Zealand J of Ophth 1996;24(3):215-22.
2. O'Doherty MA, O'Doherty JV, O'Keeffe M. Outcome of LASIK for myopia in women on hormone replacement therapy. J Refract Surg 2006;22(4):350-53.
3. Sharif K. Regression of myopia induced by pregnancy after photorefractive keratectomy. J Refract surgery 1997; 13:445-46.
4. Valde D, Ghini M, Gammi L, Passarini M, Schiavi L. Effects des contraceptifs oraux triphases sur la secretion lacrymale. Ophthalmologie 1988;2:129-30.
5. Esmaeli B, Harvey JT, Hewlett B. Immunohistochemical evidence for oestrogen receptors in meibomium glands. Ophthalmology 2000; 107:180-84.
6. Smith RE, Taylor NA, Rao NA, Young LL, Rye LL. Immunohistochemical identification of androgen receptors in human lacrimal glands. Curr Eye Res. 1999;18:300-09.
7. Akramian J, Wedrich A Nepp J, Sator M. Oestrogen therapy in keratoconjuntivitis sicca. Adv Exp Med Biol 1998;438:1005-09.
8. Baudouin C.The pathology of dry eye. Surv ophthal 2001; 45Suppl:s11-20.
9. Albietz JM, Lenton LM, Mc lennan SG. Chronic dry eye and regression after LASIK for myopia. J cataract and refractive surgery 2004; 30:675-84.
10. Schaumberg DA, Buring JE, Sullivan DA, Dana MR. Hormone replacement therapy and dry eye syndrome. JAMA 2001; 286:2114-19.
11. Chia EM, Mitchell P, Rochtchina E, Lee A, Maroun R, Wang JJ. Prevalence and associations of dry eye syndrome in an older population; the blue mountains eye study. Clinical and Exp Ophthal 31;3: 229-36.
12. Mathers WM, Stovall D, Lane JA, Zimmerman MB, Johnson S. Menopause and tear function: the influence of prolactin and sex hormones on human tear production. Cornea. 1998;17: 353-86.
13. Weinreb RN, Lu A, Beeson C. Maternal corneal thickness during pregnancy. Am J Ophthal 1988;105:258-60.
14. Ziai N, Ory SJ, Khan AR, Brubaker RF. Beta human chorionic gonadotropin, progesterone and acqueos dynamics during pregnancy. Arch ophth 1994;112:801-6(6).
15. Dougherty PJ, Wellish KL, Maloney RK. Excimer laser ablation rate and corneal hydration. Am J Ophthalmol 1994;118:169-76.
16. Fiels CR, Taylor SM, Barker FM. Effect of corneal edema upon smoothness of excimer laser ablation. Optom Vis Sci 1994;71:109-14.
17. Ediger MN, Pettitt GH, Weiblinger RP, Chen CH. Transmission of corneal collagen during ArF excimer laser ablation. Lasers Surg Med 1993;13:204-10.

Presby-LASIK in Pseudophakic Eyes with the Wavelight Allegretto

19

FREDERIC HEHN (FRANCE)

INTRODUCTION

Natural eye is a bi-optic optical system with a variable axial myopic additional power due to the crystalline lens. Because evidently along visual axis (object to macula) the vision will be the more discriminate with the best contrast sensitivity[5] and MTF (modulation of transfer function) for the both near and far vision. This bioptic system produces the best near and distant visual acuity, in using crystalline lens accommodation which can be achieve.[3] Because Presby-LASIK can not restore accommodation, it just can be a good compromise between near and distant vision.

Natural eye present some coma HOA[2] due to the difference between visual axis (object to macula) and optical axis (apex of cornea to the center of crystalline lens). That's the reason why we are thinking that presbylasik technique does not increase the natural existent coma. Then to avoid to increase coma presby-LASIK must be centered. Inspired of multifocal or bifocal soft lens for presbyopia, that's give good results in many cases, the therapeutic choice will be to place distant vision in center or not. Some authors have got good results with a small optical zone for near vision in the the very center cornea,[1] we preferred the contrary with distant vision in the very center of cornea because it's more natural like we are, shown just below.

The natural cornea has got an aspherical (that's mean non spherical) shape, which is quantified by the so called "Q value" for asphericity coefficient. Therefore in an aspherical cornea the curvature is not the same in central part than it is in peripheral part. Generally the natural cornea present a negative asphericity ($Q < 0$) where curvature is higher in the center cornea than it is in peripheral cornea.

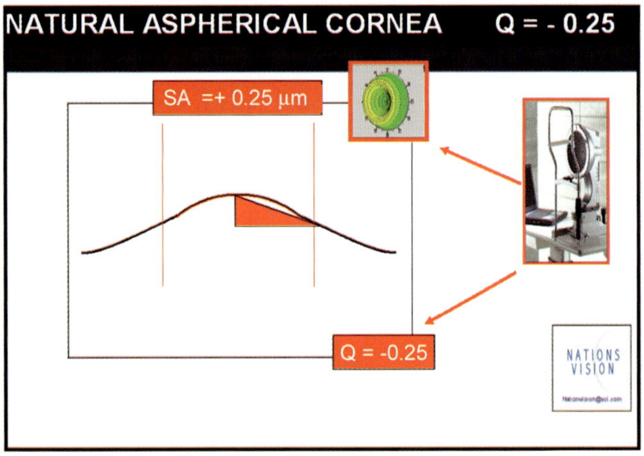

Fig. 19.1

But in fact the central part of cornea [0-6 mm OZ] is spherical,[11] like previous study shows. In one hand there are no spherical aberrations in the very central cornea [0-3 mm OZ]: that the reason why distant vision occurred in it. Then for presby-LASIK it's logical to place distant vision in the very center of the cornea; In a other hand there are positive spherical aberration in the medium cornea [3-6 mm OZ]. Due to the Descartes fresnel low some intermediate vision is possible in using medium cornea , without contact lens accommodation: that's we called the depth of focus. If we are able to gentle increase positive aberrations in this region, we increase the depth of focus in decreasing the ponctum proximum until a relax eye or a pseudophakic eye can read something without using lens accommodation. Then for presby-LASIK it's logical to place near vision in the medium part of cornea.

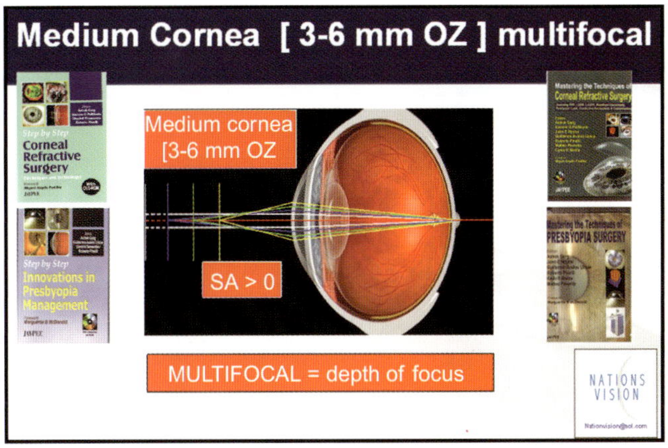

Fig. 19.2A

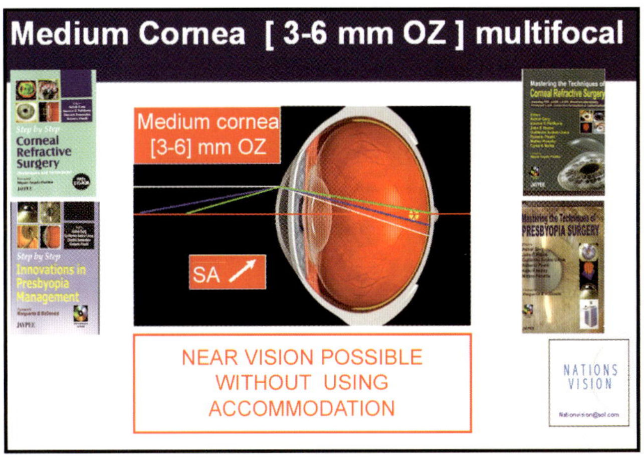

Fig. 19.2B

Patients and Methods

Presby-LASIK could be logically compensate presbyopia in emmetropic pseudophakic eye with monofocal IOL , like the MF IOL do.[6] The centered presby-lasik technique with distant vision in the center give a very good distant vision and a useful optional near and intermediate vision. The difficulties remain the necessity to get high luminance for reading a book. The goal of presby-lasik is not to completely erase spectacles but to decrease the patient's glasses dependency. The two figures below show ideal presby-LASIK profile.

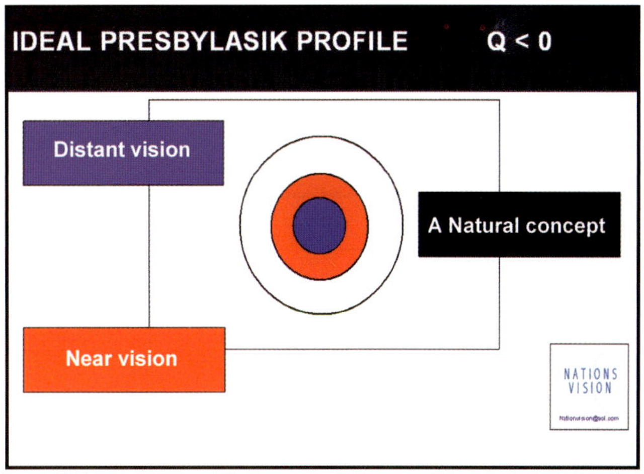

Fig. 19.3A

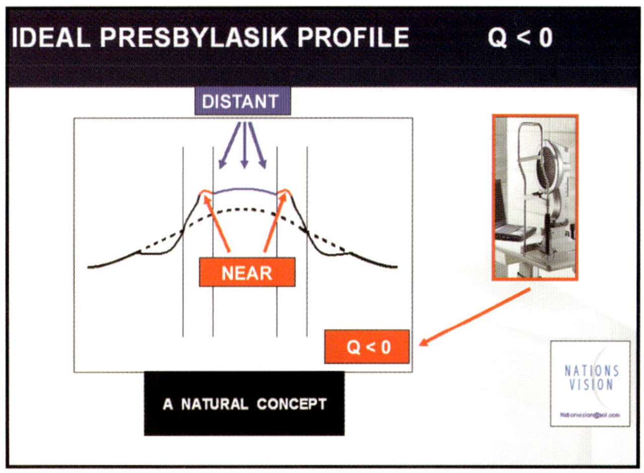

Fig. 19.3B

According to the previous refractive basements we have choice to built a presby-LASIK profile with distant vision in the very center of cornea like naturally it is. This way give excellent distant vision and an optional useful near and intermediate vision. We report a clinical study about 10 pseudophakic eyes with monofocal IOL after a previous non complicated cataract surgery. A complete check up of visual acuity in terms of BCVA and UCVA before and after surgery, slit lamp examination, orthoptist examination, and macular exploration by NMR and OCT were performed. In all cases the Nd yag capsulotomy has been made at least 6 months before LASIK surgery, to avoid any kind of HOA (high order aberrations) due to the capsule fibrosis. We practice at first a hyperopic treatment of + 3.00 diopters on a large 6.5 or 7.0 mm OZ to get a good near vision. Secondly we performed a myopic treatment of - 3.00 on a small OZ depending on pupil size,[8] to get a very good vision in central cornea as naturally it is. We measure also our results in using the TOPOLYZER topograph of wavelight.

We are using the very precise allegretto wavelight, argon fluor excimer laser, with a little flying spot of 0.8 mm diameter and a high speed delivery system of 400 Hz , and eye tracker so.

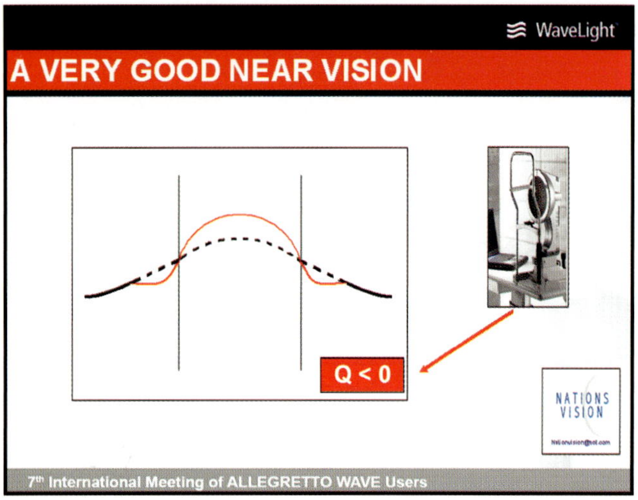

Fig. 19.4A

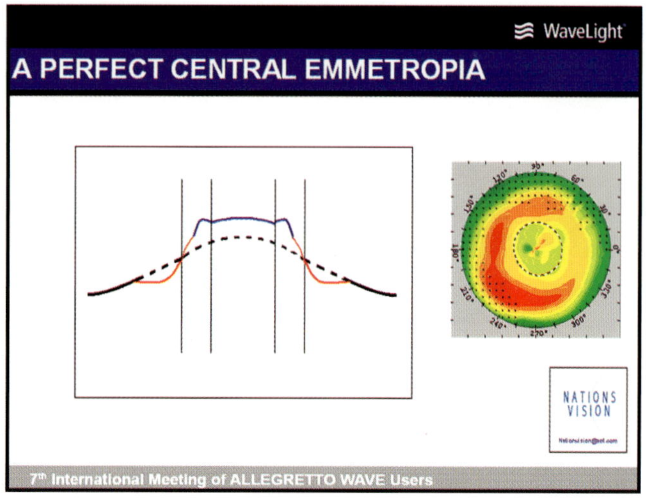

Fig. 19.4B

Results

We show results in two exemples of pseudophakic patients with monofocal IOL. the first patient a 53 years old man has got hydrophilic STABIBAG IOLTECH laboratories in the both eyes.In this case we remark some irregularities in the topographic map due to the fact in this first case studying we have not ever practice a previous A-CAT (aberrometric customized ablation treatment) treatment to make sure to get a free HOA eye before performing presby-LASIK. The second point is that this patient get in monocular vision very good results on the defocalisation curve. That's a proof of very good depth of focus with this technique as so good than with MF IOL it is.

The other one, a 50 years old man has got ACRYSOF SN60 ALCON laboratories in the both eyes. None of them present other pathology , neither glaucoma, nor retinal macular degeneration ... In this case we can see that preby-LASIK corneal shape looks like natural accommodation in terms of negative asphericity, with Q value = - 1.00

DISCUSSION

What's happens during accommodation in abrrometric measurement: the augmentation of anterior curvature of the crystalline lens give a myopic shift with an increasing of Z2,0 zernike polynoma: without myopia no near vision possible.[7] But in concern of HOA only spherical aberration C12 or Z4,0 have significant modification according to a study.[4] These authors demonstrate that during accommodation the variation of spherical aberration are always negative, and most interesting point is that variation is precisely and linearly correlated to the amount of accommodation in using a hartmann-shak aberrometer system. Variation of SA = –0.0435 μm/diopter. Therefore 3 diopters of accommodation correspond

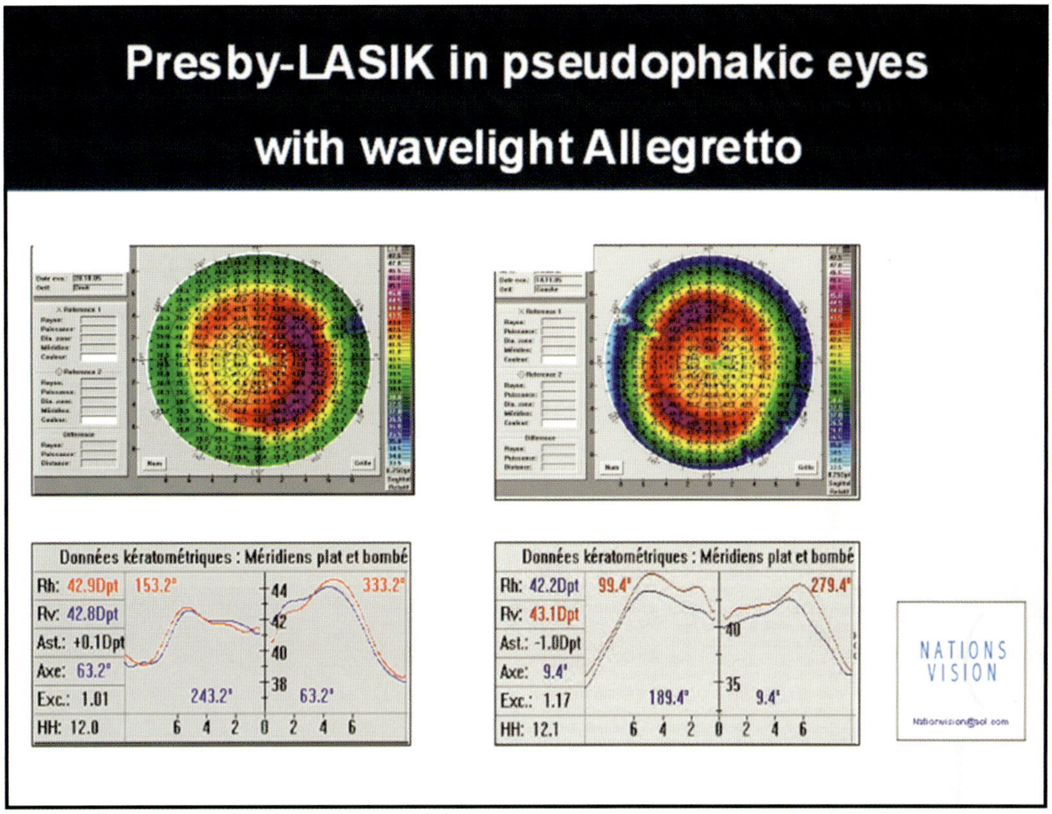

Fig. 19.5A

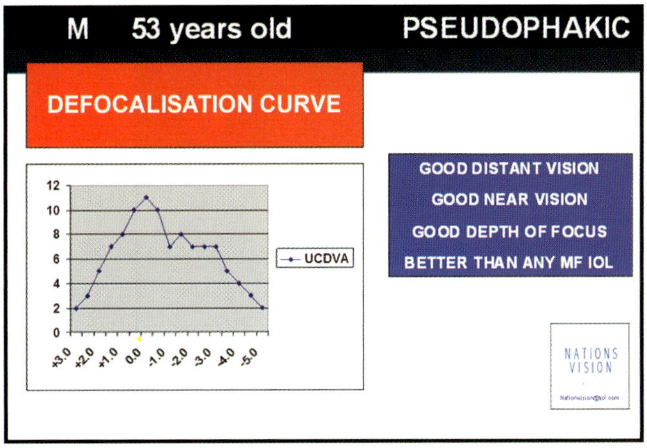

Fig. 19.5B

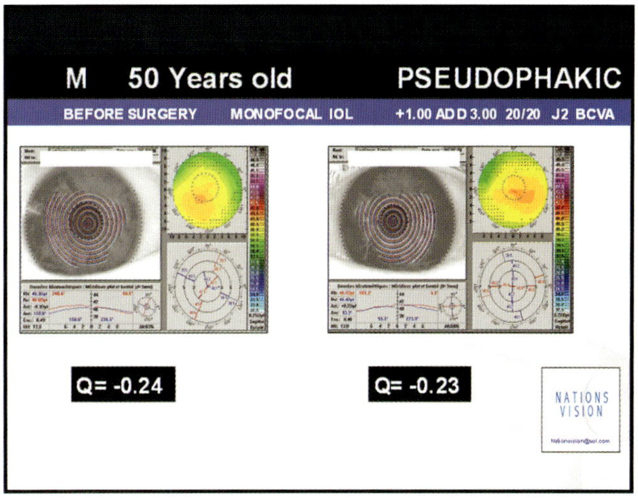

Fig. 19.6A: Q value before surgery

to a variation of - 0.130 μm in SA. Presby-LASIK technique must simulate accommodation in creating a myopic zone and also negative spherical aberration. We have verified this fact in using our wavelight aberrometer[9] system and obtain exactly the same results: we place our 16 years old son behind aberrometer and present to him myopic lens to turn he to hyperopia and force he to accommodate; we relate these results in figure just below.

Analyze of results is difficult because we must well understand what we measure and what exactly we do[10] in performing presby-LASIK. The first important point is to know that TOPOLYZER topograph measure

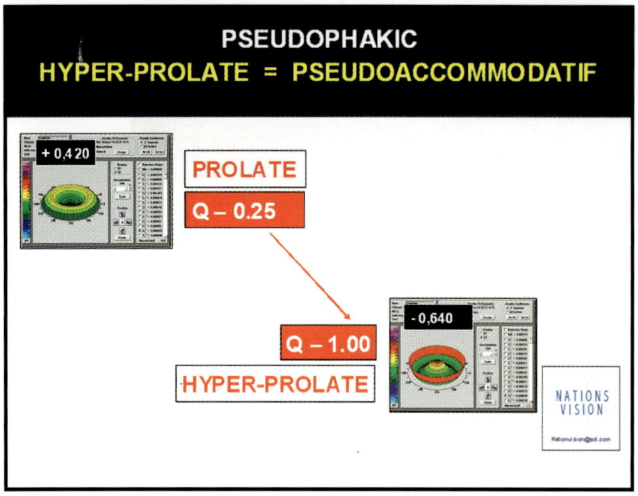

Fig. 19.6B: Q value after surgery

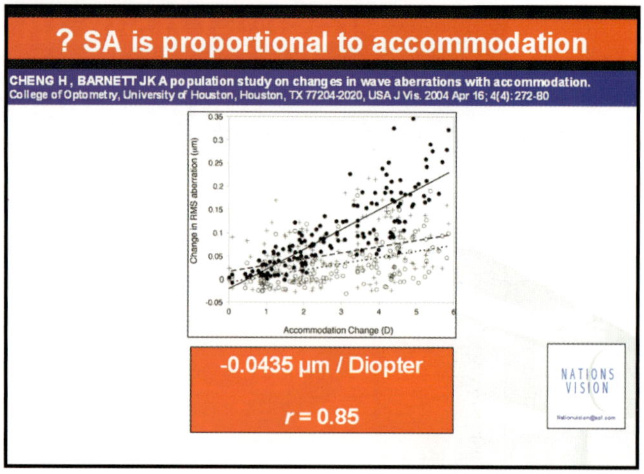

Fig. 19.7A

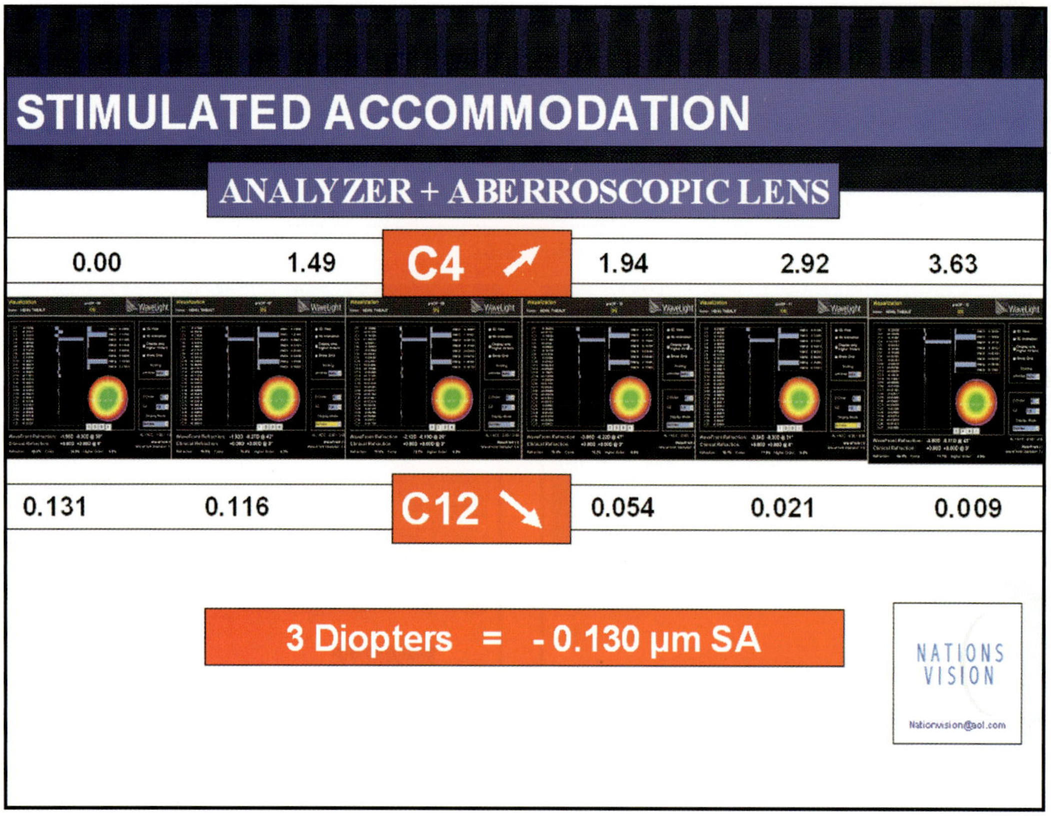

Fig. 19.7B

eccentricity then Q value asphericity of the cornea shape on a 6.50 mm OZ. Q value describe the variation of corneal shape between apex and 6.5 OZ. If curvature grows up Q becomes > 0, spherical aberration increase to become positives so and the cornea profile is called oblate. At the contrary if curvature grows down Q becomes < 0, spherical aberration decrease to become negatives so and the cornea profile is called prolate. But in fact there not only one Q value along the cornea , but a lot of variation in it from the center to the peripheral . For instance like you can see on the draw below Q is not the same if measure at 3.5 OZ than to 6.5 . in a natural cornea in the center from 0 to 6.0 mm OZ the cornea is spherical then Q = 0 with some positives SA, but at 6.5 mm OZ Q becomes negative , that's the result which is giving by the TOPOLYZER. Then Q value can not describe precisely the shape variation. In a new exemple who can see that the both black and blue line cornea shape have got the exactly same Q value for instance –1.00 because they have got the same apex corneal reference plan and the same difference curvature between center cornea for instance 43 diopters and same curvature at 6.5 mm OZ for instance 41 diopters. But with blue shape no near vision possibility instead of with black shape a paracentral near vision is possible: that's our optical profile choice for presby-LASIK.

What about comparison between natural eye system with and without accommodation; the myopic additional system give a myopia, and then the anterior prolapse of crystalline lens , looks like an hyper-prolate corneal shape with Q value < 0 and diminution of spherical aberration to negatives values. In our presby-lasik technique the TOPOLYZER measure the same things: Q < 0 and SA < 0, but in fact that's the really positives

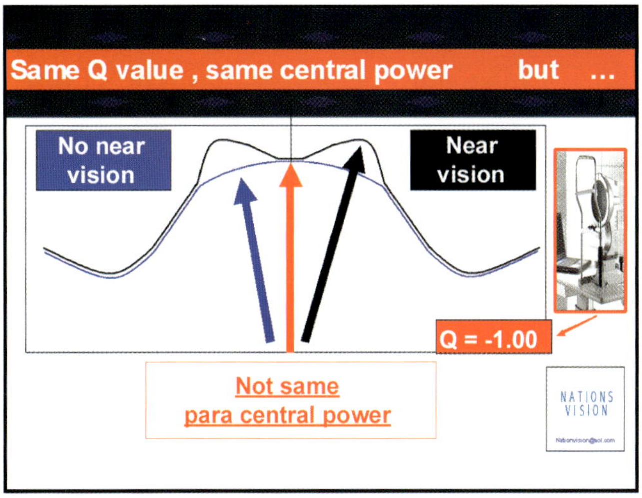

Fig. 19.8A

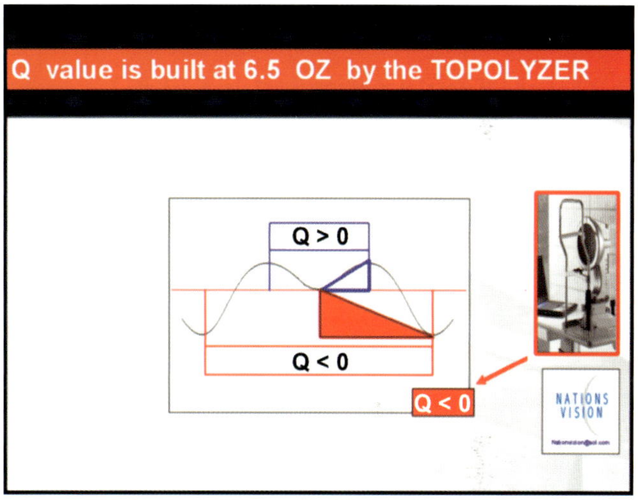

Fig. 19.8B

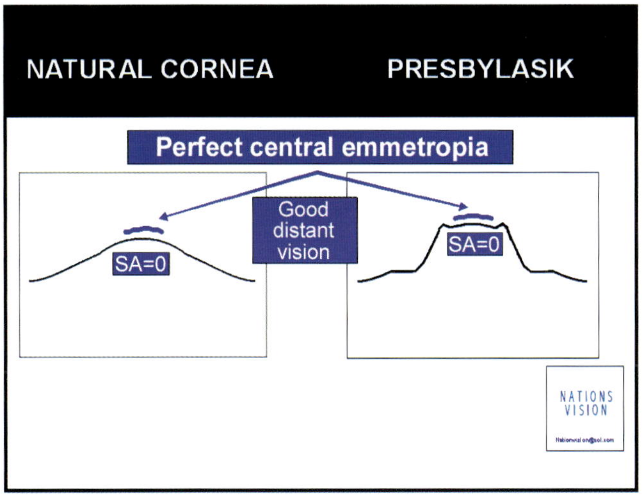

Fig. 19.9A

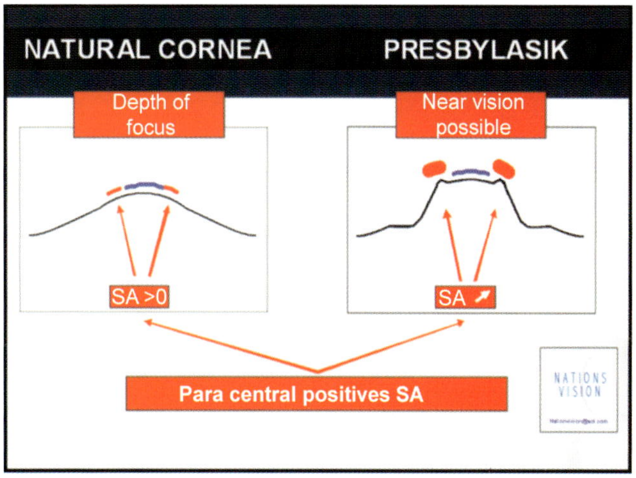

Fig. 19.9B

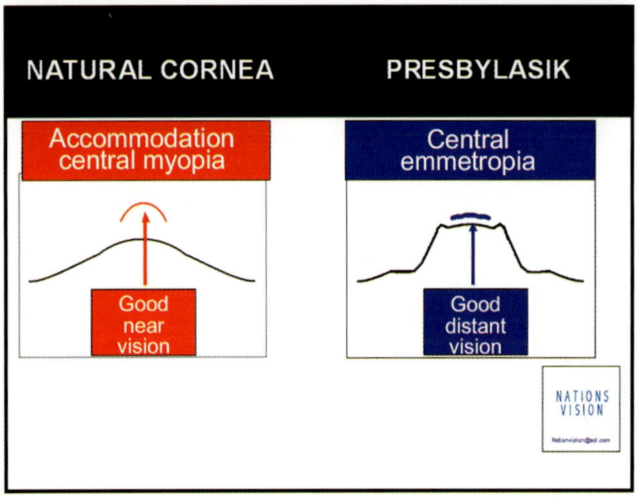

Fig. 19.10A

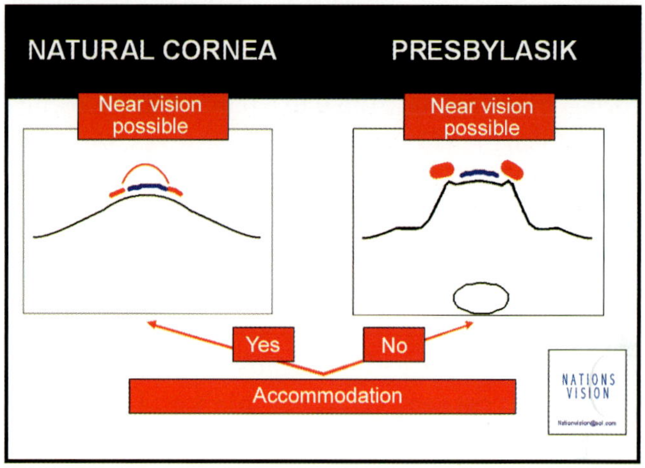

Fig. 19.10B

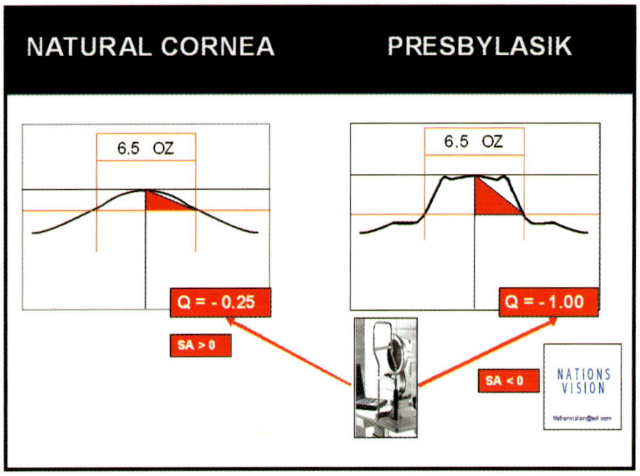

Fig. 19.11A

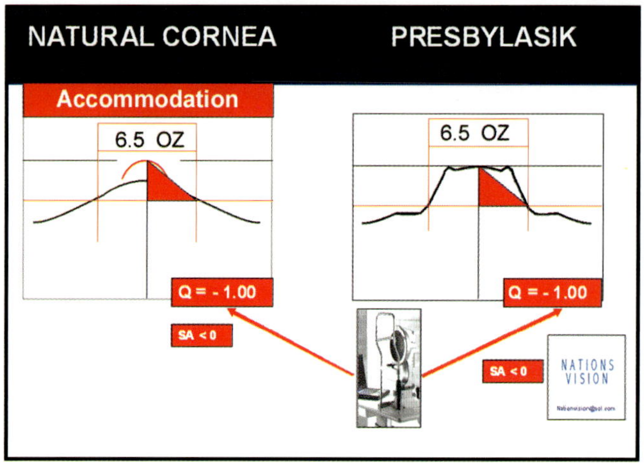

Fig. 19.11B

SA which occurred in the paracentral cornea which permit near vision without accommodation. But at 6.5 mm OZ TOPOLYZER does not measure this positives spherical aberrations.

CONCLUSION

Presby-LASIK could be logically compensate presbyopia in emmetropic pseudophakic eye with monofocal IOL , like the MF IOL do. The centered presby-lasik technique with distant vision in the center give a very good distant vision and a useful optional near and intermediate vision. The difficulties remain the necessity to get high luminance for reading a book. The goal of presby-lasik is not to completely erase spectacles but to decrease the patient's glasses dependency. Presby-LASIK seems to get as so good results as Multifocal IOL. Is presby-LASIK will become a non penetrative alternative of the clear lens exchange?

REFERENCES

1. Alio JL, Chaubard JJ, Caliz A, Sala E, Patel S. Correction of presbyopia by technovision central multifocal LASIK (presbyLASIK). J Refract Surg 2006;22(5):453-60.
2. Applegate RA, Sarver EJ, Khemsara V. Are all aberrations equal? J Refract Surg 2002 Sep-Oct; 18(5): S556-62.
3. Cantu R, Rosales MA, Tepichin E, Curioca A, Montes V, Ramirez-Zavaleta JG. Objective quality of vision in

presbyopic and non-presbyopic patients after pseudo-accommodative advanced surface ablation. J Refract Surg 2005;21(5 Suppl):S603-05.

4. Cheng H, Barnett JK, Vilupuru AS, Marsack JD, Kasthurirangan S, Applegate RA, Roorda A. A population study on changes in wave aberrations with accommodation. J Vis 2004;4(4):272-80.
5. De Brabander J, Chateau N, Bouchard F, Guidollet S. Contrast sensitivity with soft contact lenses compensated for spherical aberration in high ametropia. Optom Vis Sci 1998;75(1):37-43.
6. Dick HB, Kaiser S. [Dynamic aberrometry during accommodation of phakic eyes and eyes with potentially accommodative intraocular lenses] Ophthalmologe. 2002;99(11):825-34. German.
7. Hofer H, Artal P, Singer B, Aragon JL, Williams DR. Dynamics of the eye's wave aberration. J Opt Soc Am A Opt Image Sci Vis. 2001;18(3):497-506.
8. Howland HC, Buettner J. Computing high order wave aberration coefficients from variations of best focus for small artificial pupils. Vision Res 1989;29(8):979-83.
9. Krueger RR, Mrochen M, Kaemmerer M, Seiler T. Understanding refraction and accommodation through "retinal imaging" aberrometry: A case report. Ophthalmology. 2001;108(4):674-78.
10. Plainis S, Ginis HS, Pallikaris A. The effect of ocular aberrations on steady-state errors of accommodative response. J Vis 2005;5(5):466-77.
11. Waring GO. Refractive keratotomy "for myopia and astigmatism" Mosby year book 1992.

Wavefront Aberrometry for Irregular Astigmatism

20

JORGE L ALIÓ, ROBERT MONTES-MICÓ (SPAIN)

INTRODUCTION TO WAVEFRONT ABERRATION

Wavefront aberration is defined as the deviation between the reference wavefront that comes from a in ideal optic system and the wavefront that originates from a measured optical system. The unit used to measure it is microns of waves and it is shown as the root mean square (RMS). Wavefront analysis of the eye allows to determine the optical quality of the eye by evaluating the shape of its wavefront as wavefront aberrations.

There are several methods to evaluate the wavefront shape and are classified into the following three types:

1. Outgoing wavefront aberrometry (Hartmann-Shack sensor)[1].
2. Ingoing retinal imaging aberrometry (Cross cylinder aberroscope,[2] Tscherning aberroscope[3] and the sequential retinal ray tracing method).[4]
3. Ingoing feedback aberrometer (Spatially resolved refractometer[5] and the optical path difference method).[6]

When the wavefront shape has been obtained, using any of the previous methods, it can be analyzed by expanding it into sets of Zernike polynomials to extract the characteristic components of the wavefront shape. In the Zernike polynomial expansion, the different optical aberrations may be described by terms which are raised to different orders. First and second order terms describe tilt, astigmatism and spherical refractive error respectively; and third, fourth and higher-orders describe spherical aberration, coma and the rest of aberrations. Polynomials can be expanded up to any arbitrary order if sufficient numbers of measurements for calculations are made.

CORNEAL WAVEFRONT ABERRATIONS

Videokeratoscopes have enabled the measurement of the corneal shape and the determination of corneal first surface wavefront aberrations and their influence on visual performance.[7,8] To date, these methods have been used mainly to quantify the effects of refractive surgery on corneal aberrations and visual performance.

The corneal wavefront, which is one of the components of the total ocular wavefront, can be calculated from corneal topographic height data. The corneal wavefront can be fitted with a Zernike polynomial decomposition in the same way that total ocular wavefront is measured by aberrometry and fitted with the same polynomial decomposition. Both decompositions allow inspection of the total ocular and corneal aberrations of the human eye, considering the contribution of the cornea to the total aberrations of the eye.

Using Zernike polynomial decomposition we are able to examine the optical quality of the corneal surface generating the wavefront of the anterior surface of the cornea. Zernike analysis is a sophisticated analytical method which is ideal for representing surfaces of any shape. It is based on a set of orthonormal polynomial developed by Zernike. Using Zernike's analysis, any surface can be described as the weighted sum of typical shapes represented by the polynomials. The series of polynomial is of increasing order and potentially infinite. The greater the number of polynomials used, the more detailed the surface representation. The components chosen by Zernike are those specific for the wavefront aberrations. The orthonormal characteristics of this mathematical approach allow the analysis of the individual components of the different aberrations independently of each other, quantification of the prismatic component, the defocus component, the degree of regular astigmatism, the spherical aberration, coma and the rest of the higher order aberrations.

Figures 20.1A to E shows the procedure for calculation of the optical characteristics of the corneal surface. From a topographic map (Fig. 20.1A) it is possible to compute the corneal wavefront aberrations of the cornea, and to differentiate between second (defocus and astigmatism) and higher-order aberrations. Figures 20.1B and C represent the total

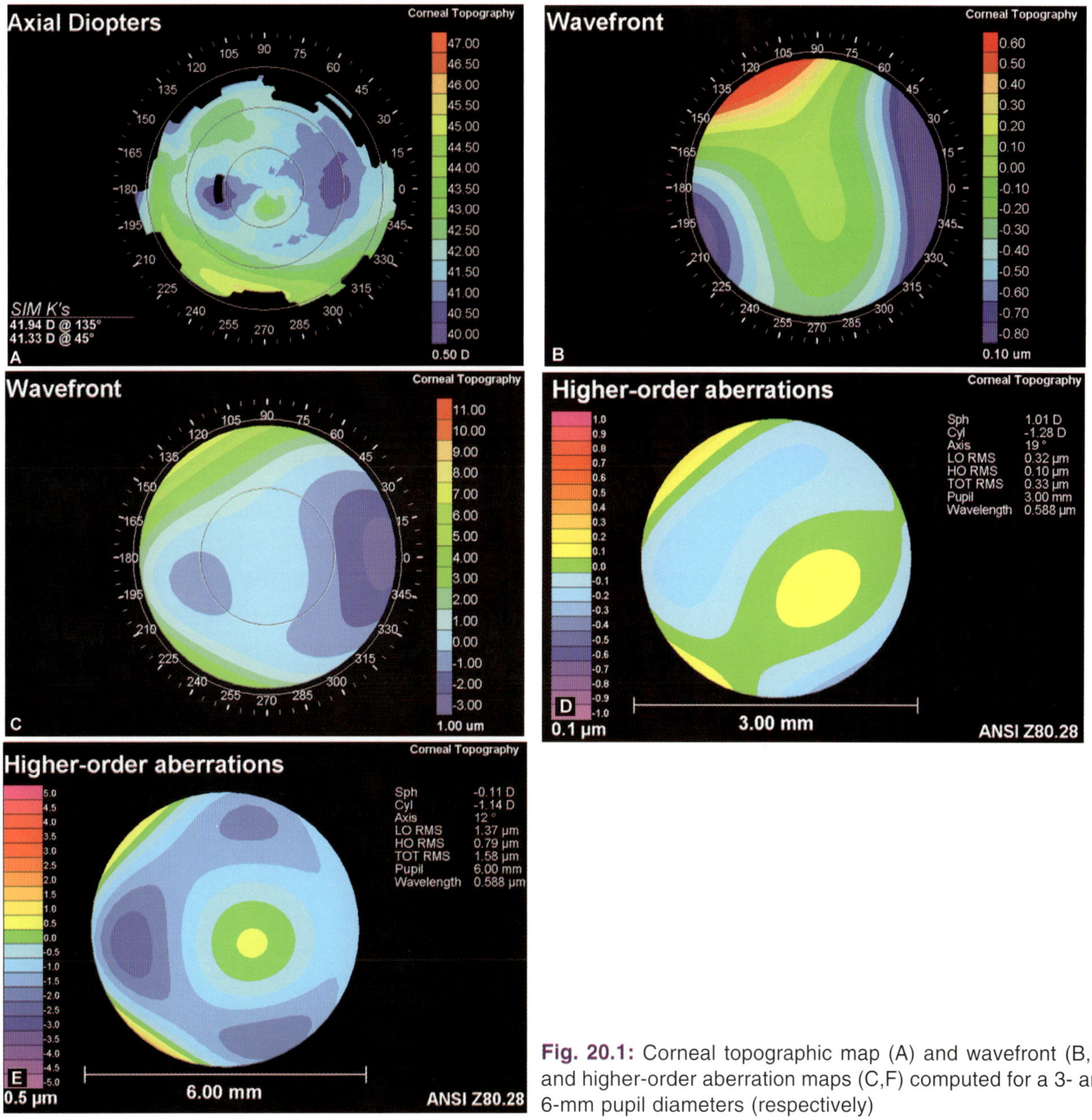

Fig. 20.1: Corneal topographic map (A) and wavefront (B,D) and higher-order aberration maps (C,F) computed for a 3- and 6-mm pupil diameters (respectively)

wavefront aberrations and the higher-order aberrations, respectively, for a 3-mm pupil diameter. In the same way, figures 20.1D and E show the same distribution but computed for a 6-mm pupil diameter. These plots show graphically the importance of the pupil diameter to calculate the optical quality of the cornea. In this specific case, the total root-mean-square (RMS) of higher-order aberrations varies from 0.10 to 0.79 microns, showing the variation in the optical quality of the cornea as a function of considering one pupil diameter.

As we have commented previously, we can compute the different Zernike polynomials and separately evaluate the contribution of the different coefficients to the final quality of the corneal surface. Figures 20.2A and B represent the corneal wavefront Zernike coefficients of the topographic map of figure 20.1 computed for a 3- and 6-mm pupil diameter. X-axis represents the coefficient number (tilt, defocus, astigmatism, spherical aberration, coma, etc...) and the Y-axis represents the value of the deviation from the reference wavefront in microns (advanced or delayed, positive or negative values). Large value of deviation indicates large deformation and poor optical quality of the corneal surface, then, from both graphs it is possible to observe an increase in the coefficient values and consequently a reduction in the optical quality of the cornea for a large pupil size (6-mm).

CORNEAL WAVEFRONT AS A GUIDE FOR THE CORRECTION OF IRREGULAR ASTIGMATISM

Basis of Treatment

The CSO topographer allows the analysis of the optical performance of the cornea. It measures a maximum of 6144 points of the cornea from the projection of 24 placido rings onto the cornea. The elevation data is computed from the ring positions and surface location measured from the video images. Corneal height is then translated into corneal wavefront and fitted into Zernike polynomials. These corneal aberrations do not depend on accommodation and pupil size.

Corneal aberrations contribute to approximately 80% of the total ocular aberrations in normal eyes and to an even greater value in corneas with irregular astigmatism. Corneal aberrometry is a revolutionary tool for the evaluation of quality of vision, and can be advantageously used to treat irregular astigmatism causes by a previous corneal refractive surgery.

For this prospective, non-randomized pilot study, we evaluated 18 patients (18 eyes): 10 males and 8 females. Mean age of the patient was 38.5 ± 7.3 years (range 25 to 63 years). All these patients had a previous uneventful corneal refractive surgery and they were diagnosed of macroirregular or mixed (macro and micro) irregular astigmatism caused by the previous corneal refractive surgery. We evaluated

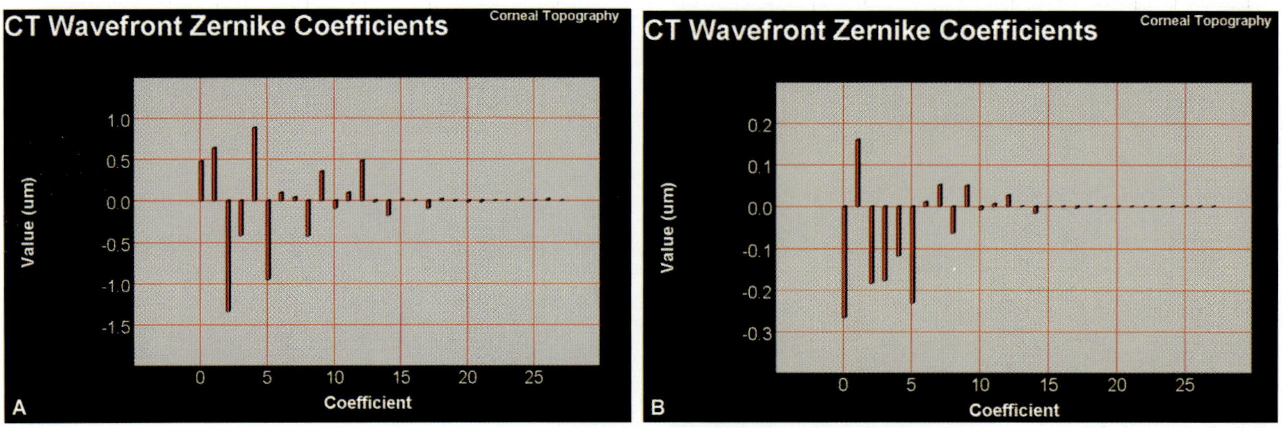

Fig. 20.2: Corneal topography Zernike coefficient values computed for a 3- and 6-mm pupil diameter (a and b, respectively)

the results obtained after a follow-up of 3 months. All surgical procedures were performed by the same surgeon (JLA) at the Instituto Oftalmológico de Alicante (Alicante, Spain).

The criteria for the selection of the patients were: corneal irregular astigmatism induced by previous corneal refractive surgery, decreased best spectacle-corrected visual acuity (BCVA), glare, ghost images and distorted vision, intolerance or absence of motivation to use contact lenses. We waited for a period of 6 months to confirm both the complete stabilization of the subjective refraction, the corneal topography and the tear film.

Clinical Examination

For each visit a comprehensive preoperative ocular examination was performed on each patient. This included previous ocular medical report, slit-lamp biomicroscopy, applanation tonometry, ultrasonic pachymetry. Subjective evaluation of quality of vision was assessed by asking the patients whether halos, glare, and monocular diplopia were reduced after surgery with best spectacle correction. Uncorrected visual acuity (UCVA) and BCVA were tested preoperatively, 1 and 3 months follow-up. Refraction was measured preoperatively and postoperatively under cyclopegia and using the high plus technique.

Corneal topography and corneal aberration is a very important diagnostic and treatment tool and was obtained under proper tear film conditions before treatment, 1 month and 3 months after treatment.

Surgical Technique

Preliminary step of the procedure included obtaining the corneal topography by means of the CSO (CSO Ophtalmics, Milano, Italy). For this process, both the alignment and the stability of the pre-corneal tear film are extremely important. As mentioned above, the CSO topographer is able to convert the elevation data in terms of Zernike Polynomials to quantify the corneal wavefront aberrometry. The root-mean-square (RMS) was used as a measure of the optical quality before and after customized corneal wavefront analysis.

After capturing and analyzing corneal aberrations up to the 7th Zernike order, this data is processed by the ORK-W software (Schwind), which transforms this corneal aberration data into an adequate ablation profile. The software enables the surgeon to take an active part in the decision-making process, selecting the best solution for each patient. The software also allows the exclusion of specific aberrations according to specific surgical criteria and the choice of wide optical and transition zone.

Finally, customized ablation is performed with the Schwind ESIRIS Excimer-Laser. It is a scanning spot laser technology with a spot of 0.8 μm and a repetition rate of 200 Hz guided by its 330 Hz video based eye-tracking system.

Results

Efficacy

UCVA improved in 81% of the patients, from 0.3 ± 0.15 (range from 0.7 to 0.1) logarithm of minimum angle of resolution (logMAR) preoperatively to 0.2 ± 0.27 (range from 0.8 to 0.00) logMAR at 3 months follow up (Fig. 20.3) with an efficacy index of 1.08 (Fig. 20.4). The mean gain of lines of postoperative UCVA was 1.81 ± 1.5 lines.

Safety

At 3 months follow up 55% gained one line of BCVA, 27 % gained two lines, 11% gained 3 lines and 11% had no change (Fig. 20.5) with a safety index of 1.16 (Fig. 20.6). The mean preoperative BCVA was 0.2 ± 0.17 logMAR (range 0.5 to 0.1) and mean postoperative BCVA was 0.10 ± 0.23 logMAR (range 0.5 to 0.0). Then mean gain of lines of postoperative BCVA was 1.09 ± 0.7 lines.

Predictability

Mean preoperative SE was -0.29 D (range 1.75 D to -2.00 D; SD 1.04); at last postoperative examination, mean SE was -0.20 D (range -0.50 D to -2.25; SD, 0.62)

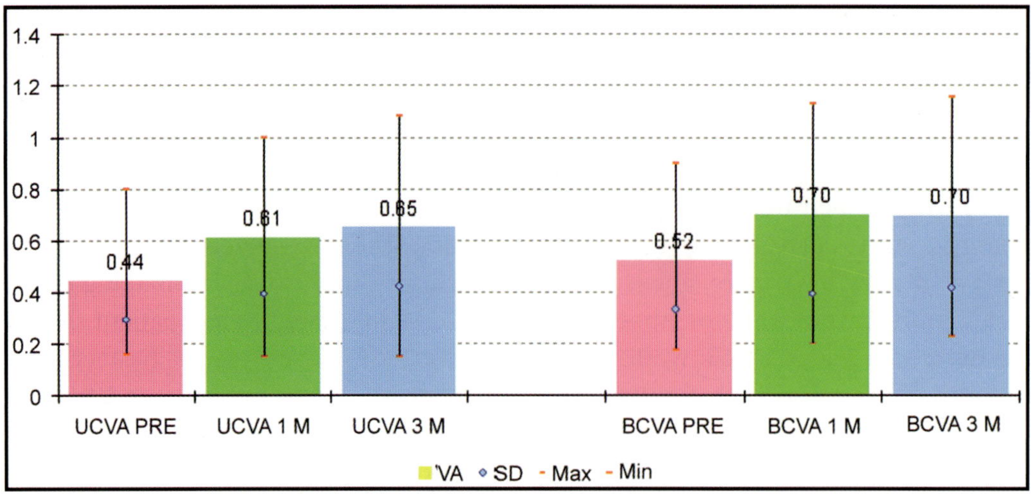

Fig. 20.3: UCVA and BCVA before an after corneal aberration oriented ablation

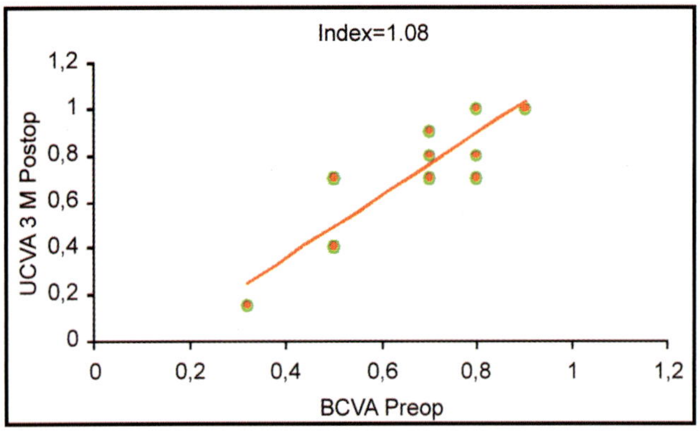

Fig. 20.4: Efficacy index

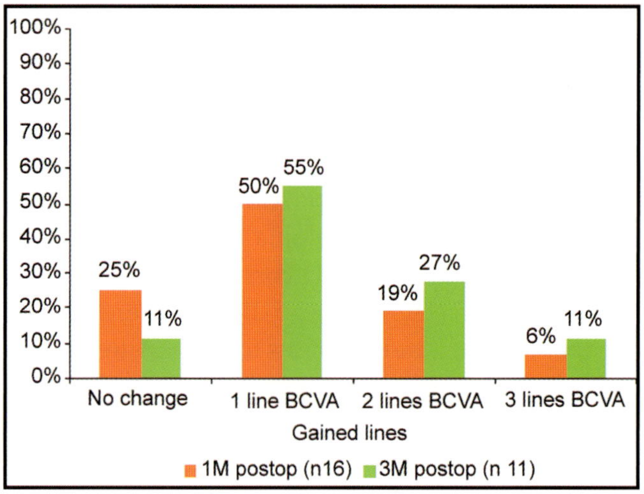

Fig. 20.5: Safety. Change in best spectacle-corrected visual acuity (1 Month and 3 months after ORK-W treatment)

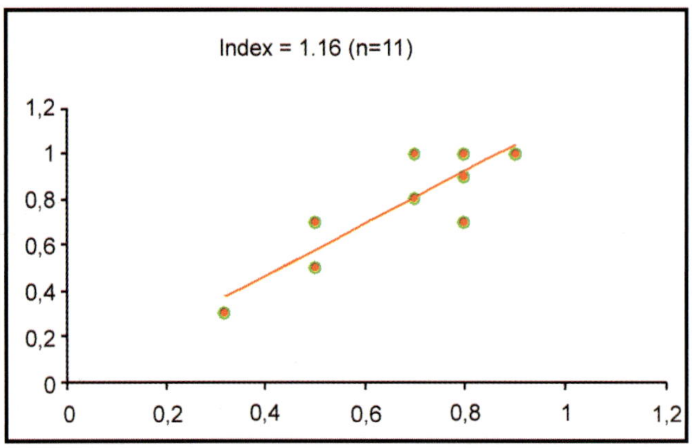

Fig. 20.6: Safety index

Higher Order Aberrations

The preoperative and postoperative changes in the root mean square values (RMS) of the corneal higher-order wavefront aberration (total, spherical and coma-like aberrations) are shown graphically in Figure 20.7. All the data was analyzed for a 6 mm pupil. After ORK-W, there was a statically significant decreased in total higher order aberration.

Total Higher Order Corneal Wavefront

After ORK-W, there was statistically significant change in total higher order corneal wavefront aberration. Total higher order aberration reduced by a factor of 1.34 and 1.45 at 1 month and 3 months of surgery respectively. (Paired t-test; $p < 0.005$ for 1 and 3 months follow-up).

First Order Aberrations

Although ORK-W treatment does not affect directly in first order aberration, all the patients have shown statically significant changes in first order aberration. First order corneal aberration reduced by a factor of 1.62 and 1.54 at 1 and 3 month after surgery respectively. (Paired t-test; $p < 0.005$ for 1 and 3 months follow-up).We may suggest that this improvement in first order aberration could be as a consequence of recentration in the ablation profile.

Coma-like Aberrations

Third order and fifth order Zernike coefficients are indicators of coma-like aberrations. For a 6 mm pupil, the root mean square (RMS) of the wavefront aberration decreased significantly at 1 and 3 months by a factor 1.34 and 1.38 respectively. In all cases the reduction in coma-like corneal wavefront aberration was statistically significant. (Paired t-test; $P < 005$ for 1 and 3 months).

Spherical-like aberration

Fourth order Zernike coefficients are indicators of spherical-like aberrations. The RMS values decreased significantly 1 and 3 month after surgery by a factor of 1.27 and 1.47 respectively.

CASE REPORT

A 33-year-old white male was referred to our clinic with an ocular history of refractive surgery in both eyes. He complained of poor quality of vision, ghost

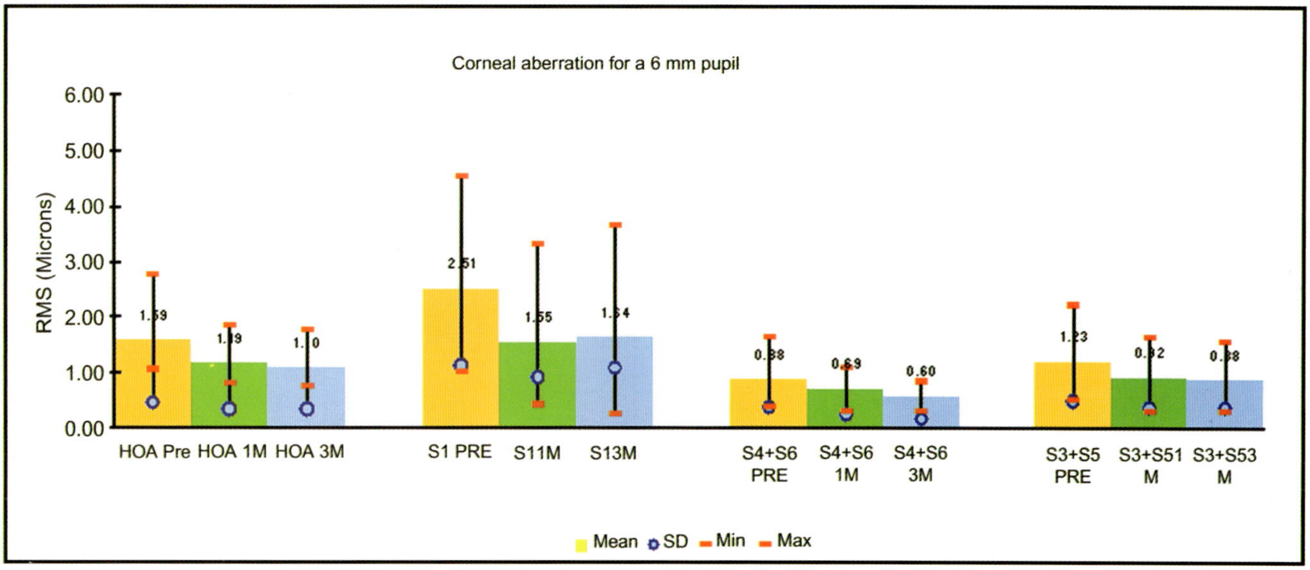

Fig. 20.7: Corneal aberrometric analysis for 6 mm pupil. Change in RMS values on preoperative day, 1 and 3 months after ORK-W treatment

images and halos especially at night in his right eye. He had a history of moderate myopia (– 3.75 – 1.00x 115°, 20/20 visual acuity) before LASIK treatment. After we examined the patient, his uncorrected visual acuity (UCVA) was 20/40 with a manifest refraction of – 1.75 – 0.75 × 170°, 20/30 visual acuity. Corneal thickness measured by ultrasonic pachymetry was 482 μm. Preoperative corneal higher order aberration revealed a RMS of 1.19 μm (largest component was coma-like aberration with a RMS of 1.12 μm). Analysis of the RMS values shows that the major improvement was for tilt and coma-like aberration (Fig. 20.8). After pre-evaluation the patient underwent corneal wavefront-guided custom ablation (ORK-W) Fig. 20.9 shows the ablation pattern used by the laser according to corneal wavefront data. The differential instantaneous map is shown in Figure 20.10 and demonstrates the efficacy of the treatment. At 6 months after ORK-W treatment UCVA was 20/20 with a manifest refraction of OD: – 0.50 × 180° (20/20). The RMS was 0.72 μm for Total HOA and 0.63 μm for coma-like aberrations.

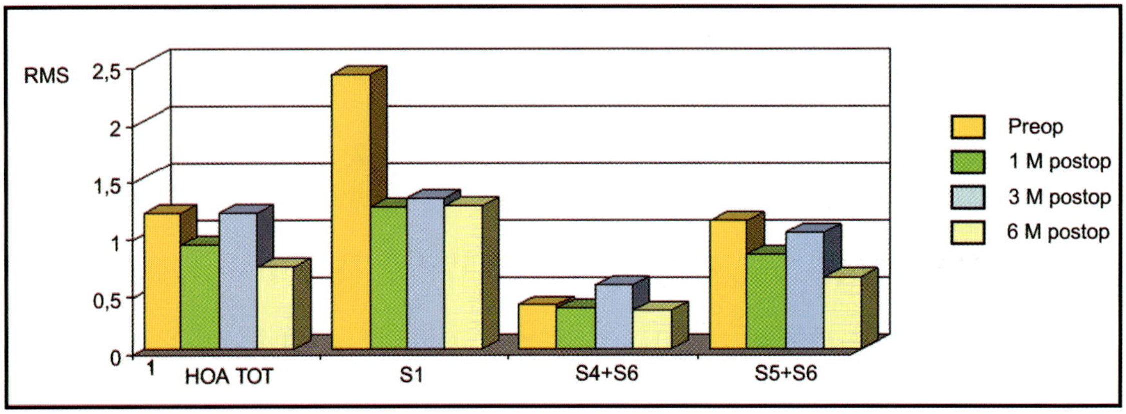

Fig. 20.8: The bar graph above shows the magnitude (RMS) of each higher order corneal aberration (total, tilt, spherical- and coma-like aberrations) for 6 mm pupil, before and after ORK-W treatment (1 ,3 and 6 months postop) for these patient.

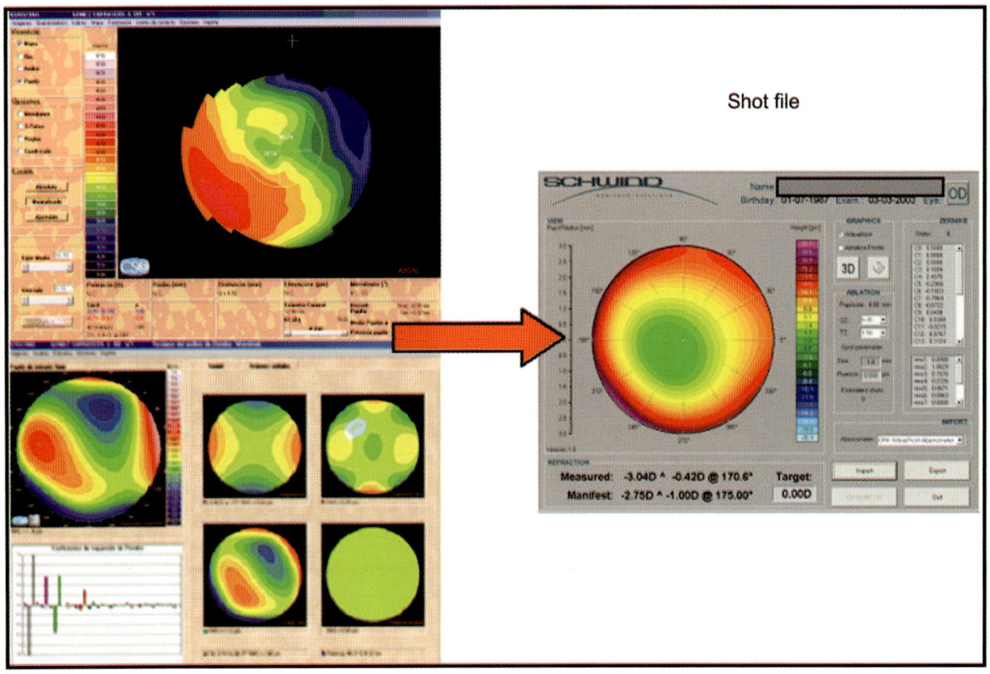

Fig. 20.9: Clinical case. Treatment ablation profile

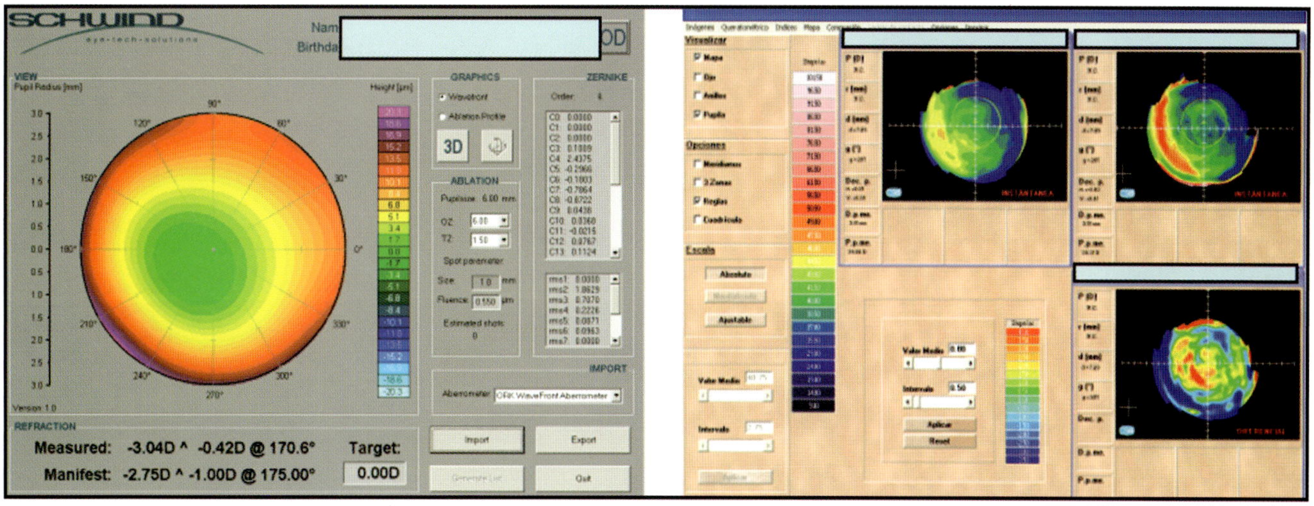

Fig. 20.10: Clinical case. Differential instantaneous map at preop an 6 months postop

CONCLUSIONS

The extensive use of corneal refractive surgery has increased the number of patients with corneal irregularities[7,8]. Correction of irregular astigmatism remains a challenge to refractive surgeons. Irregular astigmatism can be one of the most difficult and frustrating problems in refractive surgery. Treatment of irregular astigmatism oriented by corneal wavefront aberration has proved to be a successful technique. We have observed a significant improvement of uncorrected visual acuity, best corrected visual acuity and RMS values of HOA. These objective results also correlate with an improvement of patient visual symptoms after ORK-W treatment.

Corneal wavefront guided laser may be an excellent tool for correction of irregular astigmatism induce by previous corneal refractive surgery. In our hands preliminary results have shown that both visual and corneal irregularity improvements are better with corneal wavefront oriented treatment ORK-W compared to topography oriented treatment (TOPOLINK)[8].

REFERENCES

1. Liang J, Grimm B, Goelz S, Bille JF. Objective measurement of wave aberrations of the human eye with the use of a Hartmann-Shack wave-front sensor. J Opt Soc Am A 1994;11:1949-57.
2. Howland B, Howland HC. Subjective measurement of high-order aberrations of the eye. Science 1976;193: 580-82.
3. Mrochen M, Kaemmerer M, Mierdel P, Krinke HE, Seiler T. Principles of Tscherning aberrometry. J Refract Surg 2000;16:S570-71.
4. Molebny VV, Panagopoulou SI; Molebny SV, Wakil YS, Pallikaris IG. Principles of ray tracing aberrometry. J Refract Surg 2000;16:S572-75.
5. Burns SA. The spatially resolved refractometer. J Refract Surg 2000;16:S566-69.
6. MacRae S, Fujieda M. Slit skiascopic-guided ablation using the Nidek laser. J Refract Surg 2000;16:S576-80.
7. Alió JL, Artola A, Rodriguez-Mier FA. Selective zonal ablations with excimer laser for correction of irregular astigmatism induced by refractive surgery. Ophthalmology 2000;107:662-73.
8. Alió Jl, Belda JI, Osman AA, Shalaby AM. Topography-guided laser in situ keratomileusis (TOPOLINK) to correct irregular astigmatism after previous refractive surgery. J Refract Surg 2003;19:516-27.

Hyperopic Lasik for Accommodative Esotropia

21

Jairo E Hoyos, Melania Cigales,
Jairo E Hoyos-Chacon (Spain)

Accommodative esotropia is defined as a convergent deviation of the eyes associated with activation of the accommodation reflex. Donders described Refractive Accommodative Esotropia (RAE) as occurring in patients who must accommodate to clear blurred retinal images produced by high hyperopic refractive errors. This accommodation leads to excessive convergence, which eventually exceeds the patient's fusional divergence amplitude, resulting in esotropia.[1]

RAE is characterized by high hyperopia (ranging between + 3 and + 10 with an average of + 4.75 diopters), moderate deviation angle (ranging between 20 and 30 prism diopters) and an angle of esodeviation equal to, or within 10 prism diopters for distance and near (normal accommodative convergence to accommodation [AC/A] ratio).[2]

When seeing an approaching object, accommodation (through the contraction of the ciliary muscle) is required for maintaining the sharpness of the image on the foveal plane. Simultaneously, convergence (through medial recti contraction) keeps the foveae in the position required for normal retinal correspondence. In this way, keeping constant the ratio 1 unit of accommodation to 1 unit of convergence through a fixed central accommodation-convergence synkinesia, the emmetrope maintain a sharp and single image.

In the axial hypermetrope, due to the shorter lens-foveal distance, more accommodation is required, therefore the one to one ratio is not maintained. The result is one of the following. In a majority of cases the linkage is abnormal, and for the required increased accommodation there is a normal amount of convergence. While in a minority of individuals the excessive required contraction of the ciliary muscle drags the medial recti in the same one to one ratio as in an emmetrope, resulting in excess convergence, which is an accommodative esotropia, either permanent or whenever near vision is required.

Treatment of RAE is based on eliminating accommodation induced by high hyperopia, thus decreasing accommodative convergence. The standard treatment of RAE patients is optical, prescribing glasses or contact lenses for the full hyperopic refractive error, as determined under complete cycloplegia.[3] Miotic agents have also been used but they have been rejected because of their local and systemic side effects.[4]

Many patients show a decrease in their hyperopia with growth, as they approach seven years of age or more.[5] Some patients with accommodative esotropia will develop fusional divergence amplitudes sufficiently large to allow for the gradual reduction and eventual elimination of glasses or contact lenses while maintaining orthophoria or a well-controlled esophoria during accommodation. Other patients maintain orthophoria only while wearing their full hyperopic correction and do not develope sufficient fusional divergence amplitude to control their esotropia when their optical correction is decreased. Glasses are unappealing esthetically to these adult patients, and not all patients are candidates for continued contact lens wear. In addition, the esodeviation is still present when contact lenses are removed.[6]

The obvious way to permanently alleviate the excess convergence is to eliminate the need for the causative excess accommodation. We achieved this by correcting the hyperopia with LASIK.

TREATMENTS FOR ACCOMMODATIVE ESOTROPIA

The classical treatment for RAE is the use of glasses or contact lenses to correct the hyperopic error, but the esodeviation reappears when the optical correction is removed.[3] Although the hyperopic error diminishes and a fusional divergence amplitude large enough to maintain orthophoria without optical correction develops in some patients when they reach adulthood, it does not happen in all cases.[5,6]

Another form of treatment is the use of miotic agents (diisopropyl fluorophosphate and echothiophate iodide) which are thought to maintain the eyes straight by facilitating the myoneural transmission at the ciliary muscle, thus reducing the patient's need of central accommodative effort and, consequently, of the associated medial rectus contraction.[7] However, this treatment is frequently not well tolerated for long periods of time because the patient does not achieve good visual acuity and it produces undesirable ocular and systemic effects.[6,8,9]

Some authors[10-11] advocate muscle surgery in adult or adolescent patients with accommodative esotropia who wish to remove their glasses in undesired situations. This goes against traditional teaching, because with time accommodation strength lessens, thus dooming the eyes to secondary exotropia. For this reason, it is generally agreed that surgical treatment by extraocular muscle surgery for esotropia is indicated only for non-accommodative esotropias and for the correction of the non-accommodative component of mixed esotropias.[6-8]

Therefore, the mainstay of treatment of RAE continues to be the correction of the hyperopic refractive error. This has been traditionally accomplished by means of optical correction but now there are new surgical alternatives for the correction of refractive errors. Hiles et al[12] report one case of an 11-year old girl with RAE treated with bilateral phakic hyperopic epikeratoplasty where the esodeviation was successfully corrected. Bilgihan et al[13] report one 19-year old patient with RAE in whom orthophoria was achieved after the correction of the refractive error with photorefractive keratectomy (PRK). Maldonado-Bas et al[14] report 6 RAE patients ranging between 10 and 30 years of age treated with LASIK in whom orthophoria was achieved without optical correction.

Preoperative Examination

All patients underwent a thorough ophthalmological examination. Refraction was performed under cycloplegia and surgery was planned for total hyperopia in order to achieve orthophoria without optical correction. Additionally, prisms were used to measure deviation angle with and without optical correction, for distance and near fixation. A computerized corneal topography was done and the Simulated Keratoscope reading (Sim K) was used to analyze the pre- and postoperative corneal curvature. Ultrasound pachymetry was performed. Patient work-up was completed with sensory studies using red glassees, Bagolini striated lenses, Worths peripheral and macular test, Cüppers foveo-foveolar test, and Randolt stereo-test, in order to assess fixation, suppression, retinal correspondence and stereopsis.

Surgery was performed in patients older than 18 years of age with refractive accommodative esotropia and with hyperopia under cycloplegia up to +7 diopters on the flattest meridian. The following were considered to be exclusion criteria:

- Corneal pathology
- Thin corneas to allow for a stromal bed of at least 250 microns under the ablation.
- Glaucoma
- Lens opacity
- Active inflammatory or infectious ocular disease
- Presence of peripheral retinal lesions not treated prophylacticly
- Dry eye
- Profound amblyopia
- Patients with false expectations.

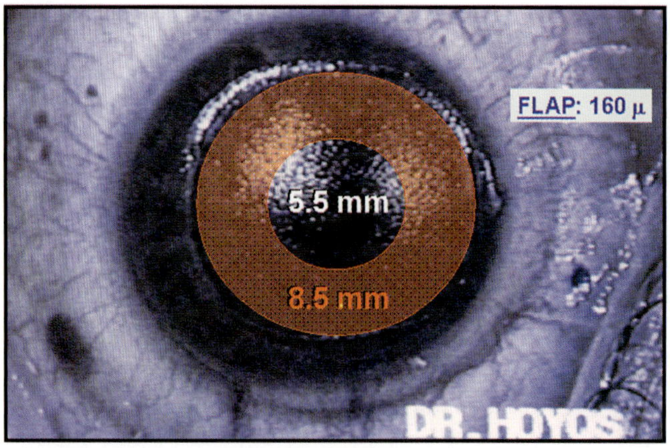

Fig. 21.1: Surgical technique: Keratectomy was performed with the ACS microkeratome using the 160 micron thickness plate and the 12 mm suction ring in order to create a nasally flap of approximately 8.5-9.0 mm. A 5.5 mm optical zone and a transition zone of up to 8.5 mm was used to do the ablation

SURGICAL TECHNIQUE

All of the interventions were performed at the *Instituto Oftalmologico de Sabadell* (Barcelona–Spain) and both eyes were operated in the same surgical session.

The cornea was marked with the 4-radii radial keratotomy marker dyed with gentian violet, plus one additional pararadial marking. The keratectomy was performed with the Automated Corneal Shaper microkeratome (ACS) using the 160 micron thickness plate; the 12 mm suction ring was placed with a 1 or 2 mm nasal displacement in order to create a nasally decentered flap of approximately 8.5-9.0 mm in diameter to avoid exposure of the hinge during the ablation (Fig. 21.1). The hyperopic ablation was done with a broad beam excimer. The surgery was planned to the cycloplegic refraction correction expressed in terms of a positive cylinder and the astigmatism was treated by steepening the flattest meridian (Fig. 21.2). A 5.5 mm optical zone and a transition zone of up to 8.5 mm was used. At the end of the ablation, the interface was thoroughly rinsed with Ringer's lactate using the irrigation-aspiration maneuver during which the flap was replaced. The reference markings were aligned and time was allowed for the flap to adhere totally to its bed, and a few drops of cyprofloxacin were instilled.

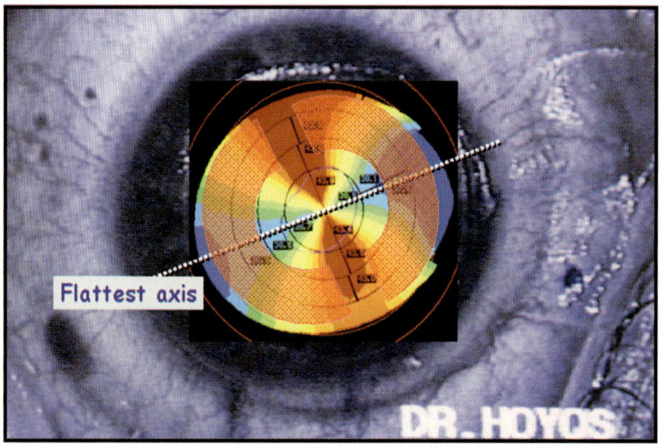

Fig. 21.2: Surgical technique: The surgery was planned to the cycloplegic refraction correction expressed in terms of a positive cylinder and the astigmatism was treated by steepening the flattest meridian

Protective shields were placed until the following day when postoperative treatment was initiated with antibiotic and steroid drops for one week and artificial tears for one month. Patients were instructed to avoid ocular trauma and rubbing during the first month and were advised to wear protective shields at night.

RESULTS

This study includes 18 eyes of 9 adult patients (age from 18 to 38 year old) with refractive accommodative esotropia who were treated with hyperopic LASIK with the objective of producing orthophoria and eliminating the need for optical correction. All patients had refractive accommodative esotropia at the time of the LASIK treatment and 3 of them had mixed esotropia and were operated on for the non-accommodative component of their esotropia in childhood. Average follow-up was 20 months (range 12 to 24).

Refraction

The average preoperative spherical equivalent was +5.01 ± 1.24 diopters (D) (range +2.50 to +7.00) and the post-operative average was +0.06±0.69 D (range – 0.75 to +1.25). Ten eyes (56%) were within ± 0.50 D of emmetropia and 16 were within ± 1.00 D (89%). Table 21.1 shows the evolution of the spherical equivalent during follow-up. The average pre-operative astigmatism was 1.41 ± 1.10 D and the post-operative average was 0.61 ± 0.65 D. Nine eyes were retreated in five patients within 3 and 5 months of the initial surgery. Those 9 eyes showed, at three months, an average residual spherical equivalent of +1.38 ± 1.04 D and an average residual astigmatism of 1.72 ± 0.93 D.

Topography

The average pre and postoperative corneal curvatures were 41.86±1.30 D and 44.80 ± 1.77 D, respectively. The average steepening was 2.94 ± 1.07 D (range 1.30 to 4.80).

Visual Acuity

The average pre-operative uncorrected visual acuity (UCVA) was 0.49±0.26 (20/40) for distance and 0.37 ± 0.22 (20/50) for near. The average postoperative result for distance was 0.83 ± 0.19 (20/25) and for near the result in all cases was 1.0 (20/20). The improvement of the UCVA after the procedure was highly significant ($p < 0.005$).

Table 21.1: Preoperative spherical equivalent and its follow-up at 1, 3, 6, 12, 18 and 24 months postoperative. Enhancement was performed between 3 and 5 months post-operative*

Spherical equivalent	*Preop) (n = 18*	*1 Month (n = 18)*	*3 Months (n = 18)*	*6 Months (n = 18)*	*12 Months (n = 18)*	*18 Months (n = 14)*	*24 Months (n = 12)*
Case 1	+7	+1	+1	+1	+1	+1	+1
Case 2	+5.5	+0.5	+1.5	+1.25	+1.25	+1.25	+1.25
Case 3	+2.5	+0.25	0	+0.25	0	0	0
Case 4	+2.5	0	–0.5	–0.25	–0.5	–0.5	–0.5
Case 5	+5	+1	+1	h –0.5	–0.5	+0.5	+0.75
Case 6	+5.5	+1.5	+0.75	h 0	–0.5	–0.5	0
Case 7	+5.5	+1.25	+1	h 0	0	0	0
Case 8	+5.25	+0.5	+0.5	h 0	0	0	0
Case 9	+4.5	–1	–0.75	–0.75	–0.75	–0.75	–0.75
Case 10	+4	–0.75	0	0	0	0	0
Case 11	+5.75	0	+0.5	–0.25	–0.5	–0.75	–0.75
Case 12	+5.5	0	-0.25	h –0.75	–0.5	–0.5	–0.5
Case 13	+4.75	+0.25	+1.75	h –0.25	–0.75	–0.75	
Case 14	+4.5	+1	+2.25	h +1.5	–0.25	–0.25	
Case 15	+4	+1.75	+1.25	+1.25	+1.25		
Case 16	+5.25	+2.5	+1.5	+1	+1		
Case 17	+7	+1.25	+2.75	h 0	0		
Case 18	+6.25	+1.25	+2.75	h –0.5	–0.5		

*Enhancement

The average preoperative best corrected visual acuity (BCVA) was 0.97 ± 0.22 (20/20-) for distance and 1.0 (20/20) in all cases for near vision. The average BCVA for distance was 0.94 ± 0.18 (20/20-) after surgery. Four eyes (22%) showed a loss of one line of visual acuity and 1 eye (6%) gained one line. There were no losses of two or more lines. Loss of lines of vision was not statistically significant ($p < 0.145$). The postoperative corrected visual acuity for near did not change as compared with the preoperative value in any of the cases. After the refractive retreatment, none of the patients required optical correction.

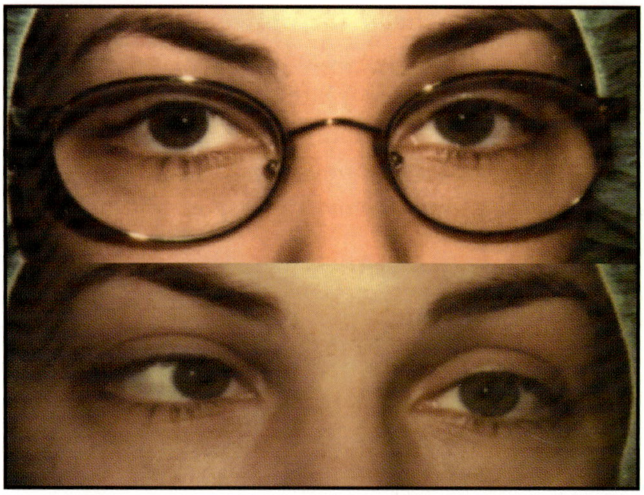

Fig. 21.3: The patient is orthophoric with glasses and shows esotropia in the left eye without glasses

Primary Position

All patients had an accommodative esotropia with the same deviation angle for distance and near, or within 10 prism diopters (PD) (normal AC/C ratio). The average preoperative deviation angle without optical correction was 36 PD (range 20 to 50); with their optical correction, 4 patients (44%) were orthophoric and 5 patients (56%) showed a microesotropia from 4 to 15 PD (average of 7.20 PD). In the immediate postoperative period (at 24 hours), all the 9 patients had orthophoria without optical correction or the same microesotropia which they already had with their optical correction before surgery. This status remained stable throughout the postoperative follow-up.

Figure 21.3 shows the preoperative appearance of a patient with RAE. Figure 21.4 shows the same patient orthophoric without optical correction a few minutes after LASIK and after two years.

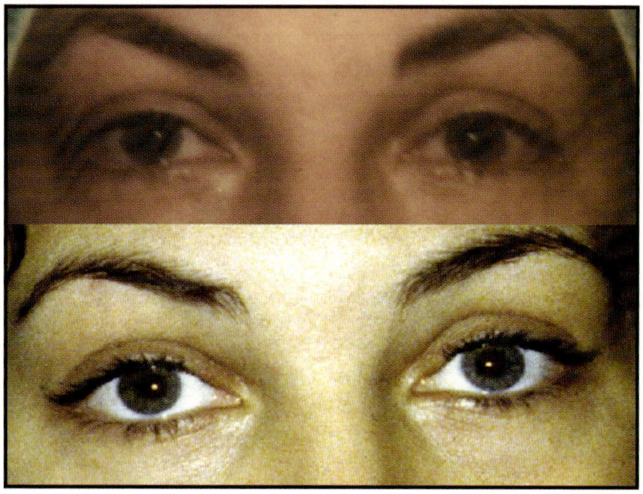

Fig. 21.4: The patient became orthophoric without optical correction a few minutes after LASIK and after two years

Sensory Tests

The fixating eye was the left one in 4 patients (44%) and the right one in 5 patients (56%). In the four patients who exhibited orthophoria with optical correction there was normal retinal correspondence, central macular fixation, peripheral and central fusion with a stereopsis equal to 100 arc seconds both pre- and post-operatively. The five patients in whom a microesotropia persisted in spite of total hyperopia correction, showed alternating central suppression, normal retinal correspondence, central macular fixation and a stereopsis equal to 400 arc seconds.

Complications

There were no serious complications during or after the surgical treatment. Three eyes (16.66%) showed topographic decentration: 0.5 mm in two eyes and 1 mm in one eye. Two eyes (11.11%) showed superficial punctate epitheliopathy during the early post-operative period which disappeared with the increased use of artificial tears. Two eyes (11.11%) showed peripheral epithelialization after reintervention; however, it was self-limiting and did not require treatment. One patient (11.11%) complained of glare and night halos, consistent with a topographic decentering of 1 mm in one eye and 0.5 mm in the other.

DISCUSSION

The correction of the hyperopic error with LASIK in our series of 9 patients over 18 years of age, resulted in the correction of the esodeviation angle previously corrected with glasses, giving rise to orthophoria or leaving the patient with the microesotropia observed with the optical correction before surgery. There is no doubt that LASIK, with the excimer laser ablation under the flap, has some advantages over other corneal surgical techniques: greater predictability, no pain, no haze, shorter use of steroids after surgery, greater corrections, and sparing of the anatomical structure of the cornea because Bowman's membrane is preserved.[15-20]

In our series, as well as in other case reports[12], the correction of the deviation angle was achieved despite the fact that there was a residual refractive error in some cases. The fusional divergence amplitude was not measured in this series, but we believe that it could explain the orthophoria achieved in spite of the undercorrection. Figure 21.5 shows the efficacy of LASIK in correcting the deviation angle in RAE, and Figure 21.6 shows the stability of the phoric status in our series after a follow-up period of 12 to 24 months.

Concerning spherical equivalent predictability, 56% of the series came within ±0.5 diopters of emmetropia and 89% were within ±1 diopter. Figure 21.7 shows the predictability in our series and Figure 21.8 shows the stability of the optical correction achieved during follow-up. The predictability at ±1 D of emmetropia reported in other LASIK series for hyperopia varies according to the attempted refraction; Ditzen et al[20] reports 85% in one group of up to +4 D and 58% in another between +4.25 and +8 D; Knorz et al[21] reports 75% in a group of up to +5 D and 60% in another between +5.1 and +10 D; Buzard

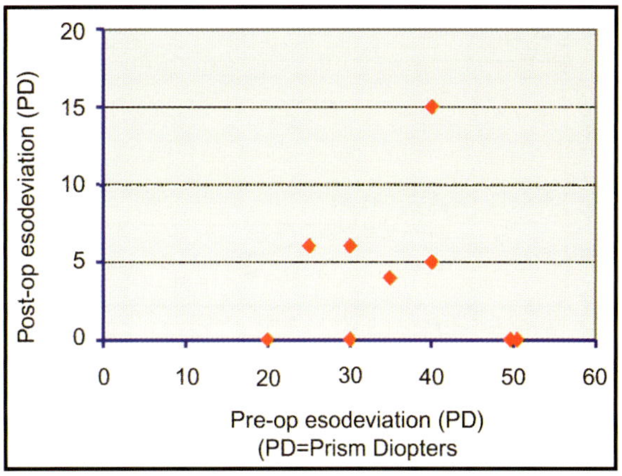

Fig. 21.5: Efficacy: Preoperative esodeviation without correction versus postoperative esodeviation without correction

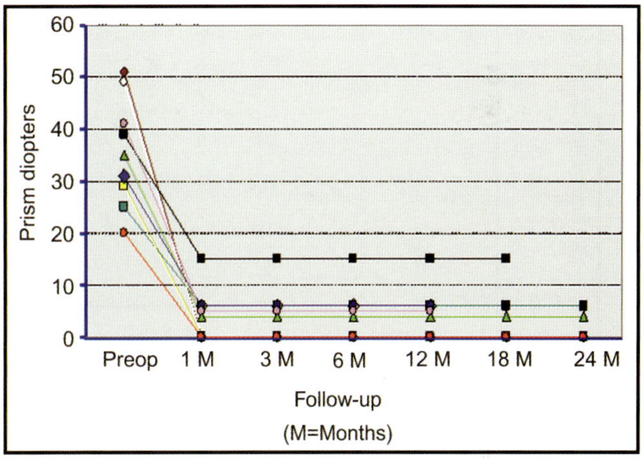

Fig. 21.6: Stability: Esodeviation follow up at 1, 3, 6, 12, 18 and 24 months

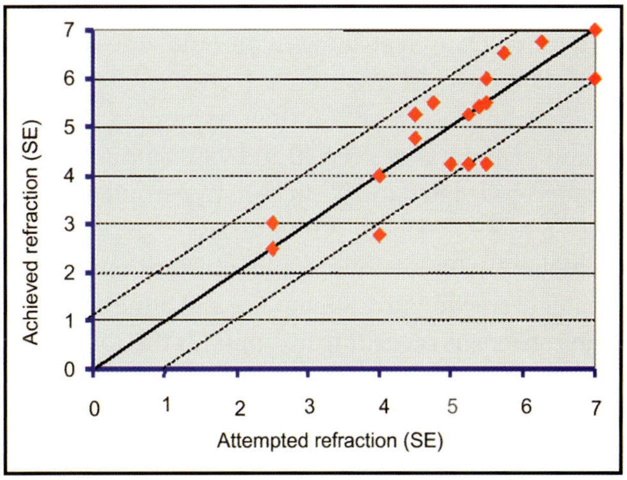

Fig. 21.7: Predictability: Attempted spherical equivalent (SE) versus SE achieved

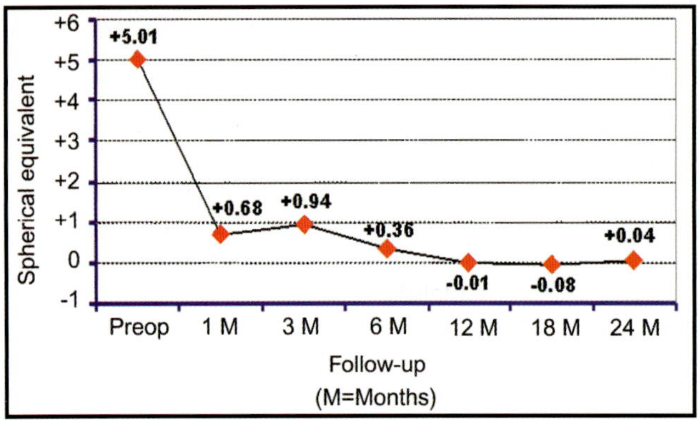

Fig. 21.8: Mean spherical equivalent over time. Data include all 18 eyes preoperatively, 18 eyes at 1, 3, 6, 12 months, 14 eyes at 18 months, and 12 eyes at 24 months

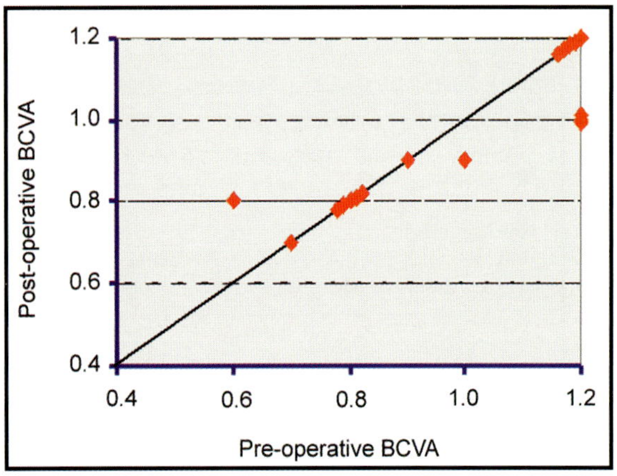

Fig. 21.9: Safety: Preoperative best corrected visual acuity (BCVA) versus post-operative best corrected visual acuity

et al[22] reports 86% in up to +4 D. The predictability of the PRK series for hyperopia shows greater variability: Dausch et al[23] in hyperopic series of up to +8.25 D reports 81% within ± 1 D of emmetropia, , whereas other series[24-26] in low hyperopia of up to +4 and +6 report between 40 and 98% within ± 1 D of emmetropia, and 0 to 17% in high hyperopia from +4 and +6 to +9.75 D. All of the series[20-26] report good predictability in low hyperopia which diminishes as greater corrections are attempted; and although there is no consensus regarding the limit for the correction, this limit appears to be between +4 and +6 diopters.

Visual acuity without optical correction showed a significant improvement ($p < 0.005$) after LASIK for distance and near vision. The average uncorrected visual acuity at the last check-up was 0.83±0.19, the best average corrected preoperative visual acuity being 0.97±0.22; patient satisfaction was demonstrated by none of the patients requiring optical correction to perform any of their daily tasks after treatment. As far as postoperative best corrected visual acuity is concerned, there was an improvement during follow-up and at the last check-up, four eyes (22%) had lost 1 line of vision. The FDA panel on excimer laser PRK for myopia has published guidelines stating that loss of best-corrected visual acuity should be limited to 5% of eyes losing two or more lines[27]. None of the eyes in our series lost 2 or more lines of vision, which speaks to the safety of the procedure. Figure 21.9 compares pre and post-operative BCVA. Some series of LASIK for hypermetropia[20,21] report losses of 2 or more lines of vision, especially in high hyperopic groups. The cause of lost visual acuity lines after hyperopic treatment is not always clear. Most of the authors attribute it to a decentered ablatión,[20,24,25,28] but mention has also been made of image minimization after LASIK as compared to the preoperative image with optical correction, and of optical aberration caused by the new corneal surface[21]. In our series, there were 3 cases of decentering, two with a slight 0.5 mm decentering in whom the best corrected visual acuity did not change and one with a 1.0 mm decentering who lost one line of vision. In three eyes from the four that lost one line of vision, the ablation was perfectly centered and no complications were observed in relation to the flap or the healing process. This leads us to consider that image minimization and the optical aberration induced by the new corneal surface could be associated with the loss of visual acuity.

The patients included in this series were adult patients (over 18 years of age) with a stable sensory status; no changes were observed in the sensory tests performed after LASIK. Other series[12,14] include younger patients (10 or 11-year old) and no sensory decompensations are reported. This surgical technique could perhaps be used in children with RAE, as if they could cooperate during a procedure performed under local anesthesia, adequate centration could be ensured and, in our opinion, as long as they were beyond the age where amblyopia could be induced in the event a serious complication were to occur. We believe that an additional problem with LASIK in children might be the placement of the suction ring given the small size of the eye and the narrow palpebral fissure characteristically found in hyperopic children. Refractive surgery treatments are indicated only for stable refractive errors and some studies[5] report that, hyperopia in accommodative esodeviation showed a mean annual decrease between ages 7 and 13 year of –0.18±0.25 D.

The most important limitation of hyperopic LASIK in patients with RAE is the degree of hyperopia. Different studies[20,21,24-26] show that, in high hyperopia, predictability is reduced and there is an increased percentage of loss of visual acuity lines. In such cases of high hyperopia, an alternative to the use of LASIK might be clear lens extraction[29,30] in patients over 45 years of age and phakic lens implantation[31-33] in younger patients. However, we must not forget that these other intraocular techniques entail a greater risk of serious complications.[34,35]

CONCLUSION

In conclusion, hyperopic LASIK proved to be an effective surgical technique for the correction of the deviation angle in RAE and in mixed esotropia after the correction of the muscle component using conventional surgery.[36] In this series, LASIK was predictable in the indicated hyperopic range and proved to be safe considering that there were no serious surgical complications and that there were no losses of two or more lines of vision. Results were stable during the 12 or 24-month follow-up. Further studies are required in order to determine the age at which this form of surgery could be used for RAE patients.

REFERENCES

1. Parks MM. Concomitant Esodeviations. In: Ocular motility and strabismus. Hagerstown: Harper and Row 1975;12:99-105.
2. Parks MM. Abnormal accommodative convergence in squint. Arch Ophthalmol 1958;59:364-80.
3. Parks MM. Management of acquired esotropia. Br J Ophthalmol 1974;58:240-7.
4. Diorio PC. The role of miotics in the management of accommodative esotropia. Am J Orthoptic 1977;27: 96-9.
5. Raab EL. Hypermetropia in accommodative esodeviation. J Ped Ophthalmol Strab 1984;21:194-7.
6. Parks MM, Mitchell PR, Wheeler MB. Concomitant esodeviations. In: Tasman W, Jaeger EA, eds. Duane's Clinical Ophthalmology, revised ed. Philadelphia: JB Lippincott 1998;1:12:1-21.
7. Preslan MV, Beauchamp GR. Accommodative esotropia: review of current practices and controversies. Ophthalmic Surgery 1987;18:68-72.
8. Von Noorden GK. Burian-von Noorden. Esodeviations. In: Binocular vision and ocular motility; Theory and management of strabismus. St Louis: The CV Mosby Company 1974;279-303.
9. Chamberlain W. Anticholinesterase miotics in the management of accommodative esotropia. Trans Am Ophthalmol Soc 1974;72:229-41.
10. Albert DG, Hiles DA. Surgical treatment of accommodative esotropia with an abnormal distance/ near relationship. South Med J 1967;60:856-58.
11. Dyer JA. Nonsurgical treatment of esotropia. In: Symposium on Strabismus; Transactions of the New Orleans Academy of Ophthalmology. St Louis: The CV Mosby Company 1971;154-59.
12. Hiles DA, Cheng KP. Bilateral phakic hypermetropic epikeratoplasty for accommodative esotropia. J Cataract Refract Surg 1990;16:361-66.
13. Bilgihan K, Akata F, Or M, Hasanreisoglu B. Photorefractive keratectomy in refractive accommodative esotropia. Eye 1997;11:409-10.
14. Maldonado-Bas A, Hoyos J. Estrabismo: componente acomodativo tratado con LASIK. Rev Bras Oftal 1998; 10:757-60.
15. Trokel SL, Srinivasan R, Braren B. Excimer laser surgery of the cornea. Am J Ophthalmol 1983;96:710-5.
16. Trokel SL. Evolution of excimer laser corneal surgery. J Cataract Refract Surg 1989;15:373-82.
17. Seiler T, Wollensack J. Myopic photorefractive keratectomy with the excimer laser: one year follow-up. Ophthalmology 1991;98:1156-63.
18. Pallikaris IG, Papatzanaki ME, Siganos DS, Tsilimbaris MK. A corneal flap technique for laser in situ keratomileusis. Arch Ophthalmol 1991;1699-1702.
19. Buratto L, Ferrari M, Genisi C. Myopic keratomileusis with the excimer laser: one year follow-up. J Refract Corneal Surg 1993;9:12-19.

20. Ditzen K, Huschka H, Pieger S. Laser in situ keratomileusis for Hyperopia. J Cataract Refract Surg 1998;24:42-47.
21. Knorz MC, Liermann A, Jendritza B, Hugger P. LASIK for hyperopia and hyperopic astigmatism – results of a pilot study. Seminars in Ophthalmology 1998; 13:83-87.
22. Buzart KA, Fundingsland BR. Excimer laser assisted in situ keratomileusis for hyperopia. J Cataract Refract Surg 1999;25:197-204.
23. Dausch D, Smecka Z, Klein R, et al. Excimer laser photorefractive keratectomy for hyperopia. J Cataract Refract Surg 1997;23:169-76.
24. Pietilä J, Mäkinen P, Pajari S, Uusitalo H. Excimer laser photorefractive keratectomy for hyperopia. J Refract Surg 1997;13:504-10.
25. Sener B, Özdamar A, Aras C, Yanyali A. Photorefractive keratectomy for hyperopia and aphakia with a scanning spot excimer laser. J Refract Surg 1997;13:620-3.
26. Jackson WB, Casson E, Hodge WG, et al. Laser vision correction for low hyperopia: an 18-month assessment of safety and efficacy. Ophthalmology 1998;105: 1727-38.
27. McDonell PJ. Excimer laser photorefractive keratectomy-the Food and Drug Administration panel speaks. Arch Ophthalmol 1995; 113:858-59.
28. Aron-Rosa DS, Febbraro JL. Laser in situ keratomileusis for hyperopia. J Refract Surg 1999; 15(suppl):S212-S5.
29. Siganos DS, Siganos CS, Pallikaris IG. Clear lens extraction and intraocular lens implantation in normally sighted hyperopic eyes. J Refract Corneal Surg 1994; 10:117-24.
30. Siganos DS, Pallikaris IG. Clear lensectomy and intraocular lens implantation for hyperopia from +7 to +14 diopters. J Refract Surg 1998;14:105-13.
31. Rosen E, Gore C. Staar collamer posterior chamber phakic intraocular lens to correct myopia and hyperopia. J Cataract Refract Surg 1998;24:596-606.
32. Davidorf JM, Zaldivar R, Oscherow S. Posterior chamber phakic intraocular lens for hyperopia of +4 to +11 diopters. J Refract Surg 1998;14:306-11.
33. Sanders DR, Martin RG, Brown DC, et al. Posterior chamber phakic intraocular lens for hyperopia. J Refract Surg 1999; 15:309-15.
34. Fink AM, Gore C, Rosen E. Cataract development after implantation of the Staar collamer posterior chamber phakic lens. J Cataract Refract Surg 1999;25:278-82.
35. Pérez-Santonja JJ, Ruíz-Moreno JM, De la Hoz F, et al. Endophthalmitis after phakic intraocular lens implantation to correct high myopia. J Cataract Refract Surg 1999;25:1295-98.
36. Hoyos JE, Cigales M, Hoyos-Chacón J, Ferrer J, Maldonado-Bass J. Hyperopic laser in situ keratomileusis for refractive accommodative esotropia. J Cataract Refract Surg 2002;28(9):1522-29.

Wide Zone Lasik for Hyperopia

22

Rishi Mohan (India)

INTRODUCTION AND BRIEF HISTORY

Keratomileusis in situ, first reported by Jose Ignacio Barraquer, was initially performed by removing layers of frozen corneal tissue with an oscillating microkeratome.[1]

Initial attempts to correct myopia with an excimer laser on the cornea (photoablation) were made by Trokel & Srinivasan et al,[2] Tuft et al[3] and Seiler et al.[4] Ruiz in 1986 developed the surgical technique of in situ keratomileusis. Pallikaris described the combined excimer laser photorefractive keratectomy and in situ keratomileusis technique (LASIK).[5]

Hyperopia or hypermetropia is a type of refractive error in which the cornea has to be made steeper to neutralize the anomaly for focusing the incident rays on the retina. High success rates and stability of outcomes were reported with myopic Lasik where the objective was to flatten the central cornea. The objective, however, in hyperopic Lasik is to steepen cornea. Traditionally, attempts to steepen the central cornea have been less successful and less stable. Non-excimer laser methods such as hexagonal keratotomies,[6,7] thermokeratoplasty with the Holmium-Yag[8,9] and epikeratophakia[10] have been tried in the treatment of hyperopia with mixed success.

Excimer laser photoablation of corneal tissue for hyperopia is performed in a concentric ring-like pattern in the peripheral cornea to produce central steepening. The ablation requires a refractive optical zone and a peripheral transition zone. In the earliest forms of surface treatments for hyperopia, the treatment zones were only 4-5 mm with peripheral blend zones of 2-3 mm making a total treatment area of 7-8 mm. Acceptable results were reported by many authors, including Dausch,[11,12] and Ditzen and Anschutz (unpublished report, German Ophthalmologic Soc, 1994). However, problems of decentration and haze were encountered frequently, especially with the higher powers.

To produce central corneal steepening, a deep peripheral ablation ring has to be created with progressive steepening of the transition zone. In surface treatments (hyperopic PRK), corneal epithelial cells tend to fill the depression created in the ablation zone, thereby leading to regression and poor stability in comparison to myopia procedures. In LASIK, with the overlying flap, epithelial filling is prevented and this tendency for regression of power is markedly reduced.

WIDE ZONE VS CONVENTIONAL (NARROW ZONE) HYPEROPIC LASIK

With narrow zone hyperopic LASIK there were certain limitations. There was a limit to the range of treatment to +3.0D only. There was more astigmatism and surface abnormalities generated due to the changed corneal profile and tear film dynamics. Proper centration was critical. Patients complained of haloes, increased glare and induced astigmatism with resultant reduction in visual quality. Lastly, there was significant regression in the correction achieved. Numerous studies are available showing the comparison of the wide-zone treatments with the narrow zone.

Portellinho, Nakano and Oliveira in their series of 31eyes with hyperopia and hyperopic astigmatism studied prospectively, evaluated the efficacy, safety and predictability of the 7.0 mm OZ/9.0 mm TZ software and presented the results at the NAVEX Symposium at the AAO in 2002. All cases were performed with the Nidek EC-5000 and flaps made with either the MK-2000 automated keratome or the Hansatome. Mean preoperative SE was +2.80D and was changed to –0.70D in the first month, -0.60D in the 3rd and –0.40D by the 6th month. 68% achieved a final SE of ± 0.50D. Further, in a comparison with their previous study employing a narrow zone treatment (5.5 mm OZ/7.5 mm TZ) with a mean pre-op SE of +2.67D, there was a mean undercorrection of 0.21D at 6 months, whereas in the wide zone treatment group there was a slight mean overcorrection. They concluded that the wide zone hyperopia treatment is safe, effective and stable.

Sulimma, Schmeidt and Kermani et al presented their series on wide zone hyperopic Lasik with zones of 7.0mm OZ (Optical Zone) and 9.5 mm TZ (Transition Zone) at the ESCRS in 2003. They performed 132 eyes with narrow zone (5.5 mm OZ and 7.5mm TZ) and 131 with wide zone treatments. Mean pre-op spherical equivalent (SE) in the first group was +2.78D + 0.99D and +2.49 ± 1.3D in the latter group, with similar age, gender and right-left distribution. At 3 months post-op, in the narrow zone group, the average SE was +0.51D with a mean regression of 0.92D from the 1st day post Lasik upto the 3rd month, whereas in the wide zone group the mean 3rd month post op SE was +0.17D and the average regression from Day 1 to the 3rd month was only 0.24D in the same period.

Initial overcorrection with a larger regression was found in the narrow zone treatment group as compared to the wide zone treatment group which had a slight overcorrection on the first day and had less regression. At 3 months, 83% had correction within ± 1D in the wide zone treatment group whereas only 73% of the narrow zone treatment group had a SE of ± 1D. Wide zone treatments were found to be significantly better than narrow zone treatment with superior efficacy, predictability, stability and excellent safety.

From India, Bharti presented his initial results with the wide zone hyperopia treatments at the Nidek 9th Refractive Sugery Conference in Barcelona in 2004. 50 procedures done consecutively were divided into 3 groups and followed for minimum 60 days; Group I with 6.5/9.0 mm treatment (30 eyes), Group II with 7.0/9.0 mm treatment (10 eyes) and Group III with Right eye 6.5/9.0 mm and Left eye with 7.0/9.0 mm treatment (5 eyes each). All patients had spherical equivalents of between +2D and +8D and assigned randomly to each group.

On Day 7, in Group I, 77% eyes were overcorrected to –1.0 D, 16% to –2.0D and 7% to more than –2.0D. In Group II, 60% were within –0.5D, 20% were having –1.0Dcyl and 20% were overcorrected to –2.0D. In Group III, 80% of the treated right eyes (6.5/9.0 mm) were overcorrected from – 0.62 to –2.0D and 20% undercorrected to +0.37D. The left eyes (7.0/9.0 mm), 60% eyes were undercorrected upto +0.37D, 20% overcorrected to –1.5D and 20% to –2.25D.

By Day 60, 76.6% eyes had regressed to +1.0D, 13% to between +1.0 and 2.0D and 3% to +2.5D in Group I. In Group II, 60% eyes were within –0.37D and –0.5D, 20% had regressed to +0.5 to +1.25D and 20% had a –1.0Dcyl. (same as in the 3rd week after Lasik). In Group III, all right eyes had regressed, 40% had regressed to +0.5D and 60% to +1.0D. Of the left eyes, 80% remained unchanged and 20% remained undercorrected upto +0.5D. BCVA recovery was more rapid in the 7.5/9.0 mm group with 90% eyes having recovered pre-op BCVA by Day 7, whereas full BCVA recovery was possible by Day 60 in the 6.5/9.0 mm treated eyes. He concluded that wide zone treatments are safe, more effective and have less regression and induced astigmatism. Patients are happier due to earlier recovery of vision and less complaints of glare and haloes.

SURGICAL TECHNIQUE

My surgical technique is as follows: The patient is explained the procedure and written consent obtained. Topical anesthesia is given with 1-2 drops of proparacaine hydrochloride on table, a minute before the procedure. The area is prepared and draped and the speculum applied. The conjunctival sac is irrigated with sterile saline and the patient made to appreciate the central fixation light on the laser (Fig. 22.1). The corneal mid-periphery is marked with the methylene blue marker.

The suction ring (9.5 mm) of the microkeratome is applied in a fashion to obtain a more nasal and superior flap and the IOP checked to exceed 60 mmHg (Fig. 22.2). A superior hinge flap with the Hansatome (160 or 180 microns; 9.5 mm dia.) is created in a fashion as to leave the smallest hinge possible to avoid hinge ablation (Fig. 22.3). The suction ring is then removed

The corneal flap is reflected, the eye tracker is activated on the machine and laser photoablation performed using the Wide-zone hyperopic nomogram (7.0 mm OZ/9.0 mm TZ) on the Nidek EC-5000CX as per the plan (Fig. 22.4). After completing the ablation, the interface is irrigated with

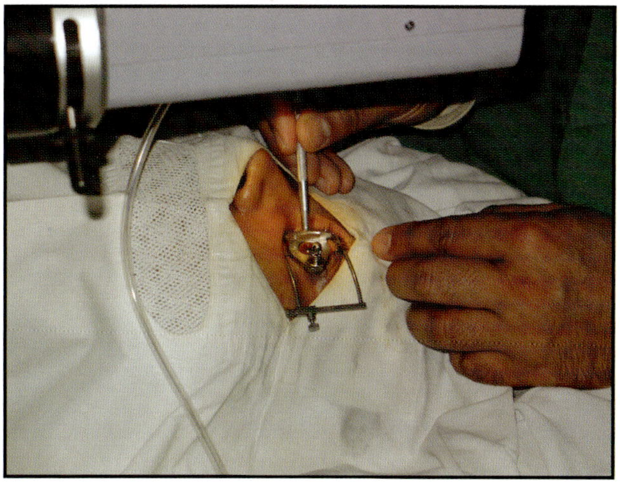

Fig. 22.2: Hansatome suction ring applied

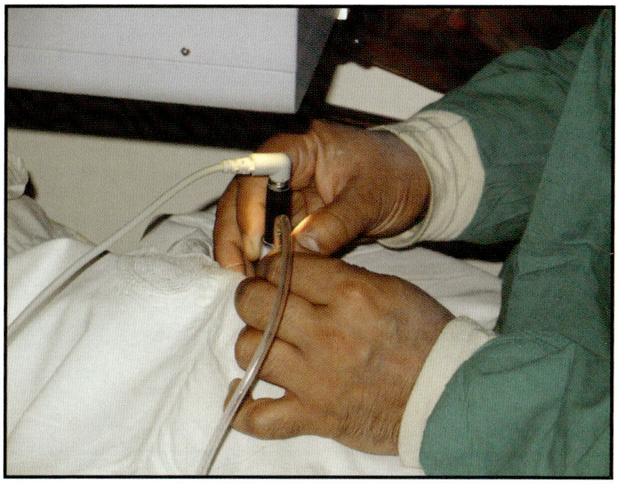

Fig. 22.3: Flap-making with Hansatome

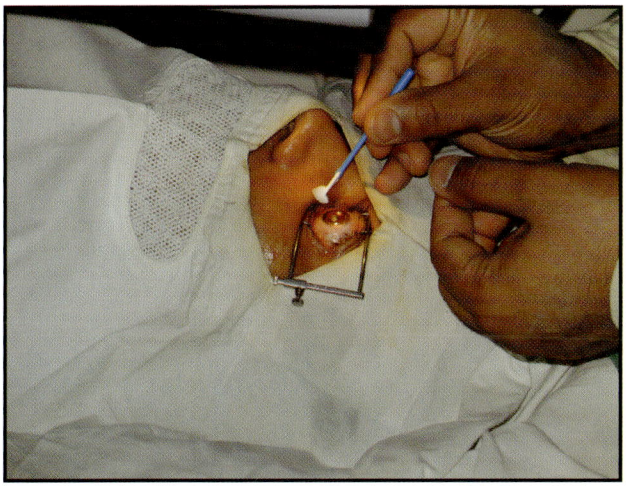

Fig. 22.1: Drying the conjunctiva with sponge

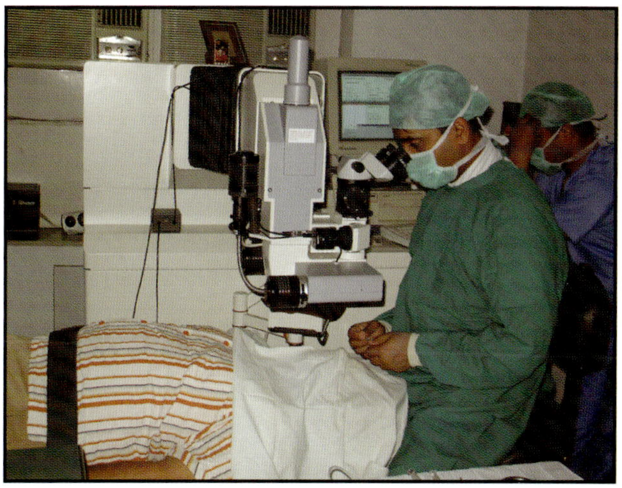

Fig. 22.4: LASIK being done on the NIDEK EC-5000CX

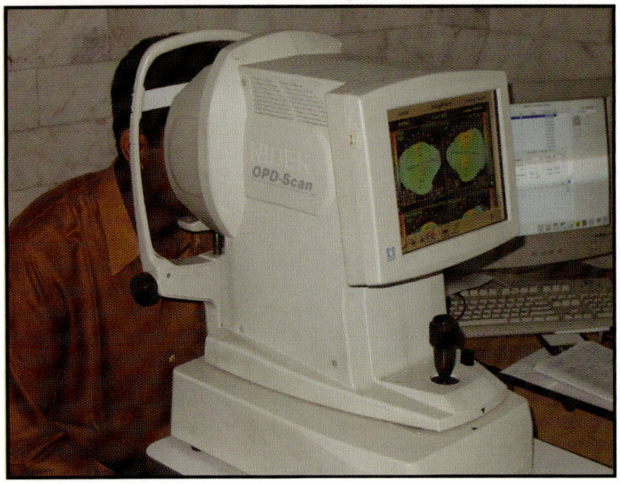

Fig. 22.5: Nidek OPD-Scan

sterile saline and the flap is floated back, repositioned and allowed to dry in position for a period of 3 minutes. Blink and Striae tests are performed. Antibiotic drops and lubricant drops are instilled and then a similar procedure carried out on the opposite eye.

Postoperatively, the patient is examined on Day 1, 3, 7 then in Week 3 and in the 2nd and 6th months (Fig. 22.5). Antibiotic, steroid and lubricant drops are administered as per assessment of need.

FUTURE ADVANCES

In the future we can expect better outcomes with the advent of iris recognition, torsion error detection and wavefront guided hyperopic LASIK (which is currently available only for myopic keratomileusis). Improved algorithms with better correction for age and corneal flatness coupled with improved designs of microkeratomes ensuring larger (10 mm) flaps and better and more efficient tracking would be useful in producing more reliable and effective outcomes for Hyperopic LASIK.

SUMMARY

Surgical correction of hyperopia and hyperopic astigmatism is still a challenge for keratorefractive surgeons. Technically, steepening procedures are more difficult and less reliable than flattening. Hyperopic Lasik requires a large flap with proper centration along the visual axis. There is a risk of hinge ablation and consequent scarring and induced astigmatism. Because of corneal biomechanics, the optical zone should never be less than 5 mm. Wide zone hyperopic LASIK offers much better safety, efficacy, predictability and reliability than the narrow zone with less regression and better patient comfort.

REFERENCES

1. Barraquer I. Keratomileusis from myopia, orientation for refractive surgery. Ophthalmology 1981;SS701-12.
2. Trokel SL, Srinivasan R, Braren B. Excimer laser surgery of the cornea. Am J Ophthalmol 1983:94;125.
3. Tuft S, Zabel RW, Marshall J. Corneal repair following keratectomy. Invest Ophthalmology Vis Sci 1989; 30:1769-77.
4. Seiler T, Kahle C, Kriegerowski M, Bende T. Myopic excimer laser (193 nm) keratomileusis in sighted and blind human eyes. J Refract Corneal Surg 1990;Sr 165-73.
5. Pallikaris IG, Papatzanaki ME, Stathi EZ. Laser in situ keratomileusis. Laser Surg Med 1990;10(5):463-68.
6. Nordan L, Maxwell W. Hexagonal keratotomy. Refract Corneal Surg 1993;9:228-29.
7. Grandon S, Sanders D, Anello R, et al. Clinical evaluation of hexagonal keratotomy for the treatment of primary hyperopia. J Catarct Refract Surg 1995; 21:109-10.
8. Durrie D, Schumer D, Cavanaugh T. Holmium:Yag laser thermokeratoplasty for hyperopia. J Refract Corneal Surg 1994;10:277-80.
9. Yanoff M. Holmium laser hyperopia thermokeratoplasty update. Eur J Implant Ref Surg 1995;7:89-91.
10. Krumeich JH. Indications, techniques and complications of myopic keratomileusis. Ophthalmology Olin 1983;23:75-92.
11. Dausch D, Klein R, Schroder E. Excimer Laser photorefractive keratectomy for hyperopia. Refract Corneal Surg 1993;9:20-28.
12. Dausch D, Landesz M. Laser correction of hyperopia. In Salz JJ, McDonald M, Flonell M (Eds). Corneal Laser Surgery. Philadelphia, PA: Mosby 1994;237-47.

Topographic and Aberrometer Guided Laser

23

AMAR AGARWAL, ATHIYA AGARWAL SUNITA AGARWAL (INDIA)

INTRODUCTION

Since as early as middle of 19th century it has been known that the optical quality of human eye suffers from ocular errors (aberrations) besides the commonly known image errors such as myopia, hyperopia and asigmatism.[1] In early 1970's Fyodorov introduced the anterior radial incisions to flatten the central cornea to correct myopia.[2] Astigmatic keratotomy,[3] Keratomileusis and Keratophakia, Epikeratophakia[4] and currently Excimer Laser[5] have been used to manage the various refractive errors. These refractive procedures correct lower order aberrations such as spherical and cylindrical refractive errors however higher order aberrations persist, which affect the quality of vision but may not significantly affect the Snellen visual acuity. Refractive corrective procedures are known to induce aberrations.[6] It is the subtle deviations from the ideal optical system, which can be corrected by wavefront and topography guided (customized ablation) LASIK procedures.[7]

Aberrations

Optical aberration customization can be corneal topography guided which measures the ocular aberrations detected by corneal topography and treats the irregularities as an integrated part of the laser treatment plan. The second method of optical aberration customization measures the wavefront errors of the entire eye and treats based on these measurements.[7] Wavefront analysis can be done either using Howland's aberroscope[8] or a Hartmann Shack wavefront sensor.[9] These techniques measure all the eye's aberrations including second-order (sphere and cylindrical), third-order (coma-like), fourth-order (spherical), and higher order wavefront aberrations. Based on this information an ideal ablation plan can be formulated which treats lower order as well as higher order aberrations.

Zyoptix Laser

Zyoptix™ (Bausch and Lomb) is a system for Personalized Vision Solutions, which incorporates Zywave™ Hartmann Shack aberrometer coupled with Orbscan™ II z multi-dimensional device, which generates the individual ablation profiles to be used with the Technolas® 217 Excimer Laser system. Thus this system utilizes combination of wavefront analysis and corneal topography for optical aberration customization.

Orbscan

The Orbscan (Bausch and Lomb) corneal topography system uses a scanning optical slit scan that is fundamentally different than the corneal topography that analyses the reflected images from the anterior corneal surface. The high-resolution video camera captures 40 light slits at 45 degrees angle projected through the cornea similarly as seen during slit lamp examination. The slits are projected on to the anterior segment of the eye: the anterior cornea, the posterior cornea, the anterior iris and anterior lens. The data collected from these four surfaces are used to create a topographic map. This technique provides more information about anterior segment of the eye, such as anterior and posterior corneal curvature and corneal thickness.[10] It improves the diagnostic accuracy and it has passive eye-tracker from frame to frame, 43 frames are taken to ensure accuracy. It is easy to interpret and has good repeatability. Three different maps are taken, and the one featuring the least eye movements is used. The maximum movements considered acceptable are 200 microns.

Aberrometer

Zywave™ is based on Hartmann –Shack aberrometry (Fig. 23.1) in which a laser diode (780 nm) generates a laser beam that is focused on the retina of the patient's eye (Fig. 23.2). An adjustable collimation system compensates for the spherical portion of the refractive error of the eye. Laser diode is turned on for approximately 100 milliseconds. The light reflected from the focal point on the retina (source of wavefront) is directed through an array of small lenses (lenslet) generating a grid like pattern (array) of focal points (Fig. 23.3). The position of the focal points are detected by Zywave™. Due to deviation of the points from their ideal position, the wavefront

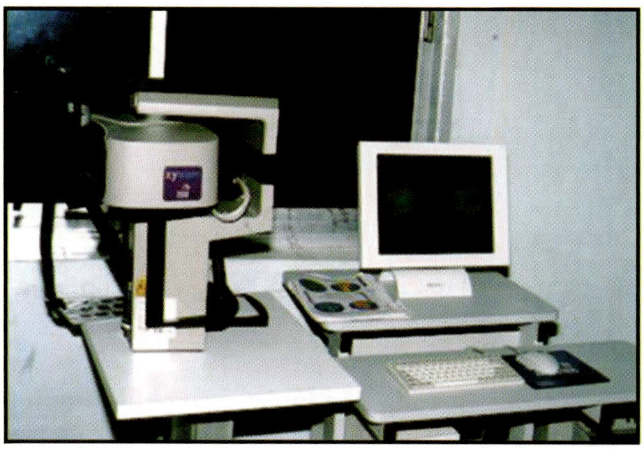

Fig. 23.1: Hartmann Shack aberrometer

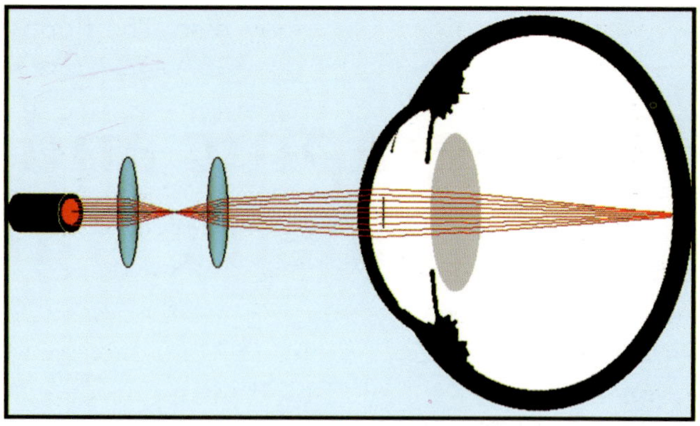

Fig. 23.2: Zywave projects low-intensity HeNe infrared light into the eye and use the diffuse reflection from the retina

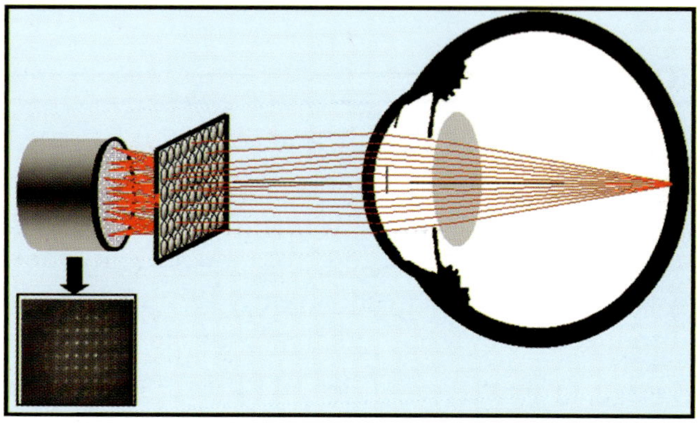

Fig. 23.3: Schematic illustration of the Bausch and Lomb Zywave aberrometer. A low-intensity HeNe infrared light is shone into the eye; the reflected light is focused by a number of small lenses (lenslet-array), and pictured by a CCD-camera. The capture image is shown on the bottom left

can be reconstructed. Wavefront display shows (a) higher order aberrations (b) predicted phoropter refraction (PPR) calculated for a back vertex correction of 15 mm (c) Simulated point spread function (PSF). Zywave™ examinations are done with (a) single examination with undilated pupil (b) five examinations with dilated pupil (mydriasis) non-cycloplegic, using 5% Phenylephrine drops. One of these five measurements, which matched best with the manifest refraction of the undilated pupil, is chosen for the treatment.

ZYLINK

Information gathered from Orbscan and Zywave are then translated into treatment plan using Zylink™

software and copied to a floppy disc. The floppy disc is then inserted into the Technolas 217 system (Fig. 23.4), fluence test carried out and a Zyopitx treatment card was inserted. A standard LASIK procedure is then performed with a superiorly hinged flap. A Hansatome™ microkeratome is used to create a flap. Flap thickness varied from 160 to 200 μm. A residual stromal bed of 250 μm or more is left in all eyes. Optical zone varied from 6 to 7 mm depending upon the pupil size and ablation required. Eye tracker is kept on during laser ablation. Post–operatively all patients are followed-up for at least 6 months.

RESULTS

We did a study comprising 150 eyes with myopia and compound myopic astigmatism. Preoperatively, the patients underwent corneal topography with Orbscan II z ™ and wavefront analysis with Zywave™ in addition to the routine pre-LASIK work up. The results were assimilated using Zylink™ and a customized treatment plan was formulated. LASIK was then performed with Technolas® 217 system. All the patients were followed-up for at least six months.

Mean preoperative BCVA (in decimal) was 0.83 ± 0.18 (Range 0.33- 1.00). Mean post-operative (6 months) BCVA was 1.00 ± 0.23 (Range 0.33-1.50). Difference was statistically significant (p = 0.0003). Out of 150 eyes that underwent customized ablation,

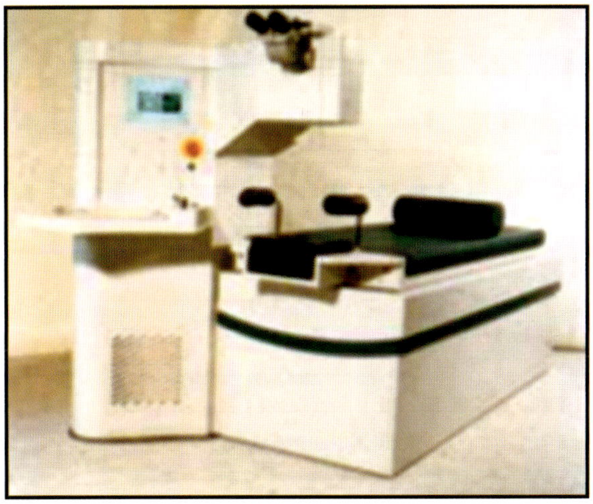

Fig. 23.4: Technolas 217 z excimer laser system

3 eyes (2%) lost two or more lines of best spectacle corrected visual acuity (BSCVA).

Safety Index = Mean post-operative BSCVA / Mean pre-operative BSCVA = 1.20 (Fig. 23.5). Mean pre-operative UCVA was 0.06 ± 0.02 (Range 0.01-0.50). Mean post-operative UCVA was 0.88 ± 0.36 (Range 0.08 – 1.50). Difference was statistically significant (p = 0.0001).

Efficacy index = Mean post-operative UCVA / Mean preoperative UCVA = 14.66 (Fig. 23.6). Pre-operatively, none of the eyes had UCVA of 6\6 or more and one eye (0.66%) had UCVA of 6/12 or more. At 6 months post-operatively, 105 eyes (69.93%) had UCVA of 6\6 or more and 126 eyes (83.91%) had UCVA of 6/12 or more.

Mean pre-operative spherical equivalent was -5.25 D ± 1.68 D (Range -0.87 to –15 D). Mean post-

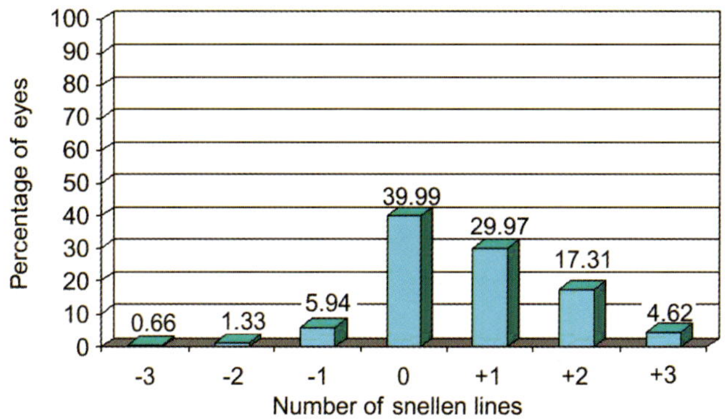

Fig. 23.5: Shows changes in BSCVA 6 months postoperatively (Safety)

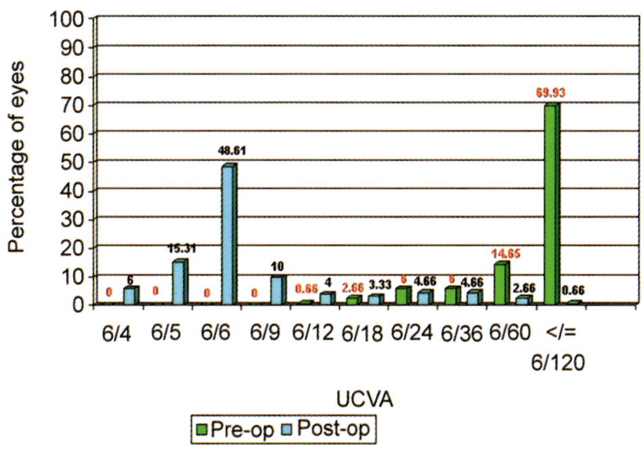

Fig. 23.6: Compares pre-op and post-op UCVA (Efficacy)

operative spherical equivalent (6 months) was –0.36 D ± 0.931 D (Range –4.25 to +1.25). Difference between the two was statistically significant ($p<0.05$) (Fig. 23.7). 132 eyes (87.91%) were within ±1.00 D of emmetropia while 120 eyes (79.92%) were within ± 0.05 D of emmetropia. 1 eye (0.66%) was overcorrected by > 0.5 D and 1 eye (0.66%) was overcorrected by >1D. The mean pupil diameter was 5.1mm ± 0.62mm. Preoperatively, 95 eyes (63.27%) had third order aberrations.42 eyes (28%) had second order aberration alone, while 13 eyes (8.65%) had fourth and fifth order aberrations. Post-operatively, 60 eyes (40%) had third order aberration.75 eyes (50%) had second order alone while 15 eyes (10%) had higher order aberrations.

DISCUSSION

Hartmann – Shack wavefront sensor was first used by Liang and colleagues to detect ocular aberrations.[11] They applied an adaptive optics deformable mirror to correct the lower and higher order aberrations of the eye. They reported a 6 times increase in contrast sensitivity to high spatial frequency when the pupil was large. This study demonstrated that correction of higher order aberrations could lead to supernormal vision in normal eyes. Figures 23.8, 23.9 and 23.10 show various aberrations.

In our series, using Zyoptix and Technolas 217 system, which is wavefront and corneal topography guided, we yielded results that are comparable to standard LASIK procedure.[12] In a series of 347 eyes, McDonald, et al [12] reported a post-operative refraction of –0.29 ± 0.45 D (-0.36 ± 0.93 D in our series) with standard LASIK. 57% of the eyes in their series had post-operative UCVA of ≥ 6/6. In our study, 70% of the eyes had UCVA of ≥ 6/6, six months post-operatively.

Higher order aberrations were reduced post-operatively in our study. Third-order aberration (coma) was most common in our series, followed by second-order (defocus and astigmatism) and fourth-order (spherical aberration). Post-operatively, after 6 months, there was considerable decrease in third-order and fourth-order aberrations. While most of the eyes had only defocus and astigmatism (i.e. second - order aberration). A slight increase in fourth-order aberration (spherical) was noted. Spherical aberration is known to increase after LASIK.[13-15] Roberts has reported that cornea changes its shape in response to ablation and this change, along with wound healing effects have to be taken into account before customized correction can nullify higher-order aberrations. Roberts and coworkers suggest that increase in spherical aberrations following LASIK may be caused by a biomechanically induced steepening and thickening that may occur in mid periphery of the cornea.[13] MacRae and coworkers have reported that simply creating a LASIK flap

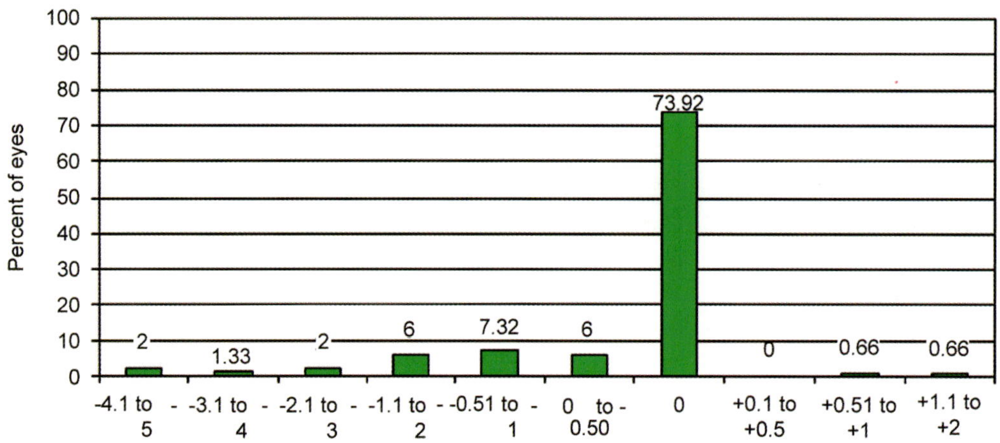

Fig. 23.7: Shows the refractive results postoperatively after 6 months

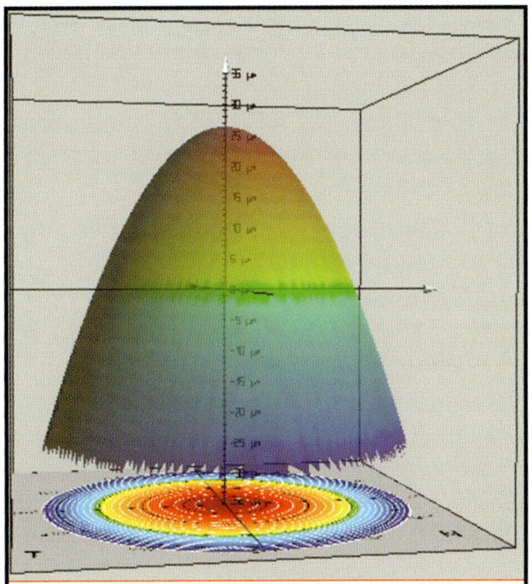

Fig. 23.8: Second order sphere

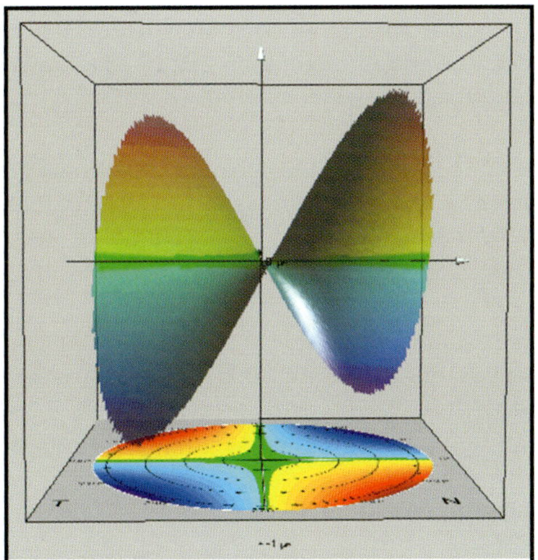

Fig. 23.9: Second order astigmatism

increases higher-order aberrations in unpredictable manner.[14] They suggest that improved results can be obtained using a surface ablation such as PRK or LASEK, or by doing a two-stage LASIK, with the second stage adjusting for the aberration created by the flap and initial ablation.

Scotopic visual complaints have been the bugbear of LASIK procedures, ranging from mild annoyance to server optical disability.[16, 17] Nighttime starbursts, reduced contrast sensitivity and haloes are the most common complaints.[16,17] Spherical aberration that is

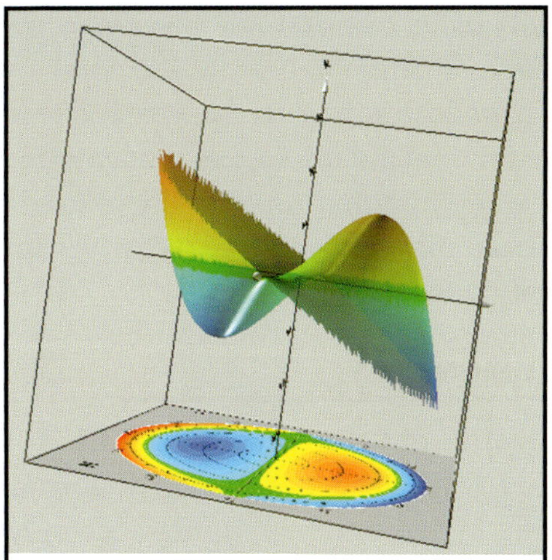

Fig. 23.10: Third order coma

induced during LASIK may account for this scotopic complaints.[14] Pupil diameter is another factor that is important. When pupil diameter is large, as in young patients, dim light vision is improved after customized correction.[18,19] In our series, 11% of the patients complained of haloes around light at night and difficult night driving. In dim light, the mean pupil diameter in these patients was 4.2 mm while it was 5.9 mm in other patients. Smaller pupil diameter and induced higher-order aberration may account for these scotopic visual complaints.

25% of the patients in our series reported improvement in bright light vision, while 40% showed improvement in dim light vision. A similar improvement was noted by Cox and co-workers (presentation by Cox IG at Zyoptix Alliance meeting, 2002 reported in *Ocular Surgery News*, July 2002 volume 13, number 7). In our series, treatment optical zone ranged from 6 to 7 mm. Treatment with larger optical zones and transition zones as compared to conventional LASIK may be possible since entire corneal topography and not just the central cornea overlying pupil along with wavefront ablation in dilated pupil are considered during treatment. This may induce lesser spherical aberration post-LASIK and account for improved scotopic vision.

Though we did not measure contrast sensitivity and glare acuity postoperatively, our results suggest improved quality of vision and fewer glare problems with Zyoptix treatment. A more temporal appraisal of the procedure has to be carried out with comparison to standard LASIK. Short-term results suggest wavefront and topography guided LASIK may be a safe and effective procedure which improves the visual performance.

CONCLUSION

Wavefront and topography guided LASIK procedure leads to better visual performance by decreasing higher order aberration. Scotopic visual complaints may be reduced with this method.

REFERENCES

1. Helmholtz H. Handbuch der physiologischen optik. Leipzig: Leopold Voss 1867;137-47.
2. Fyodorov S N, Durnev V V. Operation of dosaged dissection of corneal circular ligament.
3. Binder PS, Waring GO III. Keratotomy for astigmatism. In Waring GO III (Ed): Refractive keratotomy for myopia and astigmatism. Mosby Year Book 1992;1085-1198. in cases of myopia of mild degree. Ann Ophthalmol II: 1979;1885 -90.
4. Kaufmann HE. Correction of aphakia Am J Ophthalmol 1980;89:1.
5. McGhee CNJ, Taylor HR, Garty DS, et al. Excimer Lasers in Ophthalmology: Principles and Practice Martin Duntz: London, 1997.
6. MacRae S, Porter J, Cox IG, et al. Higher-order aberrations after conventional LASIK. ISRS: Dallas, Texas, 2000.
7. MacRae SM. Supernormal vision, hypervision, and customized corneal ablation. Guest Editorial J Cat Refract Surg 2000;Feb 26(2).
8. Howland HC, Howland B. A subjective method for the measurement of monochromatic aberrations of the eye. J Opt Soc Am 1977;67:1508-18.
9. Liang J, Williams DR, Miller DT. Supernormal vision and high-resolution retinal imaging through adaptive optics. J Opt Soc Am 1997;2884-92.
10. Fedor P, Kaufman S. Corneal topography and imaging. eMedicine Journal 2001;2(6).
11. Liang J, Williams D. Aberrations and retinal image quality of the normal human eye. J Opt Soc AM A 1997;14:2884-92.
12. McDonald MB, Carr JD, Frantz JM, et al. Laser in situ keratomilieusis for myopia up to –11 diopters with up to –5 diopters of astigmatism with summit autonomous LADARVision excimer laser system. Ophthalmology 2001;108:309-16.
13. Roberts C. The cornea is not a piece of plastic. J Refract Surg 2000;16:407-13.
14. MacRae SM, Roberts C, Porter J, et al. The biomechanics of a LASIK flap. ISRS Mid –Summer Meeting: Orlando, Florida, 2001.
15. Applegate RA, Howland HC, Klyce SD. Corneal aberration and refractive surgery. In: MacRae S (Editor). Customized Corneal Ablation. Thorofare NJ: Slack, Inc, 2001.
16. Holladay JT, Dudeja DR, Chang J. Functional vision and corneal changes after laser in situ keratomileusis determined by contrast sensitivity, glare testing, and corneal topography. J Cataract Refract Surg 1999;25: 663-69.
17. Perez-Santonja JJ, Sakla HF, Alio JL. Contrast sensitivity after laser in situ keratomileusis. J Cataract Refract Surg 1998;24:183-89.
18. Applegate R, Howland H, Sharp R, et al. Corneal aberrations and visual performance after refractive keratectomy. J Refract Surg 1998;14:397-407.
19. Oshika T, Klyce S, Applegate R, et al. Comparison of corneal wavefront aberrations after photorefractive keratectomy and laser in situ keratomileusis. Am J Ophthal 1999;127:1-7.

Presbyopic LASIK

Amar Agarwal, Athiya Agarwal, Sunita Agarwal (India),
Guillermo Avalos (Mexico), Ashok Garg (India)

24

INTRODUCTION

Presbyopia, is the final frontier for an ophthalmologist. In the 21st century the latest developments, which are taking place, are in the field of Presbyopia. In presbyopia, the nearest point that can be focused gradually recedes, leading to the need for optical prosthesis for close work such as reading and eventually even for focus in the middle distance.

PREVIOUS EXCIMER LASER TECHNIQUES

Presbyopic Photorefractive keratectomy (PRK) has been tried. In this using the excimer laser, a mask consisting of a mobile diaphragm formed by two blunt blades was used to ablate a 10-17 micron deep semilunar-shaped zone immediately below the papillary center, steepening the corneal curvature in that area.

Monofocal vision with LASIK has also been tried to solve the problem of presbyopia. The goal in such cases is to make the patient anisometropic. In this one eye is used for distance vision and the other for near vision. This is obviously not indicated in all subjects. The residual consequences are partial loss of stereopsis, asthenopia, headache, aniseikonia and decreased binocularity.

History

Guillermo Avalos[1,2] started the idea of Presbyopic LASIK. This is called the PARM technique. He held a live surgical conference in Mexico where he had invited the Agarwals to perform Phakonit and the no-anesthesia cataract surgery technique. There he discussed with them the idea of Presbyopic Lasik and when they came back they started the technique.

Principle

The objective is to allow the patient to focus on near objects while retaining his ability to focus on far objects, taking into account the refractive error of the eye when the treatment is performed. With this LASIK technique the corneal curvature is modified, creating a bilateral multifocal cornea in the treated optical zone. A combination of hyperopic and myopic LASIK is done aiming to make a multifocal cornea. We determine if the eye is Presbyopic plano, presbyopic with spherical hyperopia or presbyopia with spherical myopia. These may also have astigmatism in which case the astigmatism is treated at the same time.

PROLATE AND OBLATE CORNEA

It is important for us to understand a prolate and oblate cornea before we progress further on the technique of Presbyopic LASIK. The shape of spheroid (a conoidal surface of revolution) is qualitatively prolate or oblate, depending on whether it is stretched or flattened in its axial dimension. In a prolate cornea the meridional curvature decreases from pole to equator and in an oblate cornea the meridional curvature continually increases. The optical surfaces of the normal human eye both cornea and lens is prolate. This shape has an optical advantage in that spherical aberration can be avoided. Following LASIK the prolateness of the anterior cornea reduces but is insufficient to eliminate its spherical aberration. Thus one should remember the normal cornea is prolate. When myopic LASIK is done the cornea becomes oblate. When hyperopic LASIK is done the cornea becomes prolate.

Every patient treated with an excimer laser is left with an oblate or prolate shaped cornea depending upon the myopia or hyperopia of the patient. The approach to improve visual quality after LASIK is to apply geometric optics and use the patient's refraction, precise preoperative corneal height data and optimal postoperative anterior corneal shape in order to have a customized prolate shape treatment.

TECHNIQUE

First of all a superficial corneal flap is created with the microkeratome. The corneal flap performed with the microkeratome must be between 8.5 and 9.5 mm in order to have an available corneal surface for treatment of at least 8 mm. In this way, the laser beam does not touch the hinge of the flap. In India the Bausch and Lomb Lasik machine is used and in Mexico the Apollo machine is used. Once the flap has been created a hyperopic ablation in an optical zone of 5 mm is done (Fig. 24.1). The treated cornea now has a steepness section. The cornea is thus myopic, prolate. This allows the eye to focus in a range that includes near vision but excludes far vision.

With this myopic-shaped cornea, one now selects a smaller area of the central cornea that is concentric with the previous worked area. The size of the area is a 4 mm optical zone. A myopic LASIK is now done with the 4 mm optical zone (Fig. 24.2). The resulting cornea now has a central area (oblate) that is configured for the eye to focus on far objects and a ring shaped area that allows the eye to focus on near objects (Fig. 24.3). The flap is now cleaned and replaced back in position.

KERATOMETRY AND PACHYMETRY

Pachymetry is not important for this procedure. The pre-operative keratometry reading is extremely important. The post-operative keratometer reading should not exceed 48D. The keratometer reading should be taken from topography and not from a manual keratometer machine. For each hypermetropic diopter corrected, the corneal curvature increases in 0.89 keratometric diopters as an average. It is recommended to treat patients with keratometry

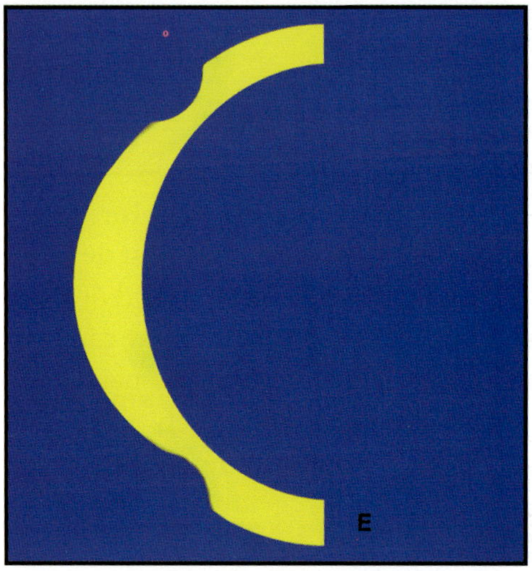

Fig. 24.1: Hyperopic LASIK done on the cornea. Myopic prolate cornea produced

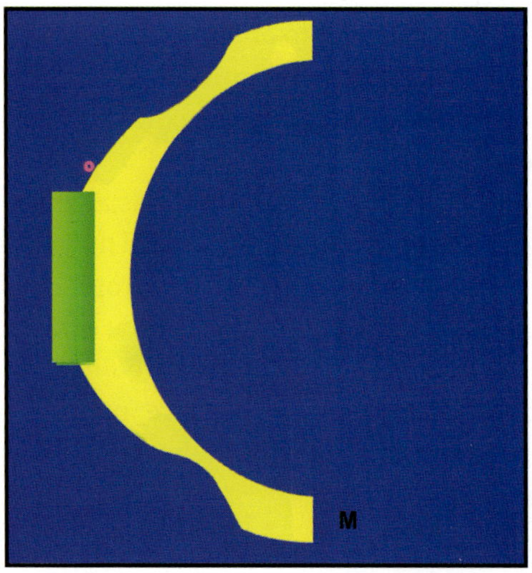

Fig. 24.2: Myopic LASIK done. Myopic ablation of 4 mm optical zone performed to create a central oblate cornea

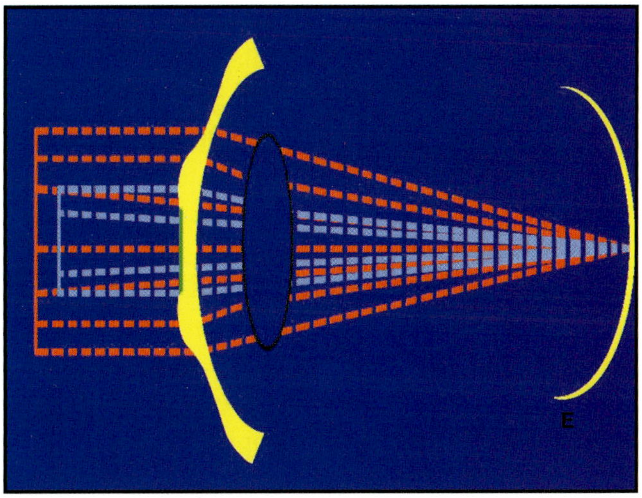

Fig. 24.3: Schematic diagram of a presbyopic cornea in which hyperopic and myopic lasik has been done. The patient can thus focus for near and distance

in the range between 41 and 43 D to obtain post-operative curves under 48 D. If the cornea is more than 48 D, it produces undesired optical alterations like glare, halos, decreased visual acuity and decreased contrast sensitivity. The preoperative and postoperative keratometer readings should be nearly the same for the patient to be comfortable.

Astigmatism

If astigmatism is present, it is recommended to use as a limit 2.5 D. One should also remember there is an induced astigmatism of 0.5 to 0.75 D created by the corneal shape after the surgery and this can decrease one or two lines of uncorrected visual acuity.

Plano Examples

Now let us look at treating presbyopic patients who are basically plano for distance.

Example 1

Let us take a patient who is plano for distance and is 20/20. For near on addition of + 2 D the patient is J1. The pre-operative keratometer let us say is 41 D.

There are three steps in the presbyopic LASIK treatment.

1 Step: For distance—No treatment is required as the patient is plano 20/20

2 Step: For near—Hyperopic LASIK is done of + 2 D. A 5 mm optical zone is taken. We have already mentioned that each diopter of hyperopia corrected changes the corneal curvature by 0.89 D, which is approximately 1 D. So the keratometer changes from 41 to 43 D (approximately)

3 Step: Myopic LASIK of minus 1 D with a 4 mm optical zone. So keratometer now becomes 42 D.

Regression occurs for hyperopia treatment to about 1 D, so we have done myopic ablation of minus 1 and not minus 2 D. The pre-op keratometer reading was 41 D and postoperative keratometer reading is 42 D, which is nearly the same.

Hyperopic Examples

Now let us look at presbyopic LASIK being performed in a hyperopic eye.

Example 2

Let us take a patient who is hyperopic for distance and is 20/20 with + 1 D. For near on addition of + 3 D the patient is J1. The preoperative keratometer let us say is 42 D.

There are three steps in the presbyopic LASIK treatment.

1 Step: For distance—Hyperopic LASIK is done of + 1 D with a 5 mm optical zone. So keratometer changes from 42 to 43 D.

2 Step: For near—Hyperopic LASIK is done of + 3 D. A 5 mm optical zone is taken. We have already mentioned that each diopter of hyperopia corrected changes the corneal curvature by 0.89 D, which is approximately 1 D. So the keratometer changes from 43 to 46 D (approximately).

3 Step: Myopic LASIK of minus 2 D with a 4 mm optical zone. So keratometer now becomes 44 D.

Regression occurs for hyperopia treatment to about 1 D, so we have done myopic ablation of minus 2 and not minus 3 D. The pre-op keratometer reading was 42 D but after making the patient plano it is 43 D. The postoperative keratometer reading is 44 D, which is nearly the same.

Though we have to correct totally 4 D for hypermetropia we take it in two steps. One should not do it in one step as that much hyperopia corrected in one step makes the central cornea too steep to perform the myopic ablation.

Example 3

Let us take a patient who is hyperopic for distance and is 20/20 with + 3 D. For near on addition of + 3 D the patient is J1. The pre-operative keratometer let us say is 44 D.

The pre-operative keratometer reading is 44 D and we have to correct 3 D for distance and 3 d for near. So if we do presbyopic Lasik we will make the keratometer reading 50 D. So, one should not treat such patients with presbyopia LASIK.

Myopic Example

Now let us look at myopic patients.

Example 4

Let us take a patient who is myopic for distance and is 20/20 with minus 2 D. For near on addition of + 2 D the patient is J1. This means the patient is plano for near. The preoperative keratometer let us say is 43 D.

There are three steps in the presbyopic LASIK treatment.

1 Step: For distance- Patient is myopic so no treatment is required.

2 Step: For near- Hyperopic LASIK is done of + 2 D. A 5 mm optical zone is taken. We have already mentioned that each dioptre of hyperopia corrected changes the corneal curvature by 0.89 D, which is approximately 1 D. So the keratometer changes from 43 to 45 D (approximately)

3 Step: Myopic LASIK of minus 3 D with a 4 mm optical zone. So keratometer now becomes 42 D.

Regression occurs for hyperopia treatment to about 1 D, so we have done myopic ablation of minus 3 and not minus 4 D. The pre-op keratometer reading was 43 D but patient was myopic by 2 D, so actually the keratometer reading should be 41 D. The postoperative keratometer reading is 42 D, which is nearly the same.

We did myopic ablation of 3 D, as patient is myopic of 2 D and presbyopic of 2 D. Regression factor taken is 1 D.

SUMMARY

This idea of presbyopic LASIK is not the end of it all. This technique needs further improvisations to become the technique of choice for one and all.

REFERENCES

1. Guillermo Avalos. Presbyopic LASIK—the PARM technique in Amar Agarwal's Presbyopia: A surgical textbook. Slack Inc, USA, 2002.
2. Agarwal T, et al. Presbyopic LASIK—the Agarwal technique in Amar Agarwal's Presbyopia: A surgical textbook. Slack Inc, USA, 2002.

Corneal Wavefront LASIK after Penetrating Keratoplasty

25

CYRES K MEHTA, KEIKI R MEHTA (INDIA)

The need for Penetrating Keratoplasty is steadily increasing. The WHO estimates that over 100,000 keratoplasties are being carried out yearly and considering that there are more than an estimated 10 million cases of corneal blindness worldwide the number of keratoplasties are still woefully inadequate.

Once keratoplasty has been successfully carried out and considering that the cornea maintains its clarity, significant visual morbidity is dependant on the residual refraction and cylinder.

Perlman, has shown that the inability to construct a perfectly similar recipient bed for the donor graft,both in shape and regularity is the main factor in inducing high astigmatism.

- Truly symmetrical, regular astigmatism is a rare condition after PK, and irregular astigmatism cannot be corrected with existing technology.
- Studies have shown that, following PK, approximately 8 to 20% of eyes have significant irregular astigmatism that cannot be satisfactorily managed with glasses or contact lenses.

In a series of 44 eyes, Pradera reports a mean astigmatism of 5.11 + /– 2.48D and a spherical equivalent of +/– 3.47 dioptres. Such Anisometropia leads to loss of binocular vision stereopsis and eventually foveal supression over time.

The advent of the excimer laser has provided us with a tool to correct the ametropic condition.

PRK has its limits Its associated with irregular astigmatism, corneal scarring, and regression along with the risk of transplant rejection (Hersh).

In 1991 Pallikaris developed LASIK which has become our procedure of choice to treatment of residual myopia, hypermetropia and astigmatism after Penetrating Keratoplasty.

In 2001Optikon, Italy released the Keratron Scout topographer which works on the Arc Step principle first proposed by Alvar Gullstrand. This unit can generate a corneal wavefront in Zernicke Polynomial format. Using the ORK–W software a shot file is generated and a corneal Wavefront LASIK(Cor-Wave) is performed with a Schwind Esiris 200Hz flying spot laser with a 330 Hz Tracker. The flap is created with a Cariazzo Pendular Microkeratome (Schwind) a brainchild of the brilliant inventor ophthalmologist, Cesar Cariazzo from Colombia. This microkeratome has certain distinct advantages over conventional straight track and rotatory keratomes in that:

1. The pivot point of the Cariazzo Pendular is nearly an inch above the cornea. So no interference from the lids, lashes drapes is possible.
2. It has a 110 micron head which for the first 2 cuts has a standard deviation of less than 14 microns, i.e. the flap will be between 95-125 microns approximately. This allows a larger thickness of the stromal bed to be available for ablation.We

need a thicker stromal bed as a corneal wavefront guided lasik generally uses more tissue as high spots are also eliminated from the stromal bed, in an effort to provide an aberration free surface. In fact cut number 3 and 4 with a 110 micron head, and the same blade resterilised with ethylene oxide gas provides us with a consistently 80-90 micron flap thickness.

3. It has a innovative spherical applanation head which applanates the corneal centre protecting it from possible buttonholes.In over 1350 eyes operated since Feb 2005 we have not had a single free flap or buttonhole. Even though the cornea may be ectatic in many cases, as the head applanates the cornea, the flap is of uniform thickness.
4. Larger diameter of suction ring on the limbus (Pressure = Force per unit area) so that the eye pressure does not have to be raised as high as other units.

TIMING OF LASIK AFTER KERATOPLASTY

- In our opinion a minimum of 6 months after suture removal is mandatory. In the literature, investigators recommend performing LASIK approximately 3 to 6 months after suture removal, and 12 to 18 months after the corneal graft procedure. Benelli and Nardi, prefer to wait a year after suture removal. Yet others have performed it just a year after PK. Thus there here is no established time interval between the initial PK and LASIK procedure, we have treated these patients a minimum of 6 months after suture removal to upto 5 years after suture removal.

We should remember that with the suction ring on the eye the IOP can rise as high as 60 mmHg. The graft host junction should be evaluated to verify that it can take such elevated pressure for nearly half a minute if necessary.

Technique

There are two ways of performing LASIK in eyes that have had prior keratoplasty.

Make the flap. Wait for a month. Then relift the flap and apply laser.

It has been noticed that after a cut with the microkeratome stresses that exist between graft and host corneas, that lead to astigmatism, are released and in some cases the cylinder can appreciably decrease. This should be greater the greater the flap thickness as a thicker and large cut (and flap) will intersect more corneal lamellae particularly in the periphery where they act like the guide wires of a suspension bridge maintaining corneal structure and stability. Marshall has shown that the peripheral corneal lamella act as guy wires to support the corneal structure and so a thinner flap or LASEK is preferable to a regular 130 to 160 micron relatively thick flap.

In "Ophthalmology" in 2000 Vajpayee and Dada have documented this phenomenon.

This is the logic in performing the cut and letting the corneal tissues realign.

However, if you use a very thin flap 80-90 microns of just 8 to 8.5 mm diameter the number of corneal lamellae transected is far less.Thus we prefer to do LASIK as a primary procedure itself and not defer it for a month. In our experience, over a 3 month period of the study there has been no reappearance of the cylinder and the correction is stable.

CASE STUDY

We carried out a study, (SLIDES) wherein 60 cases of corneal grafts were treated with corneal wavefront guided LASIK with superlative results.

IN CONCLUSION

In most cases the post LASIK refraction at 1 and at 3 months in our series of 21 eyes is stable and close to zero. However, in 3 eyes with very high cylinder (>8), BCVA was achieved with a small spectacle correction of 1-1.5 cylinder in the appropriate meridian.

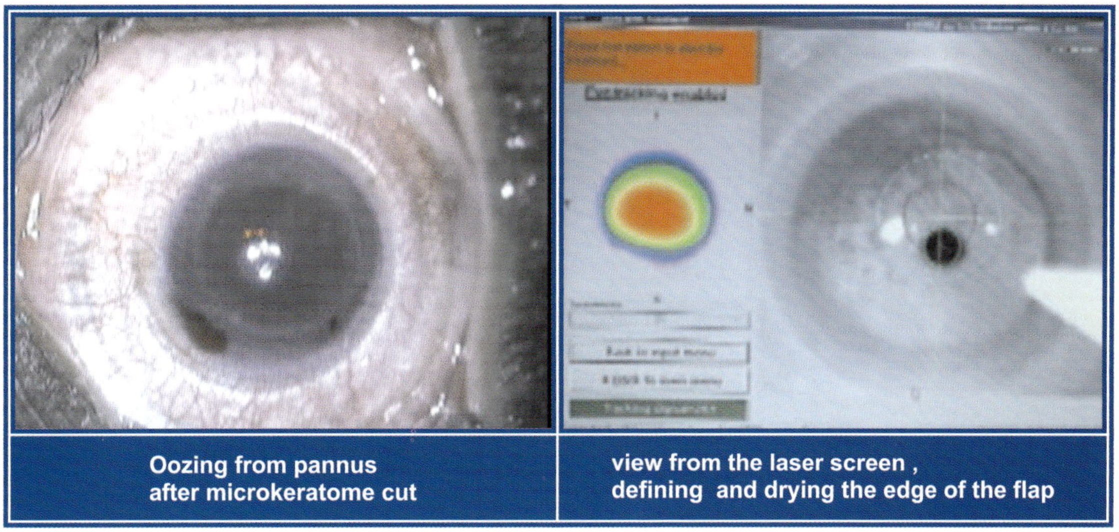
Oozing from pannus after microkeratome cut

view from the laser screen, defining and drying the edge of the flap

Fig. 25.1

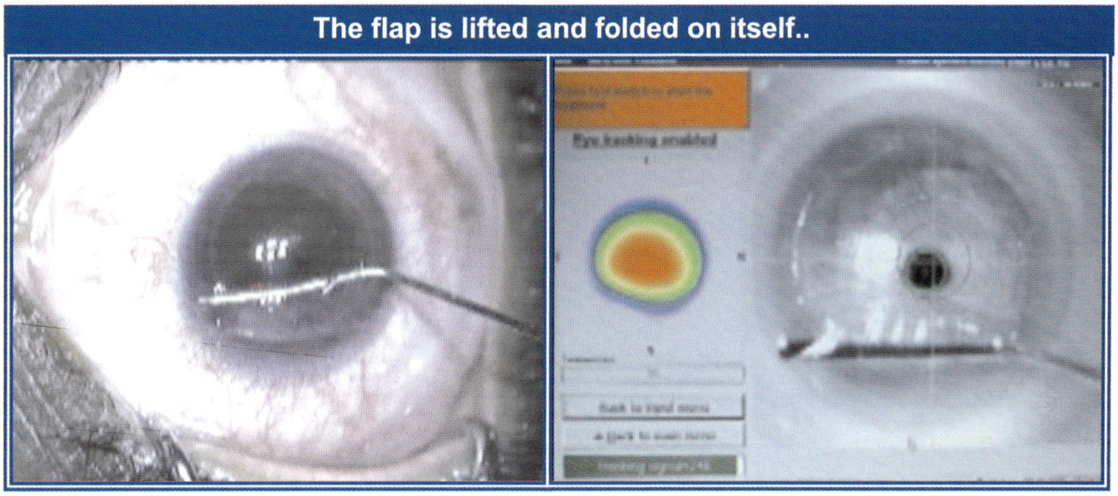
The flap is lifted and folded on itself..

Fig. 25.2

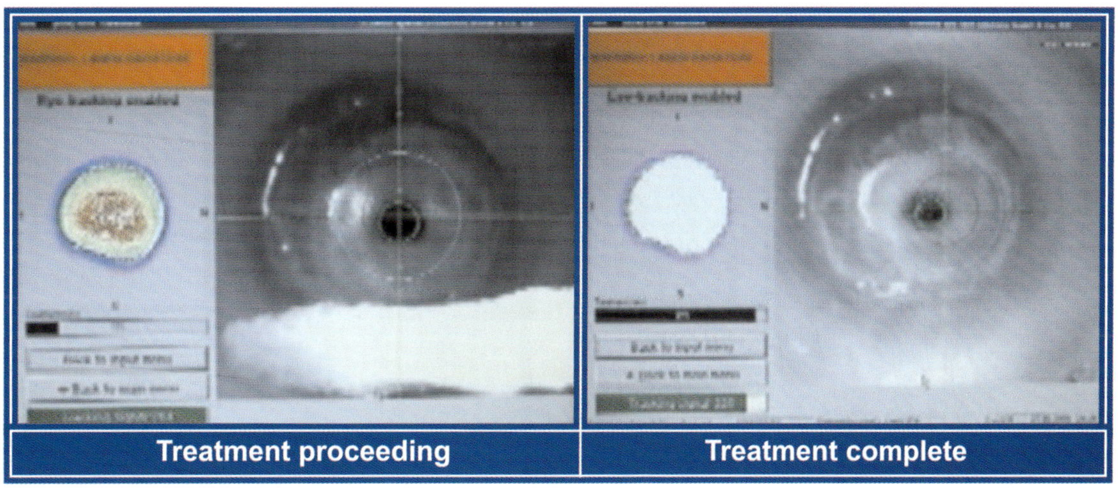
Treatment proceeding

Treatment complete

Fig. 25.3

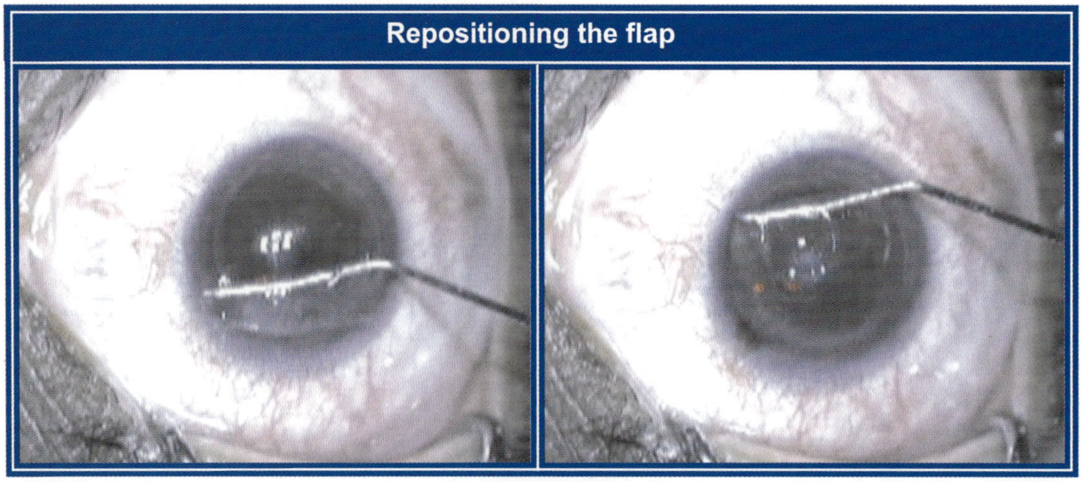

Fig. 25.4

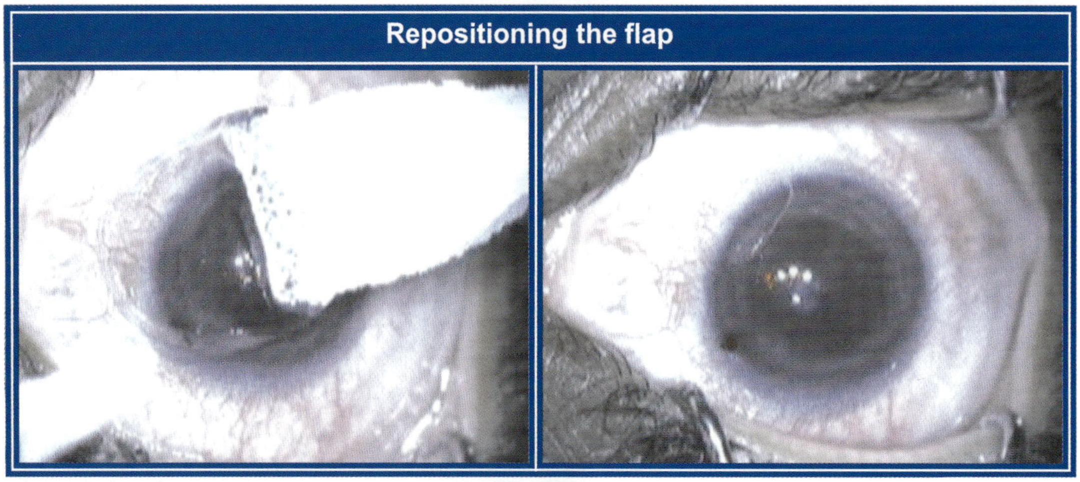

Fig. 25.5

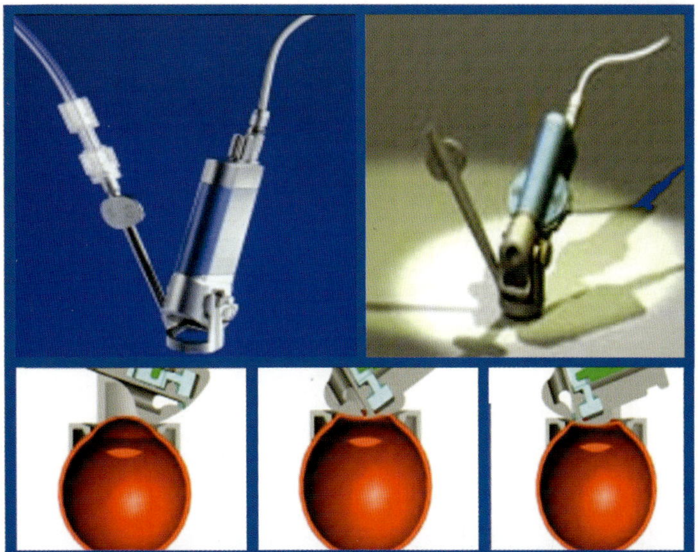

The applanation system of the cariazzo pendular microkeratome seen at various stages of the cut.this ensures a uniform flap thickness

Fig. 25.6

Case study — corneal wavefront LASIK performed for a decentered corneal graft.

- The patient was operated for penetrating keratoplasty 5 years ago. Suture removal was performed 4 years ago.
- BCVA was 6/12 -4 sph -5 cyl .
- post LASIK result -0.5 cyl (UCVA-6/6)

Fig. 25.7

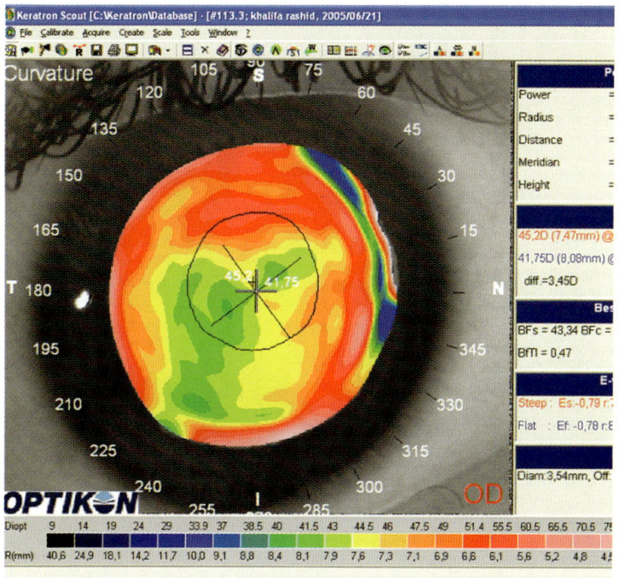

Fig. 25.8

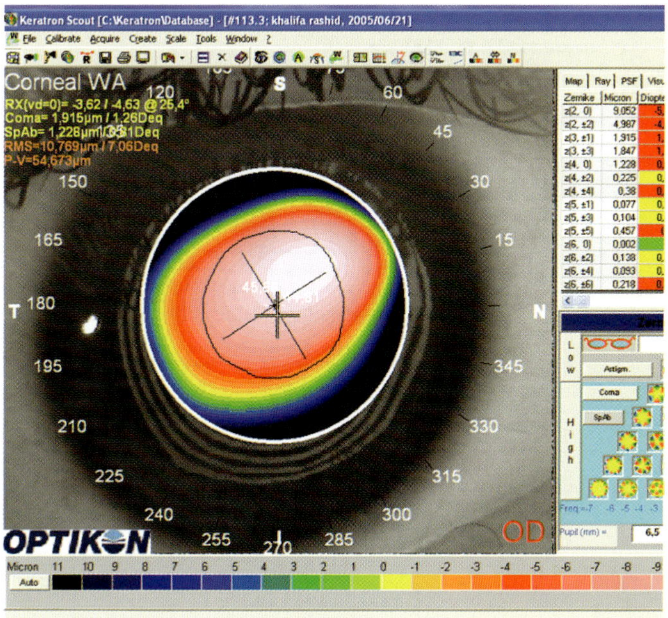

Fig. 25.9

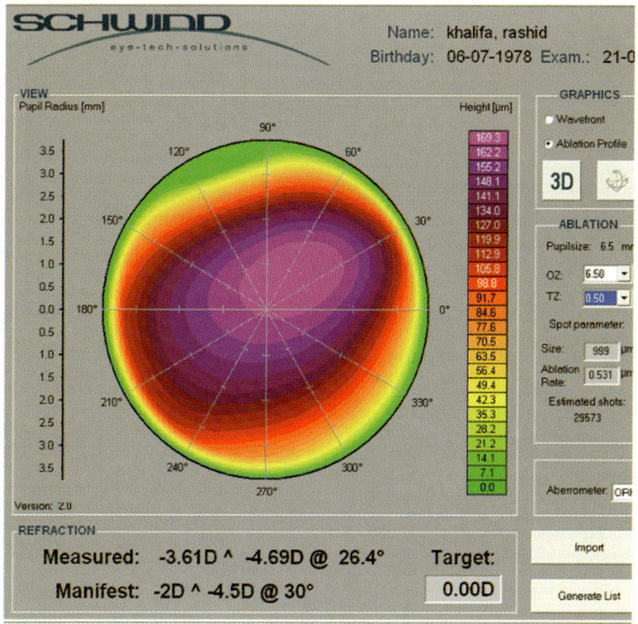

Fig. 25.10

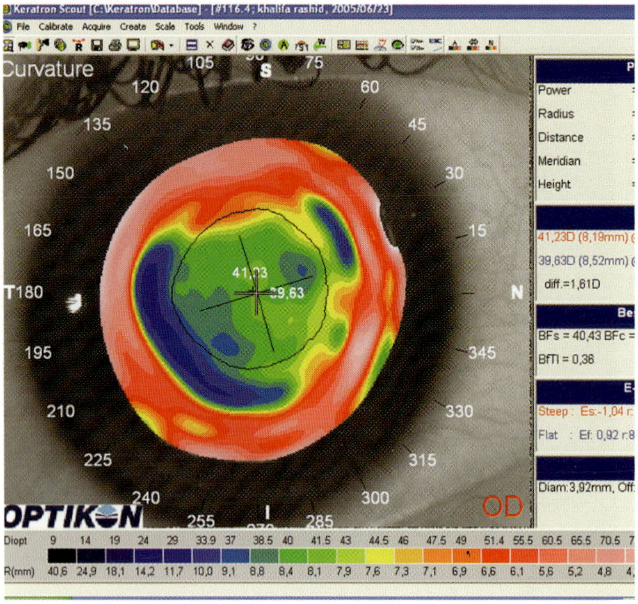

Fig. 25.11

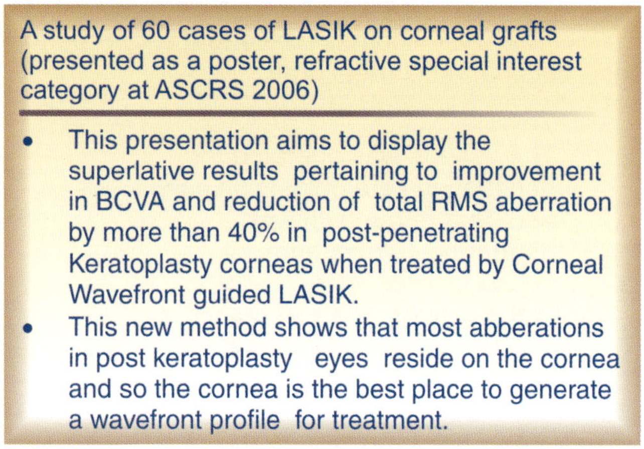

Fig. 25.12

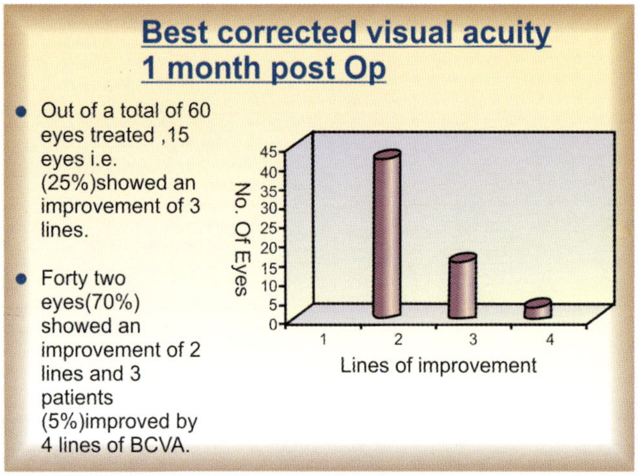

Fig. 25.13

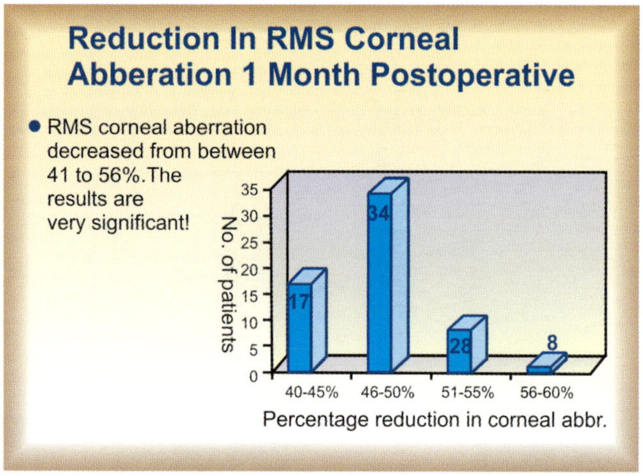

Fig. 25.14

We found that in all cases the UCVA/BCVA increased at least a line and in some cases upto 3 lines! It is our opinion that corneal wavefront guided LASIK with this system is the new standard in LASIK on Post Keratoplasty eyes and on other highly abberated eyes.

REFERENCES

1. Whitcher JP, Srinivasan M. Corneal Blindness: A global perspective. Bulletin of the World Health Organisation 2001;79:214-21.
2. Perlman EM. An analysis and interpretation of refractive errors after penetrating keratoplasty. Ophthalmology 1981;88(1):39-45.
3. Brahma A , Ennis F, Harper R, Ridgeway A, Tullo A. Visual function after penetrating keratoplasty for keratoconus: A prospective longitudinal evaluation.Br J Ophthalmol 200;84(1):60-66.
4. Dada T, Vajpayee RB, Gupta V, Sharma N, Dada VK. Mcrokeratome induced reduction of astigmatism after penerating keratoplasty. Am J Ophthalmol 2001; 131(4):507-08.
5. Epstein RJ, Robin JB. Corneal graft rejection episode after excimer laser phototherapeutic keratectomy.Arch Ophthalmol 1994;112:57.

6. Hersh PS, Jordon AJ, Mayers M. Corneal graft rejection episode after excimer laser phototherapeutic keratectomy. Arch Opthalmol 1993;111:735-36.
7. Lam DS, Leung AT, Wu JT, Tham CC, Fan DS. How long should one wait to perform LASIK after PKP. J Cataract Refract Surg 1998;24:6-7.
8. Vajpayee RB, Dada T. Lasik after penetrating keratoplasty (Letter).Opthalmology 2000;107:1801-02.
9. Arenas E, Maglione A. Laser in situ keratomileusis for astigmatism and myopia after penetrating keratoplasty. J Retract Surg 1997;13:27-32.
10. Zaldivar R, Davidorf J, Oscherow S. LASIK for myopia and astigmatism after penetrating keratoplasty [letter]. J Refract Surg 1997;13:501-02.
11. Parisi A, Salchow DJ, Zirm ME, Stieldorf C. Laser in situ keratomileusis after automated lamellar keratoplasty and penetrating keratoplasty. J Cataract Refract Surg 1997;23:1114-18.

IOL Power Calculations after Corneal Refractive Surgery

26

Srinivas K Rao, Arthur Cheng, Dennis SC Lam (China)

Cataract surgery has evolved tremendously in the past few decades and most patients expect excellent unaided vision following the procedure. Present day techniques of phacoemulsification, which disturb the corneal contour minimally and ensure in-the-bag intraocular lens (IOL) placement in a consistent fashion, have contributed considerably to such results. An improved understanding of the methods used for IOL power calculation and the precision of current technologies used to measure axial length and corneal curvature have also contributed to the increased accuracy of cataract surgery refractive outcomes.

Another procedure which has gained tremendous popularity in recent years is excimer laser corneal refractive surgery and it is currently the second most commonly performed ocular surgical procedure. Although laser in situ keratomileusis (LASIK) is the most advocated procedure, a large number of patients have undergone photorefractive keratectomy (PRK) and radial keratotomy (RK) in the past. Most of these refractive procedures have been performed in patients in the second to fourth decades of life, and as these individuals age they will need cataract surgery as well. However, initial attempts resulted in poor refractive predictability following cataract surgery in these eyes. The purpose of this article is to highlight the reasons for such poor outcomes, and to review the methods described to overcome these problems.

The two most important measurements that aid accurate IOL power calculation are the axial length of the eye and the corneal curvature. Their importance is highlighted by the fact that an error of 1.0D in keratometry would result in an equivalent error in IOL power, while a 0.33 mm error in axial length determination would cause a 1.0D error in IOL power in an eye of average axial length. In eyes shorter than 22 mm, the magnitude of the error in IOL power estimation would increase.

Another factor that has recently been recognized as important is the postoperative position of the IOL within the eye – this has been termed as the effective lens position (ELP). Previously termed the anterior chamber depth, this factor allows the surgeon to personalize the lens constant for his surgical technique, by using data from a series of patient undergoing cataract surgery with IOL implantation, and using the postoperative outcomes. Factors such as the retinal thickness have also been incorporated in more recent IOL formulae and while these do improve the accuracy of refractive outcomes, in general, they have less of an impact compared to the factors mentioned earlier. After corneal refractive surgery, the most important change is in the corneal shape – the site of the surgery. Thus, any inaccuracies in IOL power calculation in this situation arise in large part from these changes – axial length tends not to contribute much to these changes.

In this chapter, the effects of corneal changes on IOL power calculation inaccuracies during cataract surgery are explored. A better understanding of these changes and their resultant effect on the calculations has resulted in the evolution of many methods to try and counter these inaccuracies and these are described as well. Since it is important to understand the actual changes that occur in the cornea and the eye after refractive surgery, these are first described.

In RK, deep incisions in the peripheral cornea allow the intraocular pressure to shift the peripheral cornea outwards, resulting in a flattening of the central corneal curvature. There is thus, no tissue removal in this procedure, unlike in PRK and LASIK, in which the excimer stromal ablation results in tissue removal from the central cornea. In the later procedures, tissue removal would depend on the amount of myopic correction attempted. Based on a rule-of-thumb that 1.0D of refractive correction requires the removal of 10 µm of central corneal tissue, a 12.0D correction would require the removal of about 120 µm of corneal tissue. Axial length measurement using non-contact ultrasound techniques and the IOL master which uses the principle of optical coherence would detect this amount of tissue loss, when measuring the axial length. Contact ultrasound techniques may not have the sensitivity to detect this change and hence may be a source of error in IOL power calculations. This should lead to a 0.30 to 0.50D error in IOL power estimation. Studies of IOL power calculation in eyes that have undergone corneal refractive surgery have however indicated that most of the error that occurs results from inaccurate estimation of the corneal power.

Standard keratometry makes certain assumptions regarding corneal shape. The cornea is considered a regular sphero-cylindrical surface, and the measurement of its curvature is derived from points situated on a central circle which is about 3 mm in diameter. Since the central cornea within this zone is considered to be a spherical surface, this measurement is assumed to represent the power distribution within this area and at the corneal apex. Since keratometers use the first Purkinje image of the reflection target from the anterior corneal surface, what is measured is the curvature of the anterior corneal surface. Refraction at the posterior corneal surface results in a negative power, and the overall power of the cornea is the algebraic sum of these two components. Since the posterior corneal power cannot be measured using standard keratometric techniques, manufacturers use a correction in the refractive index of the cornea to account for this factor. Hence, most keratometers use a corneal refractive index of 1.3375 instead of the true value of 1.376. This allows a conversion of the measured radius of curvature of the anterior surface to the total power of the cornea. For this assumption to be valid however, a constant relationship between the anterior and posterior corneal surfaces is assumed. This assumption is violated in excimer refractive surgery, in which tissue is removed from the anterior corneal surface. This would therefore, further affect the accuracy of conversion of the measured anterior radius of curvature into corneal power in such eyes.

Since the shape of the cornea after refractive surgery, be it RK or excimer surgery, is oblate – meaning that there is a negative shape factor, or a central flattening, using a reflection-based system (standard keratometer or Placido topographer) results in errors. This is because the flattened anterior corneal surface reflects a larger image of the object in the measuring device, and hence what is used for calculation is the measurement from the paracentral cornea – and this results in an erroneously steeper value for the central corneal power. Thus, after RK and excimer surgery for myopia, the measured corneal power in the 3 to 4 mm zone is steeper than that in the central cornea which the patient uses for image formation. This results in an underestimation of the IOL power and a postoperative hyperopic refractive error.

In addition to this problem, in eyes that have had excimer surgery, tissue has been removed from the anterior cornea. This results in a change in the relationship between the anterior and posterior corneal surfaces—with a lessening of the distance between them. This causes a further inaccuracy, when the measured anterior radius of curvature is converted into total corneal power by using the effective refractive index. This reduction in the separation between the surfaces can actually result in reduced corneal power—although this is much less in magnitude compared to the change resulting from the anterior surface change. In conjunction with the initial measurement error, this conversion error can contribute further to the inaccuracy in IOL power calculations in eyes that have undergone PRK and LASIK.

In both RK and excimer surgery, there is a posterior shift in the effective and true position of the anterior corneal surface. However, the position of the crystalline lens remains unchanged and since this determines the location of the IOL after cataract surgery, it is important that IOL power calculations take into account the altered position of the anterior corneal surface. Failure to do so would result in the use of an underpowered IOL and a hyperopic refractive error after cataract surgery.

Recognition of the various factors that contribute to the postcataract refractive shift has spawned a number of strategies that try and address these issues. In this chapter, these strategies are addressed under two headings—those that can be used when the surgeon has access to the pre-refractive surgery data of the patient, and those that can be used when the patient presents with no prior data.

STRATEGIES TO BE USED WHEN PRIOR DATA IS AVAILABLE

The History Method[1]

This method derives the post-refractive surgery keratometric value from the pre- and postsurgery refractive data of the patient. This can be explained with the help of an example,

Example

Preoperative refraction	= – 8.0D
Preoperative keratometry	= 44.0D
Refractive correction attempted	= – 8.0D
Post-LASIK refraction	= – 1.0D

Calculations

Refractive error corrected	= 7.0 D
Hence, post-LASIK keratometry	= (44.0 – 7.0) = 37.0D

This method uses the post-treatment refractive error of the patient, prior to the development of the cataract. This is usually obtained one month after LASIK, or when refractive stability has been attained. Since the change in refractive error is the direct result of the corneal alterations produced by the surgical procedure, it is logical to derive the final corneal power by subtracting the refractive change attained, from the pre-treatment refractive error. Although this method works fairly well, it requires access to patient data in the pre- and early post-treatment periods. Details of the surgical procedure, including the correction attempted are also important. It is also vital that the post-refractive surgery refractive error is recorded before the development of the cataract as nuclear sclerotic cataracts often cause a myopic shift in refraction.

Whether to use the patient refraction at the corneal plane or the spectacle plane has been a point of discussion – since the changes in power are at the corneal surface, some authorities argue that it is best to use the spectacle power converted for vertex distance. In the example provided, let us see the power calculation when this approach is used.

Example

Preoperative refraction	= – 8.0D (-7.3D at corneal plane; vertex, 12 mm)
Preoperative keratometry	= 44.0 D
Refractive correction attempted	= – 8.0 D
Post-LASIK refraction	= – 1.0 D (–0.99D at corneal plane)

Calculations

Refractive error corrected	= – 6.31D
Hence, post-LASIK keratometry	= (44.0 – 6.31) = 37.69D

Hence, this results in a higher value for the postoperative corneal power, and as the IOL power calculations are best performed with the lowest corneal value, it may be preferable to use the refractive errors at the spectacle plane. However, when correcting very high errors viz., more than 10D, it has been suggested that corneal plane refractions may be more accurate, although data supporting this are lacking.

The DBR Method[2]

In this approach, preoperative patient data are essential. When the patient presents for refractive surgery, in addition to refraction and keratometry, the axial length is also measured and the IOL power required for emmetropia is calculated. Following refractive surgery, the stable refractive error prior to onset of cataract is determined and the change in refraction effected by the surgical procedure is calculated. This can be explained with the aid of the following example,

Example

Preoperative refraction	= – 5.25D
Preoperative keratometry	= 46.2D
Refractive correction attempted	= – 5.25D
Post-treatment refraction	= Plano
Axial length	= 25.0 mm
IOL power for emmetropia	= 16.8D (a constant 118.0)

Since there has been a 5.25D change in refraction at the spectacle plane following surgery (12 mm vertex distance), the IOL inside the eye should have its power increased by an equivalent amount for the post-refractive surgery eye to attain emmetropia. It is also calculated that for every diopter of change in IOL power, only 0.7 D of change in refraction at the spectacle plane will be achieved.

Example

5.25D change at the spectacle plane	= 5.25/0.7 = 7.5D change at the IOL plane
IOL power for emmetropia	= 16.8D + 7.5 D = 24.3D

Using Corneal Topography[3]

This method depends on the use of a specific topographic unit—the EyeSys device (which is not current), and the central corneal power measured from the Holladay Diagnostic Summary of the system. This value is the calculated mean refractive power of the central 3 mm of the cornea, accounting for the Stiles Crawford effect. In their study, the authors noted that the $EffRP_{post}$ (effective refractive power after surgery), tended to overestimate corneal power and this increased significantly with increasing change in refractive equivalent (SE). Hence they proposed the following regression equation to improve the accuracy of corneal power estimation.

$$EffRP_{post\text{-}adj} = EffRP_{post} - 0.15\,(SE_{post} - SE_{pre}) - 0.05$$

$EffRP_{post\text{-}adj}$ —adjusted postoperative effective refractive power of the cornea

SE_{post}—post-LASIK spherical equivalent refractive error

SE_{pre}— pre-LASIK spherical equivalent refractive error

The Double K Method[4]

In third and fourth generation IOL calculation formulae that use corneal power values to predict the effective lens position (ELP), tissue removal from the anterior corneal surface and the lesser keratometry value result in an erroneous anterior calculated ELP – this will result in underestimation of the IOL power and resultant hyperopic error postoperatively.

To overcome this fallacy, it has been suggested that the pre-refractive surgery keratometry be used to determine ELP. The post refractive surgery keratometry is then used with the previously determined ELP to calculate the IOL power. As described by Aramberri, the postoperative keratometry value is calculated using the Clinical History method. He describes in detail his method of programming the SRK/T formula into a spreadsheet so that ELP calculation algorithms used the preoperative keratometry and the vergence formula algorithms used the postoperative keratometry and interested readers are advised to refer to his article.

This insight of Aramberri has been incorporated by Holladay into his Holladay 2 formula. In this formula, the corneal power before refractive surgery can be entered for the calculation of the ELP. For patients who do not have such data available, this formula offers the option of using a standard value of 44D for the corneal power. In an editorial, Koch and Wang provide a table with precalculated values for modifying the IOL power according to the double K method.[5] However, these are based on the assumption that the pre-refractive surgery keratometry is 43D and the IOL implanted is the SA60AT (Alcon).

Theoretical Formula 2004[6]

This formula was proposed to calculate the postoperative power of the cornea after refractive surgery – and requires knowledge of the preoperative keratometry and the postoperative radius of curvature of the corneal surface (calculated using an autokeratometer)

$$K_{postop} = K_{preop} - [(N_c - 1) \times (R_{a\text{-}postop} - R_{a\text{-}preop})/(R_{a\text{-}postop} \times R_{a\text{-}preop})$$

K_{postop}— Keratometry reading after LASIK
K_{preop}— Keratometry reading before LASIK
N_c— Index of refraction of the cornea (1.376)
$R_{a\text{-}postop}$—Postoperative radius of curvature of the anterior corneal surface
$R_{a\text{-}preop}$—Preoperative radius of curvature of the anterior corneal surface

Modified Keratometry Method[3]

If the amount of refractive correction is known, Sim K or keratometry readings obtained after refractive surgery can be reduced by 0.24D per diopter of refractive correction obtained after surgery.

Corrected Keratometry[7]

The authors describe the correction factor necessary to correct the corneal power overestimation that occurs when keratometry is measured after PRK and LASIK. The table is described in their article, and the values are correlated with the amount of change in SE achieved after refractive surgery.

They caution however, that while this may be an appropriate method for eyes that have had PRK and LASIK, after RK, the Sim K value may be the most appropriate. They also suggest the use of modern keratometers with a large number of measurement points (360-420) to obtain the post refractive surgery measurement.

Back Calculated IOL Power[8]

In this method, the authors used pre-LASIK keratometry readings and axial length to derive the IOL power calculations. They then chose the IOL power that would provide the pre-LASIK SE refraction.

In another method the pre-LASIK SE refractive error and the post LASIK flattest keratometric measurement were used to adjust the power of the IOL calculated using the flattest keratometry value.[9]

Example

If a patient underwent LASIK for – 6.5D (SEQ), then the adjustment for the IOL power obtained using the flattest keratometry would be –

$$\text{Adjustment} = [-(0.47\ \text{SEQ}) + 0.85] = [-(0.47 \times 6.50) + 0.85] = +2.20\text{D}$$

Hence, if the IOL power calculated using the flattest keratometry was 17.76D, then the IOL power to be used should be 17.76 + 2.20 = 19.96D.

In another variation of this approach, the IOL power adjustment was performed using the following correction factor[10]

$$\text{IOL power adjustment} = \text{LSE} \times (-0.326) + 0.101$$

LSE—Total prior laser treatment, adjusted for vertex distance in SE

Example

- Post refractive surgery, SRK T formula suggests 16.0D IOL for emmetropia
- Prior laser correction (SE) = – 6.0D
- Adjustment = – 6.0D × (-0.326) + 0.101 = + 2.057D
- IOL power calculated as – 16.0 + 2.0 = 18.0D for emmetropia

Nomogram Based Adjustment of IOL Power[11]

Based on analysis of data using method #2, a theoretical formula was determined that allowed the estimation of IOL power underestimation, using the change in SE induced by the refractive surgery.

$$\text{IOL power underestimation} = -0.231 + (0.595 \times SE_{\text{change-spectacle plane}})$$

Using this formula, they developed a nomogram that provided the adjustment factor for IOL power based solely on post-LASIK keratometry and refractive change induced by LASIK without the need for pre-LASIK keratometry. The derived values are detailed in a table in their paper referenced above, and the example they have provided explains the method.

Example

Pre-LASIK refraction (spectacle)	= – 13.38D
Spherical equivalent (corneal plane, vertex – 12,5 mm)	= – 11.27D
Post-LASIK refraction (spectacle)	= – 2.50D
Post-LASIK SE (corneal plane, vertex – 12,5 mm)	= – 2.50D
Pre-LASIK keratometry	= 41.75/43.00D
Post-LASIK keratometry	= 35.90/33.40D
Axial length	= 30.38 mm
Desired postcataract refraction	= Plano

Step 1—The change in refraction at the spectacle plane = 10.88D

Step 2—The IOL power based on the axial length and post-LASIK keratometry with the SRK T formula is determined, aiming for plano = 13.06D

Step 3—The IOL power is adjusted according to the nomogram provided in their article,

$$13.06 + 6.31 = 19.37D$$

The IOL chosen according to this method is 19.50D (SA60AT)

Corrected Refractive Index Method[12]

The authors derived a correction factor for the effective refractive index of the cornea and suggest the use of this method to derive the post refractive surgery keratometry value.

If the pre-LASIK refractive error is known, they suggest the following new refractive indices

Pre-LASIK refractive error	*New refractive index (rN)*
< – 4D	1.3355
– 4 to – 8D	1.3286
– 8 to – 12D	1.3237
> – 12D	1.3172

The new keratometry reading is obtained by using the equation

$$K = [rN - 1/Ra]$$

Ra = anterior corneal curvature in meters, measured after refractive surgery, using an automated instrument.

The authors also describe an alternate formula to determine rN for eyes in which the change in refraction after LASIK is known,

$$rN = 0.0014SE_c + 1.3375$$

SE_c – Spherical equivalent change after LASIK

STRATEGIES TO BE USED WHEN PRIOR DATA IS NOT AVAILABLE

Corneal Topography[13]

The reasons why standard keratometry results in poor refractive outcomes after IOL implantation in eyes that have had corneal refractive surgery, have already been described. Most of the currently available computerized videokeratography units provide color-coded maps of corneal power distribution. The basic principles adopted by the Placido-based devices remain very similar to those in manual keratometers. Hence, they are subject to the inaccuracies described earlier. However, in post-RK eyes, some degree of accuracy can be attained by ignoring the simulated keratometry values provided by the machine (measured from a 3 mm zone), and deriving the value from the center of the zone of flattening indicated in the topographic map. This is more accurate since these devices use data from more points on the corneal surface including the cornea within the 3 mm zone measured by the keratometer. This method would not however be useful in eyes that have had excimer surgery, due to the inaccuracy in conversion mentioned earlier.

To further improve the accuracy of this method, Maloney suggested the following modification to the power obtained from the center of the corneal topographic map.[14]

Adjusted central corneal power = [Measured central topographic power × (376/337.5)] – 4.9

Koch et al, using data from 11 eyes suggested the use of 6.1D instead of 4.9D as the value for the posterior corneal power.

The Hard Contact Lens Method[15]

In this technique, a hard contact lens of known base curve is placed on the eye with lens changes, and refraction is performed. The subjective refraction with the contact lens in place is compared with the refraction obtained without the contact lens. These values are used to derive the corneal power, using the following relationship,

Keratometry (D) = Contact lens base curve (D) + contact lens power (D) + (refraction with the contact lens) – (refraction without the contact lens)

Example

If refraction without the contact lens (base curve 38.0D) is – 5.0D, and with the contact lens in place is plano, it means that the cornea underlying the lens is steeper than the contact lens by 5D. Hence the corneal power would be contact lens power plus 5D (assuming that the contact lens power was zero). Thus, Keratometry = 38 + 0 + (0) – (- 5) = 38 + 5 = 43.0D

This method is advantageous because it does not require access to patient data. However, it is accurate only if the cataract allows refraction and the patient has have a best-corrected visual acuity of at least 6/18 (to ensure that the refraction is accurate). If the cataract is very dense or total, and accurate refraction is not possible, or if the visual acuity in the cataractous eye cannot be improved beyond 6/24, then the accuracy of this method is open to question.

More recently, the contact lens overrefraction method was reviewed and modified by Haigis.[16] He explains that the formula described above may provide a clinically acceptable estimate of the corneal back vertex power in normal eyes without previous corneal surgery. However, in eyes that have had corneal surgery, the formula may lead to overestimation of keratometry.

To overcome this, he suggests the use of the following formula

$$PC_e = 1.119 \times P_{CLO} - 5.78$$

PC_e—Equivalent corneal power
P_{CLO}—Power from the contact lens over-refraction method

Regression Derived Clinical Method[17]

The authors used a dataset of eyes undergoing LASIK to derive the following equation using regression equations.

$$Kc.cd = 1.14Kpost - 6.8$$

Kc.cd = Clinically derived post refractive surgery keratometry
Kpost = Measured post refractive surgery keratometry

Example

If the measured post refractive surgery keratometry is 40.0D.

The value according to the above equation would be = (1.14 × 40) – 6.8 = 38.8D

Intraoperative Retinoscopy[18]

In this technique, cataract surgery is completed and retinoscopy is performed intraoperatively in the aphakic eye. From the aphakic refraction, the IOL power can be determined. Alternatively, the IOL chosen can be implanted and then retinoscopy is performed, although IOL exchange would be necessary if there was a significant error. It would also be necessary to consider the loss of aseptic technique that may occur during this intraoperative maneuver.

These issues were addressed in a recent study and the authors derived a regression equation to help determine the IOL power required using the intraoperative aphakic automated refraction obtained during surgery.[19]

$$\text{Predicted final adjusted IOL power} = 2.01449 \times \text{intraoperative SE refraction}$$

In another similar approach, the authors suggest performing a manifest aphakic refraction 30 minutes after cataract surgery and using the following equation to calculate the IOL power[20]

$$\text{Predicted final adjusted IOL power} = 1.75 \times \text{manifest SE refraction}$$

The Gaussian Optics Formula[21]

This is a theoretical approach that uses the values for anterior and posterior corneal curvatures measured after refractive surgery – using the Orbscan or the Pentacam, with the pachymetry – to derive the corneal power. The values obtained are used with the formula described below

$$\text{Corneal power} = P_1 + P_2 - [d/n_1] \times P_1 \times P_2$$

$P_1 = [1/r_1 (n_1 - n_0)]$

$P_1 = [1/r_2 (n_2 - n_1)]$

P_1 = Power of the anterior corneal surface

P_2 = Power of the posterior corneal surface

n_0 = refractive index of air (1.0)

n_1 = refractive index of cornea (1.376)

n_2 = refractive index of aqueous humor (1.336)

d = corneal pachymetry

r_1 = anterior corneal radius of curvature (mm)

r_2 = posterior corneal radius of curvature (mm)

Theoretical Variable Refractive Index Method[22]

The authors used a dataset of post PRK eyes to derive a theoretical variable refractive index correlated to axial length. This was used to derive the corrected value for post PRK keratometry using the measured value.

$$\text{Theoretical refractive index (TRI)} = [-0.0006 (AL \times AL) + (0.0213 \times AL) + 1.1572]$$

$$\text{Corneal power} = (TRI - 1) / r$$

AL – Axial length in mm

R – Corneal curvature in mm

The availability of these various techniques has resulted in improved accuracy in IOL power calculations for eyes that have had refractive surgery.[23] However, there is still scope for improvement. Concerns exist with some of the methods described – especially those that are theoretical derivations, which require verification with actual patient datasets.

With techniques that require access to pre-refractive surgery patient data, it is important that such data be accurate.[24] Especially with post-refractive surgery refractive error, it is vital that this be obtained before the onset of cataract alters the value. With methods such as the contact lens over refraction, the degree of cataract and visual function affect the accuracy of the outcome, as also the contact lens fit and centration.

Finally, even if all these are accurate, the quality of the refractive ablation is very important in determining the outcomes of these calculation techniques. If there has been a very small, irregular or decentered ablation zone, the outcomes can still be suboptimal.

Thus, in dealing with these patients, it is important to have access to as much of the available pre-refractive surgery data as possible, perform a careful preoperative examination of the eye and corneal profiles, use as many of the methods described as possible, choose the least keratometry value obtained (ensuring that it is fits with the data available), calculate the IOL power required using the third and fourth generation formulae, choose the highest IOL power determined (for eyes that have had myopic refractive surgery), and aim for a slight postoperative myopia of 0.75 to 1.0 D. Despite all this, it may be necessary also to discuss with the patient the issues involved and explain the possible need for some further procedures, should the desired result not be obtained. Finally, it is important to keep a database of these patients, to help improve our ability to improve refractive outcomes after cataract surgery.

REFERENCES

1. Holladay JT. Consultations in refractive surgery. Refract Corneal Surg 1989;5:203.
2. Feiz V, Mannis MJ, Garcia-Ferrer F, Kandavel G, Darlington JK, Kim E, Caspar J, Wang JL, Wang W. Intraocular lens power calculation after laser in situ keratomileusis for myopia and hyperopia. Cornea 2001;20:792-97.
3. Hamed HA, Wang L, Misra M, Koch DD. A comparative analysis of five methods of determining corneal refractive power in eyes that have undergone myopic laser in situ keratomileusis. Ophthalmology 2002; 109:651-58.
4. Aramberri J. Intraocular lens power calculation after corneal refractive surgery: Double K method. J Cataract Refract Surg 2003;29:2063-68.
5. Koch DD, Wang L. Calculating IOL power in eyes that have had refractive surgery. J Cataract Refract Surg 2003;29:2039-42.
6. Jarade EF, Tabbara KF. New formula for calculating intraocular lens power after laser in situ keratomileusis. J Cataract Refract Surg 2004;30:1711-15.
7. Stakheev AA, Balashevich LJ. Corneal power determination after previous corneal refractive surgery for intraocular lens calculation. Cornea 2003;22:214-20.
8. Walter KA, Gagnon MR, Hoopes PC, Dickinson PJ. Accurate intraocular lens power calculations after myopic laser in situ keratomileusis, bypassing corneal power. J Cataract Refract Surg 2006;32:425-29.
9. Latkany RA, Choksi AR, Speaker MG, Abramson J, Soloway BD, Yu G. Intraocular lens calculations after refractive surgery. J Cataract Refract Surg 2005;31: 562-70.
10. Masket S, Masket SE. Simple regression formula for intraocular lens power adjustment in eyes requiring cataract surgery after excimer laser photoablation. J Cataract Refract Surg 2006;32:430-34.
11. Feiz V, Moshirfar M, Mannis MJ, Reilly CD, Garcia-Ferrer F, Caspar JJ, Lim MC. Nomogram-based intraocular lens power adjustment after myopic photorefractive keratectomy and LASIK. Ophthalmology 2005;112: 1381-87.
12. Jarade EF, Abi Nader FC, Tabbara KF. Intraocular lens power calculation following LASIK: Determination of the new effective index of refraction. J Refract Surg 2006;22:75-80.
13. Celikkol L, Pavlopoulos G, Weinstein B, Celikkol G, Feldman S. Calculation of intraocular lens power after radial keratotomy with computerized videokeratography. Am J Ophthalmol 1995;120:739-50.
14. Wang L, Booth MA, Koch DD. Comparison of intraocular lens power calculation methods in eyes that have undergone LASIK. Ophthalmology 2004;111: 1825-31.
15. Hoffer KJ. Intraocular lens power calculation for eyes after refractive keratotomy. J Refract Surg 1995;11: 490-93.
16. Haigis W. Corneal power after refractive surgery for myopia: Contact lens method. J Cataract Refract Surg 2003;29:1397-1411.
17. Shammas HJ, Shammas MC, Gabaret A, Kim JH, Shammas A, LaBree L. Correcting the corneal power measurements for intraocular lens power calculations after myopic laser in situ keratomileusis. Am J Ophthalmol 2003;136:426-32.
18. Seitz B, Langenbucher A. Intraocular lens power calculation in eyes after corneal refractive surgery. J Refract Surg 2000;16:349-61.
19. Ianchulev T, Salz J, Hoffer K, Albini T, Hsu H, LaBree L. Intraoperative optical refractive biometry for intraocular lens power estimation without axial length and keratometry measurements. J Cataract Refract Surg 2005;31:1530-36.
20. Mackool RJ, Ko W, Mackool R. Intraocular lens power calculation after laser in situ keratomileusis: Aphakic refraction technique. J Cataract Refract Surg 2006;32: 435-37.

21. Cheng ACK, Lam DSC. Keratometry for intraocular lens power calculation using Orbscan II in eyes with laser in situ keratomileusis. J Refract Surg 2005;21: 365-68.
22. Ferrara G, Cennamo G, Marotta G, Loffredo E. New formula to calculate corneal power after refractive surgery. J Refract Surg 2004;20:465-71.
23. Cheng AC, Lam DS. Correcting the corneal power measurements for intraocular lens power calculations after myopic laser in situ keratomileusis. Am J Ophthalmol 2004;137:970.
24. Cheng AC, Rao SK, Tang E, Lam DS. Pachymetry assessment with Orbscan II in postoperative patients with myopic LASIK. J Refract Surg 2006;22:363-66.

Comparison of Methods for IOL Power Calculation after Incisional and Photoablative Refractive Surgery

27

ANTONIO CALOSSI, MASSIMO CAMELLIN (ITALY)

CORNEAL POWER AFTER KERATOREFRACTIVE SURGERY

With the advent of keratorefractive surgery, more and more patients undergoing cataract surgery with intraocular lens (IOL) implantation have previously undergone some type of refractive surgery. In these cases, no particular technical difficulty exists when performing cataract surgery; however, the IOL power is usually inaccurate.[1-13]

The problem is that after keratorefractive surgery, conventional keratometry provides incorrect corneal power values. In the specific case of refractive surgery for myopic correction, keratometry readings overestimate the corneal power. In this case, by using conventional measuring methods and calculation formulas, the resulting IOL power is too low and an unintentional postoperative hyperopic refraction results. In hyperopic refractive surgery, the reverse occurs, i.e., corneal power is underestimated and IOL power is higher than necessary with the consequence of induced myopia after cataract surgery.[14]

The origin of the error lies in a series of approximations made in the measurement of corneal power. Usually this value is an outcome of only the anterior corneal surface measured by a keratometer. This instrument measures the sagittal curvature in a small paracentral area and, by using a fictitious refractive index (variable from 1.3315 to 1.3375, according to the different manufacturers[15]) that considers the refractive effect of the corneal posterior surface of an average eye, provides the dioptric power of the measured cornea. After refractive surgery, two phenomena occur that render this method inapplicable: (1) the corneal asphericity is considerably modified: e.g. in myopic correction, asphericity is often reversed, in a more or less accentuated way, depending on the type of surgery, and the central part of the cornea is flatter than the one measured by the keratometer; and (2) in laser ablative surgery, the ratio between the modified anterior corneal surface curvature and the unaltered posterior surface changes, making the commonly utilized keratometric refractive index no longer valid.

Change of Corneal Asphericity

After keratorefractive surgery for myopic correction, the optical zone of the cornea becomes flatter. Usually, inside the pupillary area the central cornea becomes flatter than the portion of cornea that lies over the marginal zone of the pupil, so its prolate shape becomes oblate (with reverse asphericity) (Figs 27.1 and 27.2). In hyperopic correction, the cornea becomes even more prolate and asphericity increases. This phenomenon increases with the amount of surgical correction and is more evident in incisional surgery or laser ablative surgery with a small optical zone.[16-22]

Keratometers measure a portion of cornea that does not include the pupillary central area. The

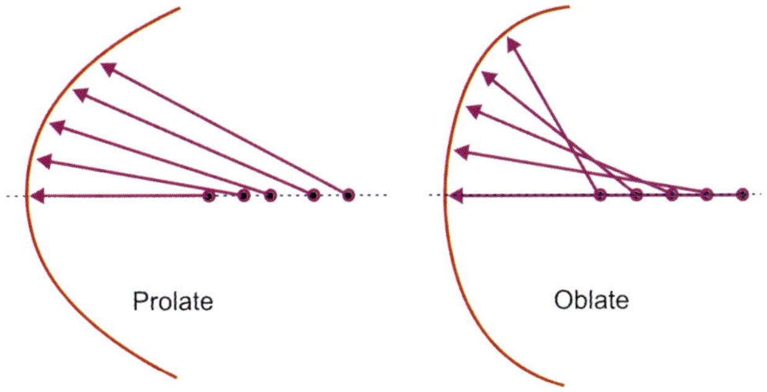

Fig. 27.1: In a prolate cornea the marginal radius of curvature is longer than the central one, while in oblate shape the marginal radius is shorter than the central one

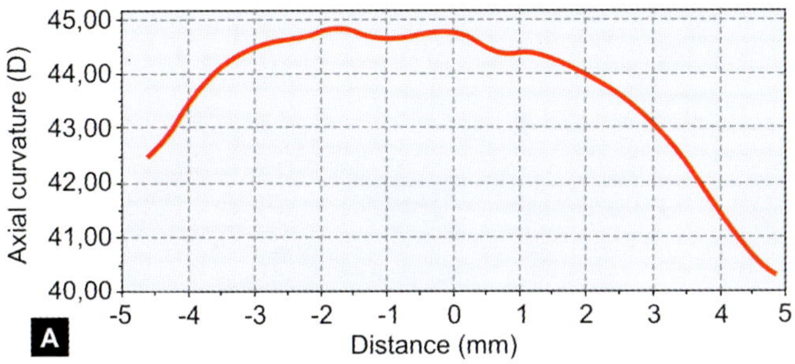

Fig. 27.2A: The graph shows the sagittal (axial) curvature profile of an unoperated normal cornea

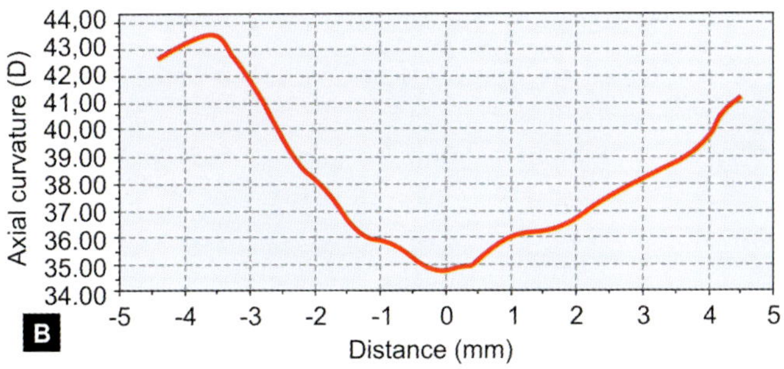

Fig. 27.2B: Post myopic LASIK sagittal curvature profile. As usually in conventional treatments, inside the pupillary area the central cornea has become flatter than the portion of cornea that lies over the marginal zone of the pupil

measured area is limited to the portion of cornea that reflects the keratometric targets; it is constituted by a circular crown with a diameter that varies between approximately 2 and 4 mm and a width that varies between 0.1 and 0.4 mm according to the constructive characteristics of the keratometer and to the measured surface curvature.[23-25] (Fig. 27.3) With the same keratometer on a steeper cornea, a portion of cornea closer to the center is measured, whereas on a flatter cornea a more peripheral zone is measured. Due to the Stiles-Crawford effect (SCE) of the first kind,[25-27] the area of the cornea that covers the central pupillary zone gives a brighter image than the one formed by the portion of the cornea that covers the marginal zone of the entrance pupil: if the central ray is perceived as having a brightness of 100%, a ray 1 mm off-center appears 93% as bright, 2 mm off-center it appears 71% as bright and 3 mm off-center only 41% as bright (Fig. 27.4), so the central cornea, which is not measured, has a more dominant role in the formation of the foveal image in respect to the portion of cornea that is usually measured by keratometers. In a normal cornea with an average asphericity this phenomena is of little impact because the sagittal curvature varies slightly from the center to the keratometer measuring area,[23] but when asphericity has high absolute values, differences between central and paracentral curvature cannot be neglected (Figs 27.5 to 27.7). In our opinion, it is for these reasons that the measurement of the corneal curvature for optical purposes should provide the average value, weighted according to SCE (i.e. a gaussian weighing),

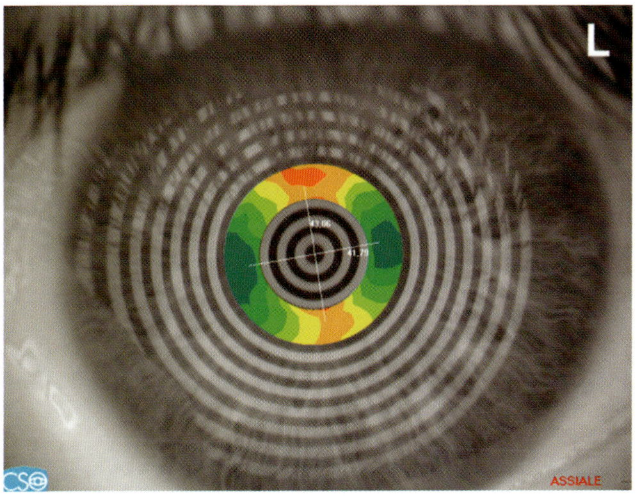

Fig. 27.3: The colored area represents the zone of the cornea utilized for keratometry measurements and for computerized videokeratography Sim-K index. As we can see, the central pupillary area is not measured

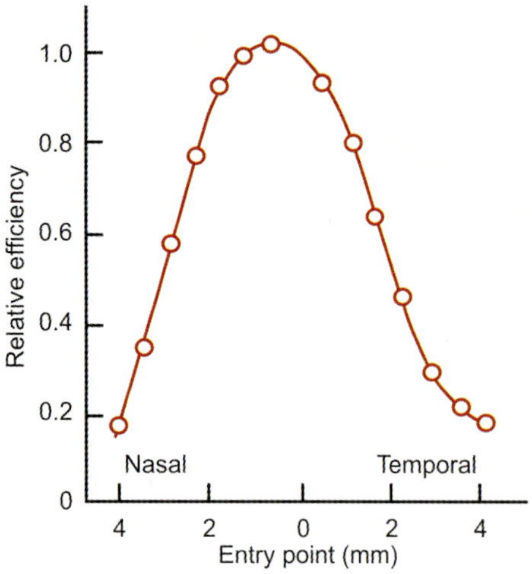

Fig. 27.4: The area of the cornea that covers the central pupillary zone gives a brighter image than the one formed by the portion of the cornea that covers the marginal zone of the entrance pupil. The graph represents the relative efficiency of the entrance pupil. (After Stiles WS and Crawford BH, 1933) [25]

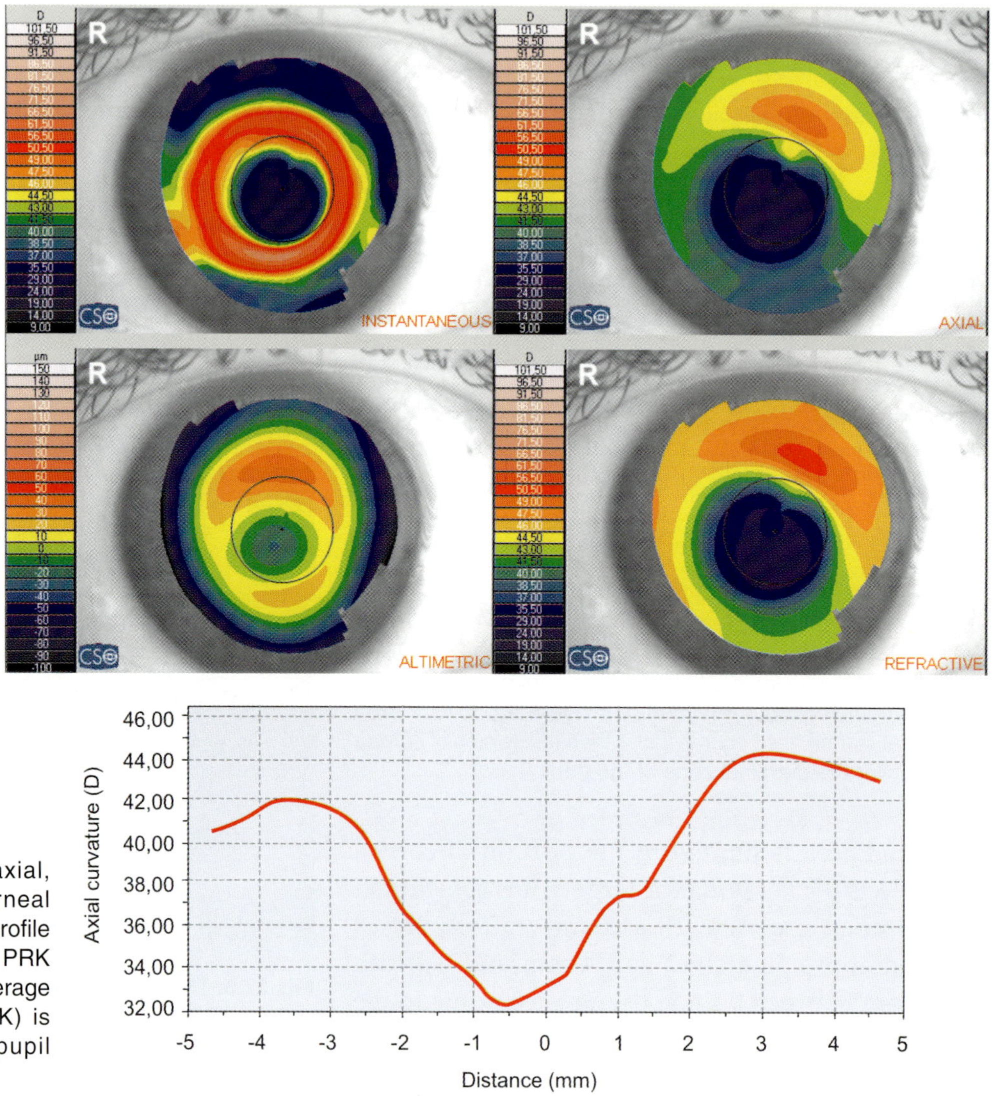

Fig. 27.5: Instantaneous, axial, altimetric and refractive corneal maps and sagittal curvature profile of a cornea post a high myopic PRK treatment. In this case the average simulated keratometry (sim-K) is 36.56 D, while the mean pupil curvature is 32.25 D

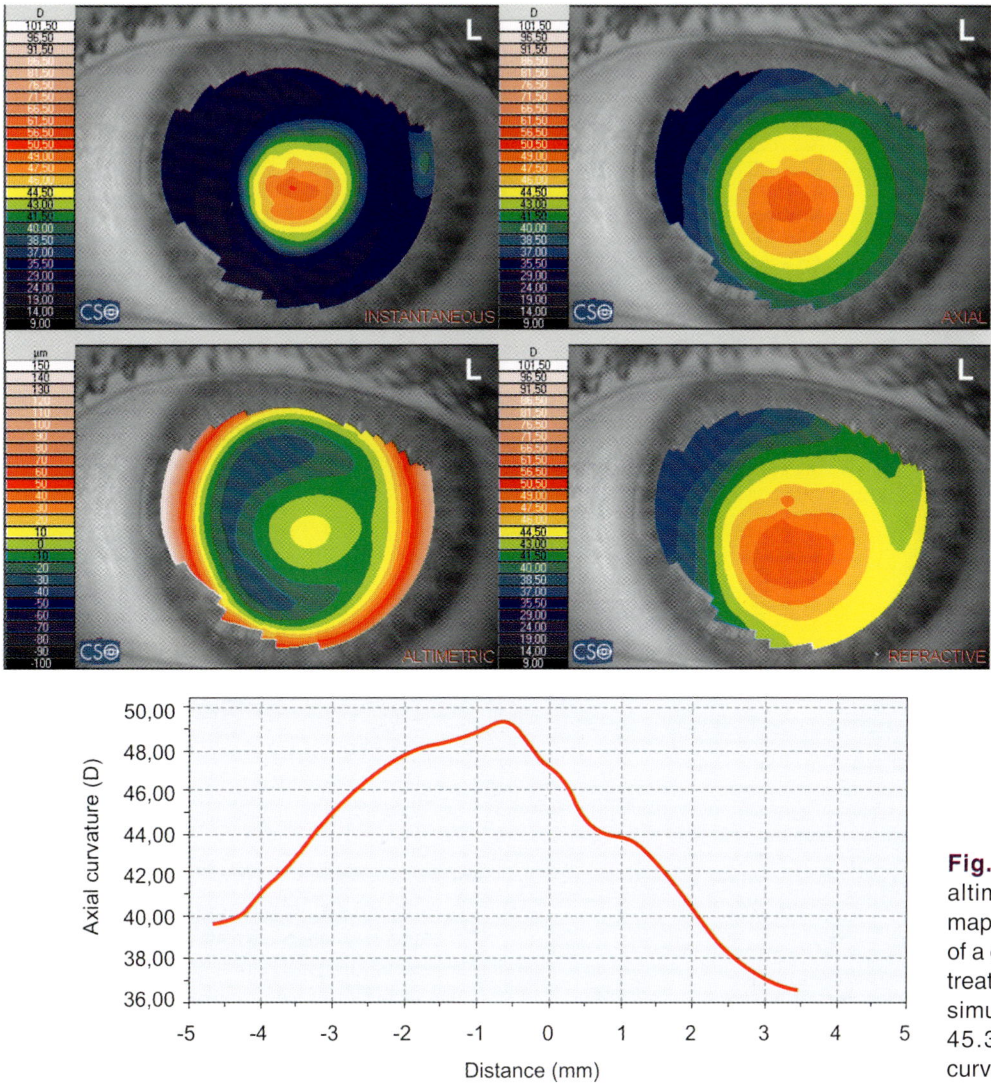

Fig. 27.6: Instantaneous, axial, altimetric and refractive corneal maps and sagittal curvature profile of a cornea post a hyperopic LASIK treatment. In this case the average simulated keratometry (sim-K) is 45.38D, while the mean pupil curvature is 46.50D

of the whole corneal area that covers the entrance pupil. For the reasons we have just described, this measurement cannot be performed by conventional keratometers, but can be obtained by computerized videokeratographs.

Change of Ratio between Anterior and Posterior Corneal Surfaces

Clinical measurement of corneal power usually is performed by instruments that do not measure the corneal power directly, in the same way that a lensmeter does for ophthalmic lenses, but only the curvature of its anterior surface, from which the dioptric power of the whole cornea is derived. Instruments such as keratometers, autokeratometers and computerized videokeratographs based on the Placido principle follow the same concept: the anterior curvature of the cornea is measured, then the radius is converted into diopters by using the following paraxial equation:

$$P = \frac{n - 1}{r} \qquad (1)$$

where P is the corneal power (in diopters)

r is the corneal radius (in meters)

l is the air refractive index

n is the corneal refractive index.

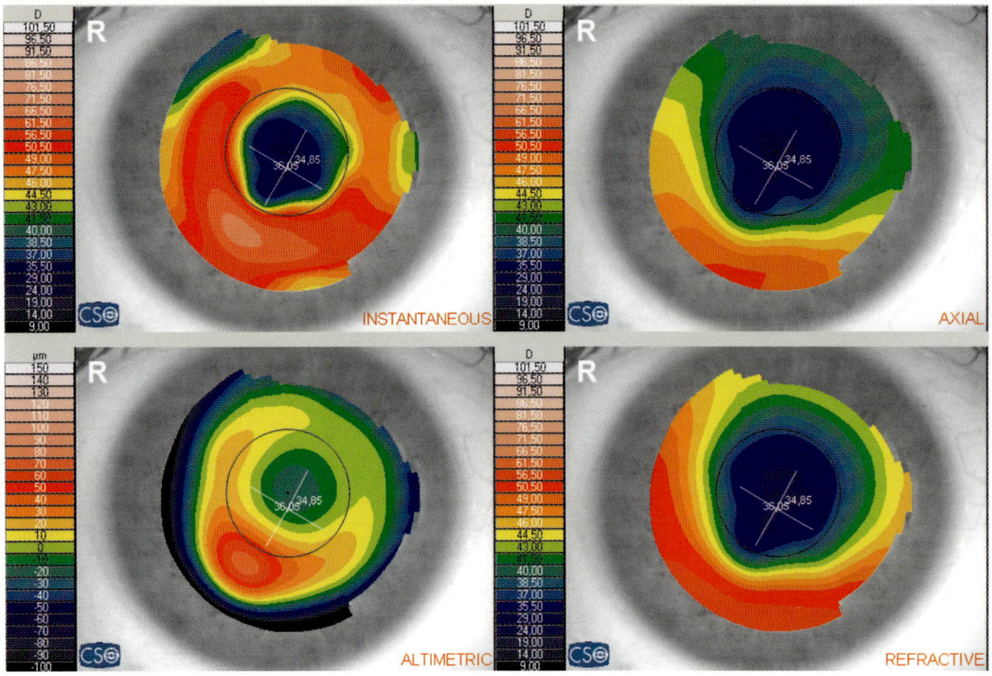

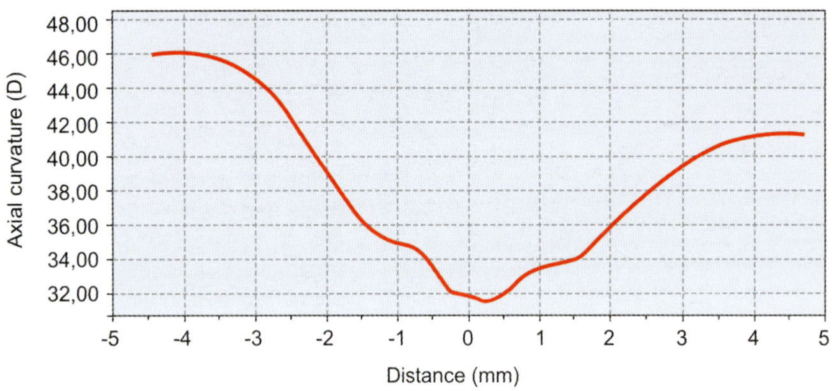

Fig. 27.7A: Instantaneous, axial, altimetric and refractive corneal maps and sagittal curvature profile of a cornea post a radial keratotomy treatment with a high central flattening effect. In this case the average simulated keratometry (sim-K) is 35.74, while the mean pupil curvature is 32.75

Because the principle of all current instruments is to consider the cornea as a single refractive surface, to compensate the effect of the posterior surface and corneal thickness, instead of using the real refractive index of the corneal tissue, a fictitious keratometric index (lower than the one of the epithelium and of the stroma) is used. The keratometric refractive index usually is considered constant for all cases and is obtained by calculating the average ratio between the anterior and posterior corneal surface of an average schematic eye.[28] This approximation is acceptable for an average normal eye but may cause intolerable errors in some cases.

Theory

Gullstrand's Schematic Eye

As in all dioptric compound systems, corneal power is function of the curvature of the surfaces that separate its optical media and of their refractive index. The optical media that condition the corneal dioptric system are: air, tear film, corneal tissue, and aqueous humor. In order to have an accurate study of corneal dioptrics, we should perform a complete ray tracing applying Snell's law:

$$\frac{\sin i}{\sin r} = \frac{n_2}{n_1} \qquad (2)$$

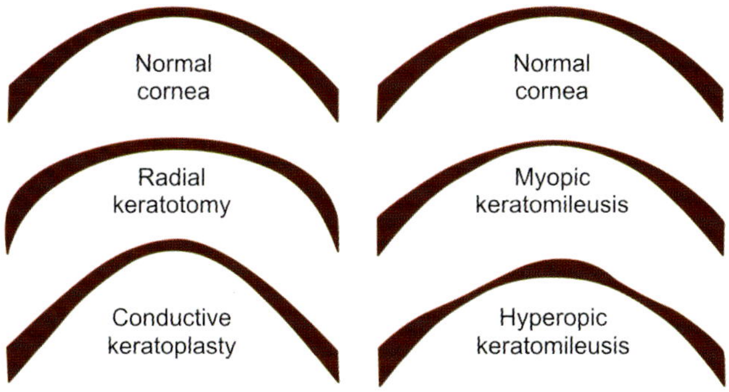

Fig. 27.7B: Schematic relationship between the anterior and posterior corneal curvature in a normal unoperated cornea and after different types of corneal refractive surgery. After RK and CK we observe an indirect change of the central anterior corneal curvature. Since no tissue is removed, it is assumed that the anterior and posterior surface of the cornea react in an analogous way, and the ratio between the anterior and posterior corneal curvature remain almost the same. The asphericity of the cornea changes proportionally to the curvature changes. After the laserablative procedures, although the central anterior curvature changes, the posterior surface should remain unchanged

where i is the angle of incidence of a light ray
r is the refraction angle
n_1 is the refractive index of the incident ray medium
n_2 is the refractive index of the refracted ray medium.

In order to apply Snell's law, we must know the refractive indexes of the various optical media, the profile of the separating surfaces, and the distance between the surfaces. Since it is not possible to measure directly all these quantities in a living eye, we can use a geometric model. This model should represent with sufficient precision the real eye, but for a simple model some approximations are needed. For simplify, we shall try to reason following Gauss's paraxial approximation, where the rays from the object to the image lie close to the principal axis and form small angles with the axis. If we accept this approximation, we can apply to the cornea the paraxial equation of the spherical diopters:

$$P = \frac{n_2 - n_1}{r} \qquad (3)$$

where P is the power of the dioptric surface (in diopters)
r is the power of the dioptric surface (in diopters)
n_1 is the refractive index of the first medium
n_2 is the refractive index of the second medium

We can therefore calculate the power of the anterior surface, of the posterior surface and, following the laws of paraxial optics, vertex and effective corneal powers.[29] In the Gullstrand "exact" Schematic Eye No. 1,[28] the cornea is schematically reproduced as a system formed by two spherical surfaces 500 μm apart, the anterior face has a curvature of 7.70 mm and the posterior surface of 6.80 mm; the refractive index of the air (n_1) is 1.000, the one of the cornea (n_2) is 1.376, and the one of the aqueous (n_3) is 1.336. The tear film is ignored, since it is like a thin lamina with parallel surfaces with power equal to zero. Applying formula (3) we obtain an anterior corneal power (P_1) of +48.83 D and a posterior power (P_2) of –5.88 D. When two dioptric surfaces of power P_1 and P_2 separated by a distance t are combined, we can calculate the equivalent power by applying the following formula:

$$P_e = P_1 + P_2 - \frac{t}{n} P_1 P_2 \qquad (4)$$

In this case the corneal equivalent power is +43.05 D.

If we subsequently simplify our corneal model approximating it to a single surface system, by resolving the inverse formula of (1) we can calculate the keratometric refractive index in order to obtain the same equivalent power of the two-surface model:

$$n = r\,P + 1 \qquad (5)$$

Being r = 7.70 mm and P = +43.05 D we obtain an equivalent refractive index (n) of 1.3315.

This keratometric refractive index value is purely fictitious and does not represent any real optical medium present in the eye, so Gullstrand proposed a simplified Schematic Eye No.2,[28] with a single corneal surface and as refractive index the one of the aqueous: 1.336. In order to maintain the same equivalent power of the exact Schematic Eye No. 1, Gullstrand modified in this model the corneal curvature radius from 7.70 to 7.80. Normally, when we perform a keratometry, we do not compensate the radius in this way, so by using a keratometric index of 1.336 we cause an average error of 0.59 D (see Table 27.1).

If in Gullstrand exact Schematic Eye No.1, instead of considering the effective power (P_e) of (4), we calculate the back vertex power (P_v), with the following equation:

$$P_v = P_2 + \cfrac{n}{\cfrac{n}{P_1} - t} \qquad (6)$$

we obtain a corneal power of +43.83 D. In this case, applying again (5) we obtain an equivalent refractive index of 1.3375. This keratometric refractive index was initially proposed by Javal and Schjötz [30] and is still nowadays probably the most diffused one. This value is very close to the real acqueous humor and tear film index and furthermore it yields the simple relation 7.50 mm = 45.00 D. Nevertheless, we must consider the focal distances from the posterior surface of the cornea and not from its anterior vertex otherwise, in an average eye, we have an error of 0.78 D (see Table 27.1).

In some cases a keratometric index of 1.333 has been proposed.[31-33] This value is equivalent to 4/3 and consents more simple calculations. This value is relatively close to the equivalent refractive index; in an average eye creates an overestimate of the real corneal power of 0.24 D.

Table 27.1: Keratometric power for radius = 7.70 mm and various keratometric refractive indexes for the Gullstrand "exact" Schematic Eye. Delta K is the difference in power in comparison with the real one calculated with index = 1.3315

Corneal radius (mm)	7.70	7.70	7.70	7.70
Keratometric index	1.3315	1.3360	1.3333	1.3375
Corneal power (D)	43.05	43.64	43.29	43.83
Delta K (D)	0.59	0.24	0.78	

We must remember that when, instead of evaluating the absolute dioptric power of the whole cornea, we must consider the dioptric effect of the anterior surface only, i.e. for ablation calculations and dioptric variation estimates due to laser ablation refractive surgery, the refractive index of the corneal epithelium or stroma of 1.376 should be used in converting radius to optical power values.[34-36]

The Real Eye

What we have until now described is true for a real eye only if the relation between its posterior corneal curvature and anterior one is equal to 6.80/7.70. In this case, utilizing a keratometric index of 1.3315 we can approximate the cornea to a model with an only surface and obtain the same power equivalent to a two surface model without adjusting the radius.[37] Between the real eyes there are individual variations in corneal thickness and ratio between posterior and anterior corneal curvature,[38-41] when this relation between the two curvatures changes in a significant way, we cannot use a constant keratometric index to convert millimeters in diopters.

A particular case is the cornea treated with laser ablative refractive surgery. In this case only the anterior curvature of the cornea is modified, while the posterior surface remains ideally unchanged (Fig.27.7). This way the relation between posterior curvature and anterior curvature is changed, so a keratometric index that would have been valid before surgery cannot be valid after the treatment. Our purpose was to verify possible differences in the dioptric power.

Keratometric Refractive Index after Laser Ablative Refractive Surgery

In order to calculate the variations of refractive index necessary to maintain a correct equivalent power, in the Gullstrand Schematic Eye, we have calculated the curvature change of the corneal anterior surface needed to obtain a certain amount of refractive correction on the spectacle plane, so, given a constant optical zone, we have calculated the change of corneal thickness consequent to curvature change due to laser ablation; maintaining the corneal posterior surface unvaried, we calculated the equivalent corneal power, and then finally obtained the equivalent refractive index as a function of the surgical induced refractive change (SIRC).

Since with this type of surgery only the anterior surface of the cornea is modified,[34] in order to calculate the change of curvature necessary to obtain a certain dioptric effect by laser ablative surgery, we considered the stroma refractive index ($n = 1.376$) and, by subtracting the SIRC from the pre-operative anterior corneal power, by means of (1) we obtained the post-operative curvature radius. The change of thickness (Δz) has been calculated with the following equation[42] which is the basis of the non approximate Munnerlyn formula: [34]

$$\Delta z = \frac{a^2(\Delta P)}{2(n-1)} \quad (7)$$

where a is the half diameter of the optical zone, ΔP is the variation of power, and n is the stroma refractive index. With these values, using (4), we calculated the effective corneal power, then using (5) the equivalent refractive index. Finally, we calculated the differences between the corneal power obtained by utilizing a fixed refractive index and the real corneal power as a function of the SIRC.

Results are reported in Figures 27.8 and 27.9. After corneal laser ablative surgery, the equivalent keratometric refractive index approximately decreases of 0.001 units per diopter of myopic correction and increases of the same amount in case of hyperopic correction. By using a constant keratometric index, in corneas treated with myopic laser ablation we have an overestimate of the corneal power, which increases with the operated correction. Vice versa, in hyperopic correction, the tendency is to underestimate. By utilizing a keratometric refractive index = 1.3315, for a surgical correction of –4.00 D, we have an error of 0.50 D, for a SIRC of –9.00 D the error is 1.00 D and reaches a 2.00 D error for a correction of –20.00D. If, as it usually happens, we use a greater keratometric refractive index, the error increases in case of a myopic correction. I.e., with a keratometric index = 1.3375 the error is 1 D for a correction of –2.00 D and goes up to 2.00 D for a correction of –13.00 D.

Our calculations show that differences between real corneal power and the power estimated using conventional keratometric procedures cannot be neglected. The possibility that corneal refractive index varies through its thickness[43, 44] and in relation to stroma hydration[45-47] could further increase the value of the errors we reported. These aspects are usually ignored when using a constant keratometric refractive index for all cases. This matter has a considerable clinical importance in calculating the power of IOL in eyes that have been previously treated with refractive surgery. Corneas that have been treated with laser ablative refractive surgery are a particular case in which errors may become particularly significant. After this type of surgery, the anterior surface of the cornea is modified while the posterior surface ideally remains unchanged (even if bio-mechanic effects may induce a slight posterior corneal change). In this case, the ratio between anterior and posterior curvature is changed, so a keratometric refractive index that could have been valid before surgery may not be the same after surgery.[48]

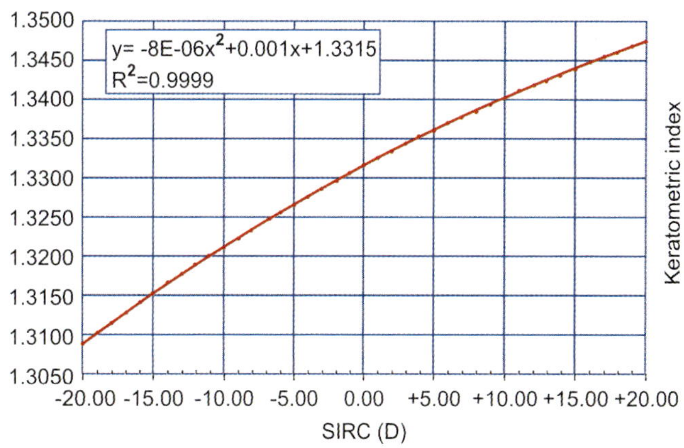

Fig. 27.8: Keratometric refractive index in function of surgically induced refractive change (SIRC). The regression curve equation reported on the graph shows that the equivalent keratometric refractive index varies approximately of 0.001 units per diopter of correction

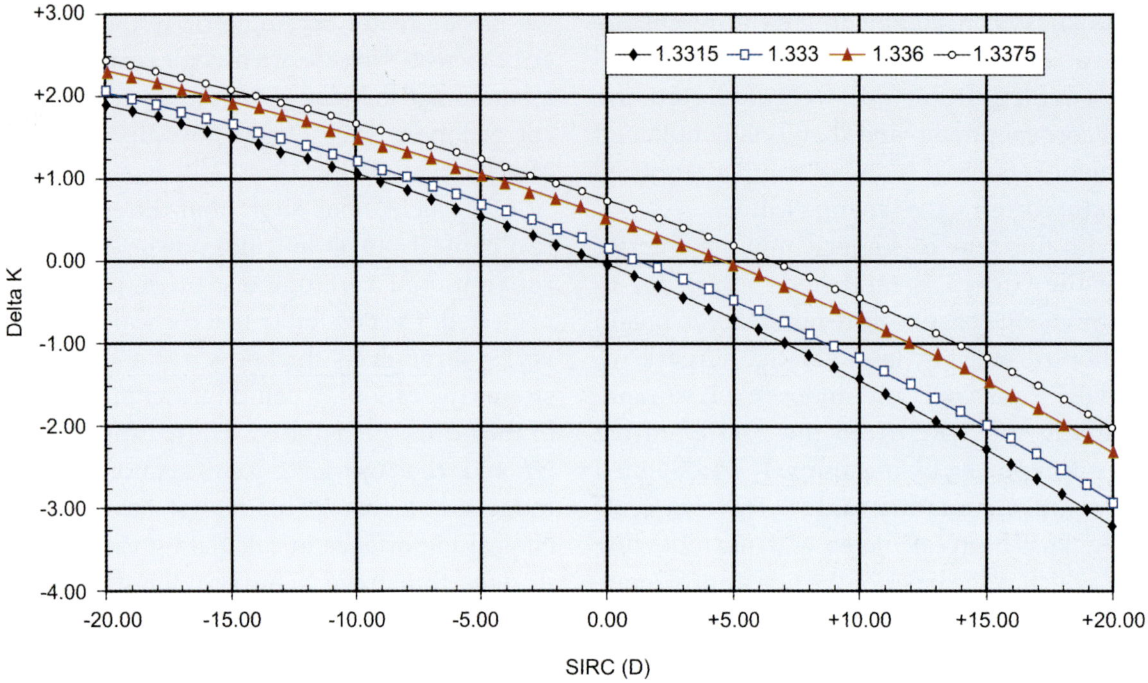

Fig. 27.9: Difference (delta K) between corneal power calculated by using a constant keratometric refractive index and the real equivalent power calculated in function of surgically induced refractive change (SIRC)

Conventional keratometric refractive index, after a myopic laser ablation causes an overestimation of the corneal power, whereas in hyperopic correction, it causes an underestimation. Unfortunately, errors due to corneal asphericity changes and those caused by variations in ratio between anterior and posterior corneal surface curvatures always go in the same direction and their effects are cumulative.

The Effective Lens Position: Another Source of Error

Until recently, the attention of cataract surgeons for the post-keratorefractive eye has mainly been focused on accurately determining the central corneal power. It is now becoming more widely understood that a flattened or steepened central cornea not only renders keratometry inaccurate, but also causes problems with many IOL power calculation formulas that in normal eyes work well.[49, 50] When it is entered into a standard IOL power formula, the post-keratorefractive surgery K readings are not only used as a measure of the corneal power but also to calculate the effective lens position (ELP) which is the estimated postoperative distance between the anterior corneal surface and of the principal plane of the IOL (Fig. 27.10a). This measurement is also referred to as the pseudophakic anterior chamber depth. Modern, 2-variable IOL power calculation formulas[51-55] use different methods to calculate the effective lens position; however, except for the Haigis formula,[56,57] which does not use corneal power readings to predict postoperative ELP, they all use the keratometric values in their calculations. In normal cases, a flatter corneal measurement signifies a shallower anterior chamber depth. With a low central corneal power the formula makes the assumption that the IOL following cataract surgery will end up sitting closer to the cornea than normal and call for less power (Fig. 27.10b). The contrary occurs with a high corneal power (Fig. 27.10c). After keratorefractive surgery, the anterior corneal surface is flattened for myopic correction, or steepened for hyperopic surgery, but the effective lens position is unaltered. And the flatter or steeper the cornea, the

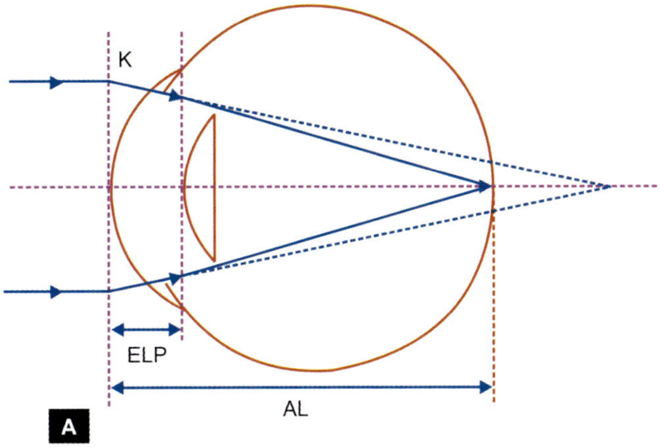

Fig. 27.10A: The 3 main variables utilized by an IOL power calculation formula: corneal power (K), axial length (AL), and the effective lens position (ELP). The effective lens position (ELP) is the estimated postoperative distance between the anterior corneal surface and of the principal plane of the IOL

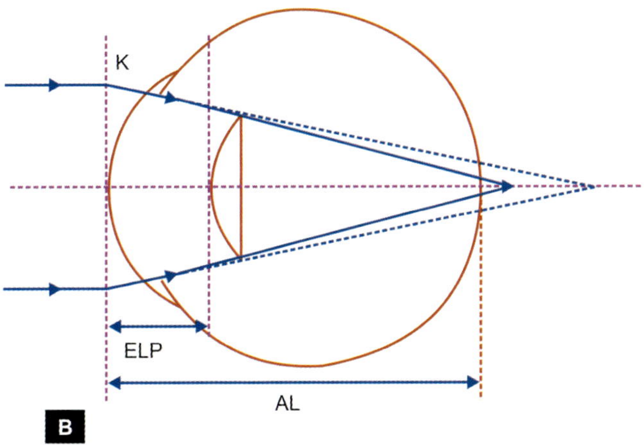

Fig. 27.10B: If the ELP is incorrectly assumed falsely shallow, a deeper post-operative ELP occurs that induced a hyperopic error

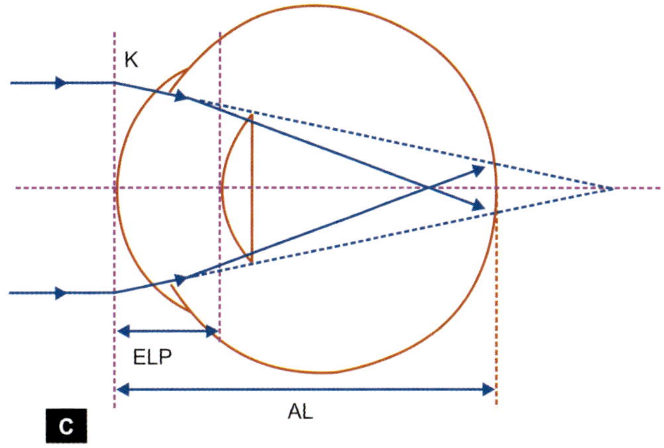

Fig. 27.10C: If the ELP is incorrectly assume falsely deep, a shallower post-operative ELP occurs that induced a myopic error

bigger a problem this becomes.[49,50,58,59] Unless a correction is made for this situation, the artifact of centrally altered Ks following keratorefractive surgery will have these formulas incorrectly assume a falsely shallow or deep post-operative ELP. The end result is that without a special correction, 2-variable formulas following keratorefractive surgery will recommend less IOL power after myopic surgery and more IOL power after hyperopic surgery than is actually required. Furthermore, its effect is cumulative to the error produced by the corneal power estimation. The Aramberri double-K method[49] was established specifically to correct for this problem.

Intraocular Lens Power Calculation after Refractive Corneal Surgery

Several methods have been proposed for calculating corneal refractive power in patients who have undergone corneal refractive surgery, including (1) empirical adjustment;[4,60] (2) refraction-derived method;[50,61] (3) clinical history method;[62-64] (4) contact lens overrefraction;[63,64] (5) computerized videokeratography (CVK);[65-72] (6) consideration of posterior corneal curvature;[48,73,74] (7) method based on correlation between axial eye length and corneal radius correcting factor;[75] (8) method based on correlation between axial eye length and a theoretical variable keratometric refractive index;[76] (9) method based on correlation between actual corneal curvature and corneal power correcting factor;[50] (10) calculating IOL power in a standard fashion and modifying the final value of the IOL as a function of the SIRC;[14,77,78] (11) using a variable keratometric refractive index that is a function of SIRC;[79-83] (12) and aphakic intra-operative refraction techniques.[84-87]

Empirical Method

On patients that have previously undergone radial keratotomy, Lyle and Jin[4] have proposed the subtraction of a fixed value of 1 D from usual keratometric readings (adjusted K)

$$K_{adj} = K - 1\text{ D}$$

where K_{adj} is the adjusted keratometric reading and K is the average of keratometric reading, moreover to use an average result between the Binkhorst and Holladay formulas. Jin, et al[60] proposed the same approach for eyes with previous myopic LASIK. Although this approach may reduce the chance of post-operative hyperopia, we believe it is over-simplified and does not allow calculation of individual differences due to the type and amount of surgery.

Clinical History Methods

This method, first published by Guyton[62] and Holladay[63] and later termed as 'clinical history method' by Hoffer,[64] consists of subtracting the changes in spherical equivalent refraction induced by the refractive procedure from the keratometric diopters measured before refractive surgery:

$$K = K_{pre} + Rx_{pre} - Rx_{post}$$

where, K is the actual value to be used; K_{pre} is the preoperative keratometry; Rx_{pre} is the preoperative spherical equivalent refraction; Rx_{post} is the postoperative spherical equivalent refraction. The refractive change must be calculated at the corneal plane with correction for the vertex distance from the spectacle plane. Both Holladay and Hoffer recommend against vertex-correcting the refractive errors due to published reports of improved results without it. In their clinical series, Odenthal, et al[88] also found not vertex-correcting more accurate. However, Seitz et al published a case report of cataract surgery after a PRK for excessive myopia of –24 D in which they demonstrated that pure subtraction of the spherical equivalent change at the spectacle plane (without vertex correction) from the corneal power value before refractive surgery has to be avoided because it results in a far too small corneal power.[89] In this case, they found that subtraction of 24% of the refractive change at the spectacle plane from the actually measured corneal power before cataract surgery gave the best IOL power prediction with the Haigis[56,57] formula.

In theory, this method is formally correct; however, sometimes it cannot be adopted because the required data are not always available. The required information is the pre-operative refractive and keratometric data and post-operative refraction data unaffected by change in lens power due to cataract. Each diopter of error in evaluating variations of refraction due only to refractive surgery causes 1 D of refractive error after IOL implantation.[90] Furthermore, in the time between refractive surgery and cataract, there should be no change in axial length.

A variant of the clinical history method was described by Ladas and Stark,[91] Walter et al[92] and by Sambare et al.[93] Following this approach, one simply calculates IOL power as if the patient had not had corneal refractive surgery, targeting the patient's original refractive error. Therefore, if the patient was spherical equivalent "8.00 before refractive surgery, simply use "8.00 as the post-implant refractive target. The results in their small series are excellent. This variant of clinical history method is, probably, more simple and do not affect the estimation of ELP described by Aramberri.[49] The limitations of this approach are the same described above: (1) pre-refractive surgery data may not be available or accurate and (2) the patient's outcome from corneal refractive surgery prior to developing the cataract may not be known or accurate.

Contact Lens Method

This method, first described by Frederick Ridley of the UK and later by Thomas Soper in the USA, determines the difference between the manifest refraction with and without a hard contact lens of known base curve and subtracts this difference from that base curve plus the power of the lens:[63, 64]

$$K = BC_{cl} + P_{cl} + ORx - Rx$$

where, K is the actual outcome keratometric value; BC_{cl} is the contact lens base curve in diopters; P_{cl} is the lens dioptric power, *ORx* is the spherical equivalent of the over-refraction over the contact lens and *Rx* the spherical equivalent of the refraction without the contact lens. The spherical equivalent of refraction and over-refraction must be calculated at the corneal plane with correction for the vertex distance from the spectacle plane. Recently, a variant of this method was proposed by Haigis.[94]

From a theoretical point of view, this method is correct, however in practice, it is a difficult application due to the inevitable difficulties of performing accurate refractions with and without contact lenses, in eyes affected by cataracts. Even with this method, each diopter of error in measurement of refraction and over-refraction causes 1 D of refractive error after IOL implant.[90] Zeh and Koch[95] analyzed this method in patients with normal corneas and found that the accuracy decreased with increasing media opacity but was still acceptable with Snellen acuity of 20/70. Following all forms of ablative keratorefractive surgery (LASIK, PRK, etc.) a review of the literature now suggests that the hard contact lens method may be less accurate than originally thought. For this reason it is no longer recommended.[59]

Topographic Data

Several authors report that analysis of corneal topography describes the changes in corneal curvature due to keratorefractive surgery better than keratometry.[65-72] Modern and up-to-date computerized video-keratographers allow us to measure the anterior surface of the cornea in thousands of points in a wide area, and after being computed, all these data give us many keratometric indices: sim-K, min-K, K at 3, 5 and 7 mm, Kc (central keratometry), ACP (average corneal power) etc. Therefore, the question becomes: which of these is the most adequate for calculating IOL power? As we have mentioned previously, our opinion is to consider the average curvature of the corneal area that covers the entrance pupil weighted on the SCE. Nevertheless, if we convert the corneal curvature in such a way, by using a conventional constant refractive index, this analysis may be sufficient for incisional types of surgery, whereas in laser ablative corneal surgery, errors due to variation in ratio between corneal anterior and posterior curvatures still remain.[13]

Consideration of Posterior Corneal Curvature

To accurately determine the total keratometric diopters of the cornea, the keratometric diopters of the anterior and the posterior surface of the cornea must be known. Seitz and Langenbucher[74] proposed two methods: (1) Consideration of posterior corneal curvature without measurement of posterior curvature. In this case, the first step is to calculate the keratometric diopters using the real refractive index of the cornea ($n = 1.376$) and add –5.90 D, which is the theoretical posterior surface power according to Gullstrand's model eye, or add –6.20 D, which has been found to be the mean keratometric diopters of the human posterior surface in vivo assessed though the scanning slit topography technique.[96] (2) Consideration of posterior corneal curvature with measurement of posterior curvature by scanning slit topography device potentially improves accuracy. As reported by the same authors, the first method may be a cause of error for inter-individual variability in posterior surface keratometric diopters ranging from –2.10 to –8.50 D. Therefore, adding only the mean value of the posterior surface keratometric diopters may cause a considerable error in a given patient. For the second method, the accuracy of presently available commercial devices to measure the corneal posterior profile by means of scanning split topography is still not completely validated.[97-101] In a recent paper Cheng and Lam[102] reported that after LASIK the K-value obtained from the Gaussian optics formula (CalK) based on postoperative corneal topography by Orbscan II (Bausch and Lomb, Rochester, NY) correlated closely ($R = 0.967$) to that obtained from the clinical history method. The limits of agreements using two standard deviations were -1.37 D and +1.63 D. Oculus Pentacam (Oculus Optikgeräte GmbH, Wetzlar, Germany), which images the anterior segment of the eye by a rotating Scheimpflug camera, would seem to increase the accuracy of this method.[103, 104]

Other authors have proposed ultrasound pachymetric methods for deducing the curvature of the posterior surface of the cornea by measuring the curvature of the anterior surface and by taking a series of measurements of the corneal thickness with an ultrasonic pachymeter.[39,40,105,106] We propose this method when the patient clinical history is completely unknown (i.e. no data about the SIRC), or in eyes that underwent lamellar keratoplasty (LK) or phototherapeutic keratectomy (PTK).[79] Emergent very high-frequency (VHF) ultrasound pachymetry[107] might further increase the accuracy of this method.

Method based on Correlation between Axial Eye Length and Corneal Radius Correcting Factor

Rosa et al[75] proposed a method, based on correlation between axial eye length and corneal radius correcting factors to find a way of calculating IOL power that may be independent of preoperative data, in eyes that have developed a cataract after refractive surgery. Prior to, and 1 month after PRK, the SRK/T [53] formula was used to calculate IOL power in 88 eyes of 65 patients. IOL power was calculated by using the spherical equivalent refraction as target both before and after PRK. The mean postoperative corneal radius that gave the same IOL power found before surgery was calculated for each patient. Then, they calculated the ratios between the calculated radius and the measured postoperative radius for each patient and correlated them with the axial eye length. They found quite a good correlation ($r^2 = 0.4597$) between axial eye length (x) and these ratios (y) with a linear correlation formula:

$$y = 0.0276\,x + 0.3635$$

They propose this linear regression formula, or a subdivision into classes derived from it, to calculate the correcting factors which, when multiplied by the measured postoperative radius, gave the new adjusted radius to use in the SRK/T formula. In our experience,[79] this method induced a significant degree of myopic error. Probably, we observed this lack of accuracy because the SIRC is not necessarily correlated with axial length, though we could expect a greater photoablation in more myopic eyes. In two eyes with the same ametropia, the axial length may be significantly different. Moreover, preoperative ametropia may be the same and the postoperative refraction may be different for intentionally planned ametropia, or overcorrection, undercorrection or regression that may occur. In our group of patients, the variance of Rosa's method is two times greater than conventional formulas without corneal power adjustment, and three times greater than the Camellin-Calossi formula; this aspect underlines the unpredictability of refractive outcome obtainable only correlating corneal power with axial length.

Method based on Correlation between Axial Eye Length and a Theoretical Variable Keratometric Refractive Index

Following a similar way, Ferrara et al[76] proposed a theoretical variable keratometric refractive index (*TRI*) that is correlated to axial length as the following regression formula:

$$TRI = -0.0006 \times AL^2 + 0.0213 \times AL + 1.1572$$

where AL is the axial length. The corneal power is calculated with: $P = (TRI-1)/r$ (r = corneal curvature in m). Using this keratometric corrected power, they suggest to calculated IOL power with SRK/T formula similar to that for emmetropia.

Also for this method, in our experience we observed a large unpredictability of refractive outcome.[108] As for Rosa approach, probably, we observed this lack of accuracy because the SIRC is not necessarily correlated with axial length, though we could expect a greater photoablation in more myopic eyes.

Method based on Correlation between Actual Corneal Curvature and Corneal Power Correcting Factor

Shammas, et al[50] described a method to calculate a corrected keratometric value after myopic LASIK when the amount of myopic correction achieved by the refractive surgery is completely unknown. This clinically-derived method uses a regression equation to modify the measured post-LASIK K reading. The calculated corneal power is labeled $K_{c.cd}$:

$$K_{c.cd} = 1.14 \times K_{post} - 6.8$$

Where K_{post} represents the post-LASIK Sim-K value obtained from a videokeratograph. Another method of post-LASIK corneal power estimation was originally described by Robert Maloney and subsequently modified by Koch and Wang.[109,110] Using this technique, the central corneal power is estimated by placing the cursor at the exact center of the axial map of the corneal topographer. This value is then converted back to the anterior corneal power by multiplying the axial map central topographic corneal power by 376.0/337.5, which is the same as 1.114. An assumed posterior corneal power of 6.1 D is then subtracted from this product.

$$K_{c.cd} = 1.114 \times CCP - 6.1$$

Where *CCP* is the corneal power with the cursor in the center of the refractive map of the Zeiss Humphrey Atlas topographer (Carl Zeiss Meditec, Jena, Germany). The results of these formulas are similar to that of the first method of Seitz and Langenbucher[74] described above.

Haigis[111-113] has proposed a similar method based on current Zeiss IOLMaster keratometry. He derived corneal power from the correlation of the actual corneal power derived from the refractive history method with the measured radii after myopic LASIK in a sample of cases. The correlation formula is:

$$K_{c.cd} = -5.1625 \times RC_{post} + 82.2603$$

Where RC_{post} is the currently measured corneal radius with the IOLMaster. Haigis combined this regression formula with a correction factor to compensate a small residual error, obtaining an algorithm – the *Haigis-L* formula – that allows IOL calculation after myopic laser surgery solely based on present IOLMaster measurements.

The advantage of these methods is that they require no historical data and have been reported to have a low variance when used with either the Holladay II[114] and Haigis[56, 57] formulas or a 2-variable formula combined with an Aramberri double K method correction nomogram published by Koch and Wang.[109] The drawback of these methods is that they do not relate to the amount of treatment obtained by LASIK; in other words, a –10.00 D and a –1.00 D treatment with the same measured postoperative K readings would have the same adjustment.

It must be emphasized that the regression formulas reported here should be applied only in eyes that have had laser photoablation, not those that have had prior RK.

Modifying the Final Value of the IOL as a Function of the SIRC

Feiz, et al[14] described an IOL power adjustment method that one can apply when good historical data is available. Using this technique, first the IOL power is calculated using the pre-LASIK keratometry as though the patient had never undergone keratorefractive surgery. There is no special formula correction that needs to be employed for the Feiz et al method. This calculated pre-LASIK IOL power is then increased by the amount of refractive change at the spectacle plane divided by 0.7. This approach is outlined as follows:

$$IOL_{post} = IOL_{pre} - (\Delta D \times 0.7)$$

Where IOL_{pre} is the power of the IOL using pre-LASIK keratometry, and ΔD is the stable refractive change after LASIK at the spectacle plane, then IOL_{post} is the estimated power of the IOL to be implanted following LASIK.

This is the method that is least likely to result in a post-operative hyperopic surprise, as the Feiz, et al method will frequently produce a myopic over-correction.[59]

Latkany, et al[77] described two methods: (1) Calculate IOL power using mean keratometry readings obtained using the Javal keratometer and modify it by –0.46x + 0.21, where x equals the surgically induced change in refraction, or (2) calculate IOL power using the flat K and modify it by –0.47x + 0.85. Masket[78] proposed a formula that is similar in approach and structure to 2 formulas devised by Latkany:

$$IOL\ Power\ Adjustment = -0.326 \times LSE + 0.101$$

Where *LSE* is the total prior laser treatment (SIRC), adjusted for vertex distance, in spherical equivalent.

With these formulas one calculates IOL power in a standard fashion and simply modifies the final value of the IOL as a function of the laser ablative-induced refractive change. The differences between these 3 formulas are relatively small, and comparisons are subject to error since K-readings were obtained differently in each (IOLMaster for Masket and Javal keratometer for Latkany, et al). However, it is interesting to look at the values they calculate. For example, for a 3.0 D laser ablative-induced change, the modification of IOL power would be 0.87 D with Masket's formula, 1.17 D with Latkany et al's average-K formula, and 0.56 D with Latkany's flat-K formula. For 8.0 D, the respective values are 2.48, 2.91, and 3.47. An advantage of this method is that there is less reliance on historical data as the laser ablative-induced change is multiplied by a factor that is 0.326 following Masket, and 0.46 or 0.47 following Latkany formulas. Therefore, if there is a 1.0 diopter (D) error in the historical data regarding the refractive change, this translates to only a 0.32, 0.46 or 0.47 D error in IOL selection.

Hill[59,104] proposed a similar, but slightly different regression formula:

$$IOL\ Power\ Adjustment = -0.4385 \times LSE + 0.0295$$

By this method, the IOL power is calculated using the Holladay I formula for axial lengths greater than 23.0 mm and the Hoffer Q formula for axial lengths less than 23.0 mm. The SRK/T formula is generally not recommended as the artifact of very flat Ks may sometimes result in an under-correction. Ks are provided by simulated keratometry. The IOL power is calculated without a double K method correction. These techniques takes advantage of the fact that there appears to be a linear relationship between the spherical equivalent of the total amount of the stable laser vision correction (SIRC) and the over- or under-estimation of central corneal power by keratometry. This works for myopic and hyperopic laser-ablative procedures. It must be emphasized that these regression formulas should be applied only in eyes that have had laser photoablation, not those that have had prior RK. The chief weakness of this method is that the amount of prior laser vision correction must be known.

Refraction-derived Method

Shammas, et al[50] described a simple method to calculate a corrected keratometric value after myopic LASIK The calculated corneal power is labeled $K_{c.cd}$:

$$K_{c.cd} = K_{post} - 0.23 \times CR_c$$

Where K_{post} represents the post-LASIK Sim-K value obtained from a videokeratograph and CR_c is the amount of correction obtained by the refractive surgery. Shammas suggests decreasing the K reading by a factor of 0.23 for each diopter of myopia corrected by the refractive surgery. Half of this error is attributed to changes in the net corneal index of refraction after LASIK and the remainder error is ascribed to sampling in the periphery of an aspherical oblate corneal surface.[48,50,61,115,116] Shammas, et al propose to use this method when the pre-LASIK K readings are not available but the amount of refractive correction is known.

Hill[59] proposed a similar regression formula where the Sim-K suggested by Shammas was replaced by the adjusted effective refractive power ($EffRP_{adj}$) of the Holladay Diagnostic Summary of the EyeSys Corneal Analysis System (EyeSys Technologies, Houston, TX) or the central corneal power value (*CCP*) obtained averaging the 1, 2, 3 and 4 mm power values of the numerical view of the Zeiss Humphrey Atlas topographer:

$$Post\text{-}LASIK\ adjusted\ corneal\ power = CCP - \Delta D \times 0.19$$

Where *CCP* = the $EffRP_{adj}$, or the averaged Zeiss Atlas central corneal power, and ΔD is the refractive change after LASIK at the spectacle plane.

As with the Latkany, Masket, and Hill methods, this technique takes advantage of the fact that there appears to be a linear relationship between the spherical equivalent of the total amount of the stable laser vision correction (SIRC) and the over-estimation of central corneal power by keratometry after myopic correction. It must be emphasized that also the regression formula reported here should be applied only in eyes that have had laser photoablation, not those that have had prior RK. The chief weakness of this method is that the amount of prior laser vision correction must be known.

Aphakic Intraoperative Refraction Techniques

Mackool et al[84, 85] described a technique in which the cataract is removed and the patient is refracted 30 minutes later. Using a nomogram developed by the authors, the power of the IOL is calculated and the IOL is then implanted. Ianchulev et al[86] described a similar approach using intraoperative automated refraction. Both Mackool and Ianchulev et al multiplied the measured refractive error by a fixed, albeit different, value: 1.75 for Mackool and 2.01 for Ianchulev et al A disadvantage of this approach, of course, is the need to return to the operating room for IOL implantation. Although this approach may reduce the chance of post-operative surprise when keratometry and ultrasonic or optical biometry are unreliable, we think that it use over-simplified refractive formulas. More sources of error may be the vertex distance dependence of a high aphakic error and the instability of refraction immediately after cataract surgery. The instability of post-operative refraction is particularly important in prior incisional refractive surgery.[6] Patients with previous 8-incision radial keratometry will commonly show variable amounts of transient hyperopia in the immediate post-operative period following cataract surgery. This is felt to be due to stromal edema around the radial incisions, producing a temporary enhancement of central corneal flattening. While this central corneal flattening is usually transient, it can be as much as +4.00 D, and is further accentuated by greater than eight incisions, an optical zone of less than 2.0 mm, or incisions that extend all the way to the limbus.[59]

Ahmed and Toufeeq[87] described a variant of this method using intraoperative retinoscopy with high plus soft contact lens in estimating corneal power and the axial length. A +10 D disposable soft contact lens was applied on the cornea to minimize retinoscopic error. They conclude that intraoperative retinoscopy with a high plus soft contact lens after phacoemulsification is useful but not accurate in estimating corneal power or axial length of the eye. It should be used cautiously in IOL power calculation as a substitute for standard keratometry or biometry machines when either of these is not available or in error.

As is always the case when there are several solutions to a problem, none is perfect. Fortunately, new methods continue to improve accuracy and, in some cases, reduce the complexity of these calculations.[117]

The Camellin-Calossi Formula

To minimize the various difficulties mentioned above, we have developed a new formula for calculating the power of intraocular lenses in eyes that have previously undergone keratorefractive surgery.[79-81] The details of this formula have been described elsewhere.[79] Our formula originates from a theoretical one that we empirically adjusted in two parameters: (1) the corneal power (D_c); (2) and the prediction of effective lens position (*ELP*).

The variable *ELP* is a function of the anterior chamber depth previous to cataract surgery (ACD_{pre}), of the lens thickness (*LThick*), of the axial length (*AL*), and of the A constant (A_{const}) of the IOL. In a different way from other third-generation formulas that often use keratometry as one of the predictors to estimate the *ELP* of the IOL, we have chosen a method independent of K,[79] since an eye with a 37 D cornea without keratorefractive surgery would not be expected to be similar to an eye with a 37 D cornea with keratorefractive surgery.[58] As described above, Aramberri proposed a method in which the SRK/T formula was modified to use the pre-refractive surgery K-value for the *ELP* calculation and the post-refractive surgery K-value for IOL power calculation by the vergence formula.[49] The K_{pre} value was obtained by keratometry or topography and the K_{post}, by the clinical history method. Double-K modification of the SRK/T formula improved the accuracy of IOL power calculation after LASIK and PRK, but it is sometimes impossible to adopt because the pre-refractive surgery K-value is not always available.

To estimate the real corneal power, we propose to use the average curvature, weighted according to SCE, of the corneal area that covers the entrance pupil. Then we calculate the real corneal power adopting a relative keratometric refractive index that is a function of the actual corneal curvature (r), of the kind of keratorefractive surgery, and of the surgically induced refractive change (*SIRC*).

Our formula follows two different procedures according to the type of refractive surgery performed on the eye for which we must calculate IOL: in incisional surgery, keratometers perform an incorrect measurement of the corneal curvature; whereas, in laser ablative surgery, the prime cause of error is the conversion from curvature radius to dioptric power of the cornea.[118]

(a) Incisional Refractive Surgery

If the eye for which IOL power is being calculated has undergone incisional refractive surgery or any other type of surgery that does not modify the ratio between anterior and posterior corneal surface, the average curvature is considered as the radius (r), weighted according to SCE, of the corneal area that covers the entrance pupil. This value can be measured with a corneal topographer that allows this possibility, e.g. CSO (CSO Ophthalmic, Florence, Italy), EyeSys (EyeSys Technologies, Houston, TX), Keratron (Optikon 2000, Rome, Italy), TMS (Tomey, Japan), etc. Then, the real corneal power is calculated using equation (1) adopting a keratometric refractive index (n) of 1.332. Our opinion, in accordance with other authors,[65,72,119] is that in eyes that have previously undergone incisional refractive surgery, the use of topographic data allows the greater precision of IOL power calculation compared with keratometric data; however, clinical experience teaches us that repeatability of measurements is lower with computerized videokeratographs compared with keratometers and that the possibilities of error increase in short distance CVK.[120] For this reason, we suggest an accurate verification of the instrument calibration; we also suggest taking more measurements of the same eye, eliminating the extremes and calculating the average of the central values. If the conventional keratometric targets have a regular appearance, it is useful to compare keratometric readings with CVK sim-K, and if these values greatly differ, new measurements should be obtained. In our opinion, after radial keratotomy (RK), conventional keratometric readings should only be used when reliable topographic measurements are not available, because after RK the measurement of the corneal radius with a keratometer is affected by errors, due to great variations of corneal asphericity and the possibility that the keratometric targets are reflected out of the optical zone, in an irregular and curved area.[72,74,119] After RK, when using keratometric readings, precision can be improved by following this procedure: consider the average of the conventional keratometric readings (R), then calculate the real corneal power according to equation (1) using an adjusted keratometric refractive index (n_{adj}), which is a function of the surgical induced refractive.

(b) Laser Ablative Refractive Surgery

When the eye for which we must calculate IOL power has previously undergone laser ablative refractive surgery or any other kind of surgery that modifies the ratio between anterior and posterior corneal surfaces, the real corneal power is calculated with equation (1) using a relative keratometric refractive index obtained as mentioned above.

The methods described above cannot be used when the patient clinical history is completely unknown (i.e. no data about the SIRC), or in corneas that have undergone lamellar keratoplasty (LK) or phototherapeutic keratectomy (PTK). To solve these particular cases, we suggest obtaining the curvature of the posterior surface of the cornea using the Camellin Formula.[105] As already stated, with this formula it is possible to calculate the radius of the curvature of the posterior corneal surface on the basis of the measurement of the curvature radius of the anterior corneal surface, central pachymetry and a series of pachymetries performed in a 3-mm circular zone. All these measurements are critical and only a few microns can affect the precision of the calculation. Once the radius of the anterior (r_{ant}) and posterior (r_{post}) curvature (in mm) is known, the real corneal power can be calculated.

To eliminate the tediousness of the calculations for our formula, a computer program was developed.[80, 81]

Clinical Data

We used our formula to calculate the IOL power in 20 eyes from 12 patients (7 male, 5 female, ranging in age from 29 to 62 years) that have previously undergone refractive surgery for myopia: 6 PRK, 6 LASIK, 3 LASEK, and 5 RK. The axial length (ranging from 25.37 to 32.10 mm, mean 28.60, SD 2.02), the anterior chamber depth (ranging from 2.00 to 3.90 mm, mean 3.13, SD 0.53) and the lens thickness (ranging from 3.00 to 5.16 mm, mean 4.21, SD 0.59) were measured with an ultrasound 10 MHz A-scanner with a solid transducer probe. The corneal curvature (ranging from 28.31 to 40.76 D, mean 36.55, SD 3.20) was measured with a computerized videokeratographer EyeTop (CSO Ophthalmic, Florence, Italy), or Keratron (Optikon 2000, Rome, Italy) as described above. All eyes underwent cataract extraction and posterior chamber intraocular lens implantation (A constant ranging from 117.4 to 119.0, mean 118.45, SD 0.57). For the majority of our patients, we were not able to calculate the IOL power by utilizing the historical method because at least one of the three necessary parameters-preoperative corneal power, preoperative and postoperative refraction before cataract onset- was unknown. The final refractive result was used as a criterion to judge the accuracy and predictability of our approach. Because we did not always aim for emmetropia, we evaluated the formulas by comparing the predicted postoperative refraction with the actual measured postoperative refraction. The postoperative measurements were obtained as part of a routine follow-up, after manifest refraction had stabilized.

In the group of laser ablative cases we obtained a small average hyperopic error (mean +0.28, SD 0.66) not significantly different from zero (p = 0.1274); 60% of absolute refractive prediction errors were within 0.50D, 80% within 1.00 D and 93% within 1.50 D. In the group of RK cases (n = 5) with our formula the average error was +0.22 D (range: –1.25 to +1.49 D), two absolute refractive prediction errors were within 0.50D, and three within 1.00 D. Without adjustment of the corneal power, the conventional formulas demonstrated a significant degree of hyperopic prediction error.[79] (Fig. 27.11).

As with other published experience,[1-13] our results confirm that conventional methods, with whatever formula, do not accurately calculate the IOL power after keratorefractive surgery. With the Camellin-Calossi formula in eyes that had undergone refractive surgery, we obtained refractive outcomes similar to the ones reported by Murphy et al[121] in normal eyes with normal cornea with no previous keratorefractive surgery.

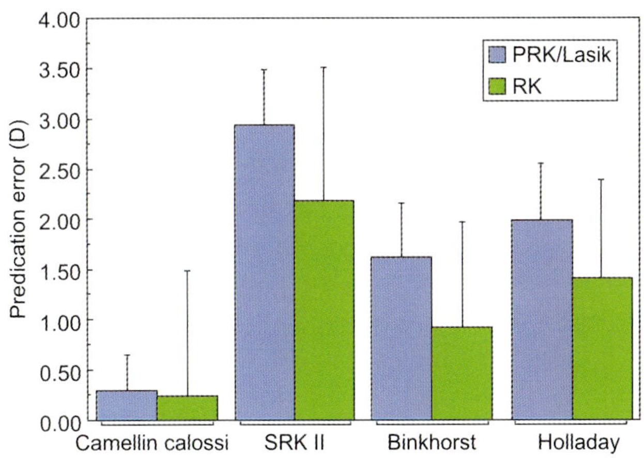

Fig. 27.11: Comparison of mean spherical equivalent prediction error for each formula split by refractive surgery procedure (error bars: 95% confidence interval). This comparison shows the entity of the errors we could have obtained using conventional formulas (empirical, theoretical, and 2-variable 3r d generation ones as well) without adjustment of corneal power

With the Camellin-Calossi formula, it has been possible to calculate the power of an IOL even in those cases in which we did not have all the necessary data to follow the clinical history method, because we did not have keratometries previous to refractive surgery or because we did not know with sufficient precision the entity of the surgical induced refractive change. Following our approach, the keratometric data before refractive surgery are not necessary, whereas even for our formula, when possible, the use of the SIRC value is recommended.

In the Camellin-Calossi formula an error in the estimate of SIRC produces an error in the refractive outcome lower than the one produced by the clinical history method, because this datum is not directly used to calculate the corneal power but is used to obtain a relative keratometric index. In this way the error in refractive outcome will be only a fraction of the error in the estimate of SIRC. In one of our cases, we knew the complete clinical history: the refraction pre PRK was: –8.75 –2.00 × 20°, BCVA 20/25, spectacle spherical equivalent –9.75 D; keratometry: 46.25/ 44.25 @ 5°. Twelve months post PRK the refraction was: –0.25 –0.50 × 180°, BCVA 20/25; K 39.25 / 39.75 @ 180. Two years later he developed the cataract; the refraction became: –2.00 –1.00 × 10°, BCVA 20/30; K 39.25 / 39.50 @ 10°; biometry was: axial length 26.70, ACD 3.10, and lens thickness 3.00 mm. Considering the refraction post PRK, before cataract, the SIRC was –9.25 D and with the clinical history method applied to Binkhorst formula the IOL power was +17.67, while with the Camellin-Calossi formula a similar IOL power of +17.29 resulted. The implanted IOL was +17.00, A const 117.5. At the four months follow-up the refractive outcome was +0.50 +0.25 × 150, BCVA 20/25. The prediction error of the history method was +0.13 D, and +0.41 D for our formula. If we had not known the real SIRC and we had considered the refraction with the cataract, the SIRC would have seemed –7.25 D: 2.00 D less then the real one. In this case, with the history method the IOL power would have been +15.21 and with the Camellin-Calossi formula +16.96; with a prediction error of +1.90 D for the history method and +0.65 D for our formula.

Our formula was conceived primarily for eyes that have previously undergone refractive surgery but may be employed in general even on non-operated eyes. In this last case, a SIRC = 0 neutralizes the personalization of the keratometric index, while the personalization of ACD remains. In this case, our formula becomes similar to the other third-generation theoretical formulas[51-53, 56] whose higher accuracy, in comparison to the previous theoretical or empirical formulas, is attributed to their improved prediction of pseudophakic anterior chamber depth, i.e. the effective lens position (ELP).[54, 122]

The issue of IOL calculation after refractive surgery is becoming an ever-increasing one, as more refractive patients are presenting for cataract surgery. Up to now, intraocular lens power calculation after corneal refractive surgery has remained challenging.[117, 123] Ophthalmologists are significantly challenged by the expectations of patients associated with any form of refractive surgery; the challenge becomes even greater when former refractive surgery patients require cataract surgery. The paradox is that, as a group, postrefractive surgery patients may have unrealistic goals for the exactness of the optical results after cataract surgery, although their outcomes have been less predictable than in routine eyes.[78] We believe that in our first series of cases, we have obtained encouraging results. With follow up of a greater number of cases, we will be able to perform further statistical empirical adjustments relative to the different types of refractive surgery in order to better improve the accuracy of calculations. The number of cataract surgeries after corneal refractive surgery is anticipated to increase. As more and more refractive patients will present for cataract surgery, more and more cases will be analyzed. In the future, it would be useful if a central data bank could be established for all eyes that had keratorefractive surgery so that details and records of previous laser treatment would be available. In this way, we shall be able to perform further statistical empirical adjustments, in order to better correct patients who, by their original decision to have vision correction surgery, have demonstrated that they have above-average refractive demands.

REFERENCES

1. Koch DD, Liu JF, Hyde LL, Rock RL, Emery JM. Refractive complications of cataract surgery after radial keratotomy. Am J Ophthalmol 1989;108:676-82.
2. Siganos DS, Pallikaris IG, Lambropoulos JE, Koufala CJ. Keratometric readings after photorefractive keratectomy are unreliable for calculating IOL power. J Refract Surg 1996;12:S278-79.
3. Kalski RS, Danjoux JP, Fraenkel GE, Lawless MA, Rogers C. Intraocular lens power calculation for cataract surgery after photorefractive keratectomy for high myopia. J Refract Surg 1997;13:362-66.
4. Lyle WA, Jin GJ. Intraocular lens power prediction in patients who undergo cataract surgery following previous radial keratotomy. Arch Ophthalmol 1997; 115:457-61.
5. Morris AH, Whittaker KW, Morris RJ, Corbett MC. Errors in intraocular lens power calculation after photorefractive keratectomy. Eye 1998;12(Pt 2):327-28.
6. Bardocci A, Lofoco G. Corneal topography and postoperative refraction after cataract phacoemulsification following radial keratotomy. Ophthalmic Surg Lasers 1999;30:155-59.
7. Speicher L, Gottinger W. Intraocular lens power calculation after decentered photorefractive keratectomy. J Cataract Refract Surg 1999;25:140-43.
8. Gimbel H, Sun R, Kaye GB. Refractive error in cataract surgery after previous refractive surgery. J Cataract Refract Surg 2000;26:142-44.
9. Gimbel HV, Sun R, Furlong MT, van Westenbrugge JA, Kassab J. Accuracy and predictability of intraocular lens power calculation after photorefractive keratectomy. J Cataract Refract Surg 2000;26:1147-51.
10. Seitz B, Langenbucher A. Intraocular lens calculations status after corneal refractive surgery. Curr Opin Ophthalmol 2000;11:35-46.
11. Gimbel HV, Sun R. Accuracy and predictability of intraocular lens power calculation after laser in situ keratomileusis. J Cataract Refract Surg 2001;27:571-76.
12. Speicher L. Intra-ocular lens calculation status after corneal refractive surgery. Curr Opin Ophthalmol 2001; 12:17-29.
13. Ladas JG, Boxer Wachler BS, Hunkeler JD, Durrie DS. Intraocular lens power calculations using corneal topography after photorefractive keratectomy. Am J Ophthalmol 2001;132:254-55.
14. Feiz V, Mannis MJ, Garcia-Ferrer F, et al. Intraocular lens power calculation after laser in situ keratomileusis for myopia and hyperopia: a standardized approach. Cornea 2001;20:792-97.
15. Bennett AG, Rabbetts RB. Clinical Visual Optics, 2nd ed. London: Butterworths 1989;468.
16. Fleming JF. Corneal asphericity and visual function after radial keratotomy. Cornea 1993;12:233-40.
17. Patel S, Marshall J, Fitzke FW, Gartry DS. The shape of the corneal apical zone after excimer photorefractive keratectomy. Acta Ophthalmol (Copenh) 1994;72: 588-96.
18. Schwiegerling J, Greivenkamp JE, Miller JM, Snyder RW, Palmer ML. Optical modeling of radial keratotomy incision patterns. Am J Ophthalmol 1996;122:808-17.
19. Holladay JT, Dudeja DR, Chang J. Functional vision and corneal changes after laser in situ keratomileusis determined by contrast sensitivity, glare testing, and corneal topography. J Cataract Refract Surg 1999;25: 663-69.
20. Holladay JT, Janes JA. Topographic changes in corneal asphericity and effective optical zone after laser in situ keratomileusis. J Cataract Refract Surg 2002;28:942-47.
21. Hersh PS, Shah SI, Holladay JT. Corneal asphericity following excimer laser photorefractive keratectomy. Summit PRK Topography Study Group. Ophthalmic Surg Lasers 1996;27:S421-28.
22. Chen CC, Izadshenas A, Rana MA, Azar DT. Corneal asphericity after hyperopic laser in situ keratomileusis. J Cataract Refract Surg 2002;28:1539-45.
23. Mandell RB. Contact Lens Pratice, 4th ed. Springfield: Charles C Thomas, 1988.
24. Layman PR. Measuring corneal area utilizing keratometry. Optician 1987;154:261.
25. Holladay JT, Waring III GO. Optics and topography of radial keratotomy. In: Waring III GO, editor. Refractive keratotomy for myopia and astigmatism. St. Louis: Mosby Year Book, 1992.
26. Stiles WS, Crawford BH. Luminous efficiency of rays entering eye pupil at different points. Proc Roy Soc Lond 1933;112:428-50.
27. Applegate RA, Lakshminarayanan V. Parametric representation of Stiles-Crawford functions: normal variation of peak location and directionality. J Opt Soc Am A 1993;10:1611-23.
28. Gullstrand A. Procedure of the rays in the eye imagery-law of first order. The optical system of the eye. In: Helmholtz Hv, Southall JPC, editors. Helmholtz's treatise on physiological optics. Rochester, N.Y.: The Optical Society of America, 1924:301-58.
29. Freeman MH. Optics, 10th ed. London: Butterworths, 1990.
30. Javal E, Schjötz H. Un ophthalmomètre pratique. Transaction of the international medical Congress. VIII.

Session. London 1881. III. p. 30. Annales d'oculistique 1881;LXXXVI:5.

31. Emsley HH. Visual Optics. London: Hatton Press Ltd., 1936.
32. Binkhorst RD. Pitfalls in the determination of intraocular lens power without ultrasound. Ophthalmic Surg 1976; 7:69-82.
33. Holladay JT. Standardizing constants for ultrasonic biometry, keratometry, and intraocular lens power calculations. J Cataract Refract Surg 1997;23:1356-70.
34. Munnerlyn CR, Koons SJ, Marshall J. Photorefractive keratectomy: a technique for laser refractive surgery. J Cataract Refract Surg 1988;14:46-52.
35. Mandell RB. Corneal power correction factor for photorefractive keratectomy. J Refract Corneal Surg 1994; 10:125-28.
36. Gobbi PG, Carones F, Brancato R. Keratometric index, videokeratography, and refractive surgery. J Cataract Refract Surg 1998;24:202-11.
37. Olsen T. On the calculation of power from curvature of the cornea. Br J Ophthalmol 1986;70:152-54.
38. Doughty MJ, Zaman ML. Human corneal thickness and its impact on intraocular pressure measures: a review and meta-analysis approach. Surv Ophthalmol 2000; 44:367-408.
39. Edmund C. Posterior corneal curvature and its influence on corneal dioptric power. Acta Ophthalmol (Copenh) 1994;72:715-20.
40. Eryildirim A, Ozkan T, Eryildirim S, Kaynak S, Cingil G. Improving estimation of corneal refractive power by measuring the posterior curvature of the cornea. J Cataract Refract Surg 1994;20:129-31.
41. Garner LF, Owens H, Yap MK, Frith MJ, Kinnear RF. Radius of curvature of the posterior surface of the cornea. Optom Vis Sci 1997;74:496-98.
42. Campbell CE. Variation in lens thickness as a function of power and radial distance from optical centre. J Br Contact Lens Assoc 1995;18:127-28.
43. Patel S, Marshall J, Fitzke FW, 3rd. Refractive index of the human corneal epithelium and stroma. J Refract Surg 1995;11:100-05.
44. Patel S, Alio JL, Perez-Santonja JJ. A model to explain the difference between changes in refraction and central ocular surface power after laser in situ keratomileusis. J Refract Surg 2000;16:330-35.
45. Fatt I, Harris MG. Refractive index of the cornea as a function of its thickness. Am J Optom Arch Am Acad Optom 1973;50:383-86.
46. Patel S, Alio JL, Perez-Santonja JJ. Refractive index change in bovine and human corneal stroma before and after lasik: a study of untreated and re-treated corneas implicating stromal hydration. Invest Ophthalmol Vis Sci 2004;45:3523-30.
47. Meek KM, Dennis S, Khan S. Changes in the refractive index of the stroma and its extrafibrillar matrix when the cornea swells. Biophys J 2003;85:2205-12.
48. Hamed AM, Wang L, Misra M, Koch DD. A comparative analysis of five methods of determining corneal refractive power in eyes that have undergone myopic laser in situ keratomileusis. Ophthalmology 2002;109: 651-58.
49. Aramberri J. Intraocular lens power calculation after corneal refractive surgery: double-K method. J Cataract Refract Surg 2003;29:2063-68.
50. Shammas HJ, Shammas MC, Garabet A, Kim JH, Shammas A, LaBree L. Correcting the corneal power measurements for intraocular lens power calculations after myopic laser in situ keratomileusis. Am J Ophthalmol 2003;136:426-32.
51. Holladay JT, Prager TC, Chandler TY, Musgrove KH, Lewis JW, Ruiz RS. A three-part system for refining intraocular lens power calculations. J Cataract Refract Surg 1988;14:17-24.
52. Hoffer KJ. The Hoffer Q formula: a comparison of theoretic and regression formulas. J Cataract Refract Surg 1993;19:700-12.
53. Retzlaff JA, Sanders DR, Kraff MC. Development of the SRK/T intraocular lens implant power calculation formula. J Cataract Refract Surg 1990;16:333-40.
54. Olsen T, Thim K, Corydon L. Accuracy of the newer generation intraocular lens power calculation formulas in long and short eyes. J Cataract Refract Surg 1991;17: 187-93.
55. Olsen T. Prediction of the effective postoperative (intraocular lens) anterior chamber depth. J Cataract Refract Surg 2006;32:419-24.
56. Haigis W. IOL calculation according to Haigis [on-line]. Available: http://www.augenklinik.uni-wuerzburg.de/uslab/ioltxt/haie.htm, last revision: 7 December 1998.
57. Haigis W. The Haigis formula. In: Shammas HJ, editor. Intraocular lens power calculations. Thorofare: Slack, 2004:41-57.
58. Holladay JT. Intraocular lens power calculation for the refractive surgeon. Operative Techniques in Cataract and Refractive Surgery 1998;1:105-17.
59. Hill WE. Determining corneal power following keratorefractive surgery. Retrieved June 02, 2006, from http://www.doctor-hill.com/iol-main/keratorefractive.htm, 2006.
60. Jin GJ, Crandall AS, Jin Y. Analysis of intraocular lens power calculation for eyes with previous myopic LASIK. J Refract Surg 2006;22:387-95.

61. Shammas HJ. Intraocular lens power calculations after corneal refractive surgery. In: Shammas HJ, editor. Intraocular lens power calculations. Thorofare: Slack, 2004:189-96.
62. Guyton DL. Consultations in refractive surgery. Refract Corneal Surg 1989;5:203.
63. Holladay JT. Consultations in refractive surgery. Refract Corneal Surg 1989;5:203.
64. Hoffer KJ. Intraocular lens power calculation for eyes after refractive keratotomy. J Refract Surg 1995;11: 490-93.
65. Celikkol L, Pavlopoulos G, Weinstein B, Celikkol G, Feldman ST. Calculation of intraocular lens power after radial keratotomy with computerized videokeratography. Am J Ophthalmol 1995;120:739-50.
66. Husain SE, Kohnen T, Maturi R, Er H, Koch DD. Computerized videokeratography and keratometry in determining intraocular lens calculations. J Cataract Refract Surg 1996;22:362-66.
67. Holladay JT. Corneal topography using the Holladay Diagnostic Summary. J Catarcat Refract Surg 1997;13:209-21.
68. Hugger P, Kohnen T, Koch DD. [Assessment of refractive difference after photorefractive keratectomy. A comparison between keratometry and computer-assisted video keratography]. Ophthalmologe 1997;94:699-702.
69. Maeda N, Klyce SD, Smolek MK, McDonald MB. Disparity between keratometry-style readings and corneal power within the pupil after refractive surgery for myopia. Cornea 1997;16:517-24.
70. McQueen BR, Martinez CE, Klyce SD. Corneal topography in cataract surgery. Curr Opin Ophthalmol 1997;8:22-28.
71. Muraine M, Siahmed K, Retout A, Brasseur G. [Phacoemulsification following radial keratotomy. Topographic and refractive analysis concerning an 18-month period (apropos of a case)]. J Fr Ophtalmol 2000;23:265-69.
72. Han ES, Lee JH. Intraocular lens power calculation in high myopic eyes with previous radial keratotomy. J Refract Surg;in press.
73. Langenbucher A, Torres F, Behrens A, Suarez E, Haigis W, Seitz B. Consideration of the posterior corneal curvature for assessment of corneal power after myopic LASIK. Acta Ophthalmol Scand 2004;82:264-69.
74. Seitz B, Langenbucher A. Intraocular lens power calculation in eyes after corneal refractive surgery. J Refract Surg 2000;16:349-61.
75. Rosa N, Capasso L, Romano A. A new method of calculating intraocular lens power after photorefractive keratectomy. J Refract Surg 2002;18:720-24.
76. Ferrara G, Cennamo G, Marotta G, Loffredo E. New formula to calculate corneal power after refractive surgery. J Refract Surg 2004;20:465-71.
77. Latkany RA, Chokshi AR, Speaker MG, Abramson J, Soloway BD, Yu G. Intraocular lens calculations after refractive surgery. J Cataract Refract Surg 2005;31: 562-70.
78. Masket S, Masket SE. Simple regression formula for intraocular lens power adjustment in eyes requiring cataract surgery after excimer laser photoablation. J Cataract Refract Surg 2006;32:430-34.
79. Camellin M, Calossi A. A new formula for intraocular lens power calculation after refractive corneal surgery. J Refract Surg 2006;22:187-99.
80. Camellin M, Calossi A. IOL Calculator: formula Camellin - Calossi. CD-rom, 1.0 ed. Firenze (Italy): CSO ophthalmic, 1999.
81. Camellin M, Calossi A. IOL Calculator 3.0: formula Camellin - Calossi. CD-rom, 3.0 ed. Canelli (AT, Italy): Fabiano ed., 2001.
82. Jarade EF, Abi Nader FC, Tabbara KF. Intraocular lens power calculation following LASIK: determination of the new effective index of refraction. J Refract Surg 2006;22:75-80.
83. Camellin M. Pachimetria topografica intraoperatoria: analisi dei dati. Atti della Società Oftalmologia Italiana, 1993:499-510.
84. Mackool RJ. The cataract extraction-refraction-implantation technique for IOL power calculation in difficult cases. [letter]. J Cataract Refract Surg 1998;24:434-435.
85. Mackool RJ, Ko W, Mackool R. Intraocular lens power calculation after laser in situ keratomileusis: Aphakic refraction technique. J Cataract Refract Surg 2006;32: 435-37.
86. Ianchulev T, Salz J, Hoffer K, Albini T, Hsu H, Labree L. Intraoperative optical refractive biometry for intraocular lens power estimation without axial length and keratometry measurements. J Cataract Refract Surg 2005;31:1530-36.
87. Ahmed I, Toufeeq A. Accuracy of intraoperative retinoscopy in corneal power and axial length estimation using a high plus soft contact lens. Ophthalmic Physiol Opt 2005;25:52-56.
88. Odenthal MT, Eggink CA, Melles G, Pameyer JH, Geerards AJ, Beekhuis WH. Clinical and theoretical results of intraocular lens power calculation for cataract surgery after photorefractive keratectomy for myopia. Arch Ophthalmol 2002;120:431-38.
89. Seitz B, Langenbucher A, Haigis W. [Pitfalls of IOL power prediction after photorefractive keratectomy for high myopia — case report, practical recommendations and literature review]. Klin Monatsbl Augenheilkd 2002;219:840-50.

90. Olsen T. Sources of error in intraocular lens power calculation. J Cataract Refract Surg 1992;18:125-29.
91. Ladas JG, Stark WJ. Calculating IOL power after refractive surgery. J Cataract Refract Surg 2004;30:2458; author reply 2458-59.
92. Walter KA, Gagnon MR, Hoopes PC, Jr., Dickinson PJ. Accurate intraocular lens power calculation after myopic laser in situ keratomileusis, bypassing corneal power. J Cataract Refract Surg 2006;32:425-29.
93. Sambare C, Naroo S, Shah S, Sharma A. The AS biometry technique-A novel technique to aid accurate intraocular lens power calculation after corneal laser refractive surgery. Cont Lens Anterior Eye 2006;29:81-83.
94. Haigis W. Corneal power after refractive surgery for myopia: contact lens method. J Cataract Refract Surg 2003;29:1397-411.
95. Zeh WG, Koch DD. Comparison of contact lens overrefraction and standard keratometry for measuring corneal curvature in eyes with lenticular opacity. J Cataract Refract Surg 1999;25:898-903.
96. Seitz B, Langenbucher A, Hoffman B, Behrens A, Kuss MM. [Refractive power of the human posterior corneal surface in vivo in relation to gender and age]. Ophthalmologe 1998;95(suppl 1):S50.
97. Iskander NG, Anderson Penno E, Peters NT, Gimbel HV, Ferensowicz M. Accuracy of Orbscan pachymetry measurements and DHG ultrasound pachymetry in primary laser in situ keratomileusis and LASIK enhancement procedures. J Cataract Refract Surg 2001;27:681-85.
98. Boscia F, La Tegola MG, Alessio G, Sborgia C. Accuracy of Orbscan optical pachymetry in corneas with haze. J Cataract Refract Surg 2002;28:253-58.
99. Du ZY, Zhang DY, Zheng Q, Chen Y, Guo H, Yin HM. [An analysis of measurement error in Orbscan topography system]. Zhonghua Yan Ke Za Zhi 2003;39:36-40.
100. Prisant O, Calderon N, Chastang P, Gatinel D, Hoang-Xuan T. Reliability of pachymetric measurements using orbscan after excimer refractive surgery. Ophthalmology 2003;110:511-15.
101. Srivannaboon S, Reinstein DZ, Sutton HF, Holland SP. Accuracy of Orbscan total optical power maps in detecting refractive change after myopic laser in situ keratomileusis. J Cataract Refract Surg 1999;25:1596-99.
102. Cheng AC, Lam DS. Keratometry for intraocular lens power calculation using Orbscan II in eyes with laser in situ keratomileusis. J Refract Surg 2005;21:365-68.
103. Holladay JT. Measuring corneal power after corneal refractive surgery. Why Cataract and Refractive Surgeons Need the Pentacam. Insert to Cataract and Refractive Surgery Today. January, 2006:4-6.
104. Hill WE. IOL power calculations following keratorefractive surgery. Cornea Day of the Annual Meeting of the American Society of Cataract and Refractive Surgery. San Francisco, California, 2006.
105. Camellin M. Proposed formula for the dioptric power evaluation of the posterior corneal surface. Refract Corneal Surg 1990;6:261-64.
106. Patel S, Marshall J, Fitzke FW. Shape and radius of posterior corneal surface. Refract Corneal Surg 1993;9:173-81.
107. Reinstein DZ, Silverman RH, Raevsky T, et al. Arc-scanning very high-frequency digital ultrasound for 3D pachymetric mapping of the corneal epithelium and stroma in laser in situ keratomileusis. J Refract Surg 2000;16:414-30.
108. Camellin M. Calcolo della IOL negli operati di refrattiva. 4th SOI International Congress. Roma, 2006.
109. Koch DD, Wang L. Calculating IOL power in eyes that have had refractive surgery. J Cataract Refract Surg 2003;29:2039-42.
110. Wang L, Booth MA, Koch DD. Comparison of intraocular lens power calculation methods in eyes that have undergone LASIK. Ophthalmology 2004;111:1825-31.
111. Haigis W. IOL calculation after myopic laser refractive surgery: the *Haigis-L* formula. Personal comunication.
112. Haigis W. IOL-Berechnung nach refraktiver Hornhautchirurgie mit aktuellen Messwerten. Ophthalmo-chirurgie 2006;18:27-30.
113. Haigis W, Lege BAM. IOL-Berechnung nach refraktiver Laserchirurgie aus aktuellen Messwerten. Klin Monatsbl Augenheilk 2006;223:S.19.
114. Holladay JT. Holladay IOL Consultant and Surgical Outcomes Assessment, 2.5 ed, 2003.
115. Budak K, Khater TT, Friedman NJ, Holladay JT, Koch DD. Evaluation of relationships among refractive and topographic parameters. J Cataract Refract Surg 1999;25:814-20.
116. Hugger P, Kohnen T, La Rosa FA, Holladay JT, Koch DD. Comparison of changes in manifest refraction and corneal power after photorefractive keratectomy. Am J Ophthalmol 2000;129:68-75.
117. Koch DD. New options for IOL calculations after refractive surgery. J Cataract Refract Surg 2006;32: 371-72.

118. Seitz B, Langenbucher A, Nguyen NX, Kus MM, Kuchle M. Underestimation of intraocular lens power for cataract surgery after myopic photorefractive keratectomy. Ophthalmology 1999;106:693-702.
119. Holladay JT. Catarct surgery in patients with previous refractive corneal surgery (RK, PRK, and LASIK). Ophthalmic Practice 1997;15:238-44.
120. Mandell RB. Everett Kinsey Lecture. The enigma of the corneal contour. Clao J 1992;18:267-73.
121. Murphy C, Tuft SJ, Minassian DC. Refractive error and visual outcome after cataract extraction. J Cataract Refract Surg 2002;28:62-66.
122. Olsen T, Corydon L, Gimbel H. Intraocular lens power calculation with an improved anterior chamber depth prediction algorithm. J Cataract Refract Surg 1995; 21:313-19.
123. Sun R, Gimbel H, Penno EE. Intraocular lens power calculation after corneal refractive surgery remains challenging. Ophthalmology 2000;107:226-28.

Epi-LASIK: An Advanced Surface Ablation Procedure

28

Vikentia J Katsanevaki, Maria I Kalyvianaki,
Ioannis G Pallikaris (Greece)

INTRODUCTION

Since the introduction of excimer lasers for photorefractive corrections the surgical trends are continuously changing in order to achieve the best possible clinical results with minimal complications. Photorefractive Keratectomy (PRK) initially introduced in the beginning of 90s[1,2] was the first technique to be used for photorefractive corrections. Despite its encouraging results for low and moderate myopia, during the evolvement of refractive surgery PRK was partially abandoned mostly due to the postoperative pain of the treated patients as well as the risk of corneal postoperative haze. Laser in situ keratomileusis (LASIK),[3,4] which involves the ablation deeper in the stroma after the creation of a corneal flap, soon became popular among refractive surgeons. Providing fast visual rehabilitation as well as the ability to correct higher degrees of ametropias LASIK is currently the undisputable leader within photorefractive treatments. However, LASIK is not without complications. Complications unique to LASIK such as those related to the use of the microkeratome,[5,6] LASIK induced diffuse lamellar keratitis[7] and the increasing reports of LASIK patients that developed corneal ectasia;[8] have set the stage for the revival of surface treatments.

Laser subepithelial keratomileusis[9] (LASEK) was the first attempt to modify surface treatments in order to control the major drawbacks of PRK, i.e. the postoperative pain and the risk of haze formation. The modification of the surgical technique as compared to the conventional PRK, was the separation of corneal epithelium as a sheet rather than its scrapping prior to the photo ablation. This epithelial sheet which is separated en toto and is replaced onto the ablated cornea, is thought to act as a natural contact lens on the operative eye[10] is expected to control the epithelial healing and thus provide better postoperative results as compared to PRK.

Epi-LASIK: An Evolving Technique

The separation of the epithelial sheet in LASEK as described by Camellin, requires the preparation of the cornea with a short-term exposure to a diluted (18-20%) alcohol solution. In order to avoid the probable toxic effect of alcohol on the epithelium and the underlying stroma[13,14] Pallikaris described Epi-LASIK.[11,12] With this modality, the epithelial sheet is separated mechanically with the use of a customized device (Centurion Epiedge Epikeratome, Ciba Vision Surgical, GA) without the need of prior corneal preparation with alcohol. This device has recently granted CE mark and 510K aproval for clinical use and is commercially available. Epi-LASIK,[11,12] is currently the treatment of choice for low myopia in the University of Crete and up to now has been performed in more than 400 eyes worldwide

(Fig. 28.1). Its name is derived from the Greek word "epipolis" that means superficial and LASIK.

Histological Findings of Mechanically Separated Epithelial Sheets

Transmission electron microscopy of harvested epithelial sheets in eyes that the treatments were reversed to PRK demonstrated that the cleavage plane of mechanical separation was located under the level of the basement membrane.[11] Basal epithelial cells had normal morphology with minimal evidence of trauma and edema and rested upon the prominent basal lamina, which consisted of an apparently structure less lamina lucida and an electron-dense lamina densa. Under the basal lamina an upper part on Bowman layer was evident in the epithelial sheets (Fig. 28.2). Intracellular organelles and intercellular desmosomal connections, as well as hemidesmosomal connections with the basement membrane appeared close to normal with only focal disruptions.

Alcohol assisted epithelial separations are reported to take place within the basement membrane thus affecting its integrity.[11,15,16] The presence of an intact basement membrane has been shown to be important in the control of epithelial wound healing[17] minimizing the fibrotic activation of keratocytes. Even though alcohol solutions are not reported toxic in the specific concentrations and exposure times that are advocated for epithelial separations in LASEK,[18,19] mechanical separation appears to have the advantage of a deeper cleavage plane over alcohol assisted separations thus being expected to provide better control of corneal healing within the first postoperative days.

Epi-LASIK: The Surgical Procedure

The operative eye is prepared with three drops of topical tetracaine hydrochloride 0.5% (applied every 5 minutes before the procedure) and povidone-iodine and is covered with a sterile drape. Before the epithelial separation the cornea is marked with a customized Epi-LASIK marker (Epi-LASIK marker,

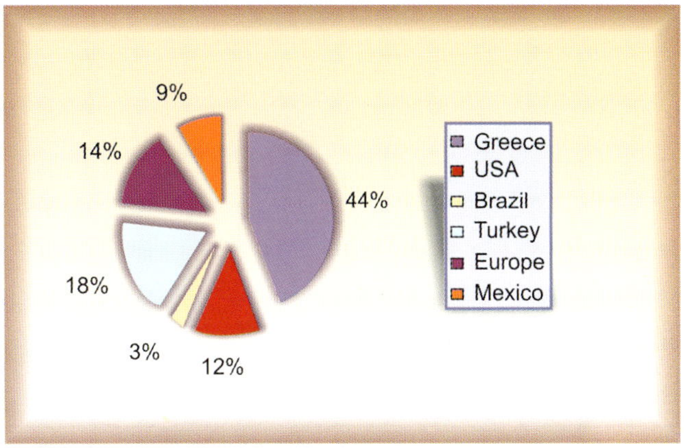

Fig. 28.1

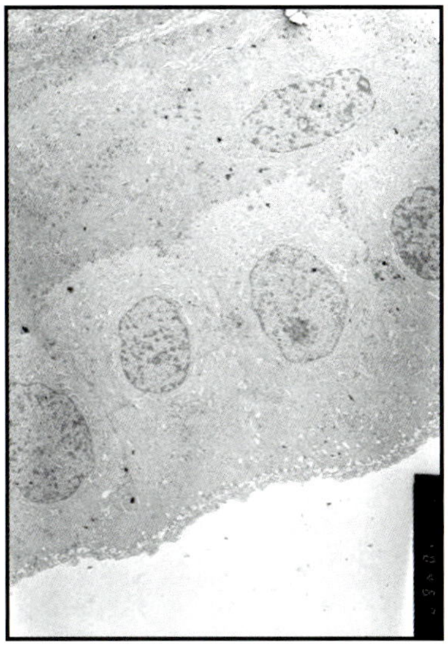

Fig. 28.2

Duckworth and Kent, Baldock, UK). This marker features two concentric circles crossed by 8 radial arms. Upon the replacement of the epithelial sheet, any deformity of the preoperative marks dictates its proper repositioning.

The Centurion EpiEdge Epikeratome is an electrically powered device (Fig 28.3) that operates under low suction similarly to a conventional microkeratome. Instead of a blade it features a disposable, oscillating polymethylmethacrylate (PMMA) separator with an advance speed of 3.5 mm/sec. The resulting separated epithelial sheet has a nasal hinge and a diameter of 9.5 to 10 mm. Any manipulations of the epithelial sheet both for its reflection and replacement, are performed with the

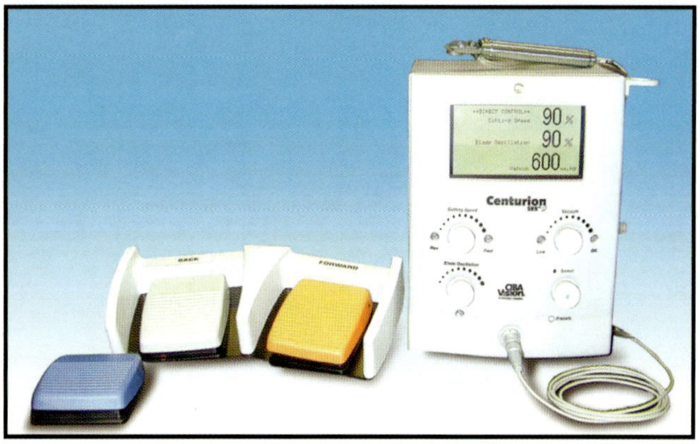

Fig. 28.3

use of a moistened sponge. The replacement of the separated epithelial sheet is often achieved with a single movement. Any inward or outward folds of its edges can be restored with the use of an anterior chamber irrigation canula under constant irrigation. Once the epithelial sheet is stuck to the underlying stroma, a therapeutic contact lens is applied onto the operative eye.

Postoperative Treatment

Postoperative treatment includes eye drops of Diclofenac sodium 0.1% qid for two days and combined eye drops of tobramycin-dexamethasone qid until the removal of the therapeutic lens. After the removal of the lens all treated eyes receive fluorometholone eye drops qid for five weeks in a tapered dose. Artificial tears are prescribed to be used at the patients' discretion.

Early Postoperative Course

At the end of the surgery, the replaced epithelial sheet often overlays its initial gutter probably due to the intraoperative mechanical stretch on the epithelial sheet upon separation. Immediately after the operation the epithelial sheet is transparent. During the healing process of the surface, slit lamp biomicroscopy reveals the borderline between the migrating epithelium and the remnants of the separated sheet. The migrating cells gradually replace the separated epithelial sheet, which is subsequently constricted in the central area. Starting from its peripheral part around the edges on the first postoperative day the sheet becomes hazy in its total area until about the third day after the treatment. At that time the hazy area measures about the central 1 to 2 mm whereas a front of newly synthesized, transparent epithelium migrates from the corneal periphery towards the centre of the corneal surface. After that stage, the transparency of the corneal epithelium is restored within 24 to 48 hours and the therapeutic contact lens is removed. The time of epithelial healing ranges from 3 to 5 days between the treated eyes.

Clinical Results

Up to date we have performed 183 mechanically assisted epithelial separations in the University of Crete. 76 eyes were left to heal as Epi-LASIK whereas the rest of the separated sheets underwent histological evaluation and the treatments were reversed to PRK. The preoperative spherical equivalent of the treated eyes was up to – 7.75 D, with cylinder up to – 2.25 D.

Postoperative pain of the treated patients was assessed subjectively with a use of a questionnaire that graded pain in a scale from 0 to 4. The patients graded postoperative pain in two-hour intervals on the operative day and once daily in the following days. No patient reported pain after the operative day.On the operative day, the mean scores remained below the threshold of pain in the reported series of eyes (Fig. 28.4). Similarly as after LASEK,[25,26]

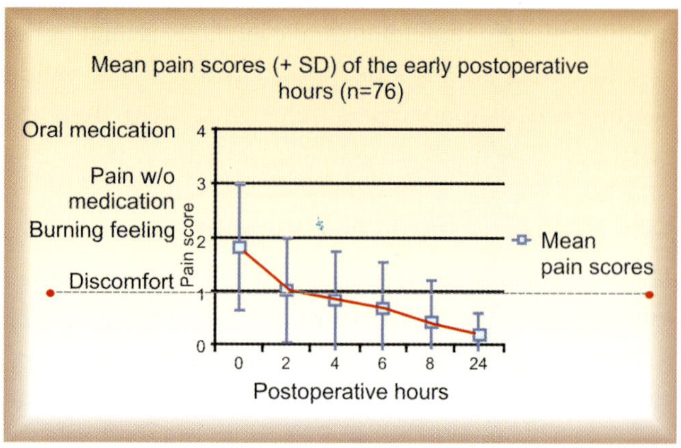

Fig. 28.4

epi-LASIK was not proved a totally pain –free procedure. We observed that discomfort or pain was mainly reported within the first postoperative hours. In order to deal with this finding we included intra operative corneal cooling in the standard treatment of the last 20 eyes. We cooled the cornea immediately before the separation and after the ablation with the instillation of pre freezed balanced salt solution. After this alteration of the technique, the reported discomfort was below the threshold of pain in all patients even in the first postoperative hours.

During the early postoperative course, the mean uncorrected visual acuity (UCVA) of the treated eyes corresponded well with the progress of the epithelial healing and the transparency of the replaced epithelial sheet. More particularly, UCVA was better on the first postoperative day, when the epithelial sheet was transparent, to decrease around the third postoperative day, as the epithelial sheet became hazy, and, finally rise again, when the epithelial healing was complete (Fig. 28.5). On the sixth month interval 94% of eyes had visual acuity of 20/25 or better whereas 48% of eyes have gained one or two (8%) Snellen lines of best-corrected visual acuity.

The vast majority of Epi-LASIK eyes had clear corneas or trace haze at three (96%) and six month's (100%) postoperative intervals.

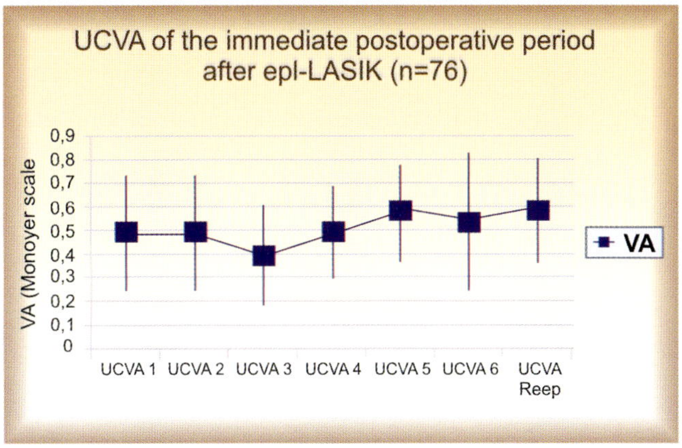

Fig. 28.5

CONCLUSIONS

Histological findings of mechanically separated epithelial sheets have shown that mechanical separation preserves the epithelial cell viability, the stratification of the sheet and the integrity of the epithelial basement membrane. In contrast to the varying solution dilutions and exposure times required for alcohol assisted separations[20,21,22] the epikeratome can achieve mechanically assisted separations in a repetitive and fully automated way with a short learning curve for experienced LASIK surgeons. Preliminary clinical results are comparable to that of LASEK[15, 21,23,24] and suggest epi-LASIK as an efficient and safe alternative surgical modality for low myopia. Given the preliminary encouraging results for low myopia the next goal will be to apply this technique for higher myopic corrections. Intra operative corneal cooling has an additive effect to the retained epithelial sheet minimizing discomfort below the threshold of pain in all the treated eyes. Future randomised comparative studies between Epi-LASIK and PRK are expected to prove the advantages of the retained epithelial sheet in surface treatments.

REFERENCES

1. Seiler T, Wollensak J. Myopic photorefractive keratectomy with excimer laser; one-year follow up. Opthalmology 1991;98:1156-63.
2. Epstein D, Fagerholm P, Hamberg-Nystroem H, Tengroth B. Twenty four-month follow up of excimer laser photorefractive keratectomy for myopia; refractive and visual outcome results. Opthalmology 1994; 101:1558-63.
3. Pallikaris IG, Papatzanaki ME, Siganos DS, Tsilimbaris MK. A corneal flap technique for laser in situ keratomileusis. Human studies. Arch Ophthalmol 1991; 109(12):1699-702.
4. Hersh PS, Brint SF, Maloney RK, et al. Photorefractive keratectomy versus laser in situ keratomileusis for moderate to high myopia; a randomized prospective study. Opthalmology 1998;105:1512-22.
5. Pallikaris IG, Katsanevaki VJ, Panagopoulou SI. Laser in situ keratomileusis intraoperative complications using one type of microkeratome. Ophthalmology 2002; 109(1):57-63.
6. Melki SA, Azar DT. LASIK complications: Etiology, management, and prevention. Surv Ophthalmol 2001(2); 46:95-116.

7. Smith RJ, Maloney RK. Diffuse lamellar keratitis. A new syndrome in lamellar refractive surgery. Ophthalmology 1998;105(9):1721-6.
8. Pallikaris IG, Kymionis GD, Astyrakakis NI. Corneal ectasia induced by laser in situ keratomileusis. J Cataract Refract Surg 2001;27(11):1796-802.
9. Camellin M, Cimberle M. LASEK technique promising after 1 year of experience. Ocular Surg News 2000;18 (1):14-17.
10. Lee JB, Seong GJ, Lee JH, Seo KY, Lee YG, Kim EK. Comparison of laser epithelial keratomileusis and photorefractive keratectomy for low to moderate myopia. J Cataract Refract Surg 2001; 27(4):565-70.
11. Pallikaris IG, Naoumidi II, Kalyvianaki MI, Katsanevaki VJ. Epi-LASIK: Comparative histological evaluation of mechanical and alcohol - assisted epithelial separation. J Cataract Refract Surg 2003;29(8):1496-501.
12. Pallikaris IG, Katsanevaki VJ, Kalyvianaki MI, Naoumidi II. Advances in subepithelial excimer refractive surgery techniques: Epi-LASIK. Curr Opin Ophthalmol. 2003 Aug;14(4):207-12.
13. Kamm O. The relation between structure and physiological action of the alcohols. J of the American Pharmaceutical Association 1921;10:87-92.
14. Kim SY, Sah WJ, Lim YW, Hahn TW. Twenty percent alcohol toxicity on rabbit corneal epithelial cells: electron microscopic study. Cornea 2002 May; 21(4):388-92.
15. Azar DT, Ang RT, Lee JB, Kato T, Chen CC, Jain S, Gabison E, Abad JC. Laser subepithelial keratomileusis: electron microscopy and visual outcomes of photorefractive keratectomy. Curr Opin Ophthalmol 2001; 12(4):323-28.
16. Espana EM, Gruetereich M, Mateo A, Romano AC, Yee SB, Yee RW, Tseng SCG. Cleavage plane of corneal basement membrane components by ethanol exposure in laser-assisted subepithelial keratectomy. J Cataract Refract Surg 2003; 29: 1192-97.
17. Stramer BM, Zieske JD, Jung JC, Austin JS, Fini ME. Molecular mechanisms controlling the fibrotic repair phenotype in cornea: implications for surgical outcomes. Invest Ophthalmol Vis Sci 2003;44(10): 4237-46.
18. Chen CC, Chang JH, Lee JB, Javier J, Azar DT. Human corneal epithelial cell viability and morphology after dilute alcohol exposure. Invest Ophthalmol Vis Sci 2002; 43(8):2593-2602.
19. Gabler B, Winkler von Mohrenfelds C, Dreiss AK, Marshall J, Lohmann CP. Vitality of epithelial cells after alcohol exposure during laser-assisted subepithelial keratectomy flap preparation. J Cataract Refract Surg 2002;28:1841-46.
20. Camellin M. Laser epithelial keratomileusis for myopia. J Refract Surg 2003;19:666-70.
21. Chalita MR, Tekwani NH, Krueger RR. Laser epithelial keratomileusis: Outcome of initial cases performed by an experienced surgeon. J Refract Surg 2003;19: 412-15.
22. Litwak S, Zadok D, Garcia-de Quevedo V, Robledo N, Chayet AS. Laser-assisted subepithelial keratectomy versus photorefractive keratectomy for the correction of myopia. A prospective comparative study. J Cataract Refract Surg 2002;28:1330-33.
23. Anderson NJ, Beran RF, Schneider TL. Epi-LASEK for the correction of myopia and myopic astigmatism. J Cataract Refract Surg 2002;28:1343-47.
24. Claringbold VT. Laser-assisted subepithelial keratectomy for the correction of myopia. J Cataract Refract Surg 2002;28:18-22.
25. Shahinian L. Laser-assisted subepithelial keratectomy for low to high myopia and astigmatism. J Cataract Refract Surg 2002;28:1334-42.
26. Rouweyha RM, Chuang AZ, Mitra S, Phillips CB,Yee RW. Laser Epithelial Keratomileusis for myopia with the Autonomous Laser. J Refract Surg 2002;18:217-24.

Excimer Laser Subepithelial Ablation (ELSA) or LASEK Offers Return to Surface Ablation

29

CHRIS P LOHMANN (GERMANY)

Refractive surgery is a field that is constantly changing with new technologies being developed and introduced routinely. Currently excimer laser photorefractive keratectomy (PRK) and excimer laser in situ keratomileusis (LASIK) are the surgical procedures most commonly been used to treat myopia. PRK makes changes in the corneal curvature by ablating part of Bowman's layer and anterior corneal stroma tissue after removing the epithelium. In contrast, LASIK does not remove the epithelium, Bowman's layer, or anterior stroma tissue but does remove deep stromal tissue after making a cut into the cornea stroma at approximately 160 micron using a microkeratome. Various peer reviewed studies have shown that the refractive results and long time visual outcomes are good and similar for PRK and LASIK in low to moderate myopia up to – 8 diopters (D).

A new keratorefractive technique, laser assisted subepithelial keratectomy (LASEK), was introduced by Massimo Camellin in 1999. LASEK is based on the detachment of the epithelium using an alcohol solution, creating an epithelial flap that is then repositioned after the laser ablation. The epithelium regenerates itself within a few days and in the meantime the existing flap protects the ablated corneal surface. This technique has the potential to eliminate or reduce many disadvantages of PRK (i.e. postoperative pain, slow visual recovery and corneal haze) and LASIK (i.e. flap complications, interface problems and possibly attenuated long time biomechanical stability of the cornea) and combine their advantages. Early studies suggest that refractive and visual results, stability and safety of LASEK are comparable to those of PRK and LASIK, but haze levels and pain seem to be lower than PRK. Visual recovery seems to be relatively faster after LASEK; approximately two third of the treated eyes have an uncorrected visual acuity (UCVA) of 20/40 or better at day three.

As there is some degree of similarity in pronouncing the names LASEK and LASIK and therefore confuse both the ophthalmic community and the patients we have re-named this procedure to ELSA (**E**xcimer **L**aser **S**ubepithelial **A**blation).

The Surgical Procedure

Although various types of LASEK procedures have been described the majority of surgeons are using the alcohol assisted classical Camellin technique which is illustrated in Figures 29.1A to E. The surgery is performed under topical anesthesia. After a lid speculum is applied to the patients eye the surgery consists of the following steps:

1. An incision of the corneal epithelium is performed using a 8.0 mm cornea trephine with a 70 micron depth calibrated blade. The trephine is designed to create a 280-degree epithelial incision leaving a blunt section of 80 degrees at the 12-o'clock

position for the formation of a hinge. The trephine is placed centrally on the papillary axis and downward pressure of the trephine is evenly applied to the blade and slight rotation of the blade (approximately 5 degrees in both directions) is used to create the incision.

2. An 8.5 mm LASEK alcohol cone is placed on the corneal surface encircling the epithelial incision. This cone is filled with 20% ethanol (in distilled water) and left for 30 seconds. After this time the alcohol is absorbed with a small sponge, the alcohol cone is removed and the cornea is thoroughly washed with BSS to remove all remaining alcohol. The area of epithelial incision is then dried with a small sponge.
3. To create the epithelial flap the pre-cut margin of the epithelium is lifted using the sharp side of a special epithelial peeler, starting at the edges of the epithelial incision and the epithelial flap is gently detached and folded-up at the 12-o'clock position using the blunt side of the epi-peeler.
4. If the epithelium shows strong adherence, the corneal surface is re-exposed to the alcohol for additional 10 to 15 seconds.
5. Then the laser ablation is performed and we are using the normal LASIK normograms.
6. After the laser ablation the cornea is flooded with BSS and the flap is repositioned with the blunt side of the epithelial peeler. A 14.0 mm soft bandage contact lens (we recommend Pure Vision Bausch and Lomb or Ciba Vision daily focus) is applied for protection of the epithelial flap for 3 days.

Surgical Instruments

Almost all ophthalmic instrument companies have LASEK instruments in their portfolio. The original ones were from Janach (Como, Italy) which are shown in Figure 29.1. The set of instruments usually consists of a epithelial trephine and alcohol cone, and a peeler or microhoe to mobilize and push back the epithelium.

For astigmatic correction there are elliptical instruments distributed by Geuder (Heidelberg, Germany) which are shown in Figure 29.2.

Just recently they have been disposable instruments introduced to the ophthalmic community. These are also been distributed by Geuder (Heidelberg, Germany) and are shown in Figure 29.3A to Z. The main advantage of these disposable instruments that they are disposable and therefore reduces the risk of infection. There is no need for sterilization which maybe of importance for high volume clinic. You will always have an ultrasharp trephine for a good quality of the epithelial incision. This is of importance for a reduced rate of postoperative pain and haze.

Postoperative Medication

A bandage soft contact lens is of critical importance to keep the epithelium in place after the surgery. This contact lens should not be removed before the third postoperative day. Until the removal of the bandage contact lens the postoperative therapy should consist of a topical antibiotic agent and a corticosteroid 4 times daily and lubrication (we prefer carbomer 2.0 mg) 5 to 8 times a day. As there is a contact lens on the eye we recommend the use of non-preserved eye drops. After the removal of the contact lens the eyes should be treated with carbomer 2.0 mg 4 times daily and with topical corticosteroids 4 times daily for 2 weeks and twice a day for 2 weeks. All medications should be withdrawn after 4 weeks.

Clinical Results

So far there have been very few clinical studies published in peer-reviewed journals. In the following we have summarized the results

Myopia

Up to a myopic correction of 8 D (spherical equivalent, SE) between 81 and 97% are within +/– 0.5 D after 6 months. Uncorrected visual acuity of 20/20 are between 73 and 92% of the treated eyes, and between 96 and 100% are within 20/40. None of the eyes have lost more than 1 line of Snellen visual acuity.

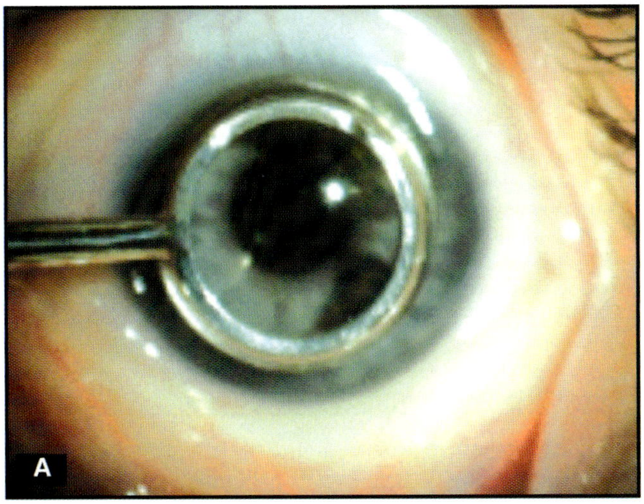

Trepanation of the epithelium

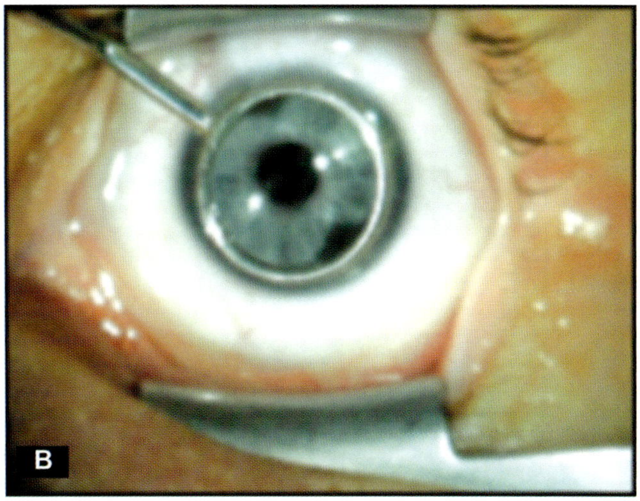

30 sec alcohol

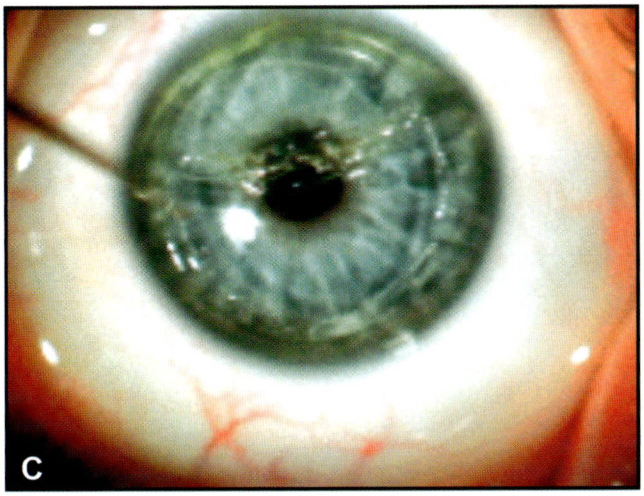

Mobilisation of the epithelium

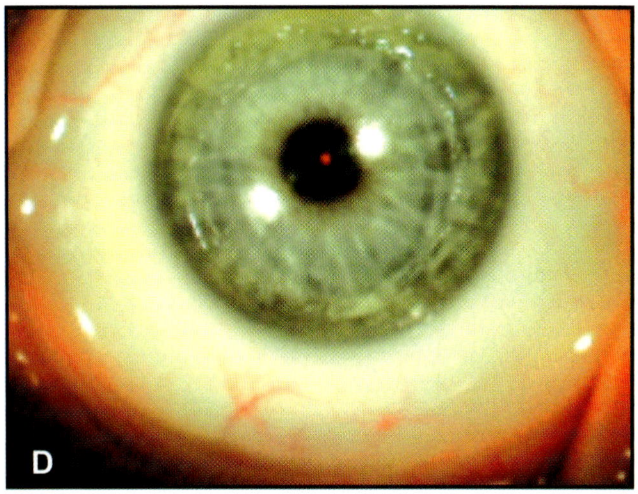

Excimer laser ablation

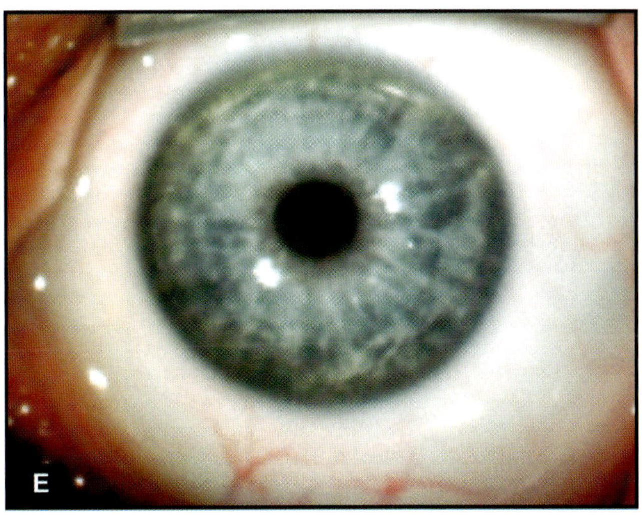

Re-positioning of the epithelium

Figs 29.1A to E: The LASEK procedure (Camellin's technique)

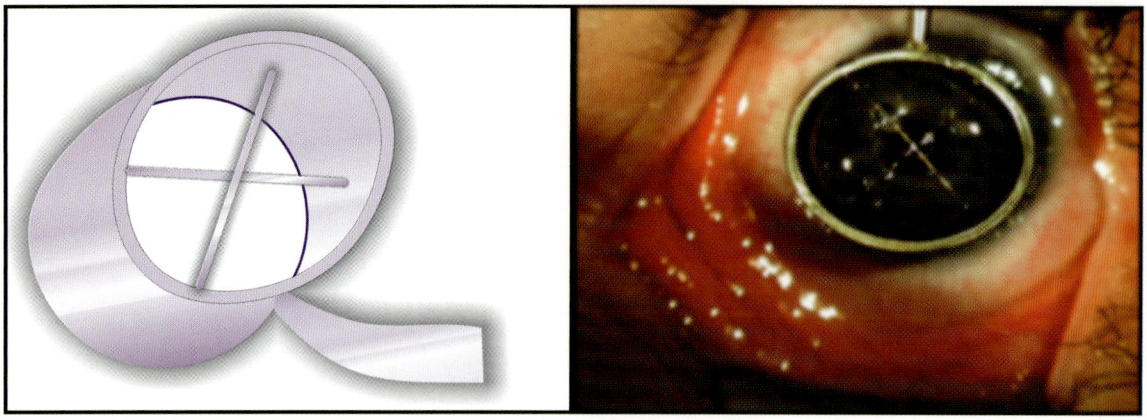

Fig. 29.2: Elliptical LASEK instrument for astigmatic corrections

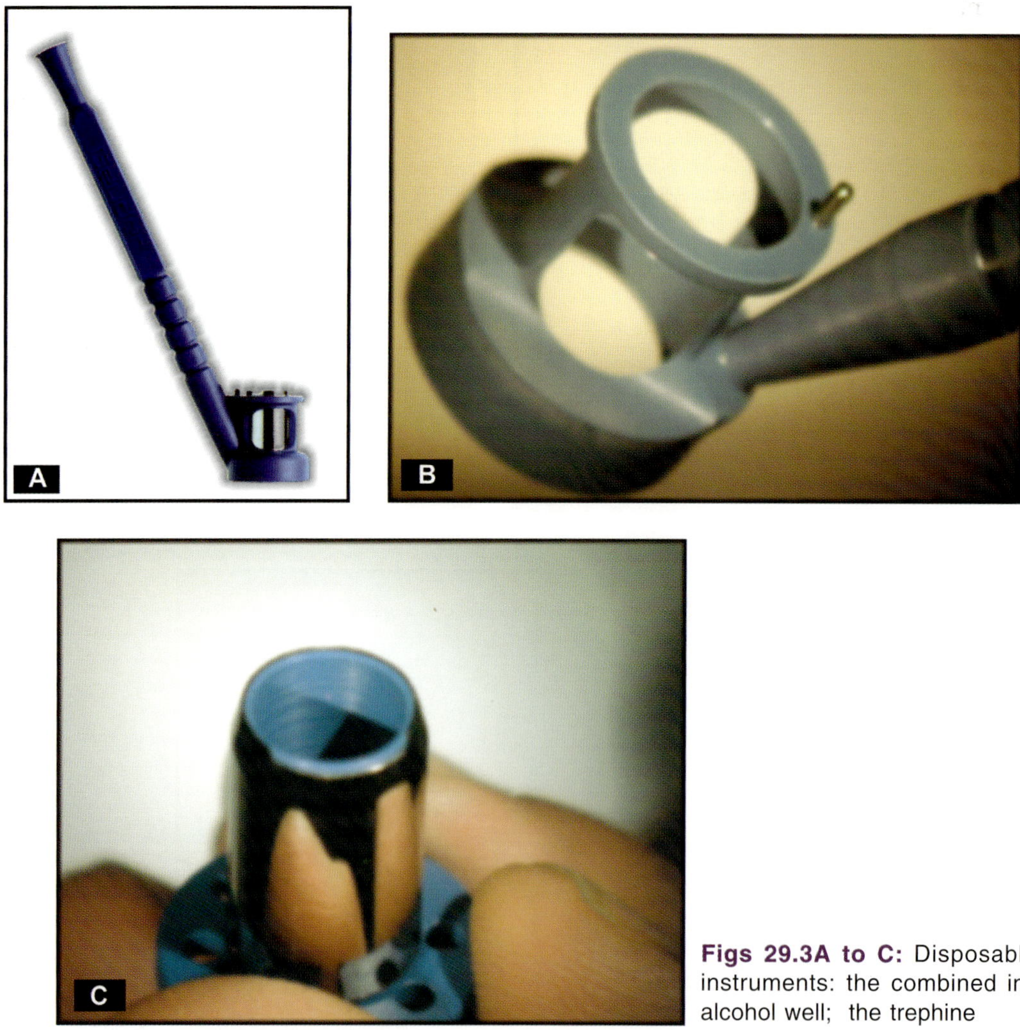

Figs 29.3A to C: Disposable LASEK instruments: the combined instrument; alcohol well; the trephine

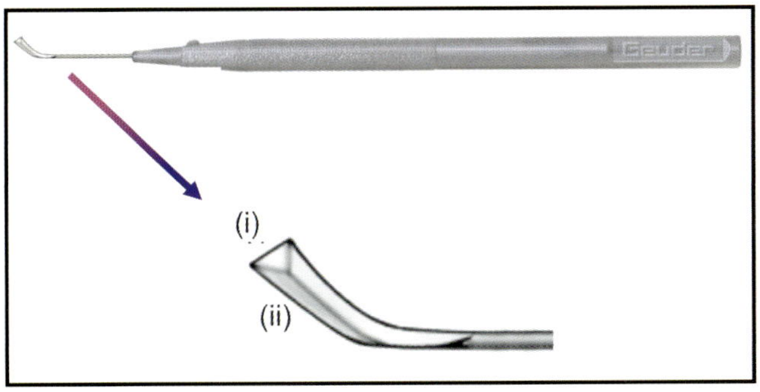

Fig. 29.3D: Disposable epi-peeler (i) Sharp part to mobilize the epithelium; (ii) Blunt part to push back the epithelium

Astigmatism

Today there is only one larger studies of the treatment of astigmatism. This have been performed by our group. We have treated 60 eyes with a myopic astigmatism between - 1 and – 4.5 D with a follow up of 12 months. All of these eyes were postoperatively within +/- 0.75 D of SE with an astigmatic correction with less than 0.5 D. None of the eyes lost more than 1 line of visual acuity, in contrast 39% gained 1 or 2 lines of visual acuity. No significant haze of greater 0.5 was seem in these eyes.

Hyperopia

So far no studies have been published in peer-reviewed journals on the treatment of hyperopia using LASEK.

Advantages and Disadvantages of LASEK

LASEK or ELSA is not as comfortable as LASIK but much less painful than PRK. In our experience 17% of our treated eyes have some kind of pain within the first 4 hours which there after disappears. Visual rehabilitation is faster in LASIK than in LASEK or ELSA. But it seems to us, that using the new LASEK microkeratom from Ciba or Gebauer (the procedure called Epi-LASIK) postoperative visual recovery is not much slower than in LASIK. The main advantage of LASEK or ELSA is that it does need a cut in the stroma as with LASIK. Therefore the LASIK flap related complications like diffuse lamellar keratitis, free flaps, button holes, incomplete flap, flap wrinkles, epithelial ingrowth, microbiological infections, biomechanical problems, and an increase in higher order aberrations are excluded with LASEK or ELSA. In particular we think of customized ablation just like wavefront- or topography-guided ablations LASEK or ELSA is obviously superior than LASIK.

CONCLUSIONS

LASEK or ELSA is a very good alternative for LASIK corrections for myopia up to – 8.0 D and astigmatism up to – 5.0 D. In particular for customized ablations it is superior to LASIK.

Tear Film Function, Ocular Surface Integrity and Corneal Sensation After Laser-Assisted Subepithelial Keratectomy

JUTTA HORWATH-WINTER (AUSTRIA)

30

INTRODUCTION

Recently, a new technique called laser-assisted subepithelial keratectomy (LASEK) has been introduced by Camellin in 1999.[1] LASEK is a modification of photorefractive keratectomy (PRK) that is based on the creation of a hinged corneal epithelial flap after the exposure to 20% alcohol solution. This epithelial flap is repositioned to its original location after anterior stromal ablation with the excimer laser so that the stromal wound is covered immediately.[1, 2]

In PRK, refractive surgical ablation is performed on the corneal surface after epithelial debridement. The disadvantage is that the epithelium is lost during this procedure with potential problems of delayed visual improvement caused by epithelial defects, significant postoperative pain, and formation of stromal haze due to the healing process.[3-7] These issues contribute to the lack of acceptance of PRK.

Laser in situ keratomileusis (LASIK) is still the most common refractive surgical procedure performed,[8] because it offers prompt visual recovery, only mild discomfort and minimal chances of corneal haze.[9, 10] During LASIK, a hinged lamellar corneal flap is raised with a microkeratome followed by ablation in the stromal bed and repositioning of the flap. Unfortunately, the incidence of problems related to the corneal flap can lead to complications such as wrinkles, epithelial ingrowth and diffuse lamellar keratitis.[11-15] In addition, the corneal flap in LASIK surgery can lead to unpredictable biomechanical corneal changes and to corneal ectasia.[16, 17] These issues have led to a regained popularity of surface ablative procedures.

LASEK has become popular for correcting refractive errors in the last years. Advantages of this method are a smoother and more regular surface than after the mechanical debridement in PRK[18, 19] and that the ablated corneal surface is covered by a full thickness epithelium immediately after surgery. Combining elements of LASIK and PRK in LASEK, flap-related complications of LASIK and the haze risk, pain, and slow visual recovery of PRK should be avoided.

Although in several reports PRK and LASEK findings were similar in relation to pain and visual outcomes,[20-22] other clinical studies have shown a reduction in postoperative pain, faster visual rehabilitation, and decreased haze in LASEK-treated eyes than in PRK-treated eyes.[2, 23-28]

Reduced postoperative pain in LASEK is probably because the epithelial flap protects the ablated stromal area. Retention of the epithelial flap acts as a smooth refractive surface, allowing better visual acuity post surgery.[23-25]

The exact mechansim for less corneal haze noted in LASEK is open to debate in the literature. It is speculated that the epithelial flap seals up the bare surface of the stroma and prevents the influx of inflammatory cells from tears, which reduces the initial inflammatory damage to the corneal stroma.[23, 25]

Various cytokines including keratinocyte growth factor and transforming growth factor β (TGF-β) are known to regulate the corneal stromal wound-healing process after excimer laser keratectomy. Among these cytokines, TGF-ß is proposed to be key in inducing corneal stromal fibrosis after excimer laser keratectomy. The upregulation in the expression of TGF-ß1 in the tear film in the early postoperative period induced by a greater epithelial trauma during PRK than during LASEK[29] may play a role in the increased myofibroblast transformation observed in PRK at higher attempted correction.

Ethanol-mediated flap repositioning during LASEK induced less keratocyte loss and a slower wound-healing process than mechanical scraping[30] and replacement of the epithelial flap after the ablation may also decrease the loss of stromal keratocytes.[31] Zhao et al demonstrated that tears may be a major factor in the induction of keratocyte loss after de-epithelialization in the mouse cornea.[32] In a rabbit model it was observed that in eyes with higher attempted corrections, there was a significant increase in keratocyte apoptosis, myofibroblast transformation and expression of chondroitin sulfate in the PRK group compared to the LASEK-treated eyes.[33]

Other factors that modulate corneal wound healing and cell migration are substance P, calcitonin gene related peptide, acetylcholine or norepinephrine.[34] The corneal substance-P-ergic innervation after LASEK and PRK was investigated in rabbits.[35] In the LASEK group an accelerated recovery of SP-immunoreactive nerve fibers in the subepithelial layer and anterior corneal stroma was found. This could promote wound healing in the acute phase after laser photoablation.

According to the data of the above mentioned studies, epithelial coverage alters the wound healing response of the cornea. Therefore, the theory that LASEK, as a modified surface ablative procedure potentially combines the advantages of PRK and LASIK is further supported.

Tear Film Function and Ocular Surface Integrity

Dry eye is known to occur commonly after refractive surgery.

Several mechanisms appear responsible for tear film and ocular surface disruption seen after this kind of surgery. Changes in the corneal curvature alter tear wetting as the lids move over a modified ocular surface. Damage to the ocular surface caused by epithelial toxic antibiotics and preservatives may induce transient dry eye.

The high level of pressure induced by the suction ring during LASIK may damage the conjunctival goblet cells, compromising the mucin layer of the tear film.[36]

The most important reason leading to the development of dry eye is consistent with the understanding that refractive surgery destroys the sensory innervation of the cornea.

The ocular surface and lacrimal glands function as an integrated unit. Communication between the ocular surface and lacrimal glands occurs through a sensory/autonomic neural reflex loop.[37] The sensory nerves innervating the ocular surface connect with efferent autonomic nerves in the brainstem that stimulate secretion of tear fluid and proteins by the lacrimal glands.

Aqueous tear production and clearance decrease in conditions when corneal nerves are damaged[38] and may induce increased inflammation on the ocular surface.[39]

Reduced corneal sensation also reduces blinking rate.[40] Regular blinking and continuous tear fluid production are vital to prevent dehydration, which can cause trophic damage to the cornea.[41]

The amputation of corneal nerves during LASIK is a risk factor for the development of a neurotrophic keratopathy due to a loss of trophic factors with severing of the sensory nerve trunks.[42]

Corneal denervation by refractive surgery not only disrupts the reflex controlling the lacrimal gland but also disrupts the reflex controlling the meibomian gland and, as mentioned before, eyelid blinking, the latter indirectly controling meibom secretion.[43] Lipid tear deficiency was demonstrated as a cause of dry eye in a subgroup of patients after LASIK.[43] This is in agreement with the concept of neuroanatomic integration of external adnexa and eyelids to maintain a stable tear film.[44]

Depending on the kind of the refractive surgical procedure, the effects on tear dynamics and ocular surface may vary.

A decrease in tear flow and tear film stability was observed 6 weeks after PRK and was found reduced up to 6 months later.[45-47] LASIK has also been shown to decrease breakup time (BUT) and Schirmer test values significantly.[38, 48-51] Basal tear secretion was reduced up to 12 months.[48] BUT was decreased 3 to 6 months after LASIK.[48, 51, 52]

In a comparative study of tear function changes after PRK and LASIK, Lee et al showed a significant reduction in Schirmer and BUT scores and a significant increase in tear osmolarity 6 months after both procedures.[52] However, a greater decrease in these tear film factors in LASIK patients was found.

There was a significant increase in punctate corneal fluorescein staining at 1 week post-operatively.[38] Increased punctate epithelial erosions and corneal epithelial rose bengal staining developed after LASIK within a few days to weeks of LASIK and typically persisted for 6 to 8 months following surgery.[42]

Since a modified wound healing after LASEK may also influence tear film and ocular surface function, these factors have been studied after LASEK.[53, 54]

The tear film breakup time was found reduced up to 1 month after LASEK and fluorescein staining of the cornea was significantly increased 3 days and 1 week after LASEK.[53, 54] Whereas Horwath-Winter et al[53] did not observe a significant decrease in reflex secretion, Hermann et al[54] noted that Schirmer test values without local anaesthesia were decreased 2 and 3 months and basal secretion was decreased 3 months after LASEK in a 6 month follow-up period. No significant changes were found in lissamin green staining postoperatively.[53]

Although there are currently no published reports detailing the course of ocular surface integrity and tear film function after LASEK in comparison to PRK, these studies mentioned above provide first results. LASEK induces shortterm effects on ocular surface and tear film. Epithelial flap repositioning in LASEK seems to have a positive influence on tear film and ocular surface factors.

Corneal Sensation

The cornea is one of the most densely innervated and highly sensitive tissues in the body. Corneal sensation is provided by the long ciliary nerves of the ophthalmic division of the trigeminal cranial nerve. The long ciliary nerve trunk runs in the suprachoroidal space, where it branches several times before entering the cornea at the limbus. The large nerves enter the limbus predominantly at the 9 o'clock and 3 o'clock positions. They then bifurcate and move toward the 12 and 6 o'clock positions. After a second bifurcation, they again run toward the 9 and 3 o'clock positions. The nerves initially enter the cornea in the middle third of the stroma, but course anteriorly as they branch, eventually forming a plexus in the sub-Bowman's layer that densely innervates the central cornea.[55-57] The nerves next penetrate Bowman's membrane and terminate in the epithelium at the wing cell layer.

All types of refractive surgery alter the corneal sensory nerves. The time course and pattern of nerve regeneration after refractive surgery is expected to depend in part on where and at which content the nerves are severed.

During PRK, those superficial nerve endings are damaged that terminate in the corneal epithelium that is removed by mechanical scrape.

In LASIK the microkeratome makes a tangential cut through the stroma, which induces a more proximal transection of the posterior corneal nerve trunks that enter the cornea at the 3 and 9 o´clock positions except in the area of the flap hinge.[58]

A superior hinge on the corneal flap severs both arms of the neuroplexus, whereas a nasal hinge transects only the nerves from the temporal side. The high level of pressure, induced perilimbally by the suction ring may also cause trauma to the corneal nerves that diverge just proximal to the limbus from those destined for the ciliary body, iris and sclera. This implies that sensory deprivation could be severe after LASIK.

The pattern of nerve damage during LASEK is similar to that in PRK. Sensory nerve endings are injured that terminate in the corneal epithelium that is removed by topical alcohol during this procedure.

In all three refractive surgery techniques PRK, LASIK and LASEK, there is additional damage to the nerves in the stroma removed by laser photoablation.

Reports showed that the return to full sensitivity of the central cornea after PRK was achieved between 3 and 12 months.[59-63] In LASIK clinical studies reported that corneal sensation after LASIK reached preoperative levels 3 to 16 months after the procedure.[38, 48, 58, 64] The severed nerves grow back slowly over months and up to even a year.[65, 66] Evidence derived from confocal microscopy suggests that a population of these nerves never return to their original state.[66, 67]

Comparing LASIK and PRK, corneal sensitivity was more depressed after LASIK than after PRK during the first 3 months.[63, 68] Studies have suggested that the extent and duration of corneal hypoesthesia is dependent on ablation depth.[60, 61, 69, 70, 71] In contrast, Chuck et al concluded that ablation depth did not seem to affect the initial level of decrease in corneal sensation.[72]

In LASEK the intraepithelial nerves are severed with lifting of the epithelium and the superficial nerves are destroyed in the area of photoablation but the deeper stromal nerves and their trunks are spared.

In a comparative study recovery of corneal sensitivity was faster after LASEK (recovered at 3 months) than after LASIK in myopic eyes with less than 6.0 diopters.[73] Ablation depth was related to the recovery of corneal sensitivity after LASEK but no correlation was found after LASIK.

As demonstrated by a study of Horwath-Winter et al, corneal sensation recovered 3 months after LASEK in a 6 month-follow up period.[53] Hermann et al observed that during the first month after surgery the depressed corneal sensation improved and subsequently went back to preoperative values, staying stable 3 and 6 months after surgery.[54, 74] They found no significant association between the depth of ablation and the postoperative sensation.[74]

Based on the findings of these studies, the restoration of corneal sensitivity seems to be comparable[53, 73] to reported results or even faster[54, 74] after LASEK than after PRK.

A possible reason for the faster recovery of corneal sensation after LASEK than after PRK is the repositioned epithelial flap that may decrease inflammation[23, 25] and enhance nerve regeneration by providing a natural matrix for the outgrowth and orientation of regenerating subepithelial nerves. Studies in rabbits[35] have shown that substance-P-ergic innervation recovers faster in the subepithelial layer and the anterior stroma after LASEK than after PRK. Moreover, it is possible that in the hinge of the epithelial flap some epithelial nerves might withstand the surgical trauma and contribute to a fast recovery of corneal sensation. Regenerating nerve fibres after refractive surgery derive from deeper stromal nerve fibres and from the subepithelial nerve plexus adjacent to the wound margins.

In conclusion, comparing the recovery of corneal sensation after different kinds of excimer laser refractive surgery, the superficial ablation in PRK and LASEK results in less damage to corneal nerves and leaves deeper stromal nerves untouched.

CONCLUSIONS

The indications for LASEK have generally been the same as those for patients with PRK, and include patients with thin corneas, occupations that predispose to ocular trauma, and patients with anatomic abnormalities, such as flat corneas, steep corneas, and deep-set eyes; to those who have had filtering blebs or retinal detachment surgery.

Because LASEK is a modified procedure of PRK the results concerning tear film, ocular surface and corneal sensibility should be similar to PRK. Concerning corneal sensibility the results of the above mentioned studies[53, 73] seem comparable to the results described in the literature[60-63, 68] or even better.[54, 74] The results concerning tear film and ocular surface function[53, 54] seem to be better than the results described in the literature.[45, 47, 52] The reason for this difference could be a modified wound healing due to the reattached epithelial flap. LASEK surgery causes only a transient decrease of corneal sensation, and dry eye signs revert to the preoperative level after a few months.

Therefore LASEK surgery should be considered in patients with reduced corneal sensation and pre-existing dry eye who are undergoing refractive surgery.

REFERENCES

1. Camellin M. LASEK may offer the advantages of both LASIK and PRK. Ocular Surgery News, International Edition, March 1999.
2. Shah S, Sarhan ARS, Doyle SJ, Pillai CT, Dua HS. The epithelial flap for photorefractive keratectomy. Br J Ophthalmol 2001;85:393-96.
3. McCarty CA, Garrett SK, Aldred GF, Taylor HR. Assessment of subjective pain following photorefractive keratectomy. Melbourne Excimer Laser Group. J Refract Surg 1996;12:365-69
4. Verma S, Marshall J. Control of pain after photorefractive keratectomy. J Refract Surg 1996;12: 358-64.
5. Lohmann CP, Gartry DS, Muir MK, Timberlake GT, Fitzke FW, Marshall J. Corneal haze after excimer refractive surgery: objective measurements and functional implications. Eur J Ophthalmol 1991;1: 173-80.
6. Ramirez-Florez S, Maurice DM. Inflammatory cells, refractive regression, and haze after excimer laser PRK. J Refract Surg 1996;12:370-81.
7. Kim JH, Sah WJ, Hahn TW, Lee YC. Some problems after photorefractive keratectomy. J Refract Corneal Surg 1994;10:226-30.
8. Duffey RJ, Leaming D. US trends in refractive surgery: 2002 ISRS survey. J Refract Surg 2003;19:357-63.
9. Esquenazi S. Comparision of laser in situ keratomileusis and automated lamellar keratoplasty for the treatment of myopia. J Refract Surg 1997;13:637-43.
10. Esquenazi S, Mendoza A. Two-year follow-up of laser in situ keratomileusis for hyperopia. J Refract Surg 1999;15:648-52.
11. Alio JL, Perez-Santonja JJ, Tervo T, Tabbara KF, Vesaluoma M, Smith RJ, Maddox B, Maloney RK. Postoperative inflammation, microbial complications, and wound healing following laser in situ keratomileusis. J Refract Surg 2000;16:523-38.
12. Gimbel HV, Penno EE, van Westenbrugge JA, Ferensowicz M, Furlong MT. Incidence and management of intraoperative and early postoperative complications in 1000 consecutive laser in situ keratomileusis cases. Ophthalmology 1998;105:1839-47.
13. Wang MY, Maloney RK. Epithelial ingrowth after laser in situ keratomileusis. Am J Ophthalmol 2000;129: 746-51.
14. Asano-Kato N, Toda I, Hori-Komai Y, Takano Y, Tsubota K. Epithelial ingrowth after laser in situ keratomileusis: clinical features and possible mechanisms. Am J Ophthalmol 2002;134:801-07.
15. Shah MN, Misra M, Wilhelmus KR, Koch DD. Diffuse lamellar keratitis associated with epithelial defects after laser in situ keratomileusis. J Cataract Refract Surg 2000;26:1312-18.
16. Seiler T, Koufala K, Richter G. Iatrogenic keratectasia after laser in situ keratomileusis. J Refract Surg 1998;14:312-17.
17. Geggel HS, Talley AR. Delayed onset keratectasia following laser in situ keratomileusis. J Cataract Refract Surg 1999;25:582-86.
18. Browning AC, Shah S, Dua HS, Maharajan SV, Gray T, Bragheeth MA. Alcohol debridement of the corneal epithelium in PRK and LASIK: an electron microscopic study. Invest Ophthalmol Vis Sci 2003;44:510-13.
19. Helena MC, Filatov VV, Johnston WT, Vidaurri-Leal J, Wilson SE, Talamo JH. Effects of 50% ethanol and mechanical epithelial debridement on corneal structure before and after excimer photorefractive keratectomy. Cornea 1997;16:571-79.
20. Litwak S, Zadok D, Garcia-de Quevedo V, Robledo N, Chayet A. Laser-assisted subepithelial keratectomy versus photorefractive keratectomy for the correction of myopia; a prospective comparative study. J Cataract Refract Surg 2002;28:1330-33.
21. Pirouzian A, Thornton JA, Ngo S. A randomised prospective clinical trial comparing laser subepithelial keratomileusis and photorefractive keratectomy. Arch Ophthalmol 2004;122:11-16.

22. Lee HK, Lee KS, Kim JK, Kim HC, Seo KR, Kim EK. Epithelial healing and clinical outcomes in excimer laser photorefractive surgery following three epithelial removal techniques: mechanical, alcohol, and excimer laser. Am J Ophthalmol 2005;139:56-63.
23. Lee JB, Seong GJ, Lee JH, Seo KY, Lee YG, Kim EK. Comparison of laser epithelial keratomileusis and photorefractive keratectomy for low to moderate myopia. J Cataract Refract Surg 2001;27:565-70.
24. Claringbold II TV. Laser–assisted subepithelial keratectomy for the correction of myopia. J Cataract Refract Surg 2002;28:18-22.
25. Autrata R, Rehurek J. Laser-assisted subepithlial keratectomy for myopia:Two-year follow-up. J Cataract Refract Surg 2003;29:661-68.
26. Saleh TA, Almasri MA. A comparative study of post-operative pain in laser epithelial keratomileusis versus photorefractive keratectomy. Surgeon 2003;1:229-32.
27. He TG, Wang LJ, Sun ZY, Shi XR. Comparison of laser subepithelial keratomileusis and photorefractive keratectomy for the correction of myopia. Zhonghua Yan Ke Za Zhi 2004;40:579-82.
28. Carones F, Fiore T, Brancato R. Mechanical vs. alcohol epithelial removal during photorefractive keratectomy. J Refract Surg 1999;15:556-62.
29. Lee JB, Choe CM, Kim HS, Seo KY, Seong GJ, Kim EK. Comparison of TGF-beta1 in tears following laser subepithelial keratomileusis and photorefractive keratectomy. J Refract Surg 2002;18:130-34.
30. Song IK, Joo CK. Morphological and functional changes in the rat cornea with an ethanol-mediated epithelial flap. Invest Ophthalmol Vis Sci 2004;45:423-28.
31. Shahinian L Jr. Laser-assisted subepithelial keratectomy for low to high myopia and astigmatism. J Cataract Refract Surg 2002;28:1334-42.
32. Zhao J, Nagasaki T, Maurice DM. Role of tears in keratocyte loss after epithelial removal in mouse cornea. Invest Ophthalmol Vis Sci 2001;42:1743-49.
33. Esquenazi S, He J, Bazan NG, Bazan HE. Comparison of corneal wound-healing response in photorefractive keratectomy and laser-assisted subepithelial keratectomy. J Cataract Refract Surg 2005;31:1632-39.
34. Kruse FE. Neuronal growth factors in the Cornea. Invest Ophthalmol Vis Sci 2003; e-abstract 19.
35. Tilch D, Selbach JM, Laube T, Theiss C, Steuhl KP, Meller D. Corneal substance-P-ergic innervation after laser epithelial keratomileusis (LASEK) in comparison to photorefractive keratectomy (PRK) in rabbits. Invest Ophthalmol Vis Sci 2003; e-abstract 2682.
36. Albietz JM, Lenton LM, McLennan SG. Effect of laser in situ keratomileusis for hyperopia on tear film and ocular surface. J Refract Surg 2002;18:113-23.
37. Stern ME, Beuerman RW, Fox RI, Mircheff AK, Pflugfelder SC. The pathology of dry eye: the interaction between the ocular surface and lacrimal glands. Cornea 1998;17:584-89.
38. Battat L, Macri A, Dursun D, Pflugfelder SC. Effects of laser in situ keratomileusis on tear production, clearance, and the ocular surface. Ophthalmology 2001;108:1230-35.
39. Afonso AA, Sobrin L, Monroy DC, Selzer M, Lokeshwar B, Pflugfelder SC. Tear fluid gelatinase B activity correlates with IL-1a concentration and fluorescein clearance in ocular rosacea. Invest Ophthalmol Vis Sci 1999;40:2506-12.
40. Collins M, Seeto R, Campell L; Ross M. Blinking and corneal sensitivity. Acta Ophthalmol 1989;67:525-31.
41. Beuerman RW, Schimmelpfennig B. Sensory denervation of the rabbit cornea affects epithelial properties. Exp Neurol 1980;69:196-201.
42. Wilson SE. Laser in situ keratomileusis-induced (presumed) neurotrophic epitheliopathy. Ophthalmology 2001;108:1082-87.
43. Di Pascuale MA, Liu TS, Trattler W, Tseng SC. Lipid tear deficiency in persistent dry eye after laser in situ keratomileusis and treatment results of new eye-warming device. J Cataract Refract Surg 2005;31: 1741-49.
44. Tseng SC, Tsubota K. Important concepts for treating ocular surface and tear disorders. Am J Ophthalmol 1997;124:825-35.
45. Özdamar A, Aras C, Karakas N, Sener B, Karacorlu M. Changes in tear flow and tear film stability after photorefractive keratectomy. Cornea 1999;18:437-39.
46. Siganos DS, Popescu CN, Siganos CS, Pistola G. Tear secretion following spherical and astigmatic excimer laser photorefractive keratectomy. J Cataract Refract Surg 2000;26:1585-89.
47. Hong JW, Kim HM. The changes of tear break up time after myopic excimer laser photorefractive keratectomy. Korean J Ophthalmol 1997;11:89-93.
48. Toda I, Asano-Kato N, Komai-Hori Y, Tsubota K. Dry Eye after laser in situ keratomileusis. Am J Ophthalmol 2001;132:1-7.
49. Yu EY, Leung A, Rao S, Lam DSC. Effect of laser in situ keratomileusis on tear stability. Ophthalmology 2000;107:2131-35.
50. Aras C, Özdamar A, Bahcecioglu H, Karacorlu M, Sener B, Ozkan S. Decreased tear secretion after laser in situ keratomileusis for myopia. J Refract Surg 2000;16: 362-64.
51. Albietz J, Lenton L, McLennan S. The effect of tear film and ocular surface management on myopic lasik outcomes. In: Sullivan D, Stern ME, Tsubota K, et al, eds, Lacrimal Gland, Tear film, and Dry Eye Syndromes 3, Kluwer Academic/Plenum Publishers, 2002.
52. Lee JB, Ryu CH, Kim JH, Kim EK, Kim HB. Comparison of tear secretion and tear film instability after

photorefractive keratectomy and laser in situ keratomileusis. J Cataract Refract Surg 2000;26: 1326-31.

53. Horwath-Winter J, Vidic B, Schwantzer G, Schmut O. Early changes in corneal sensation, ocular surface integrity, and tear-film function after laser-assisted subepithelial keratectomy. J Cataract Refract Surg 2004;30:2316-21.
54. Herrmann WA, Shah CP, Winkler von Mohrenfels C, Gabler B, Hufendiek K, Lohmann CP. Tear film function and corneal sensation in the early postoperative period after LASEK for the correction of myopia. Graefes Arch Clin Exp Ophthalmol 2005;243:911-16.
55. Muller LJ, Pels L, Vrensen GF. Ultrastructural organization of human corneal nerves. Invest Ophthalmol Vis Sci 1996;37:476-88.
56. Muller LJ, Vrensen GF, Pels L, Cardozo BN, Willehens B. Architecture of human corneal nerves. Invest Ophthalmol Vis Sci 1997;38:985-94.
57. Auran JD, Koester CJ, Kleiman NJ, Rapaport R, Bomann JS, Wirotsko BM, Florakis GJ, Koniarek JP. Scanning slit confocal microscopic observation of cell morphology and movement within the normal human anterior cornea. Ophthalmology 1995;102:33-41.
58. Donnenfeld ED, Solomon K, Perry HD, Doshi SJ, Ehrenhaus M, Solomon R, Biser S. The effect of hinge position on corneal sensation and dry eye after LASIK. Ophthalmology 2003;110:1023-30.
59. Murphy PJ, Corbett MC, O'Brart DP, Verma S, Patel S, Marshall J. Loss and recovery of corneal sensitivity following photorefractive keratectomy for myopia. J Refract Surg 1999;15:38-45.
60. Campos M, Hertzog L, Garbus JJ, McDonnell PJ. Corneal sensitivity after photorefractive keratectomy. Am J Ophthalmol 1992;114:51-54.
61. Lawrenson JG, Corbett MC, O'Brart DP, Marshall J. Effect of beam variables on corneal sensitivity after excimer laser photorefractive keratectomy. Br J Ophthalmol 1997;81:686-90.
62. Ishikawa T, Park SB, Cox C, del Cerro M, Aquavella JV. Corneal sensation following excimer laser photorefractive keratectomy in humans. J Refract Corneal Surg 1994;10:417-22.
63. Matsui H, Kumano Y, Zushi I, Yamada T, Matsui T, Nishida T. Corneal sensation after correction of myopia by photorefractive keratectomy and laser in situ keratomileusis. J Cataract Refract Surg 2001;27:370-73.
64. Benitez-del-Castillo JM, del Rio T, Iradier T, Hernandez JL, Castillo A, Garcia-Sanchez J. Decrease in tear secretion and corneal sensitivity after laser in situ keratomileusis. Cornea 2001;20:30-32.
65. Kauffmann T, Bodanowitz S, Hesse L, Kroll P. Corneal reinnervation after photorefractive keratectomy and laser in situ keratomileusis: an in vivo study with a confocal videomicroscope. Ger J Ophthalmol 1996;5: 508-12.
66. Lee BH, McLaren JW, Erie JC, Hodge DO, Borune WM. Reinnervation in the cornea after LASIK. Invest Ophthalmol Vis Sci 2002;43:3660-64.
67. Tervo T, Moilanen J. In vivo confocal microscopy for evaluation of wound healing following corneal refractive surgery. Prog Retin Eye Res 2003;22:339-58.
68. Perez-Santonja JJ, Sakla HF, Cardona C, Chipont E, Alio JL. Corneal sensitivity after photorefractive keratectomy and laser in situ keratomileusis for low myopia. Am J Ophthalmol 1999;127:497-504.
69. Kohlhaas M. Corneal sensation after cataract and refractive surgery. J Cataract Refract Surg 1998;24: 1399-1409.
70. Kim WS, Kim JS. Change in corneal sensitivity following laser in situ keratomileusis. J Cataract Refract Surg 1999;25:368-73.
71. Nassaralla BA, McLeod SD, Nassaralla JJ Jr. Effect of myopic LASIK on human corneal sensitivity. Ophthalmology 2003;110:497-502.
72. Chuck RS, Quiros PA, Perez AC, McDonnell PJ. Corneal sensation after laser in situ keratomileusis. J Cataract Refract Surg 2000;26:337-39.
73. Wu Y, Chu RY, Zhou XT, Dai JH, Qu XM. Recovery of corneal sensitivity after laser in situ keratomileusis and laser-assisted subepithelial keratectomy. Zhonghua Yan Ke Za Zhi 2005;41:972-76.
74. Herrmann WA, Shah C, Gabler B, Winkler von Mohrenfels C, Hufendiek K, Lohmann CP. Corneal sensation after laser epithelial keratomileusis for the correction of myopia. Graefe's Arch Clin Exp Ophthalmol 2005;243:33-37.

LASEK (Laser Assisted Subepithelial Keratectomy)

31

SANJAY CHAUDHARY (INDIA)

WHY IS LASIK LOOSING ITS GLORY?

With the introduction of LASIK, PRK was immediately pushed to the background. The main reasons for LASIK's popularity with the patients and the ophthalmologists were the quick recovery often termed the 'wow' factor, and the no corneal haze scenario. With the increasing numbers of LASIK, problems about this procedure started showing up. As ophthalmologists got down to correcting higher degrees of myopia and greater degrees of tissue ablation, cases of corneal ectasia began to get reported from all over the world. Initially a safe standard was set as a residual corneal bed of 300 mic. However, in a normal thickness cornea of 530 mic, and after making an allowance for a 160 mic flap, 70 mic was just sufficient tissue to correct about 5 D of refractive error. Customized LASIK and demands for prolate cornea, meant more ablation of the corneal tissue. This also meant that another one to two diopter was reduced from our capacity to correct the refractive errors. And what if the cornea was slightly thin and in the range of 500 mic. Would this mean depriving the person from the benefits of LASIK and a major loss of revenue for the ophthalmologist by increasing his rejections. Add to this the unpredictability of the flap thickness. It was demonstrated that the best of the microkeratomes, which talked of a 160 mic flap, would actually cut a flap in the range of 90 to 230 mic. Thus, with a lot of debate, the safe standard was set to 250 mic of residual corneal bed. And this gave the much-needed flexibility to the refractive surgeon to treat a mild to moderate myopia in routine clinical practice. So myopia of 1 to 8 could be handled in most of the situations. But what about the high myopes. Enterprising ophthalmologists started reducing the corneal bed further to 200 mic. As more and more cases of corneal ectasia got reported, there was a major concern for this man made complication even though the cases reported are few and far between. Doctors wanted to fell safe both for the patients and for themselves and this led to the transition to LASEK.

LASEK Gains Popularity

The more the residual stromal bed one leaves behind, the less the chances of ectasia was what makes LASEK ride the crest of popularity.

LASEK has the following advantages to offer:

1. More residual corneal bed thickness, so less chances of ectasia
2. No flap to be lifted, so
   a. No flap related complications like buttonhole, partial cut, free caps, flap wrinkling, epithelial down growth, etc.
   b. Another 90 mic of stroma available for corneal ablation thereby enhancing the limit of correction by approx. another 5D over LASIK.
   c. Less costly because the expense of a keratome and blades eliminated.

d. In a better position to handle thin cornea. A person with a corneal thickness of 490 mic may still have an option of a 6D myopia correction.
e. Large zone treatments for better corneal prolacity and in hyperopia are now possible. This essentially means that in LASIK the flap size was a restricting factor to the size of treatment. And it was seldom possible to go over a 9 mm treatment. The flap size was further reduced in a flat cornea which was a catch situation in hyperopic patients who had a flat cornea, a small flap and a need for a large treatment zone. With LASEK there is no limitation to the zone of treatment.

Surgical Considerations

LASEK involves the stripping of epithelium from the Bowman's membrane in a form of a hinged flap.

An epithelial trephine of the required size in placed on the center of the cornea after anesthetizing the eye with 0.5 percent proparacaine eyedrops. A 4 mm segment of the trephine at the 12 O'clock is blunt. By placing on the cornea with pressure, the trephine cuts through the epithelium sparing the underlying stroma and the 12 O'clock epithelium. The diameter of the trephine could vary from 8.5 to 10.5 mm. A similar sized alcohol well is now centered on the cornea. Twenty percent ethyl alcohol is filled in the well and kept in position for 60 sec. It is then removed with a cellulose sponge, the well taken off the eye and the epithelium washed with BSS. After waiting another minute to allow the alcohol to weaken the epithelial Bowman's adhesions, a micro hoe is used to pick up the epithelium from the edges of the trephine marks. A hockey shaped spatula is now used to roll the epithelium slowly towards the hinge exposing a clean Bowman's to work on. Excimer laser is delivered to the cornea surface to make a correction for the refractive error. The corneal surface is washed thoroughly and scrapped to rid of the debris and the condensed plume. The epithelium is carefully rolled back with the help of an irrigating cannula. Because of the loose elasticity of the tissue, the replaced epithelium usually crosses over the natural edges to overlap some of the healthy epithelium. A bandage contact lens is now placed over the epithelium where it rests for the next five days. The patient is sent home after instilling a preservative free lubricating eye- drop, an antibiotic and a NSAID eyedrop. These are used for the next five days. Systemic antibiotic and strong pain killers are prescribed for the next three days.

LASEK with Mitomycin C

Here, all the above steps are the same. After corneal ablation the treated area of the cornea is exposed to 0.02 percent Mitomycin C for 30 seconds. The corneal surface is then thoroughly washed with BSS for a minute to remove all traces of Mitomycin and then the epithelium is reposited back. Mitomycin C is useful in containing fibroblastic activity and thereby reducing and delaying the chances of corneal haze, more so when attempting to treat high myopia.

Follow-Up

The bandage contact lens is removed when the old epithelium is replaced by the new epithelium generated from the edges of the wound. This usually coincides on the fifth postoperative day. After removing the Bandage Contact Lens, FML eyedrops are started to replace NSAID drops to contain the tissue edema and the subsequent fibroblastic reaction. In our clinical practice we use FML six times a day for a week, and then taper it off by a drop every week over the next six weeks. Antibiotic drops are used for two weeks and lubricating drops for at least two and a half month or more as per requirement.

Disadvantages of LASEK

These are similar to PRK with minor modifications:

Postoperative Pain

This is a major setback for LASEK. The pain is intense on the day of LASIK and reduces over the next 2 to 3 days. This may be accompanied with hyperemia, chemosis of the conjunctiva, and lid edema. Strong analgesics and anti-inflammatory are required over the first 2 to 3 days. The intensity of pain is definitely less than what is encountered in PRK. This is also in sharp contrast to LASIK where there is no pain and only an occasional irritation and watering on the day of the procedure.

Buttonholing

Excess exposure to alcohol does help in easily picking up the flap, but the resultant chemical trauma to the epithelium results in greater tissue reaction, more haze, pain and tissue edema. Less exposure to alcohol or less percentage of alcohol used prevents proper loosening up of the epithelium resulting in single or multiple buttonholing. Excessive breaks in the continuity of the epithelium make the flap useless and have to be discarded. The situation then mimics a PRK.

Blurred Vision

The patient encounters blurred vision for a week. This is a result of epithelial haze as the new epithelium coming in from the sides replaces the old alcohol treated epithelium. The vision clears up in a week's time. This is in stark contrast to LASIK where the patient has good vision within a few hours and has total clarity by next morning.

Corneal Haze

This has become the most feared complication in a long-standing follow-up of LASEK. The haze is similar to the one encountered in PRK and can be graded from I to IV. The use of Mitomycin C in our routine clinical practice for myopia of over 4 D seems to have helped in the following ways:

1. Haze is usually not encountered in myopia of up to 7.0 D as compared with PRK where it could be encountered after 4 D
2. Myopia of 8 to 12 usually results in Grade I haze while 12 and above may result in Grade II to III haze

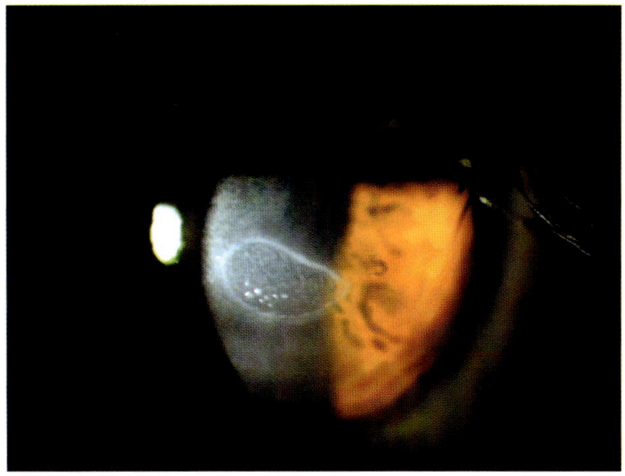

Fig. 31.1: Delayed epithelial healing with corneal haze on 9th postoperative day after LASEK with Mitomycin C. The eye was patched with an antibiotic and lubricating ointment and the defect healed over the next 3 days

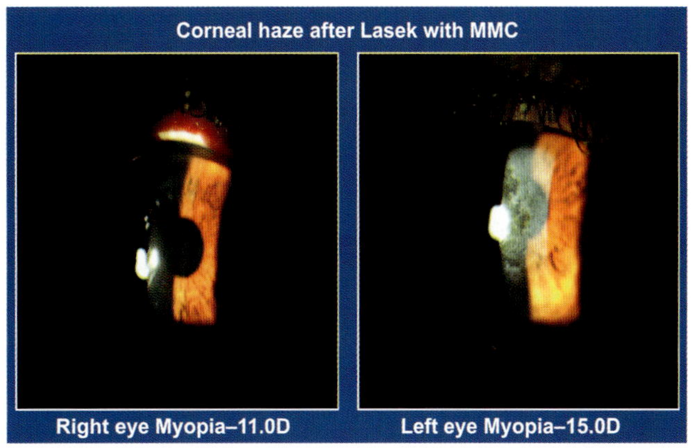

Fig. 31.2: The patient developed a Grade I corneal haze in the right eye and a Grade II haze in the left eye after one and a half year of simultaneous LASEK with Mitomycin C in both eyes

3. There have been situations where even –18 D has had no haze and on the other hand, even a –5 developed a mild haze
4. Haze usually develops after 6-9 months of the procedure
5. Haze results in a regression of the refractive error and the degree of regression depends on the severity of haze
6. Haze usually regresses spontaneously over a period of 2-3 years. Low dose topical steroids could assist resolution

7. The regression of haze sometimes results in some reversal of regression of the refractive error and improvement in refractive error and vision.

The above observations are not a rule but an indication of the surgeon's experience with PRK of over 10 years and of LASEK with and without Mitomycin on over 400 eyes in 4 years.

LASEK in Relation to PRK and Epi-LASIK

PRK, LASEK and now Epi-LASIK involve the removing or stripping of the epithelium from the Bowman's membrane. In PRK, it is mechanical scrapping, in LASEK it is alcohol assisted while in Epi-LASIK, it is again separation with a blade. Since the three are essentially similar, they carry the same advantages and disadvantages with minor modifications. The postoperative pain has definitely reduced from PRK to LASEK to Epi-LASIK. This is attributed to a healthier flap over the cornea and less alcohol injury. The rate of epithelial healing has improved favoring Epi-LASIK. This has also reduced the blurring of vision to a shorter period. However, it postulates that the effect on corneal haze may be similar in LASEK and Epi-LASEK. More experience is required to understand the long-term difference between the two. Epi-LASIK is prone to buttonholing, and in such a situation, the entire epithelium has to be scrapped off to continue with the procedure, and this then becomes a PRK.

BIBLIOGRAPHY

1. Autrata R, Rehurek J. Laser-assisted subepithelial keratectomy and photorefractive keratectomy for the correction of hyperopia: Results of a 2-year follow-up. J Cataract Refract Surg 2003;29:2105-14.
2. Autrata R, Rehurek J. Laser–assisted subepithelial keratectomy for myopia: Two-year follow-up. J Cataract Refract Surg 2003;29:661-68.
3. Azar DT, Ang RT, Lee J-B, et al. Laser subepithelial keratomileusis: Electron microscopy and visual outcomes of flap photorefractive keratectomy. Curr Opin Ophthalmol 2001;12:323-28.
4. Camellin M. Laser epithelial keratomileusis for myopia. J Refract Surg 2003;19:666-70.
5. Claringbold TV II. Laser-assisted subepithelial keratectomy for the correction of myopia. J Cataract Refract Surg 2002;28:18-22.
6. Espana EM, Grueterich M, Mateo A, et al. Cleavage of corneal basement membrane components by ethanol in laser-assisted subepithelial keratectomy. J Cataract Refract Surg 2003; 29:1192-97.
7. Lee JB, Seong GJ, Lee JH, et al. Comparison of laser epithelial keratomileusis and photorefractive keratectomy for low to moderate myopia. J Cataract Refract Surg 2001;27:565-70.
8. Scerrati E. Laser in situ keratomileusis vs laser epithelial keratomileusis (LASIK vs LASEK). J Refract Surg 2001;17:S219-S221.
9. Shah S, Sebai Sarhan AR, Doyle SJ, et al. The Epithelial flap for photorefractive keratectomy. Br J Ophthalmol 2001;85:393-96.
10. Shaninian L Jr. Laser-assisted subepithelial keratectomy for low to high myopia and astigmatism. J Cataract Refract Surg 2002;28:1334-42.

A New Suction Trephine for LASEK

32

JOSEPH COLIN (FRANCE)

A specially adapted trephine that works by suction could help eliminate the risk of corneal peripheral toxicity from alcohol use and ensure safe and consistent flap creation during laser-assisted sub-epithelial keratomileusis (LASEK) procedures .

In the traditional LASEK technique developed by the Italian doctor Massimo Camellin, the epithelium, or outer layer of the cornea, is cut not with the microkeratome cutting tool used in LASIK, but with a finer blade called a trephine.

The surgeon then covers the eye with an alcohol solution (20% in BSS or sterile water) for around 20-30 seconds. The alcohol solution weakens the attachment to Bowman's membrane, allowing the removal of a continuous layer of tissue. The result is a procedure with visual recovery and discomfort which are intermediate between photorefractive keratectomy (PRK) and LASIK, and one that is particularly suited to patients with corneas that are too thin or flat for conventional LASIK treatment.

Despite these advantages of LASEK, there is a risk that the alcohol solution can irritate or kill the peripheral corneal epithelium and the conjunctival epithelium. Dead cells can also slough off and impede the advance of new cells from the limbus. Alcohol-damaged cells have also been known to release apoptotic cytokines, which can lead to haze and regression.

The suction trephine can help to reduce the incidence of alcohol leakage on the conjunctiva when a patient blinks as well as eliminate the risk of toxicity on the corneal epithelial cells and limbal cells.

The trephine has been designed to be fixated onto the eye with suction. After 20 to 30 seconds, it is very easy to remove the alcohol without any risk of leakage because it is in a closed cylinder. The trephine has a pre-calibrated blade length to obtain reproducible superficial keratotomies. It has a safety stop, which means that we have only the possibility to turn three-quarters of a circle and we cut always 70 microns. The epithelial flap is easily lifted in all cases and the corneal cut was similar in all procedures without the risk of a too-deep keratectomy (Figs 32.1 to 32.6).

Refractive surgery is moving inevitably towards the concept of customized corneal ablation treatments, but that there were still many issues to be resolved as to how such customized techniques could best be carried out.

The key question now is focusing on where the treatment has to be delivered. Will it be on the surface of the cornea, using LASEK techniques, with or without topical mitomycin to prevent the risk of haze formation, or will we be concentrating our efforts inside the stroma?

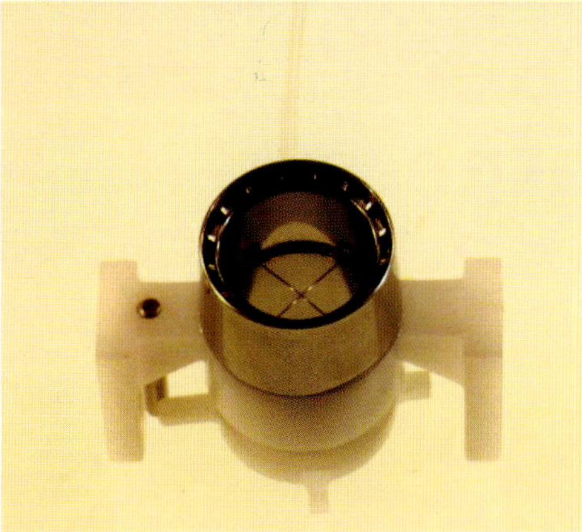

Fig. 32.1

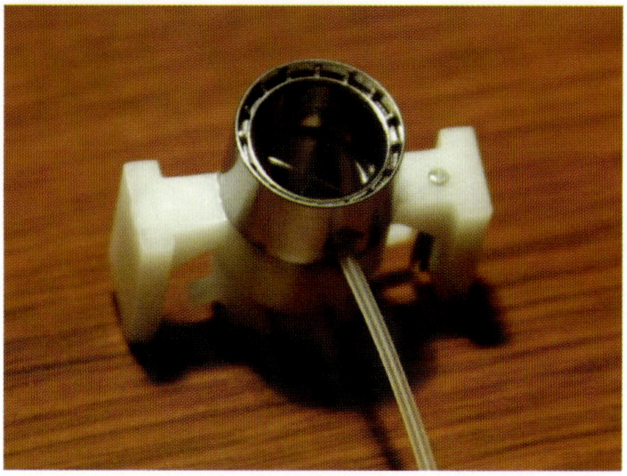

Fig. 32.4

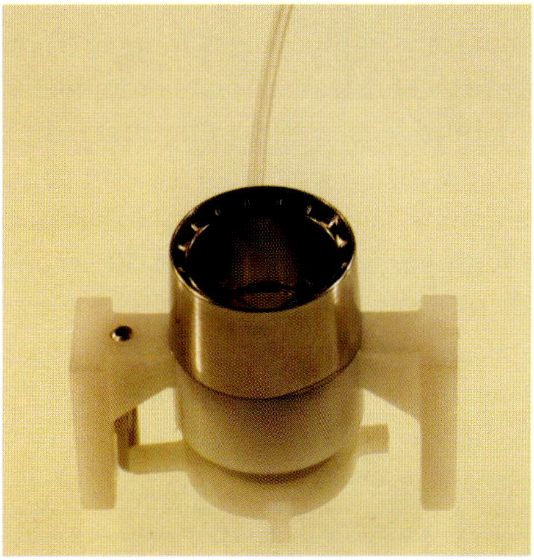

Fig. 32.2

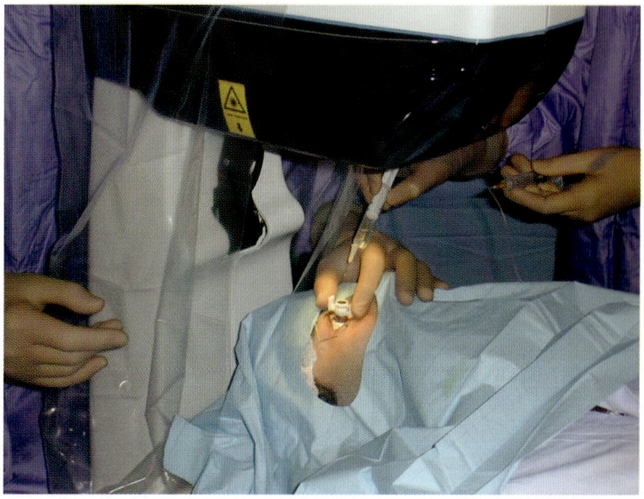

Fig. 32.5

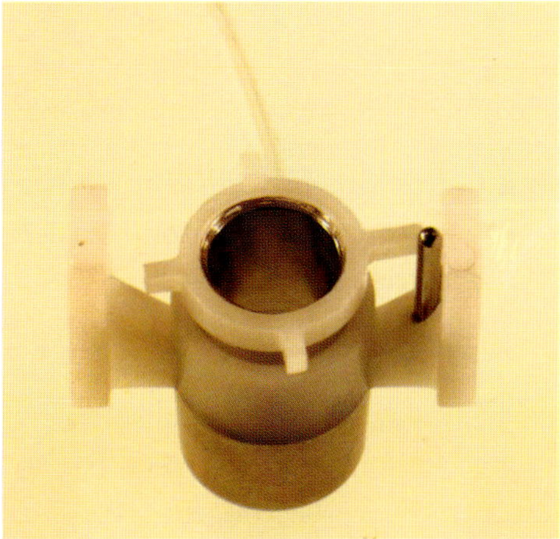

Fig. 32.3

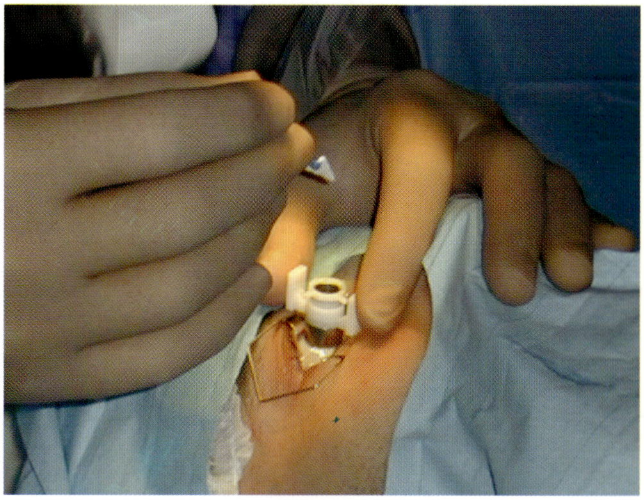

Fig. 32.6

Figs 32.1 to 32.6: Different aspects of LASEK suction trephine (Katena)

Ocular Pharmacokinetics in LASIK and LASEK Surgery

33

ASHOK GARG (INDIA)

Every since Theo Seiler in 1987 and Marguerite McDonald in 1988 did the first corneal ablation in normal sighted eye, Excimer Laser refractive Surgery has produced revolutionary changes in the field of ophthalmology. Refractive Surgery is certainly a high tech advancement in the field of ophthalmic surgery of the last decade of this millenium which has come as a great boon to spectacle weary patients all around the world.

LASIK (Laser assisted in situ keratomileusis) and LASEK (Laser assisted subepithelial keratectomy) offer a unique opportunity to provide ametropia to patients with refractive error ranging from –20.00 D of myopia to +8.00 D of hyperopia. The rapid visual recovery and decreased incidence of complications associated with LASIK and LASEK make them far superior to both excimer photoablation (PRK) and automated Lamellar Keratoplasty (ALK).

LASIK and LASEK provides an extra-ordinary accurate method of tissue removal (0.20-0.25 um tissue per pulse). The extreme pain, haze, regression and slow visual rehablitation of PRK are absent thus the minimum use of postprocedure medications specially topical steroids and its potential adverse effects.

Although pre-procedure medications are same in LASIK and LASEK as those in PRK surgery while post-procedure medications are drasticaly reduced in LASIK and LASEK surgery leading to quick visual rehabilitation of patient post-operatively.

Development of automated microkeratome Hansatome and Laser microkeratome has make LASIK and LASEK surgery more safe even in the hand of novice Refractive Surgeon. Indeed the LASIK and LASEK surgery have come of age.

Here, now I shall discuss the ocular therapeutics used in LASIK and LASEK surgery before and after the procedure.

Pre-procedure Therapeutic Medications

Pre-operatively patient is given broad range Topical antibiotic eye drops (Preferably Gatifloxacin (0.3%) or Moxifloxacin (0.5%) at 4 hourly interval starting 24 hours prior to surgery.

A mild oral sedation (diazepam 3-10 mg) is given in all cases. Bilateral simultaneous surgery is done in all cases.

Topical Anesthesia

For LASIK/LASEK Surgery, refractive Surgeon prefer to give topical anesthesia because of rapid onset of action and lesser irritation to the patient.

2-5 minutes prior to the surgery any of the following topical anesthetic agent can be safely used.

- Proparacaine HCl - 0.5%
- Benoxinate HCl - 0.4%
- Tetracaine HCl - 0.5%

Proparacaine is most commonly used anesthetic agent followed by Benoxinate and tetracaine. Other topical agent like Xylocaine (4%) is less commonly used due to problems of irritation, allergy etc.

Proparacaine, benoxinate and tetracaine have rapid onset of action and cause little tingling sensation and irritation to the patient.

Onset of anesthetic action starts with in 15-20 seconds with these agents and effects last for 15-20 minutes sufficient for the completion of LASIK/LASEK Surgery. Proparacaine or Benoxinate are given topically in the dosage of 2 drops in each eye 2-3 times repeated at the interval of one minute.

After topical anesthesia some refractive surgeon prefer to instill Pilocarpine 1% in the eye to aid in marking the optical axis.

Pachymetry is performed and patients is carefully centred and eyelids are cleaned with betadine solution (Iodine solution) and operative eye is given a sterile plastic ophthalmic drape to cover the eyelid margins and the cilia.

Post Procedure Therapeutic Medications

The biggest advantage of LASIK and LASEK over PRK is the minimum use of ocular therapeutic in post-operative phase. The visual recovery in LASIK and LASEK is virtually immediate owing to the preservation of the epithelium of the cornea. Typically recovery is painless and post-procedure refractions and vision are remarkably stable during the post-operative period. Postprocedure medications are quite significant for early visual rehabilitation and recovery of the patient. During the initial active post-operative phase. Refractive Surgeons prefer to give:

a. Oral antibiotic (Gatifloxacin 400 mg OD or Levofloxacin 500 mg OD for 5 days).
b. Topical Fluorometholone (FML, 0.1%) eye drops four times a day for two weeks.
c. Topical lubricant like Polyvinyl alcohol liquifilm tear drops 4 times a day for two weeks.
d. Topical antibiotic (Moxifloxacin 0.5%). QID for a week. Immediately after LASIK/LASEK procedure some surgeon prefer to give patch for 2-3 hours. While other view is to ask the patient to wear a clear eye shield nightly for a week.
e. Oral analgesic (Tab. Diclofenac 75 mg SR BD for three days if needed but not in routine).

Patient operated for LASIK/LASEK surgery is called for follow up on:

- 2nd day post procedure
- 1st week
- 2nd week
- 3rd week

One each follow up following examination are done

- Vision check up
- IOP with noncontact tonometer
- Slit Lamp Examination for Haze
- Topography to see corneal profile.

Corneal wound healing and its modulations after LASIK/LASEK surgery have multiple components. LASIK/LASEK is a refractive surgical procedure that is performed in several steps and each step involved a different structure of cornea.

Phases of Healing

Following LASIK/LASEK injury healing occurs in several phases. The earliest phase involves the healing of epithelial injury and is characterised by the migration of epithelium which occurs 12-24 hrs after prcedure 2.3 days after the insult, epithelial cell proliferation is evident. Six months after the surgical insult the development of fibrous metaplasia is complete. Throughout these phases of healing the types of cytokine communication are operating to create an integrated repair of injured corneal areas.

Although LASIK/LASEK is safe and reliable procedure yet it is susceptible to all the complications noted in PRK procedure which includes overcorrection, undercorrection, decentration, infection, loss and displacement of flap, central islands and epithelial in growth.

Cornea healing following LASIK/LASEK should be considered as a combination of events involving the response to injury of the epithelium and stroma.

Understanding these events and the molecules that regulate the wound healing response should enable the refractive surgeon to induce fewer complications and aid in developing therapeutic modalities to alter would healing precisely.

Close follow up and attention to post-operative medications and surface lubrication will enable the surgeon to achieve better results.

FURTHER READING

1. Agarwal Amar, Textbook of ophthalmology, Jaypee Brothers Medical Publishers, New Delhi 2002;1.
2. Bartlett JD. Clinical Ocular Pharmacology, Boston: Butterworth-Heinemann 2001;4.
3. Bartlett JD. Ophthalmic Drug facts: Lippincott – William and Wilkins, 2001.
4. Crick. RP, Trimble RB. Textbook of clinical ophthalmology: Hodder and Stoughton, 1986.
5. Duane TD. Clinical ophthalmology, Butterworth – Heinemann, 1999;4.
6. Duvall. Ophthalmic Medications and Pharmacology: Slack Inc, 1998.
7. Ellis PP. Ocular Therapeutics and Pharmacology, CV Mosby, 1985;7.
8. Fechner. Ocular Therapeutics: Slack Inc., 1998.
9. Fraunfelder. Current Ocular Therapy, WB Saunders, 2000;5.
10. Garg Ashok. Current Trends in ophthalmology, Jaypee Brothers Medical Publishers, New Delhi 1997;1.
11. Garg Ashok. Manual of Ocular Therapeutics, Jaypee Brothers Medical Publishers, New Delhi 1996;1.
12. Garg Ashok. Ready Reckoner of Ocular Therapeutics, New Delhi 2002;1.
13. Goodman. LS, Gilman A. Pharmacological basis of Therapeutics, New York: Macmillan 1985;7.
14. Havener's, Ocular Pharmacology, CV Mosby, 1994;6.
15. Kanski. Clinical ophthalmology, Butterworth–Heineman, 1999;4.
16. Kershner. Ophthalmic Medications and Pharmacology: Slack Inc., 1994.
17. Olin BR, et.al. Drugs Facts and Comparisons: Facts and Comparisons, St. Louis, 1997.
18. Onofrey. The Ocular Therapeutics; Lippincott–William and Wilkins, 1997.
19. Rhee. The Wills Eye drug Guide: Lippincott–William and Wilkins, 1998.
20. Steven Podos. Textbook of ophthalmology, Jaypee Brothers Medical Publishers, New Delhi 2001.
21. Zimmerman. Textbook of Ocular Pharmacology: Lippincott & William and Wilkins, 1997.

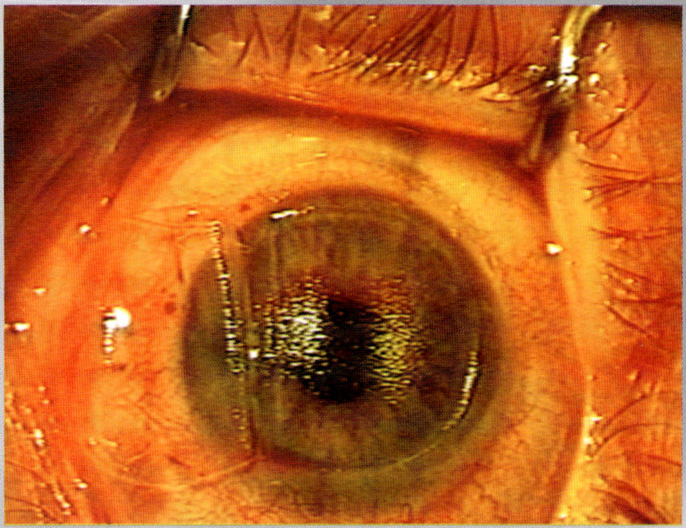

Complications and their Management

SECTION THREE

LASIK Complications and Management

34

Melania Cigales, Jairo E Hoyos,
Jairo Hoyos-Chacón (Spain)

In the last few years, owing to the speed of surgery and visual recovery along with a good visual outcome, LASIK has become the most popular refractive technique. However, like all surgical procedures, LASIK is not without its possible complications. These complications can be intraoperative, arising while creating the flap with the microkeratome or during ablation with the excimer laser. The incidence of these complications diminishes throughout the surgeon's learning curve and with each technological development. However, even when surgery is successfully undertaken, complications may also appear in the postoperative period. Herein, we discuss the most common complications of LASIK and their management.

MICROKERATOME COMPLICATIONS

One of the most important steps when performing LASIK surgery is creating the corneal flap using the microkeratome. A good corneal flap needs to be smooth and even, of an appropriate thickness including the epithelium, Bowman's membrane and anterior stroma, and of a diameter that allows the exposure of sufficient stromal bed to perform the ablation. At times, the characteristics of flap obtained are not those desired, and we should be very aware of the possible complications that can arise while creating the flap using the microkeratome. In this way, we will be able to prevent them or suitably resolve any complications that do occur.

Free Cap

To create the flap, we must stop the motion of the microkeratome before it completes its full stroke, or alternatively use a stopper. When the corneal disc finishes up unattached to the cornea by a hinge, then we have what is called a free cap (Fig. 34.1). Perhaps the most frequent cause of a free cap is, however, a very flat cornea. Patients with flat corneas and a mean keratometry of less than 41 diopters present a higher risk of a free cap occurring.[1] A flat cornea will

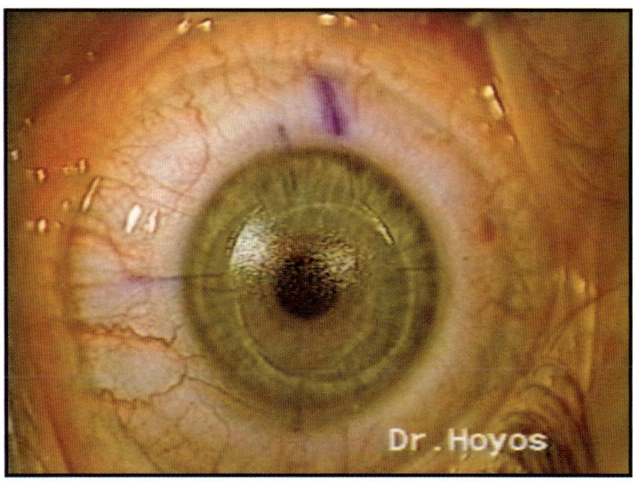

Fig. 34.1: Free cap

protrude relatively less into the suction ring compared to a steep cornea, and this will give rise to a smaller diameter disc and a free cap. This problem only affects primary flat corneas since a flat cornea secondary to refractive surgery will behave exactly as the original cornea curvature. Some microkeratomes include calibration lenses that help calibrate the stopper depending on the diameter predicted for the flap. Other instruments have several suction rings and stoppers which are selected according to the keratometric readings.

When a free cap is obtained, we are confronted with two potential complications during the surgical procedure. The most serious of these is that it is often impossible to differentiate between the epithelial and stromal sides of the disc.[2] If the disc is replaced with the epithelial side face-down, there is a risk of epithelialization of the interface and loss of the disc. A further complication arises from the difficulty of repositioning the disc in its exact position. If the disc is rotated on the stromal bed, this commonly gives rise to astigmatism. Every LASIK surgeon must be aware of the possibility of a free cap and must be prepared for this complication by always using the epithelial reference markings.

When a free cap occurs, we can continue with the surgical procedure and place the disc in an anti-desiccation chamber with the epithelial surface facing downwards[3] during the ablation step. Once the ablation is complete, the disc can then be repositioned and the markings aligned until the disc has attached to its bed.

Incomplete Flap

During a keratectomy, the microkeratome can stop before completing its stroke and give rise to an incomplete flap and a corneal bed of insufficient size to perform an ablation (Fig. 34.2). Some microkeratomes have a protection mechanism whereby they automatically stop if there is a loss of suction pressure while conducting the keratectomy, designed to impede continuous cutting and greater complications.[4] However, at times the driving motor of the instrument may fail.[4] One of the most common reasons for an automatic microkeratome with an electric motor to break-down is entry of the water used to help the instrument slide. It is, therefore, recommended that we have the microkeratome checked by the manufacture on a routine basis. In other cases, the microkeratome becomes blocked by the blepharostat, the eyelashes or eyelids.[1] It is thus essential that we prepare the surgical field well, covering eyelids and eyelashes with adhesive strips so that they do not interrupt the microkeratome stroke. Also, only use blepharostats that open the eye widely.

The size of the exposed corneal bed can be measured with callipers to check whether it will be large enough for the ablation. We could even perform the ablation by slightly decreasing the optical zone and protect the hinge to avoid its ablation. However, when the exposed bed is insufficient for ablation, surgery should be suspended; we should not attempt to prolong the keratectomy by manual dissection because this induces irregular astigmatism which is not easily resolved.[5] A few months later, a slightly deeper keratectomy can be attempted. If we make it shallower and part of the first flap remains on the bed, during ablation, tissue might be moved and lost

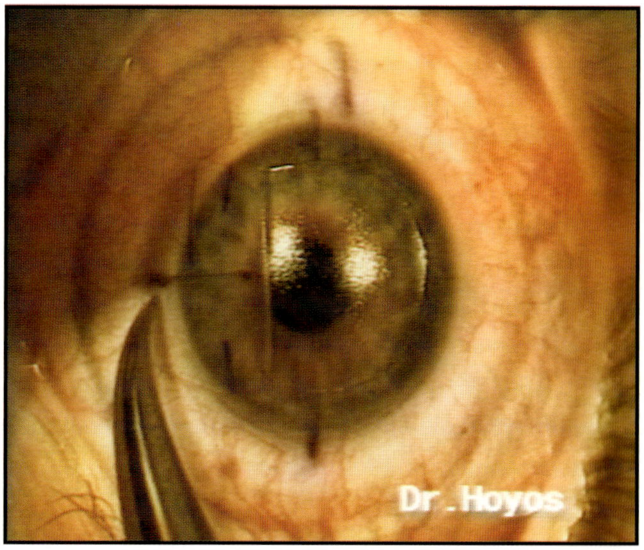

Fig. 34.2: Incomplete flap

provoking irregular astigmatism and intense hyperopization.[6]

Thin Flaps, Buttonholes and Irregular Cuts

It is widely accepted by LASIK surgeons that the ideal flap thickness is 130 to 160 microns. This measure is determined by the plate in the microkeratome head. However, most microkeratomes generally produce thinner cuts than expected and several pachymetric studies have indicated a high degree of variability in the thicknesses achieved.[7] Thin flaps are commonly associated with the complication of a central hole known as a buttonhole (Fig. 34.3). The most common causes of thin flaps, buttonholes and irregular cuts are: inadequate suction, poor blade quality, steep corneas and microkeratome malfunction.[8]

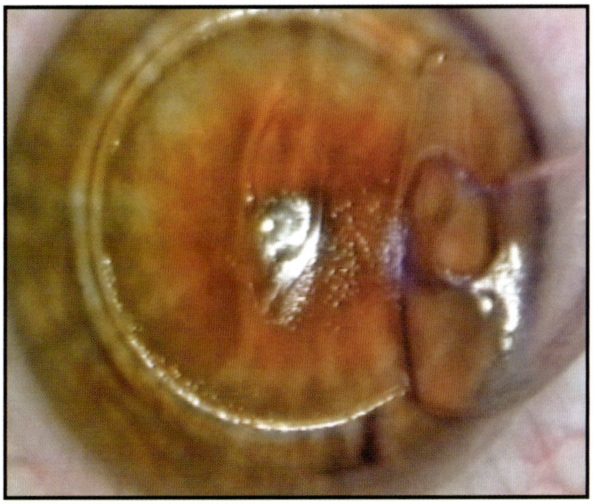

Fig. 34.3: Buttonhole

The suction ring induces an ocular hypertension above the 70-100 mm Hg required to perform the keratectomy. A lack of pressure may be due to inadequate fitting of the suction ring on the eyeball. This commonly occurs in the case of small sunken orbits or astigmatic eyes, over which it is difficult to place the ring.[8] If suction is completely lost and the microkeratome continues to function, we will obtain a free, irregular and small cut possibly affecting the pupillary area[1] (Fig. 34.4). Most of the new instruments have a protection mechanism to stop cutting when there is a loss in suction pressure. These models at most will give rise to an incomplete flap.

A dull blade creates a thin and perhaps irregular cut.[9] Sometimes, remnants of Bowman's membrane can be seen on the stromal bed (Fig. 34.5). Blade quality varies considerably and for this reason it is crucial to check and calibrate the blade in order to reject those with an irregular edge or a small gap (the distance between the blade and plate correlates with the thickness of the keratectomy).[8] Many surgeons reuse the same blade on 4 or 6 eyes. After each pass, the blade looses its sharpness creating a thinner cut each time. We therefore recommend using a new blade for each patient.

Corneal curvatures greater than 46 diopters cause thin and large diameter discs and carry a risk of buttonhole formation due to corneal buckling during

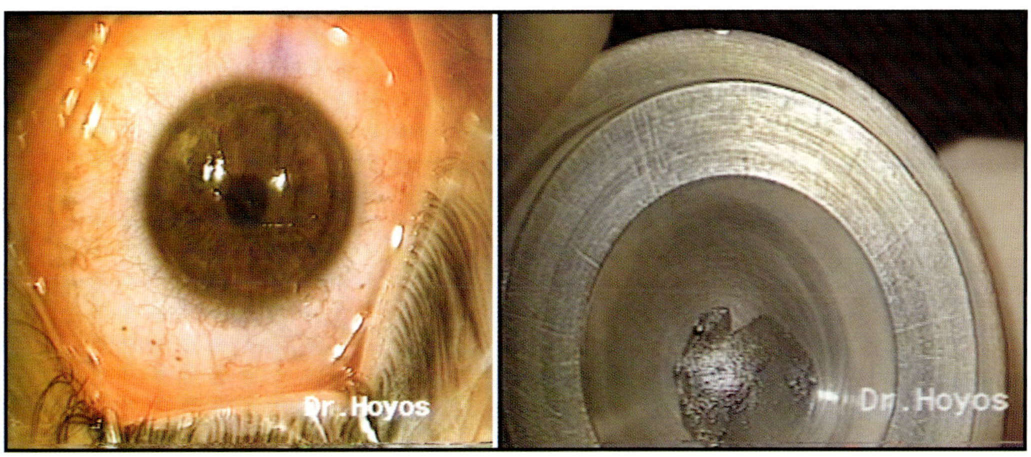

Fig. 34.4: Lost suction

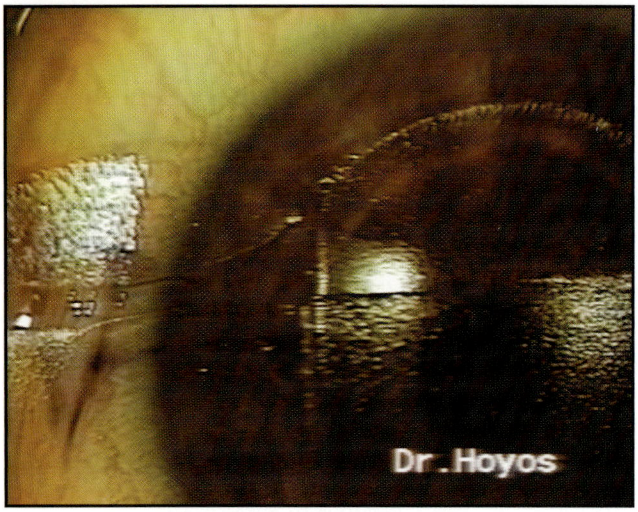

Fig. 34.5: Thin, irregular flap

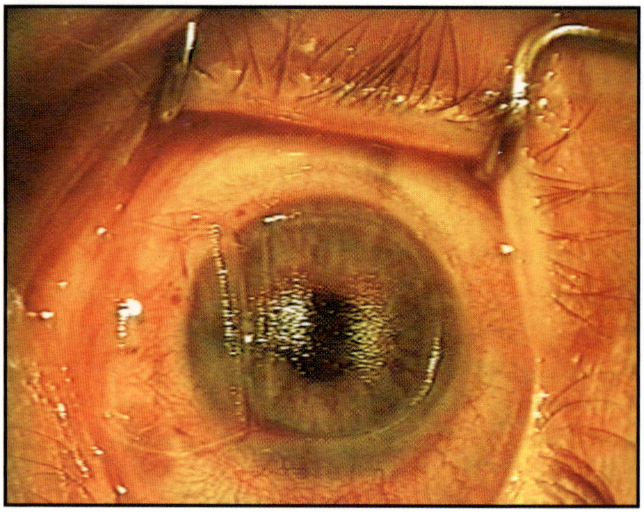

Fig. 34.6: Irregular cut

the microkeratome pass.[2] In the case of a steep cornea, we recommend the use of a 180-micron plate or a blade with a larger gap.

While performing the keratectomy, the microkeratome should be guided such that it undergoes uniform movements to achieve a smooth, even corneal bed. Any malfunction of the automatic microkeratome, or slipping of the manual instrument, preventing a uniform stroke can give rise to an irregular resection leading to an uneven stromal bed (Fig. 34.6) and thus to irregular astigmatism.

We believe than whenever one of these complications occurs at the time of creating the flap, the best thing is to interrupt the procedure and replace the flap, and then attempt another keratectomy 3 or 6 months later using a thicker plate.

Epithelial Defects

The epithelium of the corneal flap can become damaged during the keratectomy causing late and painful visual recovery. This complication is more common in diabetic or elderly patients or in those with dystrophy of the Bowman's membrane since the corneal epithelium is more fragile.[10] In this subset of patients, both eyes may show epithelial alterations. However, there are also certain intraoperative conditions that will induce damage to epithelial cells such as excessive topical anesthetic, which can be toxic for this delicate layer, or a keratectomy performed on a dry epithelium.[4] Anesthetics should be kept to a minimum and if possible should be free of preservatives. Moreover, the cornea should be moistened at the time of the keratectomy to help the microkeratome slide over the cornea and try to prevent abrasion of the corneal epithelium.

If the corneal epithelium is damaged, we should be careful when handling the flap and should meticulously wash the interface to avoid seeding epithelial cells causing its epithelialization.[2] We prefer to reposition the altered epithelium, but if this is not possible we carefully remove it. To avoid a painful postoperative course, it is best to include a mydriatic in the patient's normal medication and cover the eye or use a therapeutic contact lens until the cornea becomes re-epithelialized. The postoperative course of these cases is usually good, although there are reports of recurrent erosion syndromes,[11] which could be caused by a pre-existing dystrophy of the Bowman's membrane going unnoticed in the preoperative examination. A further possible cause is the transient corneal denervation that occurs after LASIK.

Corneal Bleeding

Corneal bleeding usually occurs in contact lens wearers, who often have more corneal neovessels (Fig. 34.7).[4] To prevent corneal bleeding in such cases, the keratectomy may be slightly decentered downwards to avoid cutting neovessels. Bleeding also occurs when the diameter of the corneal flap is excessive and almost practically reaches the limbus.[4] This frequently happens when the cornea is very steep and can sometimes be prevented using a suction ring that yields a smaller flap diameter. This complication is commonly related to the use of certain microkeratomes such as the Hansatome.

Every effort should be made to stop bleeding and we should try to avoid the blood invading the interface during ablation since this might cause uneven ablation. We can wait a few minutes without lifting the flap until the hemorrhage resolves. Compression maneuvers or the use of a sponge with vasoconstrictor over the area of blood loss may be useful.[2] Once ablation is complete, we should make sure we leave no blood remnants at the interface, which should be carefully washed to avoid triggering an inflammation process.

Corneal Perforation

Corneal perforation is the most serious complication related to the use of the microkeratome which occurs when we forget to position the plate in the instrument head or when it is not properly adjusted.[12] Due to an increased intraocular pressure during keratectomy, corneal perforation is usually associated with the partial or total loss of the iris and crystalline lens and even with the loss of eye contents (Fig. 34.8). The management of this complication is complex and stressful, but we should try to remain calm and attempt to recompose the globe with the help of viscoelastic, followed by suturing the cornea. At a later date, we will select the best surgical option to restore the patient's vision.

To avoid this devastating complication, new microkeratome models do not have interchangeable plates; their have different heads to obtained different cutting depths.

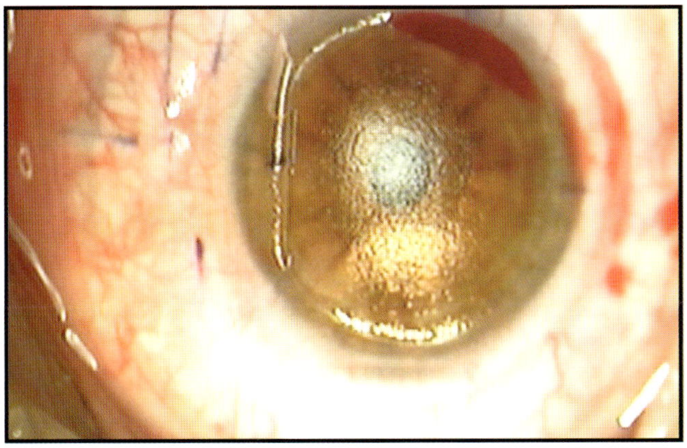

Fig. 34.7: Corneal bleeding

LASER COMPLICATIONS

Since the first excimer laser was designed in one of IBM's laboratories in 1987, there have been numerous technical advances that have induced the rapid development of laser technology. This has meant a rapidly declining incidence of complications caused by applying the excimer laser on the stromal bed, which are also ever less serious. We propose several therapeutic options for the treatment of these complications.

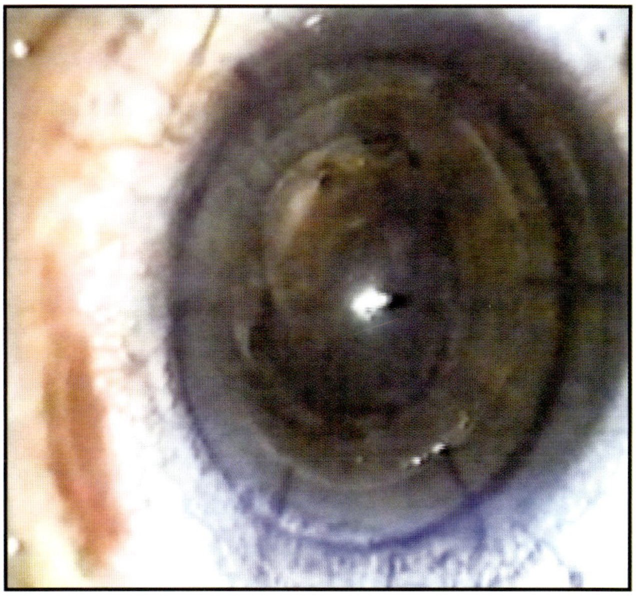

Fig. 34.8: Corneal perforation

Decentered Ablation

A decentered ablation may give rise to irregular astigmatism (Fig. 34.9) and to symptoms such as glare, ghosting, monocular diplopia, impaired night vision, reduced contrast sensitivity and even loss of best corrected visual acuity.[13] Although small decenterations are usually asymptomatic,[14] symptoms are exacerbated when treatment involves small optical zones or correcting high refractive errors.[15]

The surgeon should first ensure that the laser beam is correctly centered before initiating the laser session and the patient must be correctly positioned under the excimer laser. It is helpful to constantly encourage the patient to fix his/her sight on the fixation target. Finally, it is the surgeon's task to adequately center refractive treatment, although there is a lack of consensus concerning the point over which an ablation should be centered: at the corneal reflex or center of the pupil.[16] Most modern lasers have a built-in eye-tracking device which, despite avoiding severe decenteration, cannot ensure perfect centering.[17]

Several surgical treatments have been proposed for decentered ablations over the last few years. Pallikaris[18] suggests relaxed corneal incisions in the steep zone. Pallikaris[19] and Talamo[10] also advocate smoothing the corneal surface using a viscous solution and performing a phototherapeutic ablation until an even optical surface is achieved. In 1995, Seiler performed an ablation on the opposite side as treatment. The procedure involved establishing the new ablation center by topography and calculating the dioptric power of the new ablation as the topographic difference between the two zones.[21,22] The development of Topolink appeared to be the solution to treating decentered ablations and irregular astigmatism.[23] The technique is based on a topographically-guided ablation using elevation topography and a previously programmed flying spot laser. In this way, the amount of ablation needed at different points on the cornea to achieve a smooth surface is calculated. The final outcome of all these treatment methods has, nevertheless, been highly inconsistent. Customized ablations based on wavefront analysis have recently emerged as the latest treatment option for this complication.

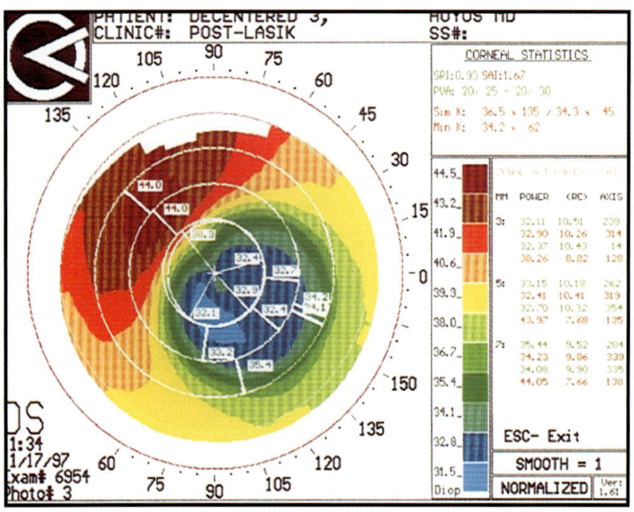

Fig. 34.9: Decentered ablation

In 1995, we treated a decentered ablation for the first time in a patient who had undergone *in situ* keratomileusis (ALK), by ablating the opposite side by LASIK retreatment.[24] Through elevation topography, we were able to establish the point at which to center treatment and the amount of tissue to be ablated according to the elevation difference in microns indicated in the topographic map. It is currently possible to simulate eccentric ablation treatment using topographic simulation programs that predict the topographic outcome before initiating treatment[25] (Fig. 34.10). We presently use the PAR Vision System topographer to measure the elevation and depression in microns at different points on the cornea with respect to a perfect sphere. Thus, points that correspond to a perfect sphere have an elevation of zero. Elevation values in microns are given a plus sign and depression values are indicated with a minus sign. The topographer determines the center of the decentered ablation and its depression. We use the 1 mm grille topographer tool to measure the distance from the middle of the decentered ablation to the visual axis at "x" and "y" axes. These measures are then used to pinpoint the opposite point ("mirror point") in the topography and the topographer measures the elevation at this point. We then use the simulation software to simulate a new ablation at the

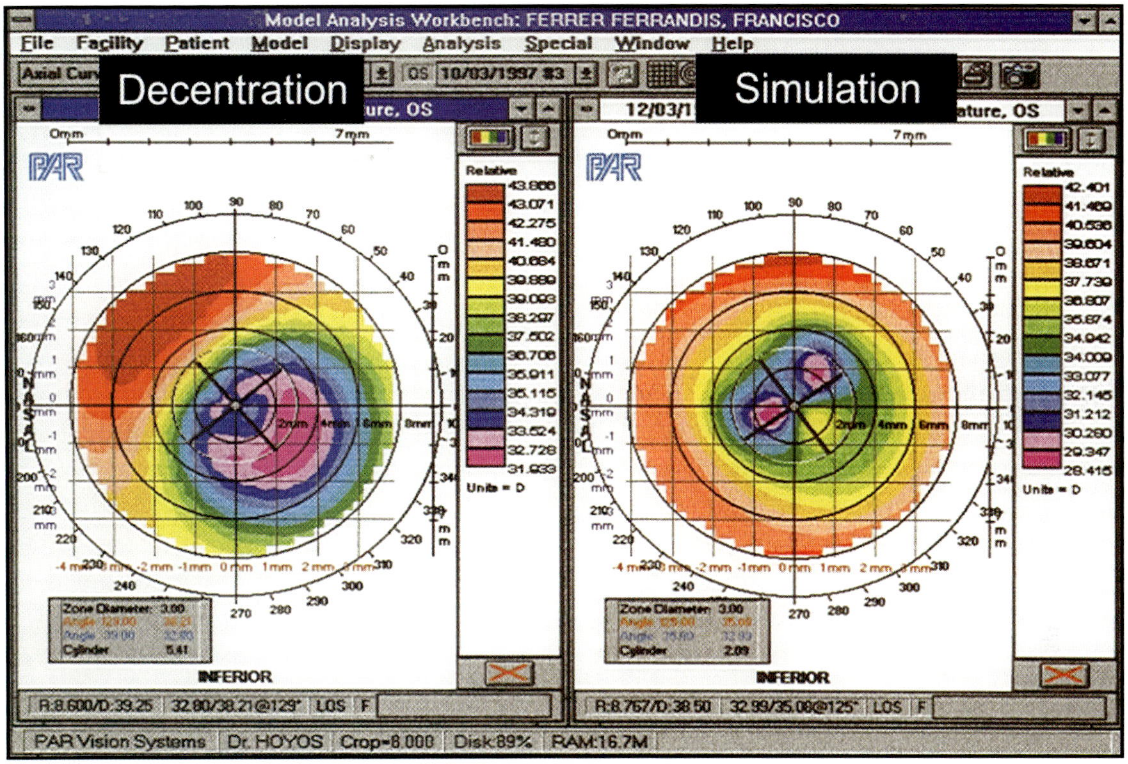

Fig. 34.10: Treating decentrations by guided topographic simulation: outcome

mirror point: the depth of the ablation is given by the sum of the elevation and depression calculated beforehand, and the optical zone corresponding to the best simulated topography is selected.

In cases of decentered LASIK, the flap is lifted using the technique normally employed in retreatments. The laser is programmed using the data obtained by guided topographic simulation (optical zone, ablation depth and mirror point). The laser then automatically decenters and focuses on the new ablation center at the established mirror point and the ablation is performed under patient self-fixation. Once treatment achieves a centered topography, the residual refractive error is retreated following a 3 month waiting period.

Central Islands

A central island is a central or paracentral steep area in the topography of 1 to 3 diopters in height and diameter 1 to 3 mm, measured at least 1 month postoperatively[26] (Fig. 34.11). Symptoms include monocular diplopia, ghosting of images, fluctuating vision and sometimes loss of lines of corrected visual acuity.[27] Central islands are more frequent when a broad beam laser is used but there are some predisposing factors[28,29] such as a moist cornea during the ablation, large optical zones, high levels of

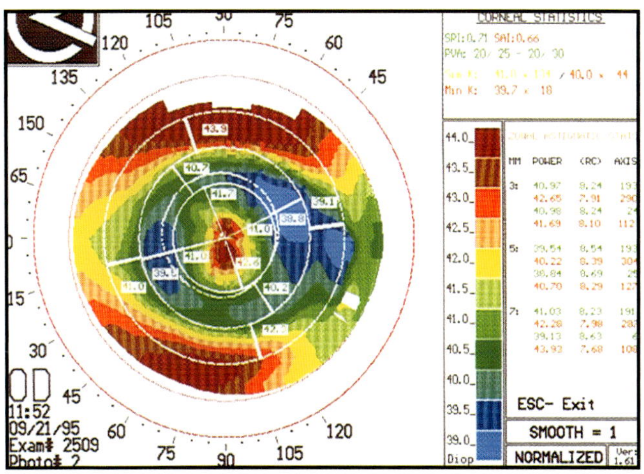

Fig. 34.11: Central island

correction, a damaged laser mirror and a laser beam cold in the center. To prevent this complication, we must check the laser mirror and laser beam homogeneity before initiating the laser session, and wipe the bed during the ablation if it is wet. The new broad-beam lasers are equipped with anticentral island pretreatment software.

LASIK central islands show modifications during topographical follow-up. Most central islands resolve spontaneously during the first 3 to 4 months and do not require treatment.[30] A variety of surgical treatments have been described to treat elevated central island areas including central reablations,[31] topographically-guided ablations,[32] Healon-assisted PTK[33] and mechanical compression in the center of the cornea (G Avalos - personal communication). We have noted that patients with persisting central islands undergo an improvement in their visual acuity after 3 to 4 months, with a low residual myopic defect left. Three to four months after LASIK surgery, we retreat these patients by lifting the flap and treating the residual myopia with an optical zone 1 mm larger than the diameter of the topographical island.

POSTOPERATIVE COMPLICATIONS

The patient who undergoes LASIK should be subjected to early and frequent follow-up examinations to be able to identify and quickly treat any postoperative complications such as infection, inflammatory or traumatic processes in the corneal flap, as well as problems in the healing process. However, even after the postoperative follow-up period, we should continue to monitor these patients since serious complications can also occur in the longer-term. Below we discuss the most common early and late complications of LASIK and options for their treatment.

Flap Folds and Wrinkles

One of the complications of LASIK is the formation of folds or striae in the corneal flap, causing irregular astigmatism and loss of visual acuity (Fig. 34.12). Striae may form during surgery due to the incorrect repositioning of the flap over the stromal bed, or in the early postoperative period if the disc is slightly displaced by blinking.[34] In the past it was thought that the nasal flap was a cause of striae formation, since it promoted displacement during blinking in the early postoperative course. Displacement is less common with a superior flap but striae still appear. We generally observe horizontal striae in nasal flaps and vertical striae in superior flaps. In the early days of LASIK, flaps created with large hinges were easily correctly repositioned. Nowadays, however, to perform ablations with large optical zones and peripheral ablations to correct hyperopia, we try to create a flap of minimum hinge. In these cases, it is important to make epithelial reference marks and correctly align these when we reposition the flap over its bed. If the reference marks are misaligned, this means that the flap is wrinkled or slightly displaced leading to the formation of folds and striae. Striae formation is also more common in the case of a thin corneal disc. It is important to check for correct alignment using the slit-lamp, and if this complication is noted, to immediately lift the flap, hydrate it and reposition it by careful alignment.[35]

The LASIK surgeon should be aware of this complication and try to avoid it. If detected, folds and striae need to be rapidly treated. Opinions vary concerning treatment, but these measures are always

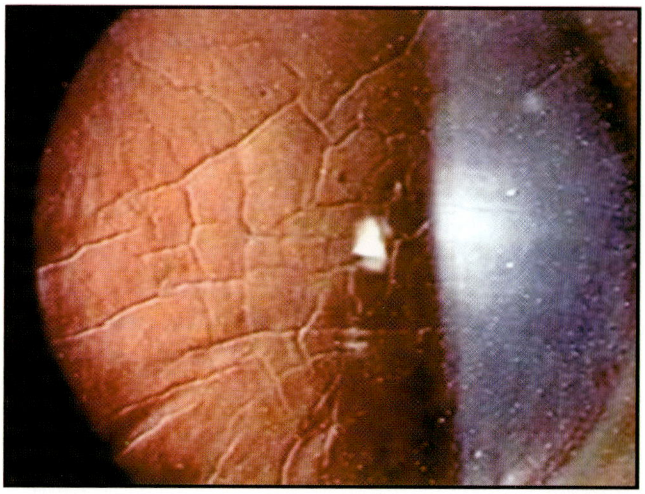

Fig. 34.12: Flap folds and wrinkles

aimed at rehydrating the disc or de-epithelialization after hydrating old folds.[36] Some years ago we presented a new technique for the treatment of flap striae with good results also for old striae.[37] The technique involves lifting the flap, hydrating, repositioning the flap over the stromal bed and massaging the flap using a spatula over a contact lens. Unlike other methods of treatment, this massaging is effective at removing flap striae as late as one month after surgery.

Flap Loss

Today, whenever LASIK is performed, we use the microkeratome to try to create a corneal flap, since this is considered the safest way of preventing disc displacement and loss. If the microkeratome does not stop at the right moment the cut may result in a free cap. The complication most feared with a free cap is the loss of the disc, such that certain precautions need to be taken before the patient leaves the clinic. First, the eyelids are closed using two crossed adhesive strips for approximately half an hour after surgery. We then check the patient and if we find that the disc has moved, we reposition it and close the lid until the next day. If the disc is found to be in the right position, the patient is sent home wearing only an eye shield and is instructed to follow the general directions for flaps. Due to the risk of losing the disc, we prefer to personally remove the eye shield or patch the next day such that we do not discard any dressing before making sure the disc is adhered to the cornea.

There have been reports of traumatic detachment of a disc despite having the security of a flap, and even cases of surgical amputation of the flap as an attempt to control an infection (Internet forum of the KM Study Group). In both these situations, some of the thickness of the cornea and the Bowman's membrane are lost. The most simple treatment option is to await the re-epithelialization of the cornea and to treat the case as we would treat a PRK to avoid haze.[38] One would think that as corneal tissue was removed, the eye would finish up with tremendous hyperopia, but the results obtain do not show any hyperopic deviations and residual defects are usually slightly irregular myopic astigmatisms.[38] We should not forget that the corneal disc has two parallel sides and therefore has no refractive power of its own. If the final visual outcome is unsatisfactory, we should move onto undertaking a lamellar keratoplasty.

Interface Debris

On slit-lamp examination, it is sometimes possible to detect small particles at the flap/stromal interface (Fig. 34.13). In general, these are of no clinical significance and they do not induce an inflammatory response, but in other cases they could give rise to Sands of the Sahara syndrome.[39] These could be metallic particles[40] from the microkeratome that are

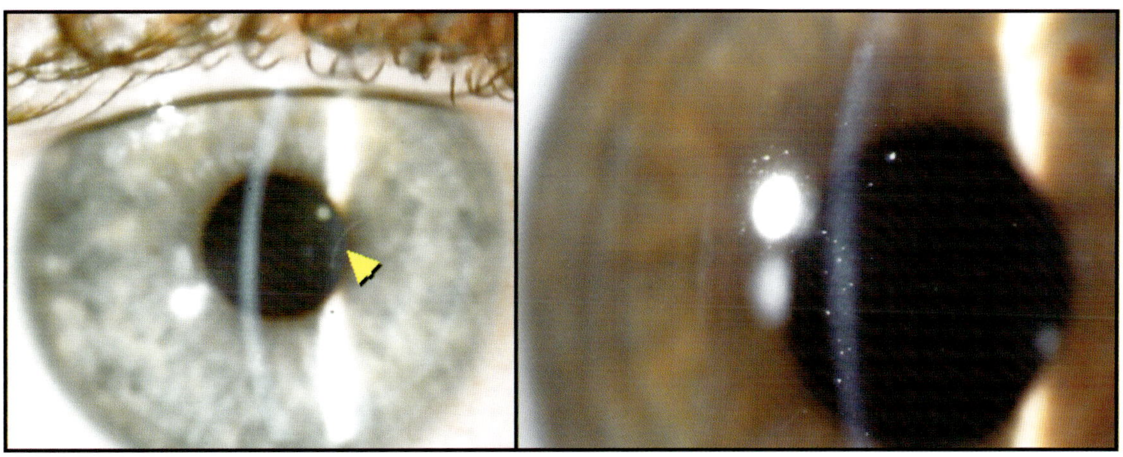

Fig. 34.13: Interface debris

difficult to remove during irrigation of the interface. Sometimes, the particles are remnants of cosmetic products, small gauze or cotton threads, talc from the gloves or even secretions that become trapped at the interface when we reposition the flap. To prevent this complication, we should try to keep our surgery free of particles using gloves without talc and avoid the use of gauze, cotton threads or fabrics.[4] Eyelids and lashes should also be meticulously cleaned before surgery and the patient should be asked to avoid the use of eye make-up a few days before surgery. A further important factor is that the stromal side of the bed and flap have to be well-cleaned using an irrigation-aspiration system when repositioning the flap. Irrigating the interface with a fine cannula after the flap has been repositioned to remove any trapped particles is also recommended.

Sands of the Sahara Syndrome

Inflammation of the interface was first described by Robert Maddox who named this phenomenon Sands of the Sahara syndrome, given its desert sand-like appearance[41] (Fig. 34.14). This complication is also known as diffuse lamellar keratitis (DLK) and starts within the first 24 to 48 hours following surgery with the appearance of a diffuse infiltrate at the interface, reduced visual acuity, pain, red eye and topographical irregularity.[39] Microscopy studies have demonstrated the presence of inflammatory cells at the interface.[42] The causes of this inflammation are not clear, but it has been related to the presence of particles at the interface,[39] particles on the microkeratome blades,[41] methods of cleaning the surgical instruments,[43] etc. The risk of this complication is multiplied when there is an epithelial defect[44] and cases have been reported both in primary LASIK surgery and retreatments. Possible causes should be kept in mind to try to avoid this complication in as much as possible.

An early diagnosis and treatment are essential for successfully resolving this complication. Treatment involves increasing topical corticosteroids and in cases of intense inflammation, the flap should be lifted and the interface profusely rinsed to remove the possible toxic substance.[39] These cases are generally effectively resolved with the complete recovery of visual acuity and no sequelae. However, some surgeons describe a greater difficulty in lifting the flap when retreatment is required (Internet forum of the KM Study Group). We should always establish a differential diagnosis from infectious keratitis of the interface.

Epithelial Ingrowth

The proliferation of epithelial cells at the flap/stromal bed interface (Fig. 34.15) is a complication that lessens throughout the surgeon's learning curve as the surgical maneuvers aimed at avoiding the intro-

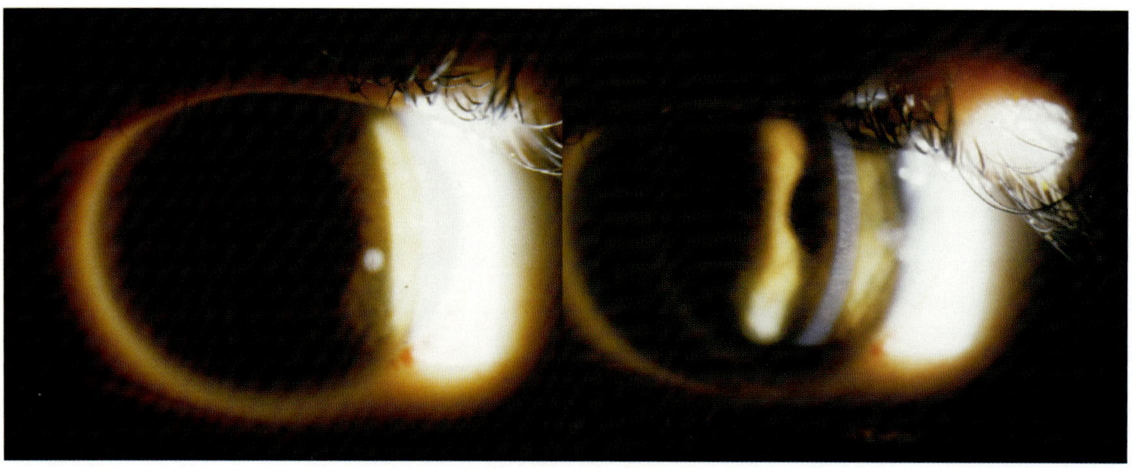

Fig. 34.14: Sands of the Sahara syndrome

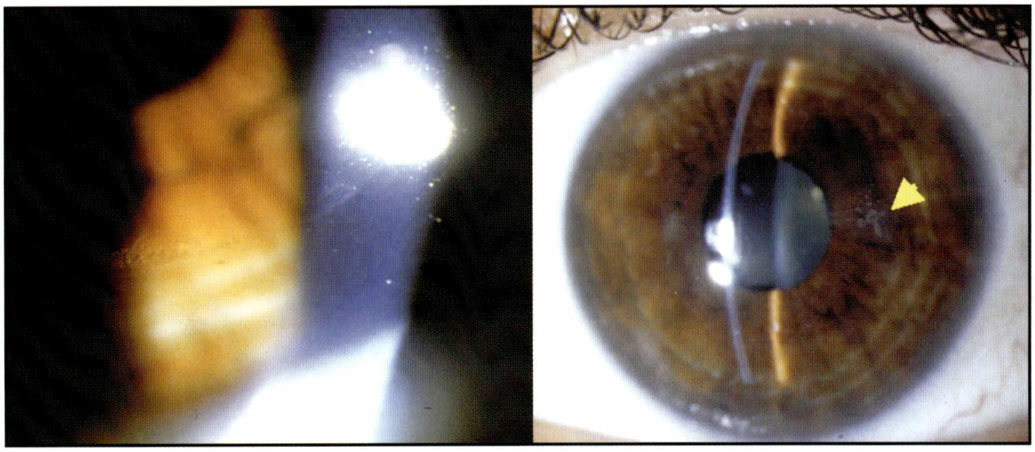

Fig. 34.15: Epithelial ingrowth

duction of epithelium under the flap improve. This complication is more common in certain situations:

- Retreatments, in which epithelial strands are produced, promoting epithelialization.[45]
- When an epithelial defect is produced during surgery because of an already altered corneal epithelial basement membrane (elderly or diabetic patients or patients with corneal dystrophy), detached epithelial cells may settle at the interface.[45, 46]
- When there is inflammation of the interface causing flap edema this induces peripheral epithelial invasion.[45]
- During hyperopic LASIK, a peripheral ablation will induce the advance of the epithelium from the stromal bed.[47]
- In the case of flaps with radial keratotomy incisions, epithelialization occurs through the insicions[48] (Fig. 34.16).

In most cases, epithelial ingrowth occurs as small self-contained peripheral islets observed at 2 to 3 weeks that do not grow nor cause any symptoms. Thus, no treatment is necessary. However, sometimes epithelial ingrowth continues and gives rise to irregular astigmatism and reduced visual acuity such that it needs to be removed[45] (Fig. 34.17). There are descriptions of cases of epithelialization causing melting of the flap, attributed to defects in the supply of nutrients to the flap or inflammatory processes secondary to epithelialization.[49] Most cases of melting are peripheral, self-contained and of no clinical significance.

The treatment of epithelial ingrowth is not always definitive and there is always a risk of recurrence. Treatment consists of lifting the flap and scraping the epithelium of the interface. Several surgical treatments have been proposed for recurrences: absolute alcohol, PTK performed on both stromal surfaces, YAG laser treatment and on some occasions, it has even been necessary to amputate the flap and perform a lamellar keratoplasty.[50] We know that

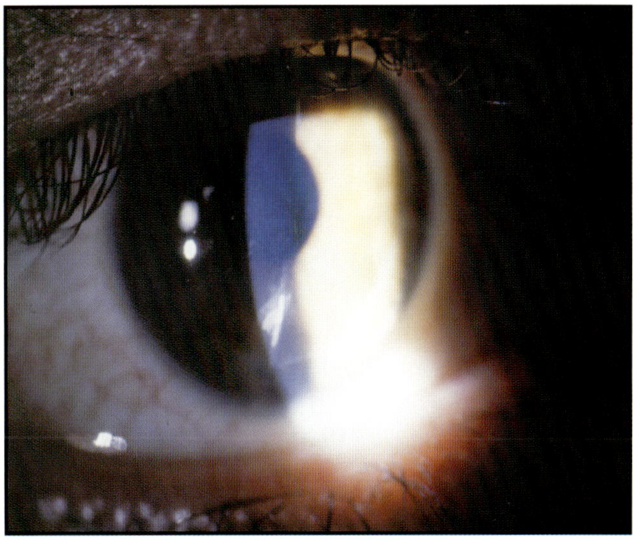

Fig. 34.16: Epithelial ingrowth through radial keratotomy incisions

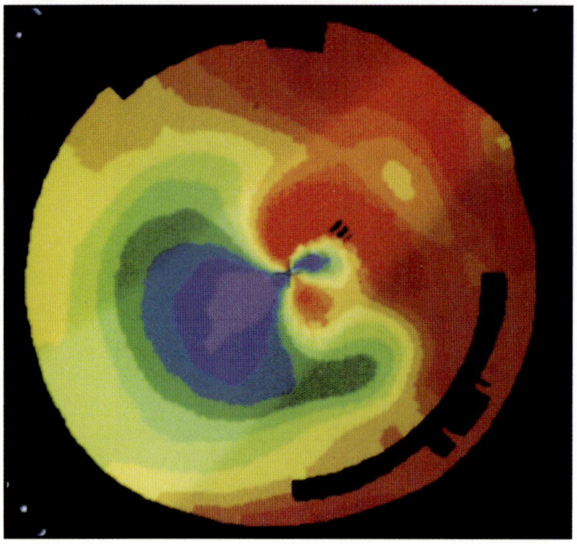

Fig. 34.17: Epithelial ingrowth causes irregular astigmatism

during the epithelial healing process of the cornea, epithelium growth from the flap and from the epithelial border of the bed, contacting in the flap border with a risk of recurrence. For this reason we scrape the epithelium of the bed until the limbus and both epithelium growth, contacting near to the limbus and far to the flap border. We should not wait until the epithelium colonizes the central zone of the cornea before embarking on treatment, since after removing the ingrowth tissue we are usually left with a leukoma at the interface which could reduce the patient's final visual acuity.

Infection

Infection is uncommon in LASIK surgery since the edge of the flap becomes reepithelialized a few hours later, thus rapidly restoring the epithelial barrier. However, when this complication arises, its effects are devastating since the focus of infection occurs at the interface and is related to a high risk of corneal perforation and endophthalmitis. Infections can be:

- Intraoperative—due to contamination of the surgical instruments or field of surgery.
- Postoperative—when the patient does not complete the antibiotic prophylaxis regime or exposes him-/herself to a risk of infection in the early postoperative period such as water sports, use of eye make-up, eye trauma, etc.

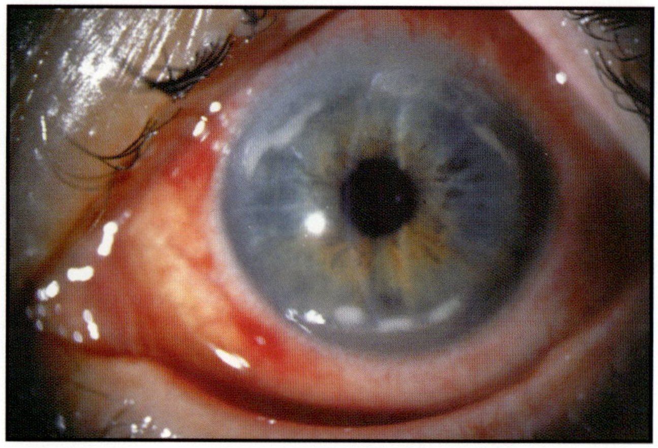

Fig. 34.18: Infection

Patients with blepharitis are at an increased risk of infection and should be diagnosed and treated before surgery.

The clinical signs of bacterial infection can appear in the first few days but when symptoms appear after several weeks, the causative agent is a fungus, an acanthamoeba or slow-growing bacterium.[51] Patients experience pain, weeping, photophobia and blurred vision, symptoms not pathognomic for diagnosis. A slit-lamp examination reveals conjunctival hyperemia, corneal infiltrates or ulcers (Fig. 34.18), flap melting, an inflammatory reaction in the anterior chamber and hypopyon.

When infection is suspected, we should first treat the patient as for a corneal abscess by topical hourly administration of wide-spectrum antibiotics against Gram-positive and Gram-negative microorganisms. This regime can then be modified according to subsequent culture and antiobiogram results.[51] Some cases require lifting the flap and irrigating the interface with an antibiotic solution.[52] The need for flap amputation[53] or a hot penetrating keratoplasty[54] have also been described. Once the infection is controlled, subsequent surgical measures to improve the visual acuity lost because of the resultant corneal opacity and irregularity will need to be considered.

Dry Eye

Refractive corneal surgery can lead to temporarily reduced tear production lasting weeks or months which appears to be related to the transient corneal denervation that occurs after surgery.[55] As the flap is cut, we also cut the nerve endings of the cornea, causing corneal hypoesthesia that gives rise to reduced tear production, taking months to resolve.[56] The highest density of nerve fibers enters the cornea through the nasal and temporal zones and it is therefore speculated that a superior flap will cause more denervation and greater tear secretion disruption than a nasal flap.[57] Although this complication does not greatly affect the final refractive outcome, over some months, patients complain of visual acuity fluctuations and transient episodes of regression and induced astigmatism which are difficult to correct with spectacles.[58] On slit-lamp examination we can observe a superficial punctate epitheliopathy (Fig. 34.19) and the topography shows an irregular cornea.

In our personal experience, these cases benefit from the use of preservative-free artificial tears and blocking the inferior lachrymal punctum. The recommended use of artificial tears during the first postoperative months is general to all patients undergoing corneal refractive surgery and attempts to avoid visual and refractive fluctuations caused by the reduced tear production. In the preoperative evaluation, we should include the Schirmer test and lachrymal BUT to identify cases of lachrymal hyposecretion that could worsen in the first few weeks after surgery. When preoperative lachrymal hyposecretion is moderate or mild, we should try to improve the quality and quantity of tears before indicating surgery using lachrymal punctum plugs, artificial tears and tear stimulating drugs. We do not recommend corneal surgery in cases of severely impaired tear secretion.

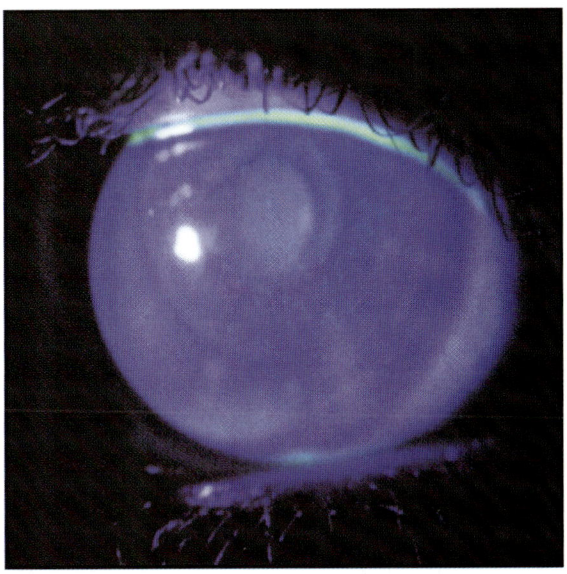

Fig. 34.19: Superficial punctate epitheliopathy after LASIK

Regression, Undercorrection and Overcorrection

The tissue repair process induced by LASIK surgery is accompanied by a regression of the effect achieved by surgery related to changes in corneal topography.[59] The scarring response varies in each patient precluding any generalizations. Regression has been associated with epithelial hypertrophy.[60] Most regression is thought to occur during the first weeks, and in this period patients describe visual fluctuations as a consequence of topographic and refractive changes.[59-61] Some authors[62] suggest that the length of the stabilizing period depends on the number of diopters corrected and estimate a month for each diopter. Accordingly, if we correct 1 diopter the stabilizing period will be one month, whereas if 10 diopters are corrected the stabilization process will last 10 months. It is true that the greater the correction the longer the period of stabilization.[61] In our routine practice, we usually wait at least a month before assessing refraction for the first time, although in the case of a residual refractive defect we normally wait 3 to 6 months before we make any decision on the possible benefits of retreatment.

Once refractive stability has been reached, there is always the possibility of a remaining refractive defect. Current nomograms have improved the predictability of refractive surgery, but residual refractive defects continue to occur. The gas in the excimer laser is highly unstable and can fluctuate with changes in humidity, pressure and temperature provoking under- and overcorrections. The environmental conditions in the surgery room should be well-controlled to avoid laser action fluctuations. Depending on the refractive and visual outcome, the degree of patient satisfaction and the limits of refractive surgery (corneal thickness and curvature), we may want to perform a retreatment. Under- and overcorrections after LASIK can be treated by the same technique, lifting the flap or recutting.[63, 64] After eight years of experience in myopic LASIK, we currently try to lift the flap whenever possible (Fig. 34.20). This is more difficult after hyperopic LASIK, and we have observed cases in which it was not possible to lift the flap after 2 years. If we create a new flap we should try to make it thicker than the first to avoid loss of tissue which would induce high hyperopia and irregular astigmatism, both being difficult to correct.[6] However, flap thickness, corneal curvature and repeat refractive surgeries pose a limit to retreatments using corneal techniques, and in some cases, the only surgical treatment option is the implant of an intraocular lens.

Corneal Ectasia

Post-LASIK corneal ectasia manifests as a progressive myopia accompanied by topographic incurving and loss of visual acuity, months or years after the intervention.[65] Topographical analysis is usually the key to detecting this complication.

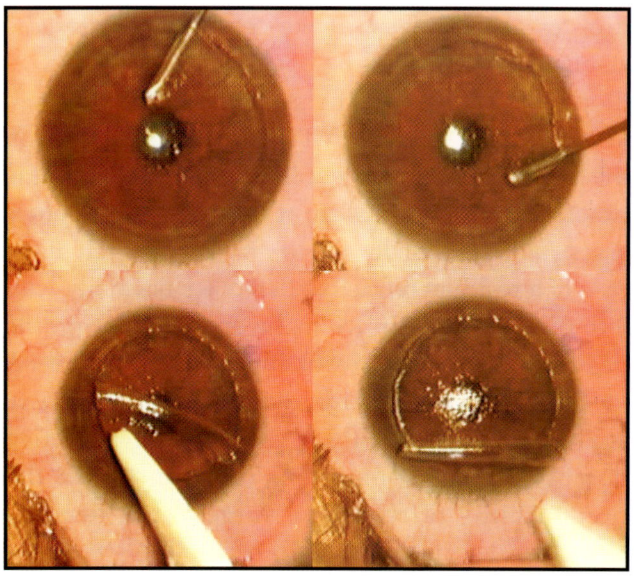

Fig. 34.20: Lifting the flap

Since the advent of keratomileusis, there have been descriptions of ectasia related to lamellar techniques, and from the beginning it was established that we should leave a residual stromal bed of 250 microns under the ablation. Some authors prefer a residual bed of 300 microns and others believe we should leave at least 50% of the corneal thickness under the ablation.[66] However, we should not forget the extensive range of microkeratome cutting depths, and after making our calculations may find the flap is too thick, highlighting the importance of intraoperative pachymetry.[7,67] Besides leaving a 250 micron residual bed, we try to leave a total corneal thickness of at least 400 microns and never ablate more than 150 microns. We should be particularly careful with retreatment LASIK. First, we should make a differential diagnosis between undercorrection and regression. We should also be aware of the thickness of the cornea so that we do not find ourselves with the surprise of an ectasia after retreating a minimal residual defect.

In some cases there can be a subclinical preoperative keratoconus (Fig. 34.21) and LASIK will enhance this corneal degenerative process. This possibility should be kept in mind and corneal surgery discouraged in patients with unstable myopia and a thinned or very steep cornea, especially if they also have some degree of asymmetric astigmatism.[68]

Treatments proposed in cases of ectasia are the use of a contact lens, intracorneal ring segments or penetrating or lamellar keratoplasty.[66,69]

Retinal Complications

There is little agreement among retinal specialists on the risks of LASIK, which include deterioration of the peripheral retina and the posterior pole in myopic patients. We believe that the suction ring used in LASIK to induce an intraocular pressure of 70 to 160 mm Hg, placed 4 mm from the corneoscleral limbus, may produce traction against the anterior vitreous and on the vitreous base provoking stretching of the anterior hyaloid and possibly also

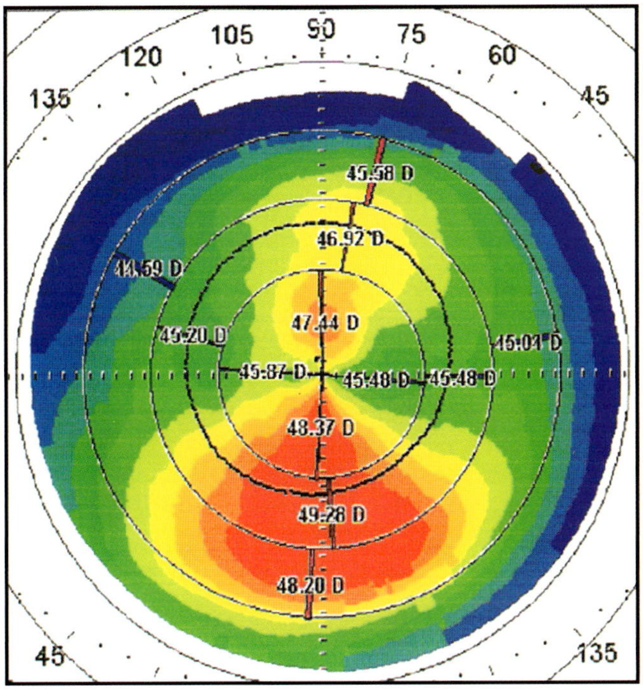

Fig. 34.21: Subclinical keratoconus

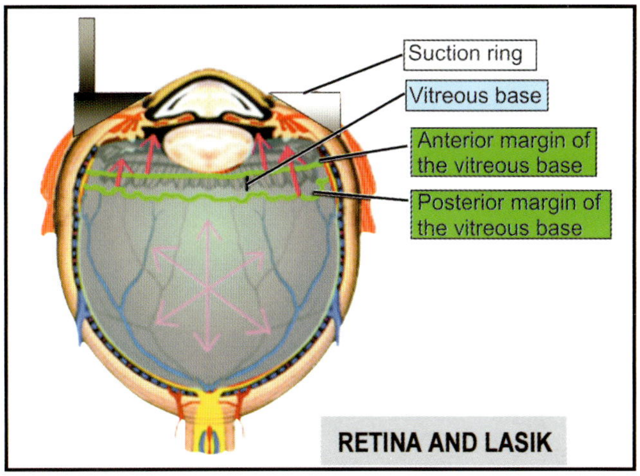

Fig. 34.22: Suction ring induces vitreous traction

of the posterior hyaloid (Fig. 34.22). The suction ring time is variable, about 12 seconds, which is the minimum time needed to create the flap, but this time depends on the difficulty of each case, the surgeon's experience and whether suction is applied only during flap cutting or also during the ablation. Suction time is longer in the learning phase of the surgeon and may also vary with the type of microkeratome used. We believe the suction time is an important factor in producing changes in vitreous anatomy.[70]

During LASIK, intraocular pressure can be 70 to 160 mm Hg. This hypertension can cause distension of the wall in an already established posterior staphyloma, with lengthening of the choriocapillaris - Bruch´s membrane - pigment epithelium complex, producing lacquer cracks which will provoke submacular hemorrhages or subretinal neovascularization in the postoperative period.[71, 72]

In a study performed on 755 eyes subjected to LASIK,[70] we detected retinal breaks in quadrants of generally low tear incidence (inferior-nasal sector), an increased intensity of white pressure-free areas, localized retinal detachment, peripheral retinal bleeding, pronounced circumferential folds, posterior extension and enhancement of the oral bays and macular hemorrhages from 12 days to two years post-LASIK. Other surgeons[71-74] have observed regmatogenous retinal detachment, partial atrophy of the optic nerve, paracentral visual field defects, the progression of previous subretinal neovascularization, giant retinal tears, increased posterior vitreous detachment, retinal branch venous occlusion and macular lacquer cracks.

The risk of further lesions post-LASIK is higher in patients with previous peripheral retinal lesions. We recommend examining and prophylactically treating predisposing retinal lesions with argon laser photocoagulation in all patients who are going to be treated with LASIK. We also recommend a further retinal examination post-LASIK, approximately one month later, carefully avoiding flap displacement during the examination.

REFERENCES

1. Jacobs JM, Taravella MJ. Incidence of intraoperative flap complications in laser *in situ* keratomileusis. J Cataract Refract Surg. 2002;28(1):23-28.
2. Slade SG. LASIK Complications and their Management. Machat JJ (Ed.). Excimer Laser Refractive Surgery. Thorofare, NJ: Slack Inc. 1996;358-400.
3. Cigales M, Hoyos JE J. Free Caps. In: Lucio Buratto, Stephen Brint (Eds). Custom LASIK: Surgical Techniques and Complications. Thorofare, NJ: SLAK Inc. 2003;226-27.

4. Buratto L, Brint S. Complications of LASIK. In: Lucio Buratto, Stephen Brint (Eds). Custom LASIK: Surgical Techniques and Complications. Thorofare, NJ: SLAK Inc. 2003;161-224.
5. Holland SP, Srivannaboon S, Reinstein DZ. Avoiding serious corneal complications of laser assisted *in situ* keratomileusis and photorefractive keratectomy. Ophthalmology. 2000;107(4):640-52.
6. Peters NT, Iskander NG, Gimbel HV. Minimizing the risk of recutting with a Hansatome over an existing Automated Corneal Shaper flap for hyperopic laser *in situ* keratomileusis enhancement. J Cataract Refract Surg. 2001;27(8):1328-32.
7. Gokmen F, Jester JV, Petroll WM, McCulley JP, Cavanagh HD. *In vivo* confocal microscopy through-focusing to measure corneal flap thickness after laser *in situ* keratomileusis. J Cataract Refract Surg. 2002; 28(6):962-70.
8. Cigales M, Hoyos JE J. Thin flaps and buttonholes. In: Lucio Buratto, Stephen Brint (Eds). Custom LASIK: Surgical Techniques and Complications. Thorofare, NJ: SLAK Inc. 2003;224-25.
9. Cummings A, Lavery F. Flap complications. In: Agarwal S, Agarwal A, Pallikaris IG, Neuhann TH, Knorz MC, Agarwal Amar (Eds). Refractive Surgery. Jaypee Bro Med Pub, New Delhi-India 2000;329-39.
10. Krüger J. Managing recurrent epithelial ingrowth. In: Lucio Buratto, Stephen Brint (Eds). Custom LASIK: Surgical Techniques and Complications. Thorofare, NJ: SLAK Inc. 2003;233.
11. Ti SE, Tan DT. Recurrent corneal erosion after laser *in situ* keratomileusis. Cornea. 2001;20(2):156-58.
12. Tabbara KF, El-Sheikh HF, Vera-Cristo CL. Complications of laser *in situ* keratomileusis (LASIK). Eur J Ophthalmol. 2003;13(2):139-46.
13. Mulhern MG, Foley-Nolan A, O'Keefe M, Condon PI. Topographical analysis of ablation centration after excimer laser photorefractive keratectomy and laser in situ keratomileusis for high myopia. J Cataract Refract Surg. 1997;23(4):488-94.
14. Verdon W, Bullimore M, Maloney RK. Visual performance after photorefractive keratectomy. Arch Ophthalmol. 1996;114:1465-72.
15. Kim WJ, Chung ES, Lee JH. Effect of optic zone size on the outcome of photorefractive keratectomy for myopia. J Cataract Refract Surg. 1996;22:197-204.
16. Uozato H, Guyton DL. Centering corneal surgical procedures. Am J Ophthalmol. 1987;103:264-70.
17. Tsai YY, Lin JM. Ablation centration after active eye-tracker-assisted photorefractive keratectomy and laser *in situ* keratomileusis. J Cataract Refract Surg. 2000; 26(1):28-34.
18. Pallikaris I, Siganos D. LASIK complications management. In: Talamo J, Krueger R (Eds). The Excimer Manual. Boston MA: Little, Brown. 1997;227-44.
19. Pallikaris I, Panagopoulou S, Katsanevaki V. The PALM technique: photoablated lenticular modulator. In: Pallikaris I, Siganos D (Eds). LASIK. Thorofare, NJ: Slack, Inc. 1997;277-78.
20. Talamo JH, Wagoner MD, Lee SY. Management of ablation decentration following excimer photorefractive keratectomy. Arch Ophthalmol. 1995;113:706-07.
21. Seiler T, McDonnell P. Excimer laser photorefractive keratectomy. Surv Ophthalmol. 1995;40:89-118.
22. Alkara N, Genth U, Seiler T. Diametral ablation – A technique to manage decentered photorefractive keratectomy for myopia. J Refract Surg. 1999;15:436-40.
23. Knorz MC, Jendritza B. Topographically-guided laser *in situ* keratomileusis to treat corneal irregularities. Ophthalmology. 2000;107(6):1138-43.
24. Hoyos JE, Cigales M. Decentration: new approach to manage it (oral presentation). IInd International Congress KM Study Group. Barcelona-Spain, September 7-9,1995.
25. Hoyos JE, Cigales M, Hoyos-Chacón J. Treating decentered ablations. In: Lucio Buratto, Stephen Brint (Eds). Custom LASIK: Surgical Techniques and Complications. Thorofare, NJ: SLAK Inc. 2003;249-52.
26. Buratto L, Brint SF. LASIK Principles and techniques. Thorofore, NJ: SLACK Inc. 1998;127-29.
27. Kang SW, Chung ES, Kim WJ. Clinical analysis of central islands after laser *in situ* keratomileusis. J Cataract Refract Surg. 2000;26:536-42.
28. Schimmick JK, Telfair WB, Munnerlyn DR, et al. Corneal ablation profilometry and steep central islands. J Cataract Refract Surg. 1997;24:899-904.
29. Haw WW, Manche EE. Large optical ablation zone using the VISX S2 Smoothscan excimer laser. J Cataract Refract Surg. 2000;26:1742-47.
30. Tsai YY, Lin JM. Natural history of central islands after laser *in situ* keratomileusis. J Cataract Refract Surg. 2000;26:853-58.
31. Manche EE, Maloney RK, Smith RJ. Treatment of topographic central islands following refractive surgery. J Cataract Refract Surg. 1998;24:464-70.
32. Knorz MC, Jendritza B. Topographically-guided laser *in situ* keratomileusis to treat corneal irregularities. Ophthalmology. 2000;107:1138-43.
33. Ambrosio R, Wilson SE. Complications of laser *in situ* keratomileusis: etiology, prevention and treatment. J Refract Surg. 2001;17:350-79.
34. Carpel EF, Carlson KH, Shannon S. Folds and striae in laser *in situ* keratomileusis flaps. J Refract Surg 1999; 15:687-90.

35. Gimbel HV, Peters NT, Iskander NG, Penno EA. Laser *in situ* Keratomileusis Flap Complications and Management. J Refract Surg. 2000;16:223-25.
36. Gutierrez AM. Treatment of flap folds and striae following LASIK. In: Buratto L, Brint SF (Eds). Custom LASIK: Surgical Techniques and Complications. Thorofare, NJ: SLAK Inc. 2003;725-27.
37. Hoyos JE, Cigales M, Hoyos-Chacón J. Treatment of flap striae. In: Benjamin F. Boyd, Sunita Agarwal, Athiya Agarwal, Amar Agarwal (Eds). LASIK and beyond LASIK – Wavefront analysis and customized ablation. Highlights of Ophthalmology Int'l. 2001;284-86.
38. Eggink FA, Eggink CA, Beekhuis WH. Postoperative management and follow-up after corneal flap loss following laser *in situ* keratomileusis. J Cataract Refract Surg. 2002;28(1):175-79.
39. Chao CW, Azar DT. Lamellar keratitis following laser-assisted *in situ* keratomileusis. Ophthalmol Clin North Am. 2002;15(1):35-40.
40. Perez-Gomez I, Efron N. Confocal microscopic evaluation of particles at the corneal flap interface after myopic laser *in situ* keratomileusis. J Cataract Refract Surg. 2003;29(7):1373-77.
41. Kaufman SC, Maitchouk DY, Chiou AG, Beuerman RW. Interface inflammation after laser *in situ* keratomileusis. Sands of the Sahara syndrome. J Cataract Refract Surg. 1998;24(12):1589-93.
42. Buhren J, Baumeister M, Cichocki M, Kohnen T. Confocal microscopic characteristics of stage 1 to 4 diffuse lamellar keratitis after laser *in situ* keratomileusis. J Cataract Refract Surg. 2002;28(8):1390-99.
43. Sandoval HP, Crosson CE, Holzer MP, Vroman DT, Solomon KD. Residual cleaner after normal cleaning of laser *in situ* keratomileusis instruments. J Cataract Refract Surg. 2003;29(9):1727-32.
44. Shan MN, Misra M. Diffuse lamellar keratitis associated with epithelial defects after laser *in situ* keratomileusis. J Cataract Refract Surg. 2000;26:1312-18.
45. Asano-Kato N, Toda I, Hori-Komai Y, Takano Y, Tsubota K. Epithelial ingrowth after laser *in situ* keratomileusis: clinical features and possible mechanisms. Am J Ophthalmol. 2002;134(6):801-07.
46. Sachdev N, McGhee CN, Craig JP, Weed KH, McGhee JJ. Epithelial defect, diffuse lamellar keratitis, and epithelial ingrowth following post-LASIK epithelial toxicity. J Cataract Refract Surg. 2002;28(8):1463-66.
47. Ditzen K, Fiedler J, Pieger S. Laser *in situ* keratomileusis for hyperopia and hyperopic astigmatism using the Meditec MEL 70 spot scanner. J Refract Surg. 2002;18(4):430-34.
48. Chung MS, Pepose JS, Manche EE. Management of the corneal flap in laser *in situ* keratomileusis after previous radial keratotomy. Am J Ophthalmol. 2001;132(2): 252-53.
49. Perez-Santonja JJ, Ayala MJ, Sakla HF, Ruiz-Moreno JM, Alio JL. Retreatment after laser *in situ* keratomileusis. Ophthalmology. 1999;106(1):21-28.
50. Domniz Y, Comaish IF, Lawless MA, et al. Epithelial ingrowth: causes, prevention, and treatment in 5 cases. J Cataract Refract Surg 2001;27(11):1803-11.
51. Karp CL, Tuli SS, Yoo SH, Vroman DT, et al. Infectious keratitis after LASIK. Ophthalmology 2003;110(3): 503-10.
52. Pushker N, Dada T, Sony P, Ray M, Agarwal T, Vajpayee RB. Microbial keratitis after laser *in situ* keratomileusis. J Refract Surg 2002;18(3):280-86.
53. Freitas D, Alvarenga L, Sampaio J, et al. An outbreak of *Mycobacterium chelonae* infection after LASIK. Ophthalmology. 2003;110(2):276-85.
54. Pache M, Schipper I, Flammer J, Meyer P. Unilateral fungal and mycobacterial keratitis after simultaneous laser *in situ* keratomileusis. Cornea. 2003;22(1):72-75.
55. Albietz JM, Lenton LM, McLennan SG. Effect of laser *in situ* keratomileusis for hyperopia on tear film and ocular surface. J Refract Surg 2002;18(2):113-23.
56. Benitez-del-Castillo JM, Del-Rio T, Iradier T, et al. Decrease in tear secretion and corneal sensitivity after laser *in situ* keratomileusis. Cornea. 2001;20(1):30-32.
57. Orfeo V, De Marco R, Loffredo L. Alteration of the tear film following photoablative refractive surgery. In: Buratto L, Brint SF, (Eds.): Custom LASIK: Surgical Techniques and Complications. Thorofare, NJ: SLAK Inc 2003;277-81.
58. Wilson SE, Ambrosio R. Laser *in situ* keratomileusis-induced (presumed) neurotrophic epitheliopathy. Opthalmology. 2001;108(6):1082-87.
59. Barker NH, Couper TA, Taylor HR. Changes in corneal topography after laser *in situ* keratomileusis for myopia. J Refract Surg. 1999;15(1):46-52.
60. Spadea L, Fasciani R, Necozione S, Balestrazzi E. Role of the corneal epithelium in refractive changes following laser *in situ* keratomileusis for high myopia. J Refract Surg 2000;16(2):133-39.
61. Magallanes R, Shah S, Zadok D, Chayet AS, et al. Stability after laser *in situ* keratomileusis in moderately and extremely myopic eyes. J Cataract Refract Surg. 2001;27(7):1007-12.
62. Probst LE. Myopic and hyperopic LASIK enhancements. In: Lucio Buratto, Stephen Brint (Eds). Custom LASIK: Surgical Techniques and Complications. Thorofare, NJ: SLAK Inc. 2003;699-708.
63. Gutierrez AM. Reoperations with the excimer laser. En: Lucio Buratto, Stephen Brint (Eds). LASIK: Principles and Techniques. Thorofare, NJ: SLAK Inc. 1998;339-50.
64. Domniz Y, Comaish IF, Lawless MA, Rogers CM, Sutton GL. Recutting the cornea versus lifting the flap:

comparison of two enhancement techniques following laser *in situ* keratomileusis. J Refract Surg 2001; 17(5):505-510.
65. Pallikaris IG, Kymionis GD, Astyrakakis NI. Corneal ectasia induced by laser *in situ* keratomileusis. J Cataract Refract Surg 2001;27(11):1796-802.
66. Moncalvi M. Corneal ectasia following LASIK. In: Buratto L, Brint SF (Eds). Custom LASIK: Surgical Techniques and Complications. Thorofare, NJ: SLAK Inc. 2003;271-74.
67. Giledi O, Daya SM. Unexpected flap thickness in laser *in situ* keratomileusis. J Cataract Refract Surg. 2003;29(9):1825-26.
68. Piccoli PM, Gomes AA, Piccoli FV. Corneal ectasia detected 32 months after LASIK for correction of myopia and asymmetric astigmatism. J Cataract Refract Surg. 2003;29(6):1222-25.
69. Lovisolo CF, Fleming JF. Intracorneal ring segments for iatrogenic keratectasia after laser *in situ* keratomileusis or photorefractive keratectomy. J Refract Surg. 2002;18(5):535-41.
70. R Paradinas R, Cigales M, Hoyos JE. Role of peripheral retina in LASIK. In: S Agarwal, A Agarwal, SJ Apple, L Buratto, JL Alió, SK Pandey, A Agarwal (Eds). Textbook of Ophthalmology. Jaypee Bros Med Pub: New Delhi, India. 2002; 4:2749-52.
71. Arevalo JF, Ramirez E, Suarez E, et al. Incidence of vitreoretinal pathologic conditions within 24 months after laser *in situ* keratomileusis. Ophthalmology. 2000;107(2):258-62.
72. Luna JD, et al. Bilateral macular hemorrhage after laser *in situ* keratomileusis. Graefes Arch Clin Exp Ophthalmol. 1999;237(7):611-13.
73. Panozzo G, Parolini B. Relationships between vitreoretinal and refractive surgery. Ophthalmology. 2001;108(9):1663-1668; discussion 1668-69.
74. Arevalo JF, Ramirez E, Suarez E, Cortez R, Ramirez G, Yepez JB. Retinal detachment in myopic eyes after laser *in situ* keratomileusis. J Refract Surg. 2002;18(6): 708-14.

A New Algorithm for Controlling Corneal Asphericity in LASIK

35

JT Lin (USA)

INTRODUCTION

Customized laser reshaping of corneal surface for supervision recently becomes available by the two combined technology of flying-spot scanning laser patented by JT Lin (Lin, US Pat. 5,144,630; 5,520,679) and the advanced wavefront devices.[1] However, the existing laser ablation algorithms are believed to rely on the parabolic approximation of the Munnerlyn formula[2,3] which provides no information about the change of the corneal asphericity (or its shape) even high-order or exact formula are used.[4-6] Discrepancy was found in measured postoperative corneal asphericities and predictions based on several proposed algorithms including the optical surface loss of laser energy and other biomechanical effects.[7-9] However, the existing theories for laser ablation profiles are based on a known preoperative asphericity and treat the postoperative asphericity as a non-correlated free parameter.[5,7,10] For customized laser ablations, a control optimized algorithm is desired to maintain a prolate cornea over the scotopic pupil, compensate for age-related changes and reduce the laser-induced spherical aberration.

To achieve the above goal, this Chapter presents a new algorithm based on the nth-order approximation of conicoid corneal surface, in which the initial and final corneal asphericity are correlated and allow us to introduce a controlled ablation profile for various applications. New strategies for controlling corneal shape with minimal ablation depth and comparisons of this study and others will be presented.

In the recent article by Cantu and associates,[11] the authors proposed an ablation algorithm to increase spherical aberration (SA) and corneal asphericity (Q) to create an improved prolate ablation profile in both myopic and hyperopic patients. A related article by Lee et al,[12] also proposed a two-step algorithm for the improvement of overall visual performance, where they use the standard Munnerlyn's formula for plano correction and followed by a second-step to eliminate the high-order aberration (HoAs) without removing too much extra corneal tissue, a strategy contrast to the zone-enlargement method which suffers the risk of thin remaining corneal bed. However, the actual ablation algorithms used in their studies were not disclosed.

This Chapter will provide a refined algorithm to analyze the strategy of controlling the postoperative asphericity and how the HoAs can be eliminated without changing the corneal surface power. An asphericity chart is provided as guidance for the prediction of post-LASIK asphericity.

ASPHERICAL PROFILE

Most of the LASIK algorithms only include the preoperative refractive error (D) and ablation radius (d). Therefore, the parabolic approximation[2] of the ablation profile given by the center depth of

$H_o = -4Dd^2/3$ (for the case of myopia) was believed to be used in the algorithms. The high-order term[4,13] requiring also the preoperative corneal anterior surface radius (R) or its keratometric power and preoperative asphericity (Q) or shape-factor (P), I believe, had not been programmed in most of the existing systems.

For an aspherical corneal surface, the ablation profile may be expressed as follows (up to the 4th-order power of d) for a myopic correction.[13]

$$H(y) = Z2 + Z4 + Hcontrol \quad (1.a)$$

$$Z2 = -(4D/3)(d2 - y2), \quad (1.b)$$

$$Z4 = 10^3[(d^4 - y^4)/8R^3](p1 - Bp2), \quad (1.c)$$

$$Hcontrol = 10^3[y^4/8R^3](p2' - p2). \quad (1.d)$$

where p1 and p2 are the preoperative and postoperative corneal shape-factor related to its asphericity by $pj = Qj + 1$ (j=1, 2); $B=(R/R')^3$ defined by the ratio of the corneal anterior surface radius R (preoperative) and R′ (postoperative); y is the distance away from the optical axis and d is the ablation radius. In the above expression, H in micron, D in diopter and R, d, y in mm.

A controlled ablation profile Hcontrol is introduced for further change of the post-LASIK asphericity or shape factor (p2). The significance of Hcontrol is that it allows us to remove a minimal corneal tissue but change substantially corneal asphericity without perturbing the plano refractive state of the post-LASIK eye.

COMPARING WITH MEASUREMENTS

One example was reported by Cantu et al[11] and second example by Lee et al.[12] However, it should be noted that when only Hcontrol is used without the Z2 and Z4 terms, that is for D=0 and B=1, one could only achieve p2'>p2, or the cornea becomes less prolate or oblate because the corneal surface tissue could only be ablated. To achieve p2'< p2, it means Hcontrol <0, or adding corneal surface tissues which is clinically not possible. In order to change the corneal asphericity in both "directions", less prolate or less oblate, one would require the first step consisting of Z2 and Z4.

The algorithm of Lee et al corresponds to the situation when all three terms included in Eq.(1.a) and Hcontrol < 0 which allows the second-step of creating more prolate profile to reduce the LASIK-induced increase of positive SA while keeping the corneal plano. Similarly, Cantu et al reported the change of initially oblate eyes (with positive Q1, or p1>1.0) to prolate (with negative Q2, or p2<1.0). However, they did not specify if any refractive powers were changed. Based on the concept presented by Eq.(1), without the Z2 and Z4 term which change the refractive power, only one direction of increasing asphericity can be achieved, that is one can only change the cornea from prolate (or oblate) to less prolate (or more oblate), but not the reversed process.

PREDICTION OF CORNEAL ASPHERICITY

The measured increasing asphericity after LASIK[7] may be easily analyzed by Z4 which is proportional to the Zernike coefficient of Z(4, 0) defined by Lee et al for spherical aberration. The role of refractive power correction (D) on the magnitude of spherical aberration is given by the B-factor in Eq.(1) which is further related to D by $B=(1+0.0204\,D)^3$ for a typical preoperative corneal radius of R=7.7 mm. However, the impact of Z4 on the ablation depth and the shape of the cornea is sensitive to the correlation ratio defined by $p1/p2=B^N$, where N=(0.66-1.0) depending on the approximation used for the conical surface function expansion. In the parabolic (second-order) approximation[5,6] N=1.0, whereas the infinity-order or asymptotic value of N is 2/3 (Lin, unpublished, see also Appendix).

Using N=2/3, Figure 35.1 shows the chart for prediction of postoperative asphericity (Q2) at any given preoperative value (Q1) given by $Q2=(Q1+1)(R'/R)^2 - 1$. The general rule is that a myopic correction produces higher Q-value or the corneal surface becomes less prolate or even oblate; whereas a hyperopic correction produces an opposite effect.

The conical shape of the anterior corneal surface may be described by the asphericity Q or the shape

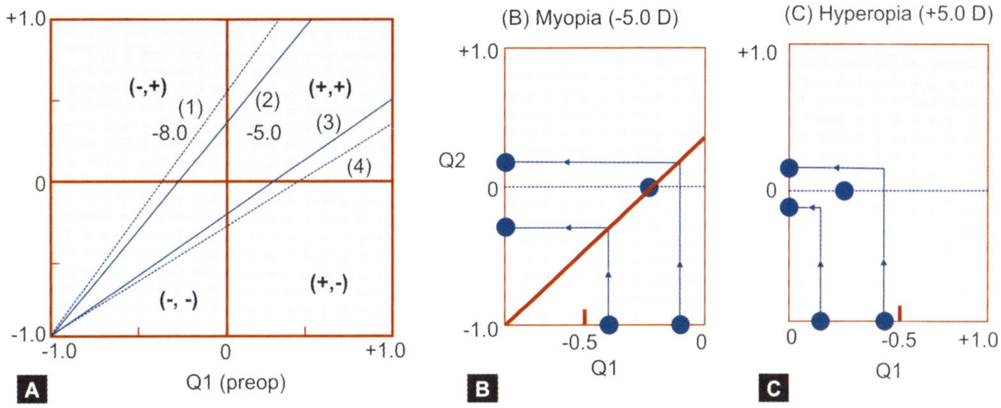

Figs 35.1A to C: A code chart for the predicted post-LASIK corneal asphericity (Q2) versus the preoperative value (Q1). Curve (1) (2) (3) (4) are for LASIK correction power of -8.0, -5.0, +5.0 and +8.0 diopter, respectively. It shows four areas defined by notations of (+, +) stands for both preop and postop surface are oblate (with Q1, Q2>0), (+, -) for preop is oblate and postop is prolate, etc. Also show are the transition points Q1* (circle dots) when Q2=0 (or a spherical surface). The possible combination of (Q1, Q2) is summarized in Table 35.1

factor p = Q+1, where Q equals – 0.18 to – 0.3 for a typical natural prolate cornea,[17,18] and about 1% of the population may have positive Q-value (or oblate surface).

The transition value is given by when Q2 = 0, or $Q1^* = (R/R')^2 - 1$. For example, Q1* = – 0.19 for D = –5.0 diopter and Q1* = +0.21 for D = +5.0 diopter. As shown in Table 35.1, an initial prolate cornea becomes less prolate when its initial Q1 < Q1*, and becomes oblate when Q1 > Q1* after a myopic correction.

Example # 1

As shown in Figure 35.1(B), for myopia of – 5.0 D correction, Q2 = 1.23 (Q1+1) – 1. Therefore an initial Q1 = – 0.1 (prolate) will result in Q2 = +0.11 (oblate); and initial Q1 = – 0.4 will result in Q2 = –0.26 (less prolate).

Example # 2

As shown by Figure 35.1(C) for hyperopia of +0.5 D Q2 = 0.826 (Q1+1) –1. Therefore an initial Q1=+0.1 (oblate) results in Q2 = –0.09 (prolate); and Q1 = +0.4 results in Q2 = 0.16 (less oblate).

Figure 35.1 and Table 35.1 provide a guideline for the prediction of postoperative corneal shape for a given preoperative shape which could be prolate or oblate. Furthermore, the controlled ablation algorithm may be used to modify corneal shape without changing its refractive power.

CENTRAL ABLATION DEPTH

The central ablation depth (in myopia) or the maximal depth (in hyperopia), in general, is proportional to B (the correlation power) and has a higher value for hyperopia than myopia. For example, a typical value of R=7.7 mm and d=3.0 mm, B=(0.724, 0.882) for myopia D = (–5.0, –2.0) diopters; B = (1.13, 1.34) for hyperopia D = (+2.0, +5.0) diopter. Hcontrol in Eq. (1.d) is proportional to R′ and the change amount (R2′-R2) and it is y-dependent. It may be easily calculated, for each 1.0 change of the controlled asphericity or

Table 35.1: Prediction of corneal surface shape after LASIK at various initial shapes

LASIK	Initial	Postoperative Q1 < Q1*	Q1 > Q1*
Myopic	PRO	less PRO	OB
	OB	more OB	more OB
Hyperopic	PRO	more PRO	more PRO
	OB	PRO	less OB

* where Q1* is a transition value defined by when Q2=0. Shorthand notations are used: PRO for prolate and OB for oblate (referred to Figure 35.1).

shape factor change, Hcontrol = 3.9 microns (at y=2.0 mm), and 19.7 micron (at y=3.0 mm). These results are consistent with the measured data of Lee et al that Hcontrol is about 10% of the total ablation depth.

EFFECTIVE ZONE SIZE

The recent articles of Holladay, Bains and El-Danasoury[15,16] reported the clinical results for excimer laser optimized prolate ablation (OPA). They claimed that new algorithms used in OPA may reduce the positive spherical aberration (SA) induced by conventional ablation due to the loss of effective fluence (Feff) in the periphery and resulted in a smaller effective optical zone (Weff). Ablation strategy was also proposed to compensate the loss of Feff to maintain its preoperative cornea shape or even for slightly more prolate to account for the decrease of negative SA of the crystalline lens by age. However, they did not present any real theory (or formulas), or quantitative analysis on how the loss of Feff is correlated to the decrease of Weff or the change of corneal asphericity.

In the following, I will present formulas to relate the decrease of Feff at the periphery of a prolate cornea to calculate Weff. These formulas may provide the basis for new algorithms for OPA and customized ablation for aged-eye.

By the definition of laser fluence F=E/Area (energy per unit area) and the simple geometry shown in Figure 35.2, Feff is derived and shown in Table 35.2, where F and Feff are the laser fluence for a flat-surface and a conicoid-surface. It should be noted that Feff is quite sensitive to both of the corneal surface radius (R) and the ablation zone (W), governed by the square of (d/R). However, Feff is not sensitive to the corneal asphericity, the high-order terms not shown in Table 35.2.

It should be noted that the absolute value of the reduced effective zone diameter (Weff) requires the actual measurement of laser ablation rate and its ablation threshold fluence which is difficult to be measured consistently due to the change of corneal conditions, surface reflection loss,[8,9] and the environmental factors such as the re-absorption of laser energy by the tissue plum. Lin's earlier formula for the central ablation depth $H=(1+C)(DW^2/3)$, with the high-order term[4] $C=0.19(W/R)^2$ is based on the Munnerlyn (or spherical) formula. For aspherical (conic) corneal surface, a revised formula is shown in Table 35.2 to include the effects of the corneal preoperative asphericity Q1 and shape-factor p1 and the postoperative values Q2 and p2.

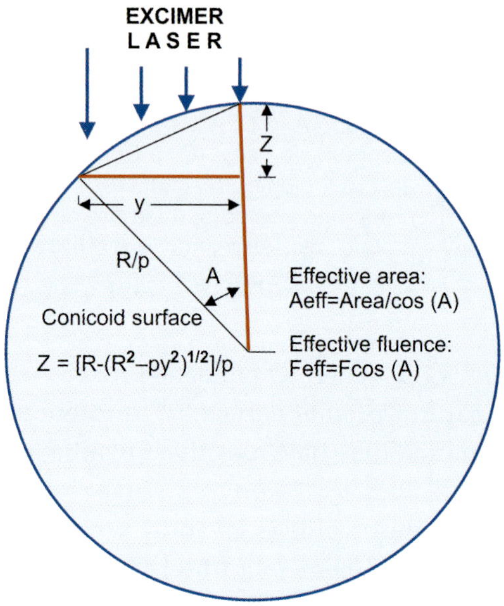

Fig 35.2: Geometry showing a LASIK laser acting on a conicoid corneal surface having a vertex radius R and a height y from the optical axis (y), where the angle (A) defines the effective fluence (Feff)

Table 35.2: Summary of formulas and notations

Feff	=	$F \cos(A)$
cos (A)	=	$1-0.5\,(y/2R)^2$
Heff	=	$(1-L1-L2)(Z2 + Z4)$
Z2	=	$-1.333D(d^2-y^2)$
Z4	=	$(1/8R^3)(p1-Bp2)(d^4-y^4)$
B	=	$(R/R')^3$

F and Feff:	the laser fluence for a flat and curved surface
L1 and L2:	adjusting factor due to surface reflection loss and reduced Feff
Z2:	ablation depth under parabolic approximation
Z4:	the 4th-power of y for an aspherical cornea
P1 and P2:	pre- and postoperative shape factor with asphericity Q1 and Q2
R and R':	pre- and postoperative anterior surface radius
y:	distance from the optical axis
d :	radius of the ablation zone (d=W/2)

Given the effective central ablation depth (Heff), one may easily calculate the effective ablation zone diameter by $Weff=(3\ Heff/D)^{1/2}$, for a myopia (or hyperopia) correction power of D (taken as its absolute value).

Most of the LASIK system manufacturers use D and H as the basis for their ablation algorithms. Therefore, for a given D and laser energy, the induced postoperative positive SA is proportional to the change of corneal surface asphericity (Q) and the decrease of the ablation zone defined by dW=(W-Weff). By further defining the effective depth decrease dH = H – Heff, one may readily obtain the following formula:

$$C1 = 1 - (1-C2)^{1/2}, \qquad (2)$$

where C2=dH/H and C1=dW/W are the percentage changes of ablation depth and zone diameter. For example, C1=(2.5%, 5%, 7.8%) for C2=(5%, 10%, 15%), that is C1 is about half of C2 as expected by the square of W in the central ablation depth formula.

To demonstrate the effect of cornea shape change on the effective ablation zone, an extra term of Z4 (see Table 35.2) was included in the effective ablation depth Heff. This nonlinear term is the fourth-power expansion of the conicoid surface defined by the shape-factor p1 and p2, and the B-factor given by the ratio of the preoperative and postoperative corneal anterior surface radius B=R1/R2. For an ablation radius of d=3.0 mm (or W=6.0 mm), R1=7.7 mm and D = – 5.0 diopter, the central depth (at y=0) Z4=0.37 (p1-0.724 p2) Z2, which contributes about 2.5% of Z2, for p1 = 0.8 (or prolate cornea of Q1 = –0.2) and p2 = 1.2 (or oblate cornea with Q2 = +0.2). The contribution from the reflection loss[9] is about 4%. Therefore, the overall reduction of Heff is about (4% – 2.5%) = 1.5% comparing to that of the parabolic approximation (PA) of a spherical corneal surface.

SURFACE ABERRATION

For a given final state asphericity (Q') and corneal anterior surface radius R2, the PSA is given by:[8,18]

$$Sj = Wjb^4, \qquad (3.a)$$

$$W1 = -0.046\ (0.535 + Q')/R2^3, \qquad (3.b)$$

where j=1, 2, 3, 4 stands for the PSA of anterior and posterior surface of the cornea and lens, b is the ray height on the corneal surface. Therefore, the change of corneal PSA is given by:

$$dS1 = 0.046(b^4/R2^3)(dp'), \qquad (4)$$

where the change of shape-factor in (p'=Q'+1) is related to the ablation depth change (dH) by:[8]

$$dp' = dH/M' \qquad (5.a)$$

$$M' = 0.263B(d^4-y^4), \qquad (5.b)$$

which may be easily obtained by the differentiation of Eq.(1.a) with respect to p2. As an example, for d=3.0 mm and D1= – 2.0 diopter, B = 0.882, M'= (16.4, 13.3) microns at y = (1.0, 2.0) mm. Therefore, the PSA change due to corneal shape change at y = 2.0 mm, and for R2 = 8.15 mm as an example, dS1 = 0.244(dH), or a positive PSA increase of 0.244 microns per 1.0 micron corneal surface ablation which changes the corneal asphericity. This is in consistent with the reported data that induce positive PSA were found in myopic LASIK procedures.[6,8] The calculated value of M' is also consistent with that of Manns et al.[10] However, formula Eq.(5.b) of this study is more accurate than the approximated one derived by Manns et al.

APPLICATIONS

It was known that in normal eyes, the aberration of the cornea tend to balance with that of the lens, particularly during youth.[17, 18] When one ages, the surface aberration of the lens changes from about – 0.25 micron to about +0.25 micron and results in an increased total positive PSA. One application of this study, therefore, is to calculate and control the postoperative anterior corneal shape (or its asphericity) with aberrations that can either compensate the LASIK-induced increase of PSA or slightly more prolate than necessary to account for age effects of the lens. A controlled ablation algorithm can also produce the desired corneal shape to compensate the aberrations resulted from other optical factors such as laser power reflection loss, reduced laser fluence due to abnormal incidence, and other tissue related factors such as wound healing, epithelial hyperplasia and other biomechanical effects.[7, 8]

Application # 1

One application of this study is to use the combined myopia-hyperopia ablation profile to create either a central myopia with peripheral for distance vision or a peripheral-myopia with center for distance vision. Either of these bifocal profiles would provide pseudo-accommodation for an aged patient to see both near and far. As demonstrated earlier based on the calculated value of M′, the LSP of myopia and hyperopia with the same amount of power correction, or D1 = – D2, results in a central ablation depth slightly larger than the depth (Z_0) under a parabolic approximation. Furthermore, the peripheral of the LSP profile depends on the approximations used and determined by the correlation between the initial and final shapes factor, p1, p2 and p3 as shown by Eqs.(9) to (12). Calculations based on Eq.(15.b) show that a change of only 1.3 to 1.7 microns in ablation depth for each of 0.1 change of the shape factor. Therefore, the defocusing effects associated with the shape factor change, or the 4th-power of y, are less than 4% for a five diopter corrections, or only 0.2 diopters.

Application # 2

Another application of the correlation Eq.(A4) is to determine the final state asphericity for a given initial corneal surface which could be prolate for most normal corneas, or oblate for some corneas. Knowing that $p_1 = Q_1+1$ and $p_2 = Q_2+1$, Eq.(4) with N = 2/3 readily gives us the threshold value for the initial asphericity $Q_1{}^* = B^{2/3}-1$ which results a final corneal surface being a spherical, or $Q_2 = 0$. Furthermore, the B-factor may be calculated from Eq.(A2) and (A3.e) for various refractive power corrections (D), B = (0.59, 0.724, 1.34, 1.57) for D = (–8, –5, +5, +8) diopters and the corresponding threshold values $Q_1{}^*$ = (–0.29, –0.19, 0.21, 0.35). Therefore, a 5.0 diopter myopic correction on an initially prolate cornea, for example, will result a less prolate cornea when $Q_1 < -0.19$, whereas a final oblate cornea will be expected when $Q_1 > -0.19$. Furthermore, a cornea will become more oblate, if it is initially oblate for all Q_1. In comparison, a cornea after hyperopic correction will become more prolate for all Q_1, if it is initially prolate; whereas an initially oblate cornea will become less oblate when $Q_1 > +0.21$. These features are summarized in Table 35.1.

Most of the previous studies treat the final state asphericity (Q_2) as a freely adjustable parameter to make a general statement of increases in the shape factor (p_2) for myopes and decreases for hyperopes[5-7] without specifying the threshold values of $Q_1{}^*$ (or $p_1{}^*$) as introduced in this study. Furthermore, the correlation power of N = 1 reported earlier[6] results in $Q_1{}^*$ = B–1 or $Q_1{}^*$ = (–0.28, +0.34) versus (–0.19, +0.21) of this study based on N = 2/3 for D = (–5, +5) diopters. The high-order Munnerlyn formula [6] on the other hand, having a correlation of $Q_2 = Q_1/B$ which gives $Q_1{}^* = 0$, a conclusion conflicting with clinical measurements.[7]

Application # 3

The above analytic formulas may be further modified to include the effects due to reflection loss, non-normal laser incidence, would healing and other biomechanical factors which were reported as the predominant factors in explaining the discrepancy between the clinical findings and the theoretical calculations.[7-9] Taking the difference of the ablation profile, Eq.(1.a), up to their 4th-power of y and d, one obtains the change of ablation due to the change of the final shape factor from p_2 to p_2'.

$$\Delta H = -C_2\,(B'p_2' - Bp_2). \tag{7}$$

Using the approximate expression of:

$$B'p_2' - Bp_2 = B(\Delta p_2) - p_2(\Delta B), \tag{8}$$

Eq.(7) may be further simplified as:

$$\Delta H = (1 + 0.5p_2/d^2)\,[10^3 B\,(y^4 - d^4)/8R_1{}^3], \tag{9}$$

where "H in micron and R_1 and d in mm. Above formula reduces to that of Manns et al,[10] if the $p_2(\Delta B)$ term, about 6%, is ignored. However, it is substantially different from that of Gatinel et al,[5] in which the authors assumed B = 1.0 and ignored $p_2(\Delta B)$ term.

As calculated earlier, B=(–0.59 to 1.57) for D = (–8 to +8) diopter, significant errors (over 50%) are expected in the results of Gatinel based on B = 1.0 and independent to D. For example, they predicted

7.0 micron of central epithelial-hyperphasia to induce an oblate final corneal contour which is about 34% overestimated comparing to that of our new formula, only needs about 5.2 micron using a +5.0 diopter hyperpic correction. The sources of error of Gatinel et al may come from two factors, their Eq.(5) approximated $(R_1/R_2)^3=8R_1D/1000$ which should be $(8R_1D/1000)(1+0.02D)$, an error of 10% for D = –5.0 diopter; and their Eq.(9) assumed B=1, or R_2 approximated by R_1 which results in additional errors as shown above.

Application # 4

Several authors have reported that optical factors such as surface reflection loss and reduced laser fluence (or energy density) on curved corneal surface would result in a decrease of ablation depth.[11,12] and an adjusted factor including these losses in the ablation algorithm will predict a better postoperative corneal shape. Alternatively, enlargement of the ablation zone or the use of greater depth of central ablation were proposed to pre-empt the oblate shift after myopic LASIK.[11,12] However, they are all involved with the risks of excessive corneal tissue ablation.

A better ablation algorithm would be based on the change of the postoperative asphericity (or shape factor) without deeper central depth ablation. This can be achieved by adding a controlled term to the non-controlled profile H(y) of Eq.(1.a) for further change of the non-controlled final shape factor (p_2) $\Delta p' = p_2' - p_2$.

$$Hcont(y) = H(y) + M\Delta p', \quad (10.a)$$
$$M(y) = 10^3By^4/(8R_1^3), \quad (10.b)$$

where Hcont, H and M all are in micron, y and R_1 in mm. It should be noted that M(y = 0) = 0 which does not change the central ablation depth and only change the controlled corneal shape. In comparison, the ΔH of Eq.(9) affects both the central depth and the corneal shape to account for the effects due to optical factors such as surface reflection loss and tissue factors. Depending on $\Delta p' < 0$ or $\Delta p' > 0$, the final (postoperative) corneal surface could be more prolate (increase negative Q_2 or $p_2' < p_2$) or more oblate ($p_2' > p_2$) than the non-controlled ablation.

Given the controlled change of $\Delta p'$, the controlled corneal shape factor may be calculated:

$$p_2' = B^{-N} p_1 + \Delta p', \quad (11)$$

where he non-controlled p_2 correlates to the initial shape factor (p_1) by the power factor B^{-N} in which N=2/3 for correlated case, and N=1 for non-correlated second-order approximation.

Applications of the controlled ablation algorithm shall include the following. It may be used to reduce the increase of positive spherical aberration (SA) after a cornea refractive surgery to compensate for the reduced depth due to optical factors such as reflection loss; to compensate for the age-related increase of positive SA from the lens by producing a slightly more prolate cornea than necessary.

For example, for D = –5.0 diopter, B = 0.724 and a typical corneal radius of R_1=7.7 mm, Eq.(10.b) gives $M = 0.198y^4$. The non-correlated shape factor $p_2 = p_1/0.806 = 0.992$, for an initially prolate cornea with Q_1= –0.2 or p_1=0.8. The controlled profile Hcont = H – 0.64 micron at y=2 mm is required to achieve a final shape factor of $p_2' = 0.8$, or $\Delta p' = -0.2$ to maintain the original prolate surface. In comparison, Hcont = H – 0.96 micron is required to have a more prolate ($Q_2' = -0.3$) cornea for aged-eye, with a final shape factor p_2' = +1.1.

DISCUSSIONS

The calculated central ablation depth defined by Hcen = H(y = 0) of this study may be compared to that of others as follows. The second-order approximation of Eq.(A6) gives:

$$Hcen = H_0 + M_0 (1-B^{1/3})p_1, \quad (12.a)$$
$$Mo = 10^3(d^4/8R_1^3). \quad (12.b)$$

where $H_0 = 4Dd^2/3$ is the parabolic approximation[2] (PA) of Munnerlyn formula having a second-order approximation (SOA) of [4]$H_{mun} = H_0 + M'(1-B)$, which does not provide any information about the corneal shape factor even high-order or exact formula is used. Furthermore, a correlation of $Q_2 = Q_1/B$ was reported in a least-square method using SOA and Munnerlyn exact formula,[6] where the mixture of spherical ablation profile and a postoperative aspherical corneal surface result in a correlation conflicting with the measured postoperative asphericity,[7] and worse than the data predicted from PA having a correlation of $p_2=p_1/B$. In comparison, the correlation of this study, $p_2=p_1/B^{2/3}$, is based on an algorithm in which both the ablation and final profiles are aspherical to avoid the artificial effects caused by the mixture of spherical and aspherical profiles.

Eq.(12) of this study is also substantially different from that of Gatinel et al,[5] in which the authors treated the postoperative shape factor p_2 as a freely adjustable parameter non-correlated to its preoperative value p_1. The non-correlated central depth may be derived from Eq.(1.a) as follows (upto the 4th power of d)

$$Hcen = H_0 + M_0 (p_1 - Bp_2), \qquad (13)$$

which may underestimate the central depth in comparing to the correlated formula of Eq.(12), since p_2 is a free parameter. For example, for R_1=7.7 mm, d=3.0 mm, p1=0.8 and D= –5.0 diopter, M_o=22.18 μm, B = 0.724, $B^{1/3}$=0.9, Δ = Hcen – H_0 =1.8 μm for the correlated case from Eq.(12); and $\Delta = 22.18 (0.8 - 0.724 p_2)$=3.3 μm, for p_2 = 0.9 in non-correlated case of Eq.(13); and $\Delta = 22.18 (1 - 0.724) = 6.12$ μm (independent to p_1) for the SOA of Munnerlyn formula.

The above examples demonstrate that the central depth changes are governed by the B-factor, the correlated values of p_1 and p_2 at a given ablation zone size (d) and intended refractive correction power (D). However, the significant contribution from the second term of Eq.(12) and (13) is on the change of corneal shape or its asphericity, rather than the ablation depth, only about 2 to 5% of H_0 as shown in the above examples. These features allow us to control or optimize the postoperative asphericity with a minimal change of its central depth which affects the intended power correction and ablation size.

CONCLUSION

The new algorithm of this Chapter based on Z4 term to account for the asphericity change was totally ignored in parabolic approximation (PA) or the exact formula of Munnerlyn. The relationship between p1 and p2 given by the correlation power N depends on the ablation algorithm and the Z4 value may be significantly affected by the choice of this relationship. For example, p1= $(R1/R2)^2$P2 (or N = 2/3) when an exact conicoid surface is used in the ablation depth, whereas N=1/3 in PA. The significant impact of the Z4 term is on the change of the corneal shape (or its asphericity) rather than the ablation depth which is only about 1.5 to 3.0 microns per 0.1 change of the shape factor p2.

Customized ablation of prolate (or oblate) corneal surface requires the accurate information of the laser fluence (or energy per unit area) and spot size, the corneal anterior surface curvature, and its preoperative asphericity (Q1) or shape factor (p1). The conventional Munnerlyn formula can not account for the change of asphericity even a high-order approximation or exact equation is used.

REFERENCES

1. Mackee SM, Krueger RR. Applegate RA. In Customized Corneal Ablation. SM Mackee, RR Krueger, RA Applegate (Eds). Thorofare, NJ: SLAK Inc. 2001;3-9.
2. Lin JT. "Critical review on refractive surgical lasers", Opt. Engineer 1995;34:668-75.
3. Twa MD, Lemback RG, Bullimore MA, Roberts C. A prospective randomized clinical trial of laser in situ keratomileusis with two different lasers. Am J Ophthalmol 2005;140:173-83.
4. Lin JT. A new formula for ablation depth in 3-zone LASIK. J Refract Surg 2005;21:413-14.
5. Gatinel D, Joang-Xuan T, Azar D. Determination of corneal asphericity after myopia surgery with the excimer laser: a mathematical model. Invest Ophthalmol Vis Sci. 2001;42:1736-42.
6. Jimenez JR, Anera RD, Diaz JA, Perez-ocon F. Corneal asphericity after refractive surgery when the Munnerlyn formula is applied. J Opt Soc Am (A) 2004;21:98-103.
7. Marcos S, Cano D, Barbero S. Increase in corneal asphericity after standard laser *in situ* keratmileusis for myopia is not inherent to the Munnerlyn algorithm. J Refract Surg. 2003;19:S592-S96.
8. Mrochen M, Seiler T. Influence of corneal curvature on calculation of ablation patterns used in photorefractive laser surgery. J Refract Surg 2001;17:S584-S87.
9. Anera RG, Jimenez JR, Barco LJ, Hitta E. Change in corneal asphericity after laser refractive surgery, including reflection losses and nonnormal incidence upon the anterior cornea. Opt Lett 2003;15:417-19.
10. Manns F, Ho A, Parel JM, Culbertson W. Ablation profile for wavefront-guided correction of myopia and primary spherical aberration. J Cataract Refract Surg 2002;28: 766-74.

11. Cantu R, Rosales MA, Tepichin E, et al. Objective quality of vision in presbyopic and non-presbyopic patients after pseudoaccommodative advanced surface ablation. J Refract Surg. 2005 (Suppl.); 21:S603-05.
12. Lee H, Oh JR, Reintein DZ, et al. Conservation of corneal tissue with wave-front-guided laser *in situ* keratomileuse. J Cataract Refract Surg. 2005;31:1153-58.
13. Lin JT. A prospective randomized clinical trial of laser *in situ* keratomileusis with two different lasers. Am J Ophthalmol. 2006; [Correspondence] (in press).
14. Anera R. Jimenez JR, Barco LJ. Equation for corneal asphericity after corneal refractive surgery. J Refract Surg. 2003;19:65-69.
15. Holladay JT, Bains HS. Optimized prolate ablation with the NIDEK CXII excimer laser. J Refract Surg. 2005;21:S595-97.
16. El-Danasoury, Baines HS. Optimized prolate corneal ablation: case report for the first treated eye. J Refract Surg. 2005;21:S595-602.
17. Jenkins TCA. Aberration of the eye and their effects on vision. Br J Physiol Opt 1963;20:59-91.
18. Atchison DA, Smith G. Optics of the human eye. Woburn, MA: Butterworth-Heinemann; 2000;14-16: 143-47, 160-62.

APPENDIX

THE LINS'S N=2/3 POWER FACTOR

The laser ablation profile (algorithm) for myopia correction may be described by the difference in sagittal height between the final and initial corneal anterior surface having a conicoid section as follows: [18]

$$H(y) = H_2(y) - H_1(y) + H_d, \quad \text{(A1.a)}$$

$$H_j(y) = [R_j^2 - (R_j^2 - p_j y^2)^{1/2}]/\, p_j, \quad \text{(A1.b)}$$

where $H_1(y)$ and $H_2(y)$ are the initial and final corneal surface defined by their apical radius R_1 and R_2, and the shape factor p_1 and p_2 which are related to the asphericity by $p_j=Q_j+1$. The central ablation depth $H_d = H_1(y=d) - H_2(y=d)$, is determined by the ablation zone radius (d) and the intended refractive power correction (D) which may be calculated by a paraxial formula:[18]

$$D = 0.377\,(1/R_2 - 1/R_1), \quad \text{(A2)}$$

where $R_2 > R_1$ for myopia ($D < 0$) and corneal refractive index of 1.377 is used.

Using the nth-order Taylor expansion of Eq.(1.b), the ablation profile becomes:

$$H(y) = Z_1 + Z_2 + Z_3 + \ldots Z_n, \quad \text{(A3.a)}$$

$$Z_n(y) = C_n\,[p_1^{\,n-1} - B^{(2n-1)/3}\,p_2^{\,n-1}]Y_n, \quad \text{(A3.b)}$$

$$Y_n(y) = (y^{2n} - d^{2n})/R^{2n-1}, \quad \text{(A3.c)}$$

$$C_n = 1.3.5.7\ldots(2n-3)/(2^n n!), \quad \text{(A3.d)}$$

$$B = (R_1/R_2)^3. \quad \text{(A3.e)}$$

To maintain the conicoid shape of the corneal anterior surface after the laser ablation, one should expect that the shape factor of final and initial surface are correlated by:

$$p_2 = B^{-N} p_1. \quad \text{(A4)}$$

Substituting Eq.(A4) to Eq.(A3.b), the nth-order term becomes:

$$Z_n(y) = C_n\,(1-B^k)p_1^{\,n-1}Yn, \quad \text{(A5)}$$

where $k = (2n-1)/3 - (n-1)N$, therefore the $(n-1)$th-order approximation of the ablation profile function H(y) is given by when $Z_n=0$, or when $B^k=1$, for n>>1, or the asymptotic value N=2/3. Noting that this correlation power N=2/3 gives k=1/3 for all the finite-power terms, Eq.(A3.a) becomes:

$$H(y) = (1 - B^{1/3})[c_1 + c_2 p_1 + c_3 p_1^2 + \ldots], \quad \text{(A6)}$$

where $c_n(y) = Y_n(y)C_n$ with the correlation power factor N=2/3, one may easily see that the final and initial conicoid surface defined by Eq.(1.b) are related by $H_2(y) = B^{1/3}H_1(y)$ which may be used to calculate the $(n-1)$th order approximation for the ablation profile given by Eq.(A1.a).

The N=2/3 power factor may be also deduced from the following truncation method. By letting $Z_n(y)=0$, for n=1, 2, 3, 4..., one obtains the power factor N=1, 5/6, 7/9, 9/12, 11/15,..which approaches to its asymptotic value 2/3 for n>>1. These N values also correspond to the second, third, fourth... and $(n-1)$th order approximation of the profile in Eq.(A3.a). The previous reported value of N=1, derived from the least-square methods.[6] Based on the parabolic approximation of Munnerlyn formula, corresponds to the second-order approximation of Lin's formula, that is when N=1 given by $Z_2=0$ in Eq.(A3.b).

Critical Issues Affecting LASIK Outcomes

36

JT Lin (USA)

INTRODUCTION

Three main refractive surgical procedures LASIK, LASEK and epiLASEK have become the choice of vision corrections for myopia, hyperopia and astigmatism, whereas other methods such as laser sclera ablation, bifocal profiles and monovision have been used for presbyopia. Customized ablation, aspherical ablation and advanced microkeratomes are targeting for supervision with minimal surface aberration. However, some critical issues still remain and limit the performance of the procedures. As summarized in Table 36.1, the issues affecting the procedure outcomes are governed by laser parameters and system design, ablation algorithms, preoperative calibrations and microkeratomes, in addition to the clinical aspects relating to the surgeon's techniques, stroma hydration and surface condition and the managements of the flap, complications and postoperative medications.

This chapter will address the above issues and provide possible solutions to improve the procedure outcomes performed by LASIK.

Table 36.1: Critical issues affected LASIK outcomes

Laser System
- Spot size (0.5 – 2.0 mm)
- Repetition rate (100 – 500 Hz)
- Energy per pulse (1.0 – 4.0 mJ)
- Laser fluence (120 – 250 mJ/cm^2)
- Eye tracking (50 – 5,000 Hz)

Microkeratome
- Flap size (8.5 – 10.5 mm)
- Flap thickness (120 – 200 um)
- Flap orientation
- Stroma surface quality

Ablation algorithm
- Ablation zone (5.0 – 7.5 mm)
- Transition zone (1.0 – 1.5 mm)
- Multizone (2, 3, 4 zones)
- High-order ablation depth
- Corneal asphericity (Q-factor)
- Random scanning (for minimal thermal)
- Customized profiles (for minimal aberration)

Preoperative calibration
- Keratometry power (K-reading)
- Corneal surface radius (r1, r2)
- Ablation rate (PMMA-reading)

Clincial aspects
- Surgeon's techniques
- Stroma conditions (hydration level)
- Flap management
- Postoperative management
- Retreatment and enhancement

Laser System and Parameters

Other than the semiscanning broadbeam system (used in Visx system), almost all the existing LASIK systems have used the flying spot scanning method (patented by Lin in 1996) which uses a typical spot size of 0.5 to 2.0 mm. For low repetition rate (R) systems (20 to 50 Hz), a larger spot size about 1.5 to 2.0 mm would be required to achieve a reasonable procedure rate of about 3 to 5 seconds per diopter of correction. For system with high R=(300 to 500) Hz, spot size of 0.5 to 0.8 mm may be the optimal for both procedure, time and ablation precision. It should be noted that spot size larger than 1.5 mm may speed up the procedure and obtain smoother surface, however, it would lose the accuracy in ablating "fine profile" having structure smaller than 1.0 mm, or for the correction of localized high-order surface aberration or irregularity in customized procedures. A system with adjusted spot size method (Lin, patent pending) was proposed to overcome the above drawbacks, where large spot (about 1.5 to 2.5 mm) is proposed for regular large area profile, whereas small spot (0.2 to 0.5 mm) for irregular or surface aberration corrections.

The procedure time (T) is also governed by the ablation rate (A) defined as tissue depth removed per laser pulse. Basically, T is inverse proportionally to A which is proportional to the tissue absorption coefficieny (B) and may be approximated by ln (F-F*), where F* is a threshold fluence for stroma tissue to be removed. The currently used systems use a typical fluence of F=(120 to 250) mJ/cms (cms=cm^2). Higher F would speed up the procedure, however, it also slightly suffers the ablation accuracy. It should be noted that A is governed only by (F-F*) rather than E (the laser energy per pulse). Therefore, one would expect the ablation rate for a spot size of 2.0 mm having E=5.2 mJ and a smaller spot of 1.0 mm with E=1.3 mJ, assuming the threshold F*=20 mJ/cms or E*=0.3 mJ (for a 1.0 mm spot) and E*=1.2 mJ (for 2.0 mm spot).

The ablation rate is very sensitive to the hydration level of the ablated stroma (for LASIK) or corneal surface (for LASEK). A possible uncertainty of 10% to 20% could occur under a noncontrolled condition. However, this may be overcome by adjusting the PMMA calibration which translates the "actual" tissue ablation rate to the PMMA by empirical factor. Greater detail will be discussed in the CALIBRATION section.

Systems use higher fluence (F) and higher repetition rate (R) may also result in greater thermal effects on the ablated tissues. In modern algorithms, these effects may be overcome by using a so-called "random scan" method which effectively reduces the "frequency of visit" on the same treatment spot. For example, R=200 Hz is reduced to an effective rate of R'=50 Hz under a random visiting rate of ¼ (1 visit per 4 spots). This may be easily achieved under a typical beam overlap of 50% to 80%.

Eye movement during the procedure, which may not be an issue in broadbeam (6 mm spot) systems, becomes a critical issue in small spot scanning system. Eye tracking with a track-rate comparable to or slightly faster than the laser repetition rate would overcome this problem. However, one of the commercial systems using KHz tracker is an overshoot of this issue.

It would be also useful for the LASIK surgeons to be aware of the above technical issues in addition to the clinical issues to be addressed later.

Microkeratome

The existing microkeratomes are designed to cut a flap thickness about 120 to 180 um with about 5% uncertainty resulting from the conditions of preparing the flap such as vacuum pressure and initial corneal surface curvatures. Stroma bed margin thickness of about 200 to 250 um is recommended. Therefore the 120 to 130 um setting would be preferred for high diopter corrections, considering that the central ablation depth (H) is about $Weff^2/3$ microns per 1.0 diopter of correction, where Weff = (4.5 to 6.5) mm is the adjustable effective zone diameter in multizone method, or H=(6.8 to 14.1) microns per diopter. Another possible issue relates to the "matching" of the microkeratome cutting edge which may be alternated by the laser ablation "transition zone". The healing of the mismatched flap might affect the effective zone Weff postoperatively, in addition to its surface quality.

In this regard, a new method using ultra short pulse IR laser (made by Intralase) was also on the market as an alternative of microkeratome. Better surface quality is expected, however, the flap thickness uncertainty may be greater in the laser-flap method.

ABLATION ALGORITHMS

High-order Term

A new formula for the corneal central ablation depth (H) in a myopic three-zone LASIK is given by Lin:

$$H = (RF)\ (DW^2/3)\ (1+C). \quad (1)$$

where H in microns, LASIK correction power D in diopters and the ablation zone diameter W in mm. RF is a reduction factor when a 3-zone-ablation is used in comparing to single-zone depth. C is a high-order correction term. Depending on the software design of manufacturers, RF ranges from 0.75 to 0.85. For example, in a 3-zone distribution design of: 100% ablation within 0.5W, 50% within 0.75W and 25% within the transition zone of 0.25W, RF=0.78.

The high-order correction term C is introduced to account for the effect of preoperative corneal anterior radius of curvature (r1) which is related to the measured preoperative keratometry reading (Kpre) by Kpre=337/r1, therefore

$$C = 0.19\ (W/r1)^2 = 0.19\ [W(Kpre/337)]^2 \quad (2)$$

The above correction term is important particularly for high-myopic (or steep cornea with r1<7.5 mm) and when large ablation zone is used (with W > 6.5 mm). Lin's calculation shows that the commonly used first-order formula (with C=0) underestimates the ablation depth by 10% to 16% in comparing to the new formula. For examples: For r1=7.8 mm (or Kpre = 43.2 D), C = (11.2, 13.2, 16.4)% for W = (6.0, 6.5, 7.0) mm; for W=7.0 mm, C= (16.4, 13.2, 11.1)% for r1 = (7.0, 7.8, 8.5) mm or Kpre = (48.1, 43.2, 39.6) D. That is the high-order correction becomes significant (about 16% deeper than the first-order formula) for steeper cornea (Kpre > 45D) and large ablation zone.

Therefore, a refined ablation algorithm should include the following as the "input" parameters:

a. The preoperative K-reading (Kprep) for individual eye, particularly for those having Kprep values substantially different from the mean value of 43 D.
b. If the personalized Kprep is not available, then the mean value may be used.

However, Eq.(1) must be used to include the high-order correction (C).

For the same LASIK ablation depth, the first-order approximation (PA) will causes an over-correction (OC), comparing to the high-order formula, an amount of OC = 3 CH/(RF)W^2. For example, a 5.0 diopter myopic correction with a zone size of 7.0 mm and RF = 0.78, OC = 0.66 diopters; and ablation depth error of (10.4, 8.4) microns for r1 = (7.0, 7.8) mm. The new formulas show central ablation depth (per diopter correction) of 14.42 micron versus 12.74 micron in PA for the case of W=7.0 mm, r1=7.8 mm and RF=0.78 (in 3-zone design). These values may also be compared with the single-zone (or when RF=1.0) which are 28% deeper in the above example. We also note that the ablation depth (H) is proportional to the square of the ablation zone diameter (W) and 10% reduction of W will cause 19% reduction in ablation depth for a given refraction correction.

The true corneal refraction power (Dpost) after LASIK may be calculated by Dpost = 1.117Kpost –41/r2, which requires the measurements of the post-LASIK K-reading (Kpost) and the corneal posterior radius of curvature (r2). The prior work of Hamed et al using a mean value r2 = 6.8 mm in above calculation will cause a refraction error of 1.1 and 1.4 diopters for individual patient with r2 = 8.0 and 5.5 mm, respectively.

Aberration Rate Calibration

Clinical factors causing variations of ablation depth include the reabsorption of laser energy by the ablated plume nearby the corneal surface and the hydration (BSS) levels on the treated surface. Surface reflection loss and the nonnormal incidence of the laser beam (with increased effective zone size) may also contribute to about 8% to 10% reduction. For example, it was measured by Lin that the central ablation depth on a PMMA was reduced by about 25% for a testing without air blowing on the surface due to the reabsorption of the PMMA plume.

Another error comes from system manufacturers provided conversion factor (CF) or the ablation rate ratio between corneal stroma tissue and PMMA. The CF value, 2.8 to 3.5 empirically defined in various systems and based on statistical average may be the major source of error in determining the actual ablation depth. The "apparent" CF value is clinically adjusted by individual surgeons such that the errors of about 10% to 15% are "smeared" and compensated. The "true" CF value depends on accurate measurement of tissue ablation rate, which is influenced by laser energy re-absorption and corneal surface hydration conditions, and is hard to measure accurately from patient to patient.

The above PMMA calibrated CF value had been suggested by the manufacturers. However, depending on the control of corneal conditions and the feedback from treated cases, some surgeons had further adjusted these CF values by 5% to 15% based on my knowledge. The other factors may also influence the ablation rate include: how the ablated plume is removed (by air blower, or by a vacuumer); control of microscope illuminating light and the number of stops made by the surgeon in each procedure. All these factors would affect the BSS level on the ablated stroma surface and therefore the ablation rate for a given laser fluence or energy per pulse.

Most of the current algorithms perform good outcomes even they had used PA and ignored the high-order correction (C). It may be fair to state that the major reason is that the errors resulting from the ignorance of the high-order term, the surface reflection loss and other biomechanical related factors had been "balanced" by the manufacturer-provided and surgeon-adjusted CF values. These values are clinically (empirically) adjusted for accurate (at least in the average sense) refractive outcome based on the approximated (PA) algorithms and ideal spherical corneal surface. It should be emphasized that the empirically defined CF value may compensate most of the uncertainties due to algorithms or ocular conditions and therefore, provide good outcomes for normal populations. For individual subjects deviating from the normal (average) conditions, the empirical CF value would suffer inevitable errors, where only the theoretically defined CF value and a refined algorithm could provide the accurate outcomes.

Optimized Transition Zone (OTZ)

It was reported by Hori-Komai et al that using a new ablation algorithm called OTZ may offer larger effective optimal zone (EOZ) and decrease the postoperative halo, glare and reduced night vision, in comparing to the conventional multizone method. Seven types of OTZ are available (in NIDEK EC 5000 system) defined by the inner/outer zone size of 4.5/8.5 mm. For example, a myopia profile of -5.0 D has a central ablation depth (H) of about 69 um, for a conventional method having an inner optical zone of 6.0 mm and transition zone of 7.0 mm. The depth would be reduced by about 3 um when # 4 profile is used; or increased by 2.4 um in #5 profile. The # 6 and # 7 profiles offers larger EOZ but also required larger ablation depth. They also found that significantly less change of corneal asphericity after OTZ than the conventional method.

Corneal Asphericity Change

It was reported by Marcos et al, Jimenez et al and Lin that the corneal asphericity (Q) increase (decrease) after myopic (hyperopic) LASIK. According to Lin's formula, the postoperative (Q2) and preoperative (Q1) asphericity are related by

$$Q2 = a\,(Q1 + 1) - 1 \qquad (3)$$

where a=1.23 for -5.0 D myopic and a=0.826 for +5.0 D hyperopic LASIK. For example, an initially prolate cornea (with Q1= –0.1) will become oblate (with Q2=+0.11) after a myopic-LASIK. In comparison, an initially prolate cornea (with Q1= –0.26) will become more prolate (with Q2= –0.39) after a hyperopic-LASIK, which may also change an initially oblate cornea (with Q1= + 0.1) will become slightly prolate (with Q2= – 0.09).

In general, the factor a in Eq.(3) is given by $a = (R'/R)^2$, where R and R′ are the corneal preoperative and postoperative surface radius, respectively. For myopia, R′>R, a>1 and Q2>Q1 or increase of asphericity after LASIK. For hyperopia R′<R, and Q2<Q1, a decrease of Q. R′ and R are related to the refractive error (D) by

$$D = (3/8)(1/R' - 1/R). \qquad (4)$$

The above theoretical prediction providing the consistent trends with measurements by Chen et al, however, underestimated the actual change of corneal asphericity which may be further changed by the proposed factors of: Reflected/absorbed energy loss and nonnormal incidence angle of the laser; the asphericity induced by wound healing and biomechanical response of the cornea.

As proposed by Lin and others, the postLASIK corneal asphericity may be controlled to meet the need for minimal high-order optical aberration (HOA) where the postoperative corneal Q-value is required to balance the lens Q-value for minimal HOA. Greater details may be found in other chapters by Lin in this book.

Q-Factor Customized Ablation

Preoperative wave-front analysis may be used to create individualized ablation to compensate for preexisting aberrations. However, this analysis is time consuming and may not be necessary for majority of the eyes, as pointed out by Koller et al. Therefore a new algorithm based on aspheric nonindividualized profile was proposed to improve the visual outcomes.

Manns et al reported that a target Q value of –0.4 would create a minimum spherical aberration. Gatinel et al reported that for an intended value change of –0.6 (within optical zone of 6.5 mm) would require about 28.5 um more central tissue removed. Therefore, for stronger attempted asphericity correction with Q change larger than –1.0 (in myopia correction) or +1.0 (in hyperopia correction), requiring extracentral ablation, depth greater than about 60 um, would not be recommended.

CONCLUSION

The outcomes of LASIK, LASEK or epiLASIK procedures depend not only on the system parameters, ablation algorithm, microkeratome, but also on surgeon's technique in handling the ocular conditions, preoperatively and intraoperatively. Laser spot size , fluency and repetition rate affect the ablation rate and the thermal effects. For improved visual outcomes, high order aberration of the cornea must be optimized by controlling the postoperative corneal asphericity (the Q-factor) for minimum overall aberration by compensating the preexisting lens aberration. The personalized preoperative overall Q value should also include the age effect on the lens.

To improve the overall visual outcome, the improved algorithm should also consider the following "individualized" extra information, in addition to the conventional input parameters of refractive error (D) and the ablation zone (W):

- Preoperative K-reading (Kpre) and/or the corneal anterior surface radius (r1)
- Preoperative corneal and lens asphericity (the Q values)
- Adjusted effective ablation zone (Weff) to include the laser energy loss due to extrahydration on the treated surface, reflection loss, nonnormal incidence and other biomechanical effects
- Readjust the manufacturer provided PMMA calibration conversion function (CF) based on surgeon's experience and the empirical data obtained. The CF value may be affected by surgeon's handling of the treated corneal surface, the material used of PMMA and the vacuum device (or blower).

BIBLIOGRAPHY

1. Anera R, Jimenez JR, Barco LJ. Equation for corneal asphericity after corneal refractive surgery. J Refract Surg. 2003;19:65-69.
2. Anera RG, Jimenez JR, Barco LJ, Hitta E. Change in corneal asphericity after laser refractive surgery, including reflection loss and nonnormal incidence upon the anterior cornea. Opt Lett. 2003;15:417-19.
3. Atchison DA, Smith G. Optics of the human eye. Woburn, MA: Butterworth-Heinemann; 2000; pp. 14-16, 143-47, 160-62.
4. Avalos G, Silva A. Presbyopia LASIK-the PMMA technique. In: Agarwal A. ed. Presbyopia, a surgical textbook. Thorofare NJ: SLACK; 2004. pp. 139-46.
5. Cantu R, Rosales MA, Tepichin E, et al. Objective quality of vision in presbyopic and nonpresbyopic patients after pseudoaccommodative advanced surface ablation. J Refract Surg. 2005 (Suppl.); 21:S603-05.
6. El-Danasoury A, Baines HS. Optimized prolate corneal ablation: case report for the first treated eye. J Refract Surg. 2005;21:S595-02.
7. Gatinel D, T Hoang-Xuan, Azar D. Determination of corneal asphericity after myopia surgery with the excimer laser: A mathematical model. Invest Ophthalmol Vis Sci. 2001;42:1736-42.
8. Gills J, et al. Corneal topography: The state of the art. SLACK Inc: Thorofare 1995.
9. Gordon M, et al. Photorefractive keratectomy (PRK) at 193 nm using an erodible mask. Proc SPIE. 1992;1644:11-19.
10. Holladay JT, Bains HS. Optimized prolate ablation with the NIDEK CXII excimer laser. J Refract Surg. 2005; 21:S595-97.
11. Jenkins TCA. Aberration of the eye and their effects on vision. Br J Physiol Opt. 1963;20:59-91.
12. Jimenez JR, Anera RG, Diaz J, Diaz A, Perez-ocon F. Corneal asphericity after refractive surgery when the Munnerlyn formula is applied. J Opt Soc Am. (A) 2004;21:98-03.
13. Jimenez JR, Anera RG, Barco LJ. Refractive changes due to ablation parameters after photorefractive surgery. J Refract Surg. 2004;20:182-82.
14. Lee H, Oh JR, Reintein DZ, et al. Conservation of corneal tissue with wave-front-guided laser in situ kerato-mileuse. J Cataract Refract Surg. 2005; 31:1153-58.
15. Lin JT: in Program and Abstract, ISRK, pre-AAO, 1994-99.
16. Lin JT: Multiwavelength solid state laser for ophthalmic applications. Proc SPIE 1992;1644:266-75.
17. Lin JT: Mini-excimer laser corneal reshaping using a scanning device. Proc SPIE 1994;2131:228-36.
18. Lin JT. Scanning laser technology for refractive surgery. In: Garg, et al. Mastering the techniques of corneal refractive surgery. New Delhi, India, Jaypee Brothers; 2005. pp. 20-36.
19. Lin JT. Critical review on refractive surgical lasers. Opt. Engineer. 1995; 34:668-75.
20. Lin JT. A new formula for ablation depth in 3-zone LASIK. J Refract Surg. 2005;21:413-414.
21. Lin JT. Prediction and control of corneal asphericity after refractive surgery. J Refract Surg. 2006;22:(in press).
22. Lin JT. A prospective randomized clinical trial of laser in situ keratomileusis with two different lasers. Am J Ophthalmol. 2006; [Correspondence] (in press).
23. Machat JJ. Excimer laser refractive surgery: Practice and principles. SLACK Inc: Thorofare, 1995.
24. Mackee SM, Krueger RR, Applegate RA. In: Customized corneal ablation. Ed. Mackee SM, Krueger RR, Applegate RA. (SLACK, Thorofare, NJ, 2001), pp.3-9.
25. Manns F, Ho A, Parel JM, Culbertson W. Ablation profile for wavefront-guided correction of myopia and primary spherical aberration. J Cataract Refract Surg. 2002;28:766-74.
26. Marcos S, Cano D, Barbero S. Increase in corneal asphericity after standard laser in situ keratomileusis for myopia is not inherent to the Munnerlyn algorithm. J Refract Surg. 2003;19:S592-96.
27. Mrochen M, Seiler T. Influence of corneal curvature on calculation of ablation patterns used in photorefractive laser surgery. J Refract Surg. 2001;17:S584-87.
28. Niemz MH et al. Intrastromal ablation for refractive corneal surgery using picosecond infrared laser pulses. Laser Light Ophthalmol. 1993;5:149-55.
29. Puliafito CA et al. Excimer laser ablation of the cornea and lens. Ophthalmology. 1985;92:741-48.thermokerato-plasty by means of a pulsed holmium:YAG laser for hyperopic correction. Refract Corneal Surg. 1990:6:335-339.
30. Ren Q, Lin JT et al. Ultraviolet solid-state laser (213 nm) photorefractive keratectomy. Ophthalmology. 1993; 100:1828-1834.
31. Rozakis G. Refractive Lamellar keratoplasty. SLACK Inc: Thorofare. 1995.
32. Seiler T, et al. Laser thermokeratoplasty by means of a pulsed holmium:YAG laser for hyperopic correction. Refract Corneal Surg. 1990;6:335-39.
33. Sher NA. Surgery for hyperopia and presbyopia. Williams and Wilkins: 1997.
34. Srinivasan R. Ablation of polymers and biological tissue by ultraviolet lasers. Science. 1986;234:559-65.
35. Tabaoda J et al. Response of the corneal epithelium to ArF excimer laser pulses. 1981. Health Phys. 352.
36. Telando A. Pseudoaccommodative cornea: A new concept for correction of presbyopia. J Refract Surg. 2004;20(Suppl.):S714-17.
37. Trokel SL, et al. Excimer laser surgery of the cornea. Am J Ophthalmol. 1983;92:741-48.
38. Twa MD, Lemback RG, Bullimore MA, Roberts C, "A prospective randomized clinical trial of laser in situ keratomileusis with two different lasers", Am J Ophthalmol. 2005;140:173-83.

Management of LASIK and LASEK Complications (Interesting Cases)

37

SANJAY CHAUDHARY (INDIA)

CORNEAL HAZE AFTER LASEK WITH MITOMYCIN

History

A 26 year old male presented with bilateral high myopia The patient had a stable myopia for the past 3 years. The right eye had a refractive error of –11D while the left eye had a refractive error of –15 D. His corrected visual acuity was 6/9p in the right eye and 6/12p in the left eye. The fundus had myopic changes and retinal holes and lattice and an LIO was done to seal the holes with double frequency Yag laser four weeks prior to the procedure. The pachymetry was 514 mic in the right eye and 520 mic in the left eye. The average K reading was 44.5 D in right eye and 44.75 D in left eye. He was scheduled for simultaneous bilateral alcohol assisted LASEK surgery in both the eyes.

Operation Done

A simultaneous bilateral alcohol assisted lasek surgery was done in both the eyes. The epithelial flap was loosened up using 20 % ethyl alcohol. The cornea was ablated using the Nidek EC5000 laser system. After corneal ablation the cornea was cooled using chilled BSS. The treated area of the cornea was then exposed to 0.02% Mitomycin-C for 60 seconds. The corneal surface was then thoroughly washed with BSS for a minute to remove all traces of Mitomycin and then the epithelium was reposited back. A bandage contact lens was then placed on the eye.

Complication

The epithelium healed in five days time. The vision subsequently improved to unaided 6/9 in the right eye and 6/9 p in the left eye. The patient was put on FML starting at seven times a day for a week and tapering off over the next seven weeks. Follow-up at 3 months showed clear cornea and emmetropia. Mitomycin–C is useful in containing fibroblastic activity and thereby reducing and delaying the chances of corneal haze, more so when attempting to treat high myopia.

The patient returned one and a half year later with diminishing vision. An examination showed myopia of -1.25 dioptre in the right eye and -2.75D in the left eye with an associated corrected vision of 6/12 in the right eye and 6/18 in the left eye. A slit lap examination showed superficial corneal haze in the right eye grade I and left eye grade II.

Management

The patient was put on low dose steroid drops three times a day for three months and asked to report after three months. There was a slight reduction in haze in these three months. It was not considered wise to continue using steroid drops and they were taken off and patient sent back on lubricating eye drops for the next three months.

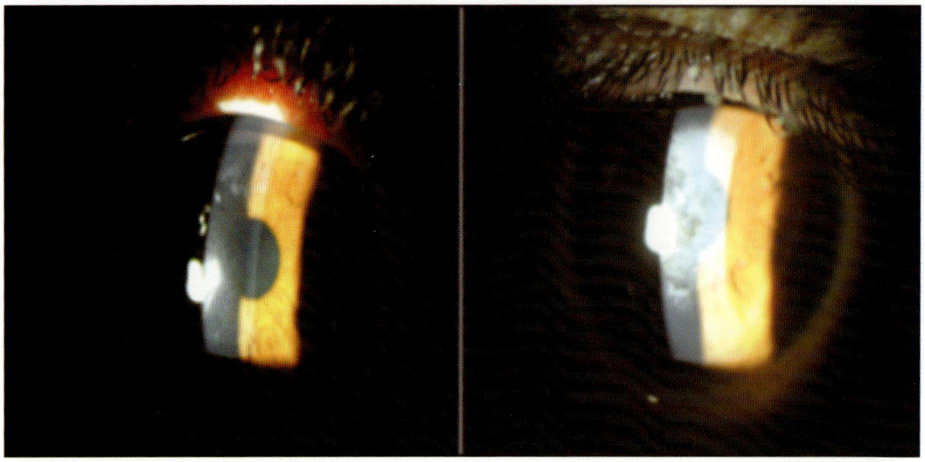

Fig. 37.1: The patient developed a gr. I corneal haze in the right eye and a gr. II haze in the left eye after one and a half year of simultaneous lasek with Mitomycin-c in both eyes. The right eye had myopia of –11D while the left eye had myopia of –15D

Discussion

Corneal Haze

This has become the most feared complication in a long-standing follow-up of LASEK. The haze is similar to the one encountered in PRK and can be graded from I to IV. It was a myth that Mitomycin prevents haze formation in LASEK while attempting higher degree of corrections. The use of Mitomycin–c in our routine clinical practice for myopia of over 4 D seems to have helped in the following ways:

1. Haze is usually not encountered in myopia of up to 7.0 D as compared with PRK where it could be encountered after 4 D.
2. Myopia of 8 to 12 usually results in Gr. I haze while 12 and above may result in Gr. II to III haze
3. There have been situations where even –18 D has had no haze and on the other hand, even a –5 developed a mild haze.
4. Haze usually develops after 6-9 months of the procedure.
5. Haze results in a regression of the refractive error and the degree of regression depends on he severity of haze.
6. Haze usually regresses spontaneously over a period of 2 to 3 years. Low dose topical steroids could assist resolution.
7. The regression of haze sometimes results in some reversal of regression of the refractive error and improvement in refractive error and vision.

The above observations are not a rule but an indication of the surgeon's experience with PRK of over 10 years and of lasek with and without Mitomycin on over 400 eyes in 4 years.

PRK, LASEK and now Epi-LASIK involve the removing or stripping of the epithelium from the Bowman's membrane. In PRK, it is mechanical scrapping, in LASEK it is alcohol assisted while in Epi-LASIK, it is again separation with a blade. Since the three are essentially similar and involve ablation of the Bowman's membrane, they carry the same advantages and disadvantages, albeit with minor modifications. Therefore, it postulates that the presence of corneal haze may be similar in PRK, LASEK and Epi-LASIK. Minor variations in the severity of haze may be achieved with the help of Mitomycin.

FLAP WRINKLES

History

A 23 year myopic male with a refraction of –6 with –1 cylinder in right eye and –6 with –3 cylinder in the left eye. He presented to our clinic for correction of his refractive error. He had not changed the

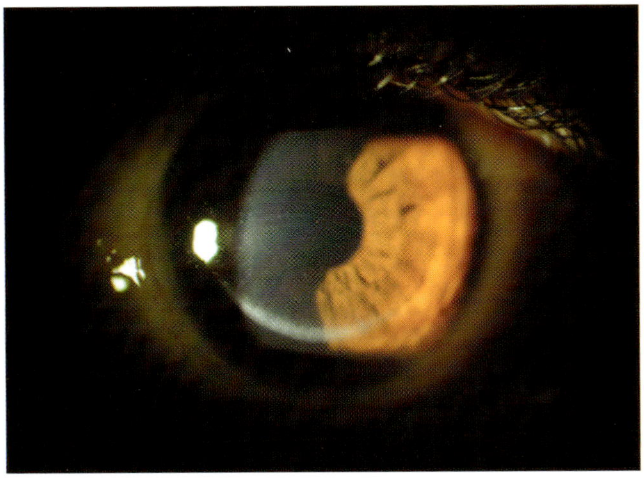

Fig. 37.2: Flap wrinkles extending into the papillary area. Note the scarring a 6'oclock due to flap displacement

power of his glasses for the last one and a half year. His visual acuity was 6/6 in both the eyes. His IOP was 18 mm Hg in both the eyes and Pachymetry was 542 mic. in right eye and 551 mic in left eye

Operation Done

He under went a bilateral LASIK procedure in both the eyes using the Nidek EC5000. The first day follow up was uneventful. The patient had an uncorrected visual acuity of 6/6 in both the eyes. The patient was advised to come for a follow-up after a week.

Complication

The first week follow-up revealed that his uncorrected visual acuity was 6/6 in the right eye and 6/18 in the left eye. Refraction of the left eye showed a cylinder correction of +1.25 and an improvement in visual acuity to 6/12. Torch light exam reveals a semicircular superficial corneal opacity at the 6 o'clock position at the point of the flap edge. Slit lamp exam showed horizontal flap wrinkles or striae in the left eye extending into the papillary area. The corneal opacity is observed to be in the area where the flap has retracted and the gap is covered by cicatrical tissue.

Management

A decision was taken to correct the flap wrinkles immediately. The patient was shifted to the OT. The flap was lifted with a micro fine iris repositer. The wrinkles become very prominent once the flap is lifted. The flap was hydrated on the epithelial and the stromal side with BSS through a 23 g cannula and stroked with this cannula in a direction perpendicular to the striae. The flap was also stretched perpendicular to the wrinkle lines with the help of a flat tipped forceps. This step was repeated several times making sure the pressure does not traumatize or avulse the flap from the hinge. The flap is repositioned back and stroked vigorously with a wet merocel sponge in a direction so as to iron out the wrinkles. This step is repeated several times. Even though the flap appears to smoothen out, the ridges persist through out the procedure. Five minutes is allowed to lapse to let the flap adhere firmly to the corneal bed. No bandage or bandage contact lens is used. The patient is asked to present for an eye examination the following day. Slit lap exam on the following day reveals that the wrinkles are almost gone and the corrected vision improves to 6/6p. Most of the cylindrical component of the refraction also disappears.

Discussion

The incidence of flap wrinkles or striae in our clinical practice is 0.6%.

Clinically they appear in the postoperative period as loss of best corrected visual acuity and irregular astigmatism. It is also sometimes associated with glare, halo's and night driving difficulties. A flap wrinkle should be treated immediately on detection if it is reaching out into the papillary area and/or causing a loss of BCVA. They are usually encountered if there is excessive intraoperative flap manipulation or excessive hydration of the flap. It could also be associated with high degree of ablation resulting in a 'flap to bed mismatch'. Postoperative squeezing or rubbing of lids especially in very thin flaps may also contribute to this pathology.

FREE FLAP

History

A 22 year old female presented with myopia of –5.0 D in both the eyes along with prominent

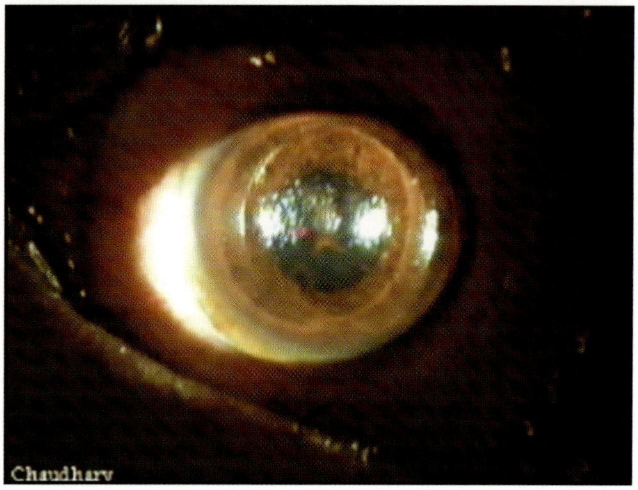

Fig. 37.3: Free cap in a patient with prominent PPM

persistent papillary membrane. The right eye pachymetry was 514 mic and the K reading was 42D and 41.75D. The patient had a stable myopia for the past 3 years. Her visual acuity was 6/9 in the right eye. She was scheduled for Lasik surgery in this eye.

Operation Done

A Moria M2 microkeratome was used and because of the flat cornea, a ring of –1 was selected which is a ring designed for flat cornea. Moria has labeled it's rings as –1, 0, +1, +2 where +2 is for steep cornea. The peripheral part of the cornea was marked with a corneal marker. The suction ring was placed on the cornea and the vacuum activated to build up the ocular pressure to 65 mm Hg. This was confirmed with a Barraquer tonometer. The head of the keratome was engaged in the ring and a forward and backward pass made. On releasing the vacuum and lifting the keratome, it was found that the corneal flap was missing and a central circular exposed area of the cornea stroma was seen.

Complication Faced

A diagnosis of a free flap or a free cap was made. The following observations were made

1. The flap was stuck in the keratome head with a small edge protruding out . This protrusion was appox. 1 mm. This protrusion belonged to the area of the hinge and in this case the 12 o'clock position.
2. The flap bed was observed to be smaller than the normal size

Management of Complication

1. Management of the flap: The corneal flap as seen protruding out of the keratome head was identified as the area which belonged to the hinge area, and in this case it was the superior hinge. The epithelial surface of the flap was marked with gentian violet pen for identification. The flap was held by a nontoothed forceps and placed in an antidesiccation chamber, epithelial surface down. A drop of BSS was placed on the tray on which the flap was placed taking care not to hydrate the stromal surface.
2. Continue lasik: The lasik ablation was continued as planned. The stromal bed was wiped clean of debris and condensed plume with BSS solution. A drop of BSS was placed on the centre of the cornea.
3. Repositioning the Flap: The flap was picked up from the antidesiccation chamber with a nontoothed forceps and placed on the cornea, epithelial surface up. The corneal markers on the flap were aligned with those on the host surface. The gentian violet epithelial surface mark comes to rest superiorly at the point of the hinge. Two BSS soaked cellulose sponges were used, one to stabilize the flap in position and the other to stroke the flap to smoothen it out. After a five minute waiting to ensure sufficient time for a good flap adherence, a striae test was done to confirm the same. A bandage contact lens was not used.

The Tricky Part of the Management is

1. It becomes very difficult to clinically differentiate the epithelial side of the flap from the stromal

side. It is therefore important to make a note of the epithelial side of the flap before pulling it out of the keratome head. In case there is a mix-up, a reference is obtained by aligning the marks on the cornea extending on to the flap. This is possible if the marks are nonsymmetrical. Placing the epithelial side on the corneal bed will result in epithelialization of the stromal bed and a subsequent loss of the flap.

2. Improper alignment of the flap: This occurs if no markers are used or the marks are so light like those made with a sharp instrument without gentian violet. This results in improper alignment resulting in astigmatism and loss of BCVA.

Discussion

The incidence of free flaps in our clinical practice is 0.5%.

Eyes with flat cornea's or high astigmatism are more prone to free flaps. Flat cornea do not protrude well in the LASIK suction ring, and therefore the size of the flap is smaller. This also results in a smaller hinge. A total loss of hinge results in a free flap. Moria keratome has a protective system where a bigger hinge can be planned by changing the position of the stopper. In my daily practice, in all flat cornea's, I place the stopper at the position of 7.5 rather than the standard 8.0 to obtain a smaller flap and consequently a larger hinge.

Corneal Ectasia Post LASIK: The Orbscan Advantage

38

Erik L Mertens (Belgium),
Arun C Gulani, Paul Karpecki (USA)

INTRODUCTION

With the advent of corneal topography and its increasing application in practice, our knowledge about the shape of the cornea has rapidly accumulated.[1] Determination of the ability of the cornea to undergo laser refractive surgery is of the utmost importance. The purpose is to avoid corneal ectasia and visual impairment in otherwise healthy eyes. First reported by Prof. Theo Seiler[2] this condition is characterized by progressive protuberance and steepening, increasing myopia and or astigmatism with distorted and decreased best corrected vision in the involved eye. Some of the reported cases can be traced back to the preoperative evaluations and lack of recognition for risk factors (Gulani A.C: Corneal Topography and Wavefront Instructional Course, ASCRS San Diego, May 2004).

CORNEAL ECTASIA

Postrefractive surgical ectasia was a planned event in automated lamellar keratomileusis for hyperopia where the corneal flap was created at 70% depth to allow for a controlled steepening. This phenomenon has been seen not only with LASIK surgery where the creation of the corneal flap is an additional contributing factor but also with surface photorefractive keratectomy wherein the depth of ablation and repetitive or multiple ablative patterns add to the risk. The most important diagnosis in this direction is that of forme fruste keratoconus.

Over several years data collected in retrospective analysis of post LASIK ectasias underscores the importance of this diagnosis. These thoughts have been repeatedly addressed but not solved (Gulani AC and Nordan LT – Personal Corresspondence). We shall need to strive to introduce newer and effective measurement criterias and combination technologies to further assist us in this field of obscure clinical findings but drastic postoperative outcomes. Through the years the Orbscan II and orbscan IIZ (Bausch and Lomb Orbtek, Salt Lake City, Utah) became more and more the standard for preoperative screening amongst refractive surgeons. It is an important diagnostic tool to help separate cases of corneal ectatic disorders like keratoconus and pellucid marginal degeneration as well as identify preclinical cases of corneal instability and forme fruste keratoconus (Gulani A.C : Advanced Diagnostics Course- B and L - AAO, Washington DC, April 2005).

SELECTION CRITERIA

A lot of these criteria are published throughout the years. Most of the parameters were empirically established by studying the unexpected postoperative ectasia patients. Some surgeons were able to find correlations with preoperative corneal maps and could even quantify abnormal preoperative corneal map findings.[3] This chapter will give you an overview of the most useful and important of these parameters.

Besides the topographical parameters never forget to look at the clinical signs (fluctuation of subjective refraction, younger patients, history of keratoconus, steep/distorted keratometry readings,...) and analyse the Orbscan maps on the Orbscan IIZ system, NOT ON THE PRINTOUT!!!

The decision to continue with refractive laser surgery is not based on a single clue, but rather on a combination of a set of criteria. When looking at the Orbscan's Quad Map you can find so called 'red flags' or 'yellow flags'. A 'red flag' definitively means a no-go situation and a 'yellow flag' is suspicious and will drive our attention to look very closely into the other corneal maps. On a typical Quad Map four corneal maps are routinely presented by the Orbscan II (Bausch and Lomb Orbtek, Salt Lake City, Utah). You will find the anterior elevation map in the upper left quadrant and the posterior elevation map in the upper right quadrant. The keratometric curvature map (power map) is located in the lower left quadrant and the pachymetry[4] map in the lower right quadrant (Fig. 38.1). In the center of these four maps a lot of statistics and useful data are displayed.

PACHYMETRY[5]

An absolute contraindication for lamellar corneal laser surgery is a thinnest point of < 470 microns. When pathological, this point is often displaced inferotemporal (Fig. 38.2). A difference of < 30 microns (yellow flag) or < 20 microns (red flag) between the central pachymetry and the peripheral thickness indicators can be seen in abnormal corneas (Fig. 38.3). A difference of > 100 microns from the thinnest point to the values at the 7 mm optical zone implies a steep gradient of thinning from the midperiphery towards the thinnest point (yellow flag) (Fig. 38.3).

POSTERIOR ELEVATION MAP (FIG. 38.4)

1. The most common reference surface for viewing elevation maps is the "best fit sphere" (BFS).

   A posterior high point > 50 microns above BFS might be indicative of an early posterior ectasia.

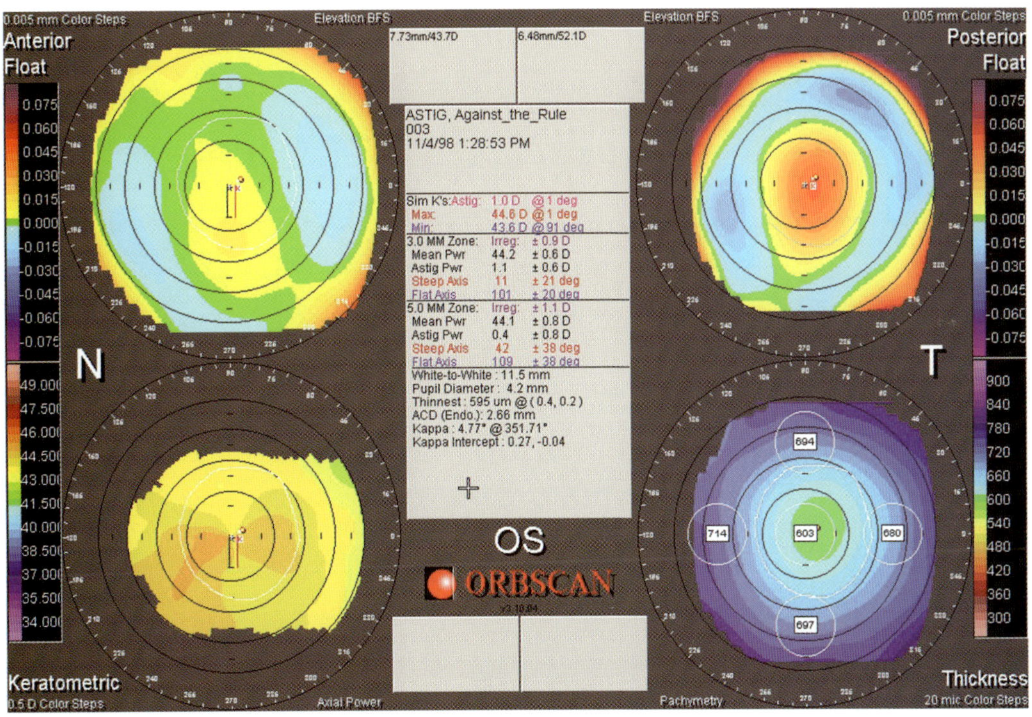

Fig. 38.1: Typical Quad Map (Orbscan II)

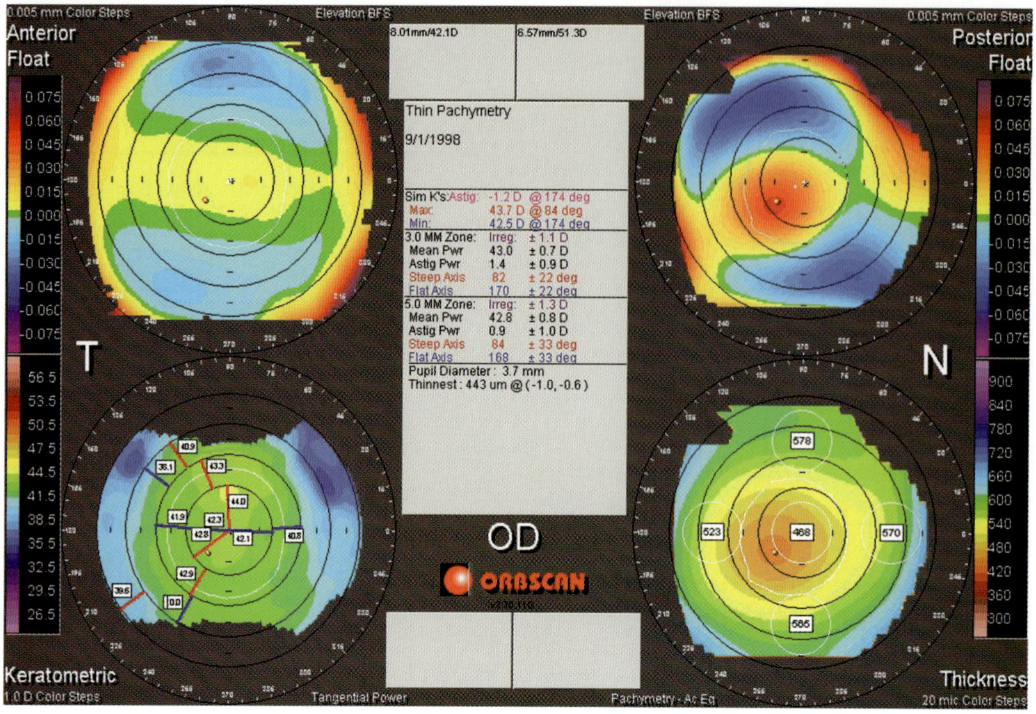

Fig. 38.2: Thinnest point (443 micron) displaced inferotemporal and a difference of >100 microns from the thinnest point to the values at the 7 mm zone

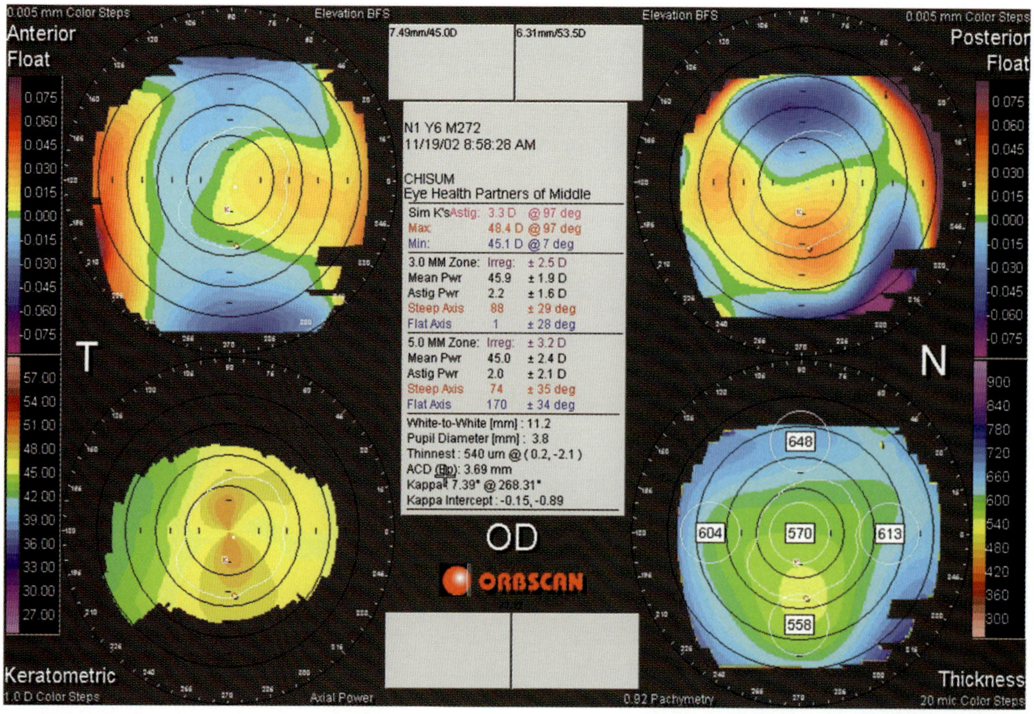

Fig. 38.3: Less than 20 microns between central pachymetry and peripheral inferior thickness

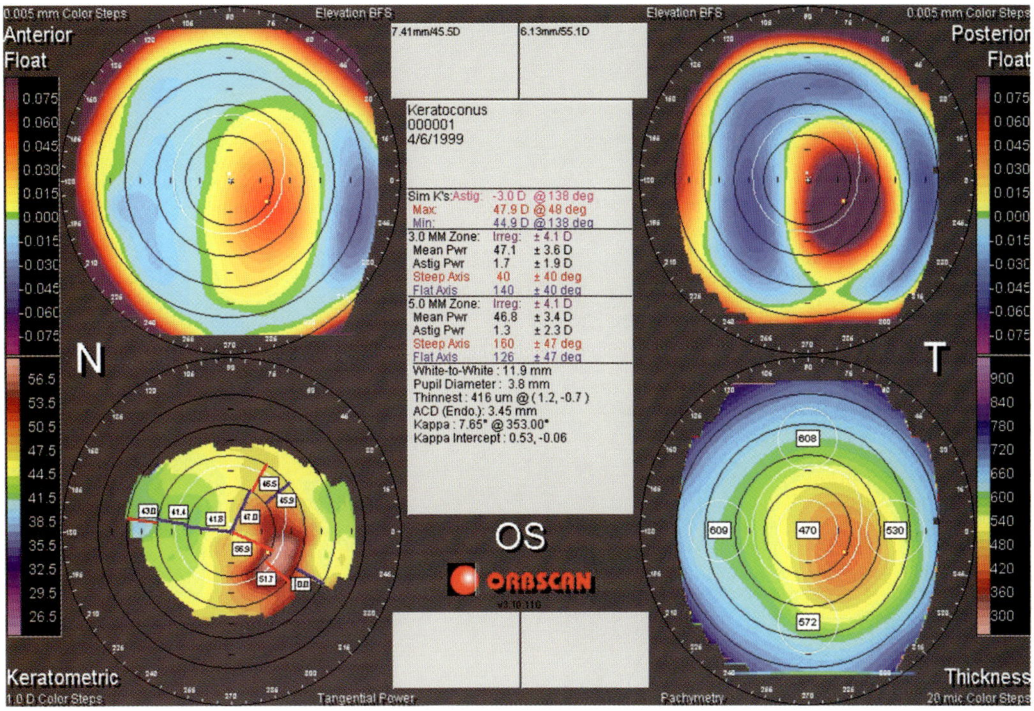

Fig. 38.4: The posterior elevation map shows multiple red flags as described in the text. The highest point on the posterior elevation coincides with the highest point on the anterior elevation, the thinnest point on pachymetry and the point of steepest curvature on the power map

However in cylindrical corneas with an astigmatism > 2.5 D this elevation can be induced by the astigmatism and needs to be checked with the other corneal maps (Fig. 38.5).

A posterior high point > 35 microns above BFS with corresponding thinning on the pachymetry map is a red flag for LASIK, but not for PRK, LASEK or epiLASIK.

2. The power of the posterior best fit sphere (BFS) is in normal corneas around 51D. A BFS with a power of more than 55 diopters (Fig. 38.4) on the posterior profile, could be indicative of early keratoconus. This criterium is not diagnostic as a sign of early ectasia[6] per se, as this may also be seen in small corneas (WTW<11 mm), very steep corneas or in Asian eyes.

   A power between 53 and 54 diopters can be suspicious, and needs to be correlated with other signs and/or symptoms.

3. Roush criterium : Indicative of early keratoconus is a relative difference > 100 microns between the highest and lowest point on the posterior elevation map (Fig. 38.4). A relative difference >70 microns is a yellow flag, except when the cornea is very symmetrical and when it is caused by a regular astigmatism.

POWER MAP

1. Steep corneal curvatures are always suspicious. Keratometric mean power map > 46 diopters or total mean power map > 45 diopters are definitely red flags (Fig. 38.6).
2. Bow-tie/broken bow-tie pattern. The so-called "lazy-C" on the axial power map is very suspicious when the astigmatism shifts > 20° from a straight line (Fig. 38.7).
3. Central corneal asymmetry. A change within the central 3 mm optical zone of the cornea of more

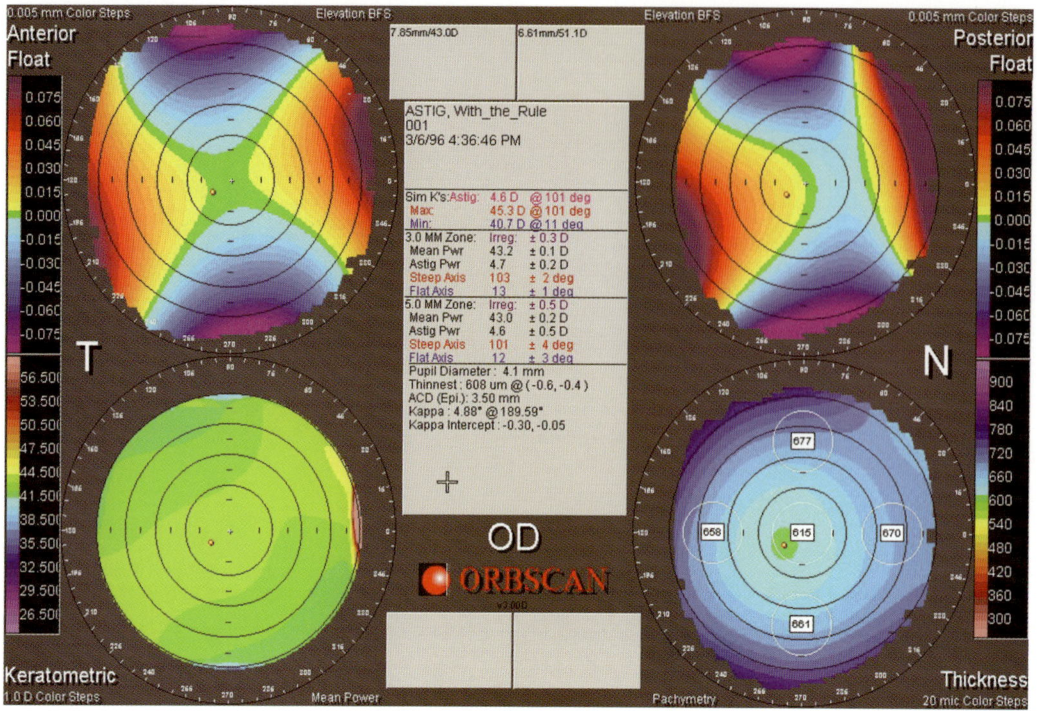

Fig. 38.5: Normal with the rule astigmatism. However the highest point on the posterior elevation map is > 50 microns

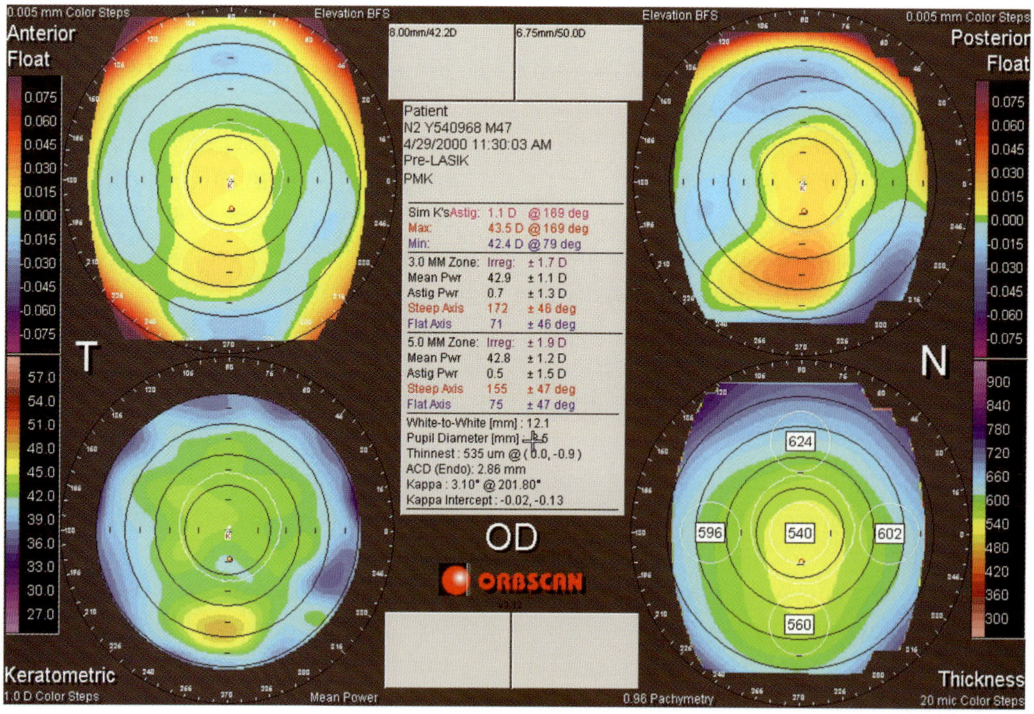

Fig. 38.6: Keratometric mean power map (lower left quadrant) showing a steepening of >46 D

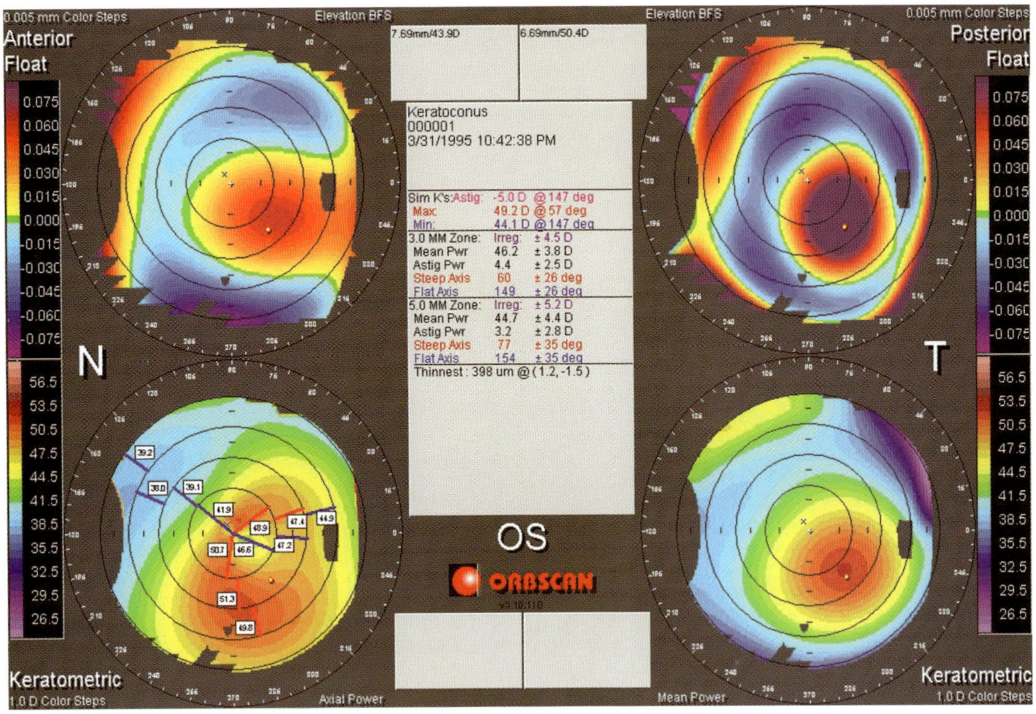

Fig. 38.7: Lazy-C associated with central corneal asymmetry

than 3 diopters from superior to inferior (yellow flag) can be correlated with the present of vertical coma (Fig. 38.7). However, this may be merely a sign of asymmetric astigmatism and is not necessarily indicative of pathology.

COMPOSITE/INTEGRATED INFORMATION

1. *Correlation of signs with the highest point on the posterior elevation.* This is probably the strongest topographic sign indicative of early keratoconus[7]. If the highest point on the posterior elevation coincides with the highest point on the anterior elevation, the thinnest point on pachymetry and the point of steepest curvature on the power map, never perform laser refractive surgery. This implies that the thinnest point represents a structural weakness, which causes a forward bending on the cornea (Fig. 38.4).
2. *Efkarpides criteria.* The ratio of the radius in mm of the anterior BFS divided by the radius in mm of the posterior BFS. Surprisingly in normal corneas this ratio will be around 1.21. Between 1.23 and 1.27 we should be suspicious and look for other abnormalities. But when this ratio is 1.27 or higher this cornea should never be treated with laser (Fig. 38.8).
3. *Bent/warped cornea.* Similarity between the anterior and posterior profiles implies a forward bending of those areas shown above BFS. If this bending is in association with the thinnest point on the cornea, it could relate to a structural weakness in the cornea. This sign needs to be evaluated within the context of the other parameters[8] (Fig. 38.9).
4. Infero-temporal displacement of the highest point on the anterior as well as the posterior elevation profile can be indicative of early keratoconus (Fig. 38.10).
5. Nature is surprisingly often very symmetrical, also our corneas. When a difference of more than 1D of astigmatism between two eyes is detected, there exists a higher risk of ectasia postoperatively.
6. Never forget to look at the information in the center of the quad maps. An irregularity of >1.5 D in the 3 mm central zone and of > 2.0 D in the

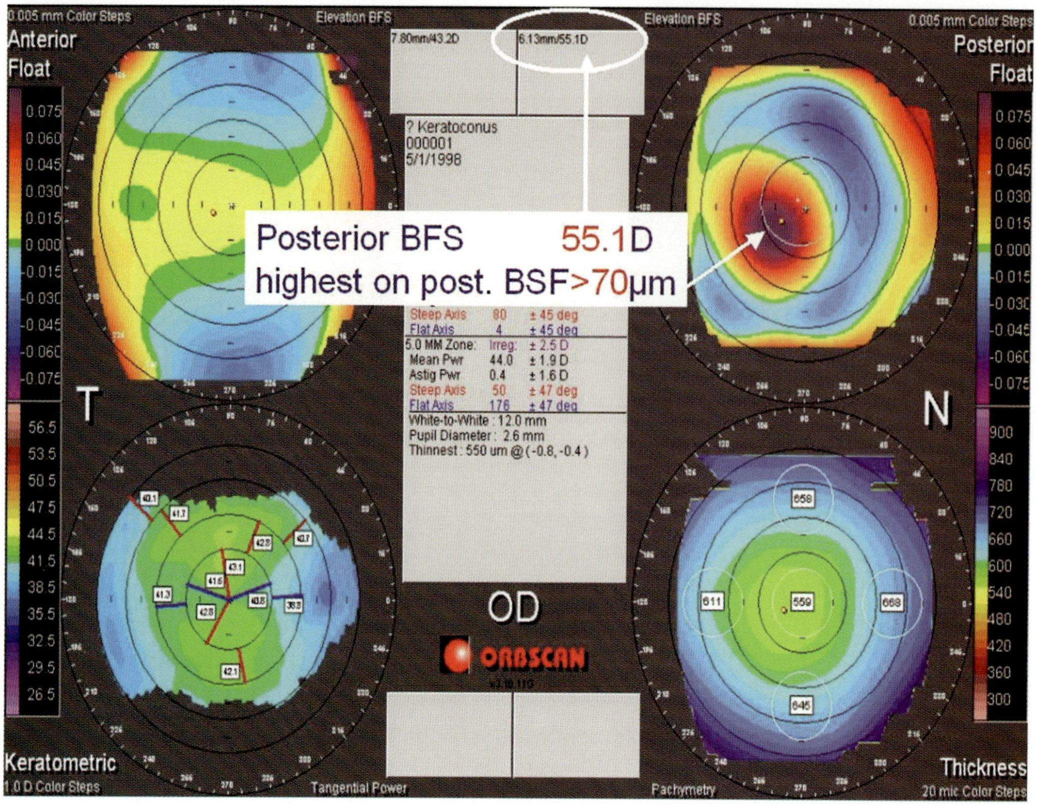

Fig. 38.8: Efkarpides : 7.8 mm/6.13 mm = 1,273. In this obvious case also other red flags appear

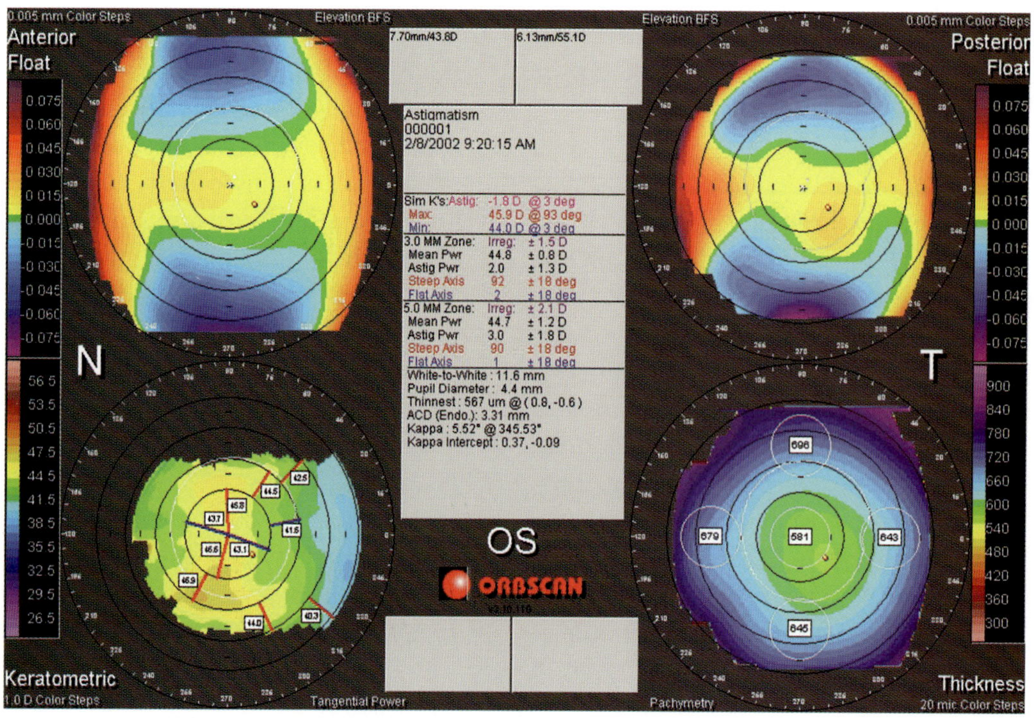

Fig. 38.9: Bent/warped cornea : Asymmetry of anterior and posterior elevation

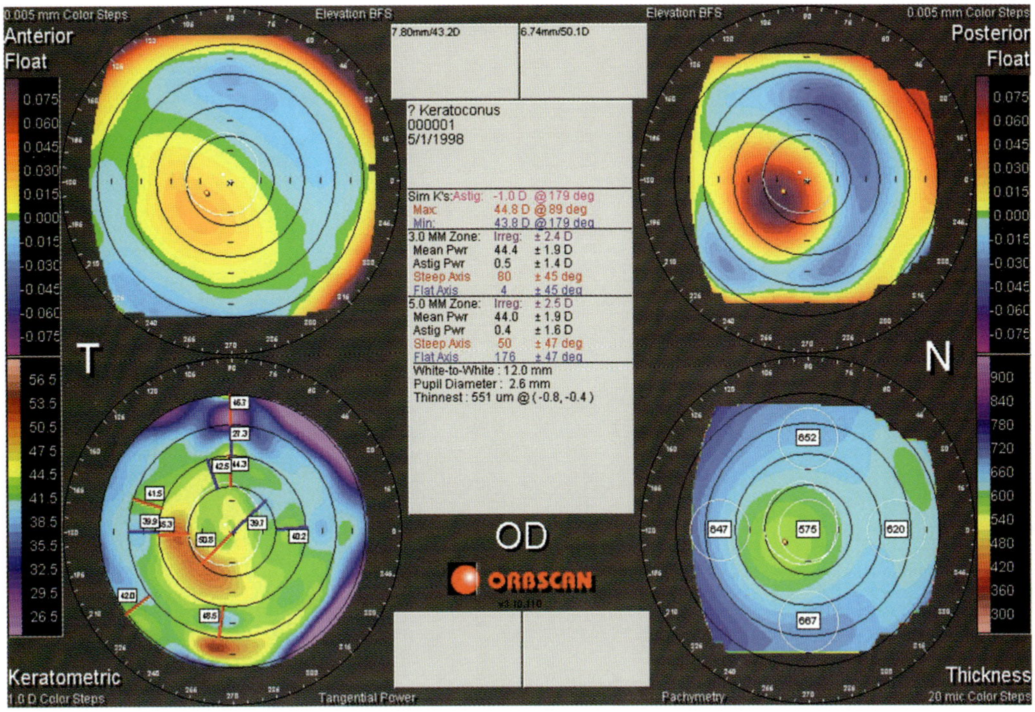

Fig. 38.10: Infero-temporal displacement of the highest point on the anterior as well as the posterior elevation profile can be indicative of early keratoconus

5 mm central zone should alert us (R. Lindstrom, MD). This sign is probably the weakest of all, but should not be ignored (Fig. 38.11).

7. *Normal band scale.* For the anterior and posterior elevation maps a normal band means an elevation within +/- 0.25 microns of the best fit sphere (BFS). The normal band for the total corneal power map is 40-48 diopters and for corneal thickness is between 500 and 600 microns. One pop-up means caution, two means concern and three pop-ups means a no-go situation (Figs 38.12 to 38.14).
8. If one eye fails on the indices but the other eye doesn't : NEVER TREAT EITHER EYE

The above mentioned indices can become useful in the armamentarium of preoperative evaluations for potential LASIK candidates towards safe and effective outcomes.

With newer technology integration using wavefront guidance (Zywave- B and L) we can detect higher order aberrations in the form of Coma and increased RMS values (Gulani AC: Wavefront principles: Simplified and Applied. Instructional course. ESCRS, Paris, Sept 2004) aiding earlier detection of keratoconus and other potential ectatic corneal conditions. Pellucid marginal degeneration is mostly the cause of corneal topographic changes when correlated with higher levels of trefoil. Keratoconus will induce most likely higher levels of coma.

FUTURE THOUGHTS

I (Gulani AC, MD) would suggest moving in a direction that will incorporate a dynamic corneal imaging system (Dynamic corneal imaging: Prof Gunther Grabner et al: University Eye Clinic, Paracelsus Private Medical University, Salzburg, Austria), video-topography for measurement of the tear film and its contour (Janos Nemeth et al from the First Department of Ophthalmology, Semmelweis University, Budapest, Hungary; the Computer and Automation Research Institute, Hungarian Academy of Sciences, Budapest, Hungary; and the Department

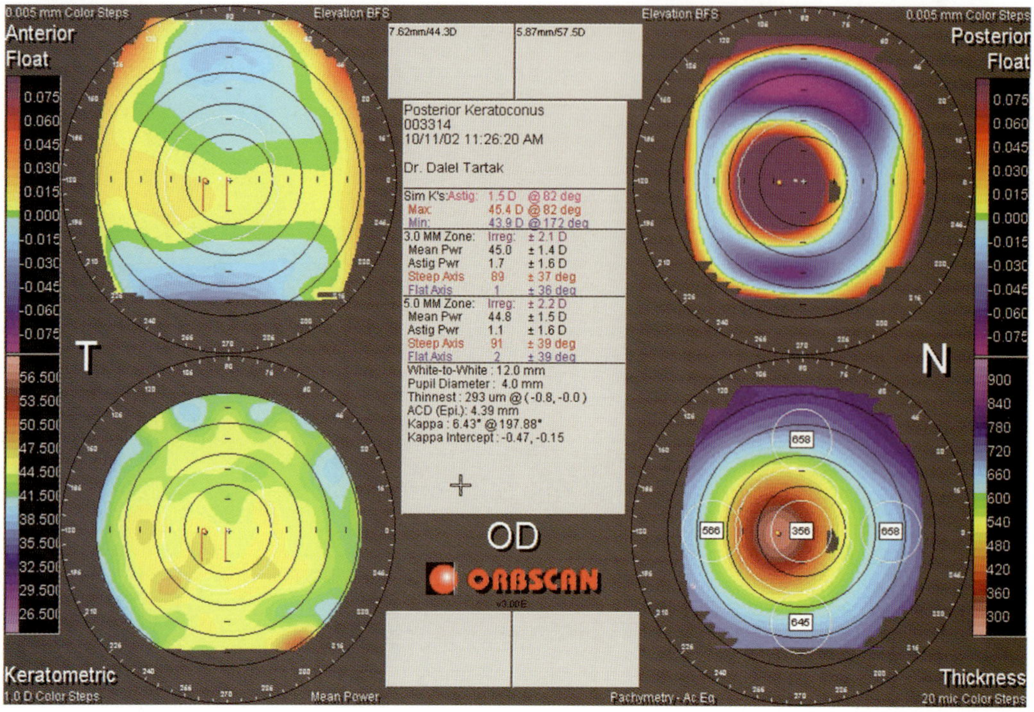

Fig. 38.11: An irregularity of >1.5 D in the 3 mm central zone and of > 2.0 D in the 5 mm central zone should alert us. This sign is probably the weakest of all, but should not be ignored

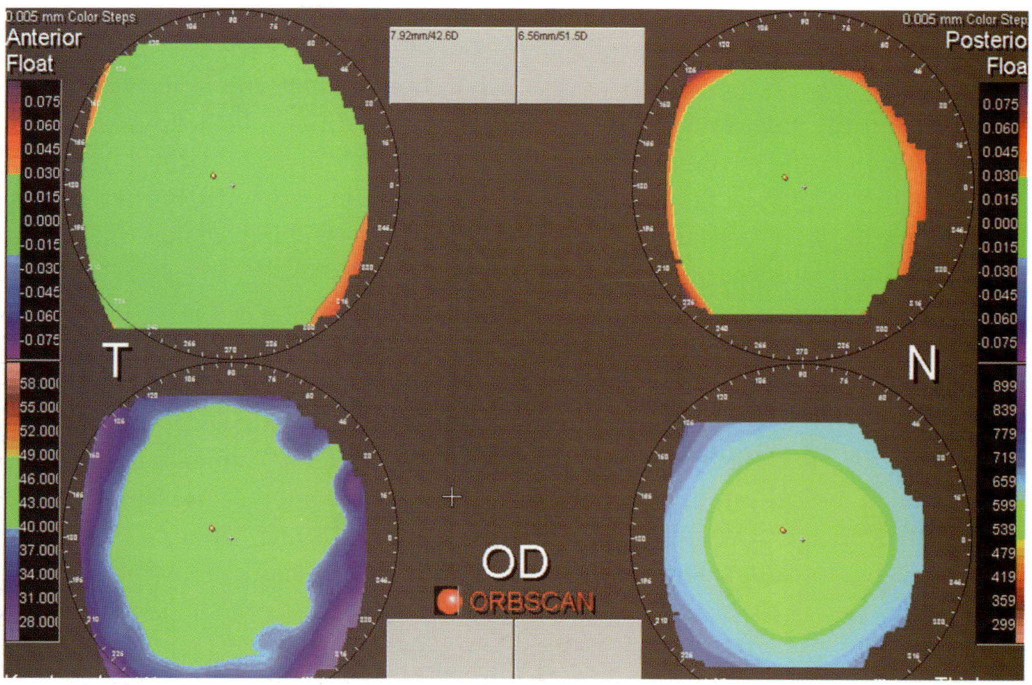

Fig. 38.12: Normal band scale : no pop-ups : Cornea within normal band

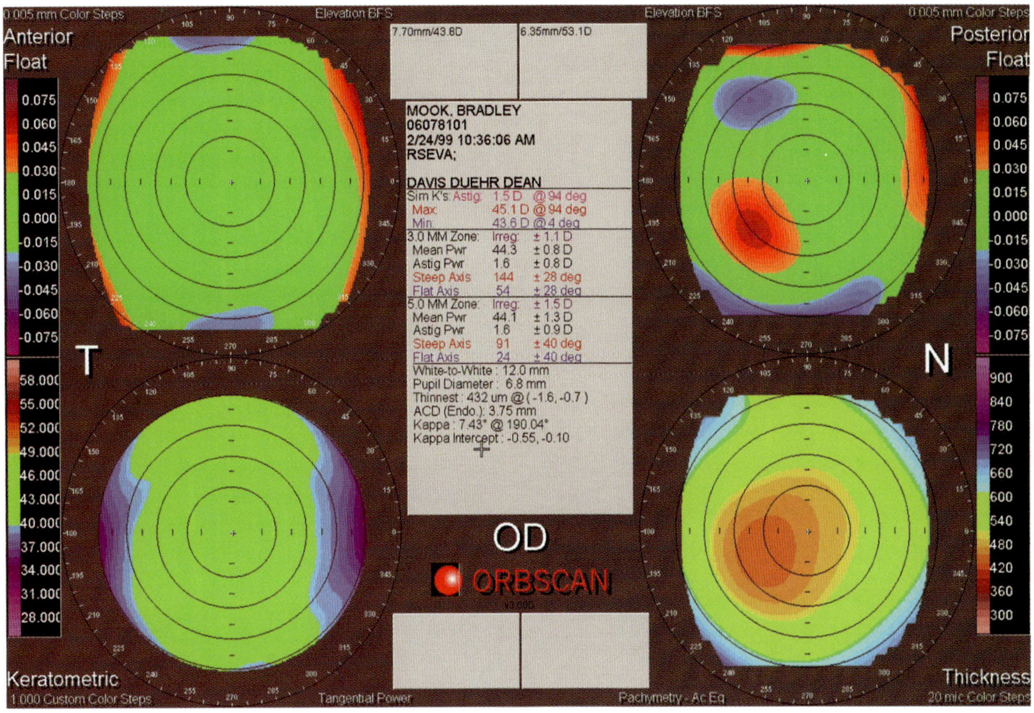

Fig. 38.13: Normal band scale with two pop-ups : One in the pachymetry map and one in the posterior elevation map : There is great concern about this corneas ability to undergo lamellar refractive surgery

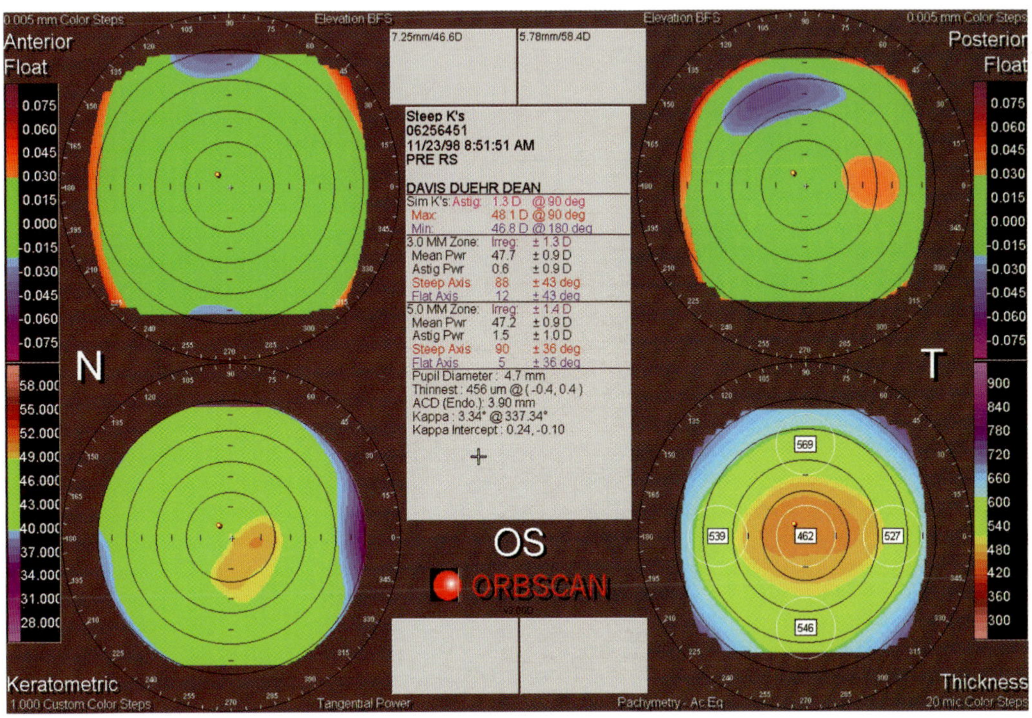

Fig. 38.14: Normal band scale with three pop-ups : Definitely a no-go situation

of Statistics, National Health Insurance Fund Administration, Budapest, Hungary). Wavefront incorporation[9] to rule out other internal optical elements keeping corneal measurement precise and noncontaminated. We could even consider confocal visiualization along with posterior corneal analysis to give clinical relevance to our findings besides artifactual assumptions.

Thus a technology that would combine, biomechanical forces, elasticity modules, wavefront analysis, confocal imaging, high-speed videography and dynamic testing even during the refractive surgery in real time would be my Gold Standard in corneal refractive surgery. I am privileged to be involved presently in this direction and shall look forward to sharing my insights in the next generation of this textbook.

ACKNOWLEDGEMENTS

The work presented above was not the achievement of any single individual, but is the result of support and encouragement by many colleagues and friends. Those who played an important role, include Dr. Frederik Potgieter, Dr. John Vukich, and our good friend, Philippe Dumarey from Bausch and Lomb, Belgium. Without their input and support, this work would not be possible.

REFERENCES

1. Charles N, Charles M, Croxatto JO, Charles DE, Wertheimer D. Surface and Orbscan II slit-scanning elevation topography in circumscribed posterior keratoconus, J Cataract Refract Surg 2005;31(3):636-9.
2. Seiler T, Quurke AW. Iatrogenic keratectasia after LASIK in a case of forme fruste keratoconus, J Cataract Refract Surg 1998;24(7):1007-9.
3. Rao SN, Raviv T, Majmudar PA, Epstein RJ. Role of Orbscan II in screening keratoconus suspects before refractive corneal surgery, Ophthalmology 2002;109(9): 1642-6.
4. Pflugfelder SC, Liu Z, Feuer W, Verm A. Corneal thickness indices discriminate between keratoconus and contact lens-induced corneal thinning, Ophthalmology 2002;109(12):2336-41.
5. Ghergel D, Hosking SL, Mantry S, Banerjee S, Naroo SA, Sha S. Corneal pachymetry in normal and keratoconic eyes: Orbscan II versus ultrasound, J Cataract Refract Surg 2004;30(6):1272-7.
6. Arntz A, Duran JA, Pijoan JI. Subclinical keratoconus diagnosis by elevation topography, Arch Soc Esp Oftalmol 2003;78(12):659-64.
7. Auffarth GU, Wang L, Volcker HE. Keratoconus evaluation using the Orbscan Topography System, J Cataract Refract Surg 2000;26(2):222-8.
8. Cairns G, McGhee CN. Orbscan computerized topography: attributes, applications and limitations, J Cataract Refract Surg 2005;31(1):205-20.
9. Gulani AC, Probst L, Cox I, Veith R. "Wavefront in Lasik": The Zyoptix. Platform. Ophthalmol Clin N Am 2004;17:173-81.

LASIK and Dry Eyes

39

Cyres K Mehta, Keiki R Mehta (India)

LASIK has a multipronged effect on corneal sensation, tear production and wound healing. As the excimer laser also alters the anterior curvature of the cornea by ablating the corneal stroma thus altering the lid interaction with the ocular surface. Post LASIK, the cornea overlying the flap is significantly anesthetic for in some cases upto 6 months, causing a drop in tear production.

Dry eye following LASIK is one of the most frequent problems facing refractive surgeons today and practically all patients experience dry eye at least transiently. Yu et al have reported that 60% of patients experienced dry eye at 1 month following LASIK, and Hovanesian et al reported that 50% of patients experienced symptoms related to dry eye at 6 months. Upto 5% experience severe dry eye that lasts at least 6 months. In most patients who are symptomatic after LASIK its found that they had a mild dry eye preoperatively. The usual complaint following dry eye is that of fluctuating vision due to tear film breakup.Fortunately, in Donnenfelds experience, the great majority of patients' dry eye symptoms resolve within a month following surgery.

Causes of Dry Eye After LASIK

The etiology is multifactorial

1. Pressure from the Suction ring at the limbus causes damage to the Goblet cells thus affecting the Mucin layer of the tear film as reported by Albietz et al.
2. Eye drops contain preservative typically Benzalkonium chloride which is epitheliotoxic. This can cause similar symptoms like those of dry eye like grittiness and irritation.
3. It's well known that corneal sensation drives tear production During LASIK, the corneal nerve trunks are severed by the microkeratome. The anterior stromal nerves are disrupted by photoablation. Both processes damage corneal innervation. The reduction in corneal neuronal feedback to the brain stem reduces brain stem innervation of the lacrimal glands. This diminishes tear production. Perez Santonja et al showed that as the nerves regenerate postoperatively the return of corneal sensation takes about 6 months. This is why the dry eye recovers eventually over 6 months or so.

EFFECT OF LASIK ON CORNEAL SENSATION

Corneal sensation is provided by the long ciliary nerves of the ophthalmic division of the fifth (trigeminal) cranial nerve. The long ciliary nerve trunk travels in the suprachoroidal space. Here it branches several times before entering the cornea at the limbus. The large nerves enter the limbus mainly at the 3 O'clock and 9 O'clock positions (Fig. 39.1). They then bifurcate and move toward the 6 O'clock and 12 O'clock positions. They then undergo a second branching and again move toward the 9 O'clock and

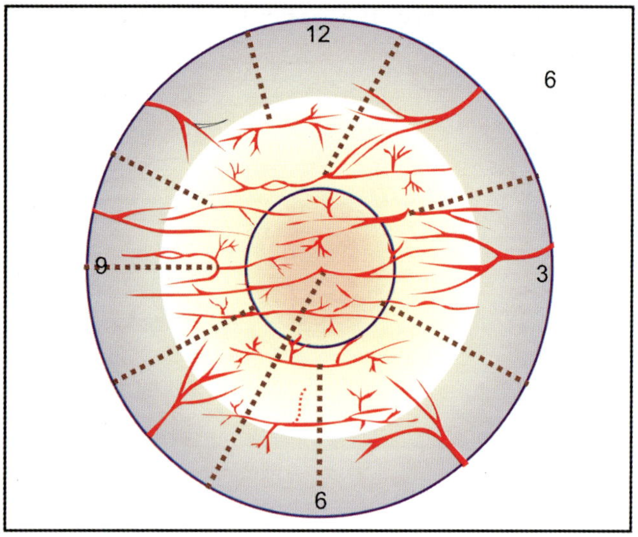

Fig. 39.1: Diagram of corneal innervation. (Reprinted from Donnenfeld ED, Solomon R, Perry HD. Prevention and management of dry eye following LASIK, in Probst L (Ed). LASIK Advances, Controversies, and Customs. Thorofare, NJ, SLACK Inc, 2004, with the kind permission of Dr Donnenfeld.)

3 O'clock positions. The nerves initially enter the cornea in the middle one third of the stroma, but course anteriorly as they branch, eventually forming a plexus in the sub- Bowman's layer that densely innervates the central cornea. The nerves next penetrate Bowman's membrane and terminate in the epithelium at the wing cell layer. Lawrenson et al using a Cohet Bonnet aesthisiometer proved that since the long ciliary nerves enter the eye at 3 and 9 O'clock positions, the corneal sensation is significantly greater at the temporal and nasal limbus than inferiorly.

Chuck et al studied the corneal sensation post LASIK and by using the technique of *in vivo* confocal microscopy showed LASIK induced alterations in the sub-Bowman's nerve plexus and that these alterations are directly related to a drop in corneal sensation. In addition they found that corneal sensation following LASIK is greatest near the hinge and decreases toward the central cornea and the peripheral cornea away from the hinge. An advantage of the hinge on the LASIK flap is that it provides a pathway or a "conduit" for corneal innervation. The corneal nerves entering through the hinge are preserved, maintaining corneal sensation in this area.

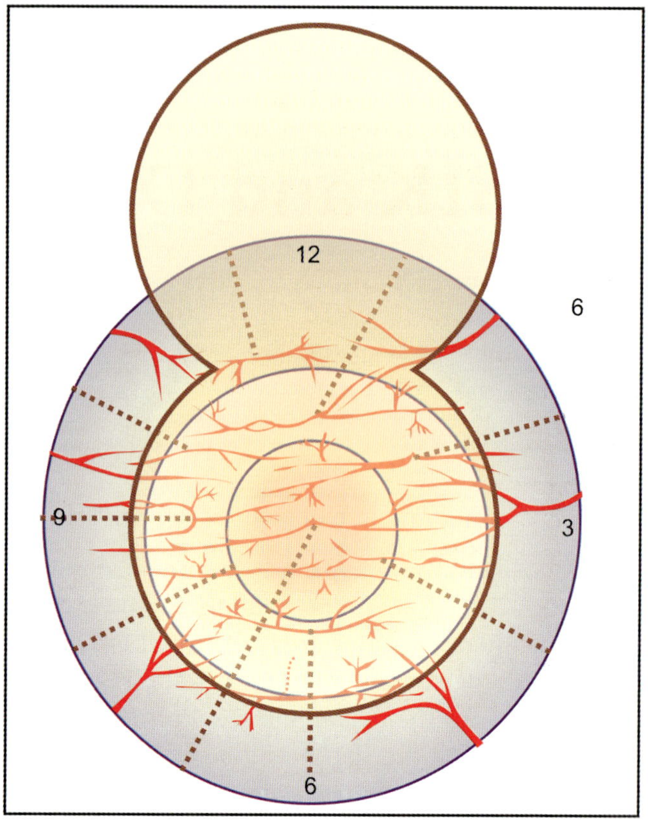

Fig. 39.2: Superior hinge corneal flap transects nasal and temporal corneal innervation. (Reprinted from Donnenfeld ED, Solomon R, Perry HD. Prevention and management of dry eye following LASIK, in Probst L (Ed). LASIK Advances, Controversies, and Customs. Thorofare, NJ, SLACK Inc, 2004, with the kind permission of Dr Donnenfeld

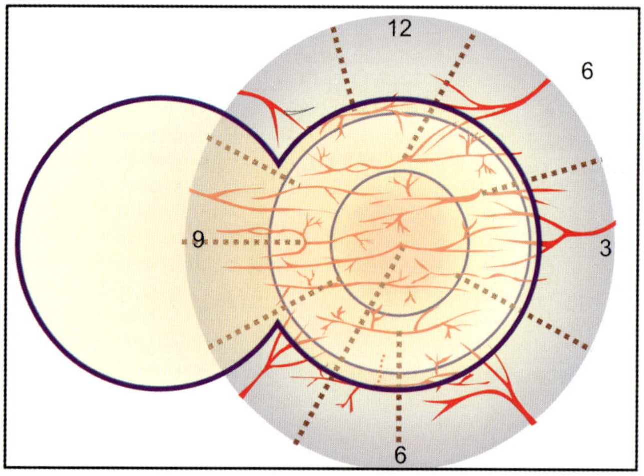

Fig. 39.3: Nasal hinge corneal flap preserves nasal innervation of cornea. (Reprinted from Donnenfeld ED, Solomon R, Perry HD. Prevention and management of dry eye following LASIK, in Probst L (Ed). LASIK Advances, Controversies, and Customs. Thorofare, NJ, SLACK Inc, 2004, with the kind permission of Dr Donnenfeld.)

Donnenfeld et al have demonstrated in a self-controlled, masked clinical study that eyes with a superior hinge flap had much greater loss of sensation and significantly increased corneal lissamine green staining compared to eyes with a nasal hinge flap. Loss of corneal sensation is always greater with a narrow flap as the "conduit" for transmission of the corneal sensation is narrower. In cases where dry eye was diagnosed before LASIK in some cases positive rose Bengal staining can be demonstrated like in a neurotrophic epitheliopathy.

MANAGEMENT OF DRY EYE AFTER LASIK

Patients who have mild dry eye symptoms can simply be treated with artificial preferably nonpreserved tears to stabilize the ocular surface prior to surgery. For patients who have meibomian gland dysfunction Donnenfeld et al recommend the addition of oral doxycycline 100 mg twice a day for 2 weeks and then daily for an additional month along with the tear substitutes

Topical cyclosporine 0.05% in a lipid emulsion (Restasis™, Allergan) has been found to produce significant improvement in both the signs and symptoms of dry eye disease, as well as to produce a decrease in the levels of inflammatory cells in the conjunctival epithelium.The connection between inflammation and dry eye is very well known where steroid topically relieves the symptoms of dry eye much quicker than tear substitutes alone. Cyclosporine A offers the advantage of immunomodulation without the risk of corticosteroid immunosuppressive side effects.

Donnenfeld et al have found that that dietary supplementation with the omega-3 fatty acids provided by eicosapentaenoic (EPA) and docosahexaenoic acid (DHA) enriched flaxseed oil is beneficial in cases of abnormal meibomian gland secretions.

They hypothesise that dietary omega-3 fatty acids are being utilized in the production of meibomian secretions (lipid layer of tear film) and are adding to the tear film oil layer.

Postoperatively, the patient uses in our setup gatifloxacin eye drops and dexamethasone eye drops postlasik four times a day for 7 days. Any patient complaining of grittiness or fluctuating vision is supplemented with carboxyethylcellulose eyedrops (Refresh Liquigel). If the patient still has symptoms of dry eye following the LASIK procedure, we an consider inserting inferior punctal plugs (SmartPlug) in an attempt to stabilize the ocular surface.

If meibomian gland disease is suspected we can try doxycycline tablets.If dry eye persists for more than 3 months we start the patient on Restasis.

In conclusion dry eye after LASIK is a manageable entity with fairly god results if diagnosed and treated early and appropriately.

(Figs 39.1 to 39.3 reproduced with permission of Dr Donnenfeld) "Donnenfeld ED, Solomon R, Perry HD". Prevention and management of dry eye following LASIK, in Probst L (Ed). LASIK Advances, Controversies, and Customs. Thorofare, NJ, SLACK Inc, 2004.

REFERENCES

1. Kanellopoulos AJ, Pallikaris IG, Donnenfeld ED, et al. Comparison of corneal sensation following photorefractive keratectomy and laser in situ keratomileusis. J Cataract Refract Surg 1997;23:34-38.
2. Linna TU, Vesaluoma MH, Perez-Santonja JJ, et al. Effect of myopic LASIK on corneal sensitivity and morphology of subbasal nerves. Invest Ophthalmol Vis Sci 2000;41:393-97.
3. Chuck RS, Quiros PA, Perez AC, McDonnell PJ. Corneal sensation after laser in situ keratomileusis. J Cataract Refract Surg 2000;26:337-39.
4. Albietz JM, Lenton LM, McLennan SG. Effect of laser in situ keratomileusis for hyperopia on tear film and ocular surface. J Refract Surg 2002;18:113-23.
5. Toda I, Asano-Kato N, Hori-Komai Y, Tsubota K. Dry eye after laser in situ keratomileusis. Am J Ophthalmol 2001;132:1-7.
6. Yu EY, Leung A, Rao S, Lam DS. Effect of laser in situ keratomileusis on tear stability. Ophthalmology 2000;107:2131-35.
7. Hovanesian JA, Shah SS, Maloney RK. Symptoms of dry eye and recurrent erosion syndrome after refractive surgery. J Cataract Refract Surg 2001;27:577-84.

8. Donnenfeld E, Solomon K, Perry H, et al. The effect of hinge position on corneal sensation and dry eye following LASIK. Ophthalmology 2003;110:1023-29; discussion, 1029-30.
9. Stern ME, Beuerman RW, Fox RI, et al. The pathology of dry eye: the interaction between the ocular surface and lacrimal glands. Cornea 1998;17:584-89.
10. Toda I, Asano-Kato N, Hori-Komai Y, Tsubota K. Laser-assisted in situ keratomileusis for patients with dry eye. Arch Ophthalmol 2002;120:1024-28.
11. Ambrosio R Jr, Periman LM, Neto MV, Wilson SE. Bilateral marginal sterile infiltrates and diffuse lamellar keratitis after laser in situ keratomileusis. J Refract Surg 2003;19:154-58.
12. Sall K, Stevenson OD, Mundorf TK, Reis BL. Two multicenter, randomized studies of the efficacy and safety of cyclosporine ophthalmic emulsion in moderate to severe dry eye disease. CsA Phase 3 Study Group. Ophthalmology 2000;107:631-39. Erratum in Ophthalmology 2000;107:1220.
13. Muller LJ, Pels L, Vrensen GF. Ultrastructural organization of human corneal nerves. Invest Ophthalmol Vis Sci 1996;37:476-88.
14. Muller LJ, Vrensen GF, Pels L, et al. Architecture of human corneal nerves. Invest Ophthalmol Vis Sci 1997;38:985-94.
15. Auran JD, Koester CJ, Kleiman NJ, et al. Scanning slit confocal microscopic observation of cell morphology and movement within the normal human anterior cornea. Ophthalmology 1995;102:33-41.
16. Lawrenson JG, Ruskell GL. Investigation of limbal touch sensitivity using a Cochet-Bonnet aesthesiometer. Br J Ophthalmol 1993;77:339-43.
17. Donnenfeld E, Ehrenhaus M, Solomon R, et al. The effect of hinge width on corneal sensation and dry eye following LASIK. J Cataract Refract Surg, In Press.
18. Stroobants A, Fabre K, Maudgal PC. Effect of non-steroidal anti-inflammatory drugs (NSAID) on the rabbit corneal epithelium studied by scanning electron microscopy. Bull Soc Belge Ophthalmol 2000;276:73-81.
19. Lenton LM, Albietz JM. Effect of carmellose-based artificial tears on the ocular surface in eyes after laser in situ keratomileusis. J Refract Surg 1999; Apr 15 (2 Suppl): S227-31.
20. Albietz JM, Lenton LM, McLennan SG, Earl ML. A comparison of the effect of Refresh Plus and Bion tears on dry eye symptoms and ocular surface health in myopic LASIK patients. CLAO J 2002;28:96-100.

Management of the Dry Eye (Ocular Surface Syndrome=OSS) after Refractive Surgery

40

JL Alio, C Feinbaum (Spain)

An eye for an eye and the world would be blind
—Mahatma Gandhi

INTRODUCTION

Refractive surgical procedures are one of the most commonly performed ophthalmic surgeries as of late. The technologies have improved over the last years and also the skill of the ophthalmic surgeons, however, complications occur albeit at a low incidence.[1]

Succesful surgery is dependent on not only the measured postoperative visual acuity or quality of vision, but also the preoperative expectations of the patients as determinants of overall satisfaction. It is therefore crucial that every refractive surgeon discuss the indications, methods, possible risks, limitations, and potential alternatives with his/her patient in advance of a planned elective refractive procedure to accurately gauge the expectations of the patient and recommend the best course, including possibly choosing an alternative or abandoning surgery.

Complications in Refractive Surgery

The most common complications in refractive surgery:[2]

1. Overcorrection
2. Irregular astigmatism
3. Ocular surface syndrome
4. Glare
5. Diffuculty with night driving
6. Corneal haze

In this chapter, it will be dealt with the so called dry eye or better Ocular Surface Syndrome complications and how to manage these after refractive surgery.

The "Dry Eye" is a generic term for a group of conditions characterized symptomatically by irritated, gritty, burning eyes and clinically by alterations in the tear film and the anterior surface of the eye and to a certain degree interference with innervation of the cornea after refractive procedures. In a classic review, this syndrome was defined as "a disorder of the tear film due to tear deficiency or excess tear evaporation which causes damage to the interpalpebral ocular surface and is associated with symptoms of ocular discomfort" (Lemp,1995). This general definition encompasses a range of dry eye states with a range of aetiologies.

Deficiencies or disturbances in the production, quality and replenishment of the pre-corneal tear film will result in dry eye conditions. Such conditions can result in ocular surface damage, and may lead to eventual corneal damage and, ultimately a loss of visual performance.

The Tear Film

The tear film is a fluid that covers the cornea (the precorneal tear film) and the conjunctiva (the preocular tear film). The roles of the precorneal tear film can be summarised as follows:

1. To protect the cornea from drying
2. To maintain the refractive power of the cornea
3. To defend against eye infection
4. To allow gas to move between the air and the avascular cornea
5. To support corneal dehydration (assisted by the tear film hyperosmolality)

As well as nurturing the cornea, the preocular tear film is necessary to protect the other epithelial tissues of the anterior surface (the bulbar and palpebral conjunctiva) from physical damage on blinking.

Under normal conditions, the tear film is of sufficient quantity and quality to fulfil the requirements outlined above.

Volume is an important issue: without a sufficient volume of tear fluid, a film cannot adequately form over the ocular surface and offer protection from exposure between blinks. An adequate volume of tears is also required if the tear film is to provide lubrication and prevent the shear forces of blinking from damaging the anterior eye.

Another important aspect is the tear film stability. The stability of the tear film is the property which allows it to maintain a confluent coverage of the ocular surface, for an adequate duration of time to protect the ocular surface between blinks. Further the tear film must also be of a sufficient quality, inherent of an adequate composition, to accomplish its numerous roles in the biophysical and bacteriostatic/bacteriocidal defence of the anterior surface.

The "Dry Eye" or the Ocular Surface Syndrome (OSS)

The "Dry Eye Syndromes" or better the Ocular Surface Syndromes have been reported as being of several classifications.[3]

A. *Aqueous deficient dry eye:* This is a partial or absolute deficiency of the aqueous phase of the tear film, and is a condition of fluctuating severity, most commonly developing in adults (especially post menopausal females). Decreased aqueous production and decreased tear drainage can compromise the anterior surface, leading to an association between aqueous deficiency and secondary infections such as bacterial conjunctivitis and keratitis.

B. *Mucus (Soluble surfactant) deficiency:* Decreased quantity or quality of surface mucus may lead to impaired surface wetting of the epithelia, and decreased lipid trapping and masking at the epithelial interface. Mucus deficiency is, like other forms of dry eye, associated with decreased tear stability. The majority of ocular mucus is produced by the conjunctival goblet cells, whose numbers are reduced by Vitamin A deficiency (which promotes epithelial keritinization) and other tear deficiencies which compromises the ocular surface.

C. *Lipid abnormalities:* While complete tear film lipid deficiency is not known in man, alterations in lipid composition (as seen in chronic blepharitis) can decrease lipid function. This can cause decreased tear evaporation control and thus decrease tear film stability.

D. *Lid surface abnormalities:* When normal lid movement (blinking) is compromised, the area of cornea and conjunctiva not adequately served shows non-wetting. This poor wetting can lead to subsequent epithelial desquamation. Loss of tonus or paresis of one or more eye lid muscles may cause abnormal blinking.

E. *Epitheliopathy:* The normal microvillous surface of the cornea is required to anchor the tear film (through interaction with the mucus phase). Any pathology or disturbance adversely effecting the integrity of this epithelial surface, decreases the tear film integrity, and thus stability.

The Cyclic Disorder by Lemp[4]

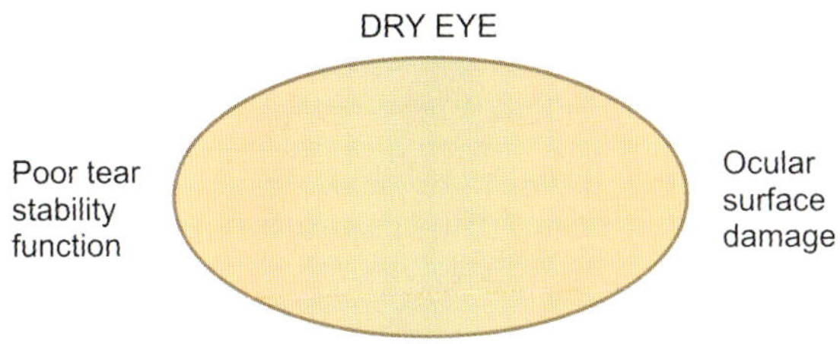

Fig. 40.1

Further in 1995 Lemp reported two major classes of dry eye:

A. Tear deificient dry eye, where deficiencies of aqueous phase tear production or distribution leads to the most common form of dry eye.
B. Tear sufficient (evaporative) dry eye, where sufficient tears are produced, but tear evaporation (due to a variety of factors) mediates dry eye signs and symptoms.

The Ocular Surface Syndrome (OSS)

The ocular surface syndrome is a term which is now used to describe a variety of conditions, sharing common symptomology and clinical signs, leading to a physical and functional break-down of the tear film.

Such tear film disorders range in severity, from the borderline dry eye, which may only be apparent under conditions such as environmental challenge, to severe (pathological) dry eye, as often found in Sjögren´s syndrome.

BASIC SCIENCES IN OSS

Corneal Innervation and the Ocular Surface Syndrome (OSS)

The cornea is one of the most densely innervated tissues in the body.

The majority of nerve fibers reaching the cornea are sensory and travel through the trigeminal nerve (the ophthalmic division of the fifth cranial nerve) to the long ciliary nerves; autonomic parasympathetic fibers from the ciliary ganglion join these nerves, and a small number of sympathetic fibers from the superior cervical ganglion are also seen.These nerves enter the cornea at the periphery in a general distribution pattern.

The nerve bundles enter radially, running parallel to the corneal surface at about two-thirds depth. About 60-80 in number, they course centrally as unmyelinated nerve bundles (Descemets membrane and the endothelium are not innervated). This network of fibers eventually heads toward the corneal surface, forming a subepithelial plexus and penetrating Bowman´s membrane. The terminal path of the corneal nerves leads to inter-and-intra-epithelial cell areas.

It has been estimated that there are between 5000 and 7000 nerve bundles present in the subepithelial plexus, with between 20000 and 40000 total axons.

The sensory receptors act as monitors directing signals via the central nervous system to afferent nerves that terminate in the lacrimal glands, ocular surface, lids and lacrimal drainage passages. Autonomic fibers ending within epithelial cells are

Dry eye classification after Lemp (1995)

			Dry eye			
	Tear Deficient			Evaporative		
Sjögren's syndrome		Non-Sjögren's tear deficient				
Lacrimal disease	Lacrimal obstruction	Reflex	Oil deficient	Lid related	Contact lens	Surface change

important for directing the normal turnover of epithelial cells and cellular healing in response to injury, surgery or disease. A healthy functioning sensory apparatus is partly essential to the maintenance of the ocular surface, and abnormalities in neurosensory transmission can lead to epithelial signs of dryness and an eventual breakdown of the ocular surface.[5]

The corneal nerves are composed of both sensory and autonomic fibers. The sensory fibers, which, with their receptors, comprise the majority of the corneal nerves, serve as monitors, responding to injury by initiating a protective blink. These fibers also act as sentinels, activating the neural loop that directs the secretory activities of the lacrimal and meibomian glands, as well as the mucin-secreting cells of the ocular surface. The composition of the pre-ocular tear film is determined by these signals.

The autonomic (predominantly parasympathetic) fibers direct basic cellular activities, including cell division and maturation (differentiation).Together, the autonomic and sensory fibers form an essential component of the tear film - ocular surface functional unit. Nerves direct cellular turnover, and they respond to injury by initiating changes in tear composition that promote healing.

The OSS is characterized by multiple break-downs of inter-related aspects of the tear film-ocular surface functional unit. Systemic initiating factors can include hormonal changes, immunological abnormalities, genetic predisposition, neurological lesions, and ageing. All of these can produce destabilizing changes in the tear film including elevated tear osmolarity, alterations in tear composition, inflammation, and refractive surgical procedures.

Hyperosmolarity is a potent stimulator of inflammation via stress kinases that promote an intracellular inflammatary escalation. Key to the tear film-ocular surface functional unit´s response to these negative changes are the sensory receptors. However, inflammation has been shown to downregulate the receptors, in effect short-circuiting the modulating response to injury. Deprived of a signaling pathway that could induce changes that might counter the destructive process of the OSS, inflammation-mediated tissue damage proceeds, leading to epithelial disruption and discomfort.

A very similar series of ocular surface events occurs in neurotrophic keratopathy. In this case, the primary lesion involves the afferent fibers of the ophthalmic branch of the trigeminal nerve. Clinical manifestations range from superficial punctate keratopathy to ulceration and perforation. These profound changes point to a central role of neural integrity in maintaining a normal ocular surface.

Surface Properties of the Normal and the Damaged Corneal Epithelium

What triggers the corneas nonwettability by the aqueous tears in a variety of ocular surface and tear film disorders? The answers are not straightforward in that they involve subtle interplays of surface-chemical and physiological factors. To address these questions in a meaningful way, a proper understanding of both the apolar and the polar (acid-base) surface properties of the corneal epithelium and mucus is required. While the early approaches[6,7] based on Zisman´s method of critical surface tension[8] did produce some limited insights, it is now generally agreed that this method lacks the requisite framework to adress the problem of polar interactions in aqueous media. Further progress in the understanding of the cornea-tear film interactions was made possible by the pioneering concepts of van Oss, Chaudhury and Good[9,10] and their applications to biological surfaces.[11,12] These developments made it possible for the first time to quantify the apolar and polar properties of various corneal and tear film components and their free energies of adhesion.[13]

An understanding of the corneal wetting by the precorneal tear film demands a small introduction to the structure and physiology of the corneal surface and the tear film.

The corneal epithelium, which is the outermost covering of the cornea, is composed of about four to six stratified cell layers, which are continuously renebwede by mitosis in the basal cell layer. The basal cells slowly move to the progressively outer layers and differentiate, until they are shed in the tear film from the superficial layer of highly differentiated and sometimes degenerating, flattened squamous cells. The surfaces of the superficial corneal epithelial cells in contact with the tear film develop a highly glycosylated glycocalix[14,15] which is a very hydrophilic extracellular matrix of the cell membrane bound glycosylated glycoproteins or MUC1 mucins.[16] At least 50-60% of their mass is carbohydrate. However, the less differentiated deeper layer cells are expected to be less hydrophillic because they lack a mature network of glycocalix[17,18] and membrane protrusion, e.g. Microvilli. The tightly bound extracellular mucins are more properly a part of the corneal surface than of the overlying tear film.

The tear film is most often described as a three-layered structure. The superficial epithelial cells are covered by an intensely hydrophillic coating of hydrated but relatively unsoluble mucous gel. Thickness of the corneal mucus layer has been shown to be in the range of about 1 to 10 µm or even higher by a variety of methods. The mucus gel covering the cornea has extra-corneal origins; it is expressed by the goblet cells of the conjunctiva as a gel froming mucin, MUC5AC[19] and smeared over the cornea by the shear exerted during blinking. Blinking assists in a slow turnover or renewal of the mucous layer by removing small quantities of superficial mucus and replenishing it with fresh supplies.

A 4 to 10 µm thick aqueous film containing electrolytes, soluble proteins and mucins completely wets the mucus coated corneal surface in normal eyes. The aqueous tears display non-Newtonian behavior; its zero-shear viscosity is high but declines close to that of pure water at very high shear rates, which may be attained during a blink[20] and also during de-wetting. A high value of zero-shear viscosity is indicative of a weak network like structure of soluble mucins in a stationary tear phase, which is readily disrupted by flow-induced stresses. The surface tension of tears is usually found to be in the range of 35 mN/m to 50 mN/m[21] which is substantially smaller than the surface tension of pure water.

Finally, the outermost layer at the tear-air interface consists largely of apolar lipids such as waxy and cholesterol esters derived from the meibomian glands. A small fraction of polar lipids such as free fatty acids are also present, which should adsorb at the aqueous-lipid interface due to their surfactant like properties, and assist in complete spreading of the apolar lipids on aqueous tears. Among other things, the superficial layer greatly retards the evaporation and flow of tears and provides a hydrophobic barrier preventing spillage of tears at the lid margins.

The normal precorneal tear film usually remains intact between consecutive blinks, but holes begin to appear and grow at random spots in about 20 to 60 seconds, when blinking is prevented. In the so called dry eye states, a much more rapid breakup on the tear film during the interblink period is usually observed, which may eventually lead to corneal dehydration and damage. In severe cases of dry eye, a complete tear film may not even reform after a blink, and dry corneal spots may be present immediately after opening of the eye-lids.

What are the factors that cause the wettability or nonwettability of the corneal surface? The most popular and the earliest view of the corneal wetting was advanced by Holly and Lemp based on the measurements of the apolar surface properties by the then widely used critical surface tension method of Zisman. It was concluded that the normal corneal epithelium without mucus is a low energy hydrophobic surface non-wettable by the aqueous tears, but the mucous gel masks its hydrophobicity and renders it completely wettable. However, it has since been argued and demonstrated that artifacts in the preparation of the corneal surfaces, use of apolar diagnostic liquids and the methods of interpretation have been responsible for these conclusions. The particle attachment method,[22] the equation method[23] as well as the use of modern "acid-base approach" have all shown the normal epithelial cells with associated glycocalix to be almost as hydrophillic and as wettable by the aqueous media as the corneal mucus. Nor is this conclusion surprising, because, like any number of cells with an extracellular coat of glycosylated glycocalyx, the corneal epithelial cells also become wettable due to a strong electron donor type of polarity which engenders copious amounts of hydrogen bonding water molecules.

The corneal surface is a mosaic of cells with varying age, morphology and degree of differentiation. The epithelial wettability should therefore also be highly variable on the cellular level. In particular, surfaces of degenerating and desquamating cells as well as the newly uncovered deeper layer cells lacking a mature network of microvilli and glycocalix, are likely to be a lot less polar and non-wettable. The function of mucous would be to mask these transient non-wettable sites of cellular dimensions, therby stabilizing the tear film. Once the mucous layer ruptures, the tear film breakup may follow on the naturally occuring non-wettable sites, or on non-wettable sites generated due to the epithelial contamination.

Very important though is that with increased dehydration and damage (surgical intervention) to the epithelium, the corneal surface becomes increasingly apolar and less hydrophillic due to the loss of its electron donating capacity. It is likely that the individual deeper layer cells, desquamating and degenerating cells, as well as cells with abnormalities of glycocalix synthesis or attachment are less polar and hydrophillic - (surgical intervention or touch).

It seems that despite a diversity of the underlying causes, the loss of epithelial polarity (and wettability) may be conceptually categorized by the following two distinct types of epithelial alterations:

1. Alterations in the physico-chemical nature and morphology of the superficial cell surfaces. This category includes loss of surface microvilli and glycocalix, damage/degeneration of the cell membranes, and abnromalities of cellular differentiation leading also to keratinization in some cases. The case of Vitamin A deficiency leading to various stages of squamous metaplasia of the corneal surface also falls in this category.[24]
2. *Abnormal loss of superficial cells:* This category includes punctate erosions and recurrent/persistent defects of the epithelium, which may be caused by the adhesion failure of cells, tear film and epithelial insults such as hyperosmolarity, drugs and preservatives, deficiencies of the epithelial maintenance/turnover and surgical corneal interventions. There is evidence that the corneal epithelial mass is maintained by a dynamic balance between rates of basal cell mitosis, cell loss and centripetal supply of cells from the peripheral "stem" cells located in the limbus. Thus in some cases, reduction of the corneal epithelial mass premature exfoliation and reduced residence time of cells and formation of superficial epithelial defects could occur secondary to the abnormalities of centripetal supply, cell mitosis and damage to the stem cell production. These alterations, in addition to encouraging the loss of epithelial surface polarity, also increase contamination of the mucus layer by the cell debris, thereby decreasing its electron donor properties.

All the above surface chemical pathways and their probable interactions leading to the tear film breakup in dry eyes are summarized in the figure below.[25]

Pre-surgical Examinations for Determination of Eventual OSS Problems in the Prospective Refractive Surgery Patient

Evaluation of the prospective refarctive surgery patient for OSS includes many of the elements of a comprehensive ophthalmological examination and a more in-depth evaluation of the ocular surface and adnexa.[26] The evaluation for ocular surface disorders includes a carefully detailed patient history, an assessment of associated risk factors, and an examination of the anterior ocular structures and their functions.

1. *Patient history:* Demographic data about the patient should be collected prior to taking the patient history. Included in the patient history is the chief complaint, ocular history, general health history (which may include a social history and an extended review of systems), and family ocular and medical history. In addition, environmental

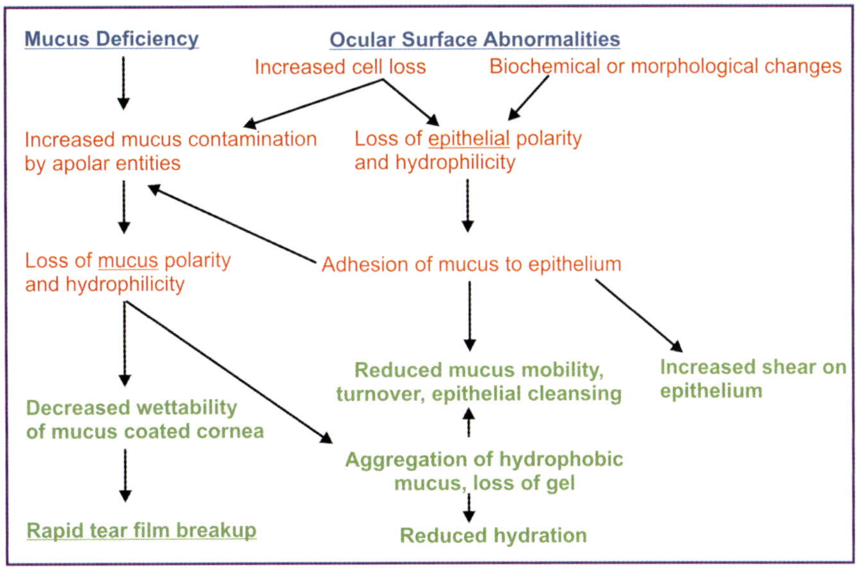

Fig. 40.3

factors relating to climate, season, vocational setting, and avocational pursuits should be reviewed.

2. *Ocular examination for OSS:* Observations, using external ocular examination techniques, both without magnification and with the biomicroscope slit-lamp, show characteristic early changes of the external eye. Evaluation for suspected ocular surface disorders should include the following:
   - External view of the eye, noting lid structure, position, symmetry, and blink dynamics
   - Biomicroscope examination of the lid margins, meibomian gland orifices and their contents
   - Biomicroscopic examination of the tear film, noting mucus, debris, interference patterns in the lipid layer, and tear meniscus height
   - Biomicroscopic examination of the cornea and conjunctiva, both with and without sodium fluorescein and rose bengal or lissamine green staining.

   Tear quantity tests are useful in conforming the diagnosis of aqueous deficient dry eyes. The most frequently utilized procedures are and will be covered in more detail further in the text:
   - Schirmer tear test
   - Fluorescein staining
   - Evaluation of the tear prism
   - Debris in tear film
   - Rose bengal staining.

Other tests which may be used to evaluate tear quantity include:
- Schirmer II (irritation)
- Lissamine green staining
- Tear volume measurements
- Lacrimal equilibration time
- Cotton thread test
- Phenol red test
- Fluorophotometry; fluorescein dilution
- Temporary punctal occlusion.

Several procedures are commonly used to evaluate tear film stability:
- Tear film breakup time (TBUT)
- Tear-thinning time
- Lactoferrin concentration tests: LactoPlate® and LactoCard®
- Lysozyme radial diffusion test: Quantiplate.

Other tests which may be used to evaluate the quality of the preocular tear film (POTF) include:
- Tear osmolarity test
- Conjunctival scraping and biopsy
- Mucin test (tear ferning)

- Specular reflection of the tear surface
- Impression cytology
- Tear protein analysis
- Lipid layer interference patterns
- Enzyme-linked immunosorbent test (ELISA) tear protein profile
- Corneal topography in wet and dry state
- Corneal hysteresis
- Water content of cornea.

3. *Ocular examination for blepharitis:* A thorough external examination of the lids and other parts of the adnexa, including comparison of the eyes, helps determining the severity of the inflammation. Differentiating among the various presentations of blepharitis requires the use of the biomicroscope to contrast the appearance of the anterior and the posterior lid margins. Evaluation of the patient with blepharitis should include:
   - External examination of the eye, including lid structure, skin texture, and eyelash appearance; and evaluation for clinical signs of acne rosacea
   - Biomicroscopic examination of the lid margins, the base of the lashes, and the meibomian gland orifices and their contents
   - Examination of the tear film for lipid layer abnormalities

   Each type of blepharitis has specific characteristics which help in making the diagnosis.

Tear Stability Tests

Tear film stability assessment techniques can be considered as invasive or non-invasive. This is an important distinction, as the non-invasive techniques are greatly superior to the invasive method.

Invasive tear breakup time (TBUT, Fluorescein break up Time): This test requires observing the cornea using a slit-lamp biomicroscope, with a broad-beam cobalt-blue light source at 10x magnification. (Norn 1969, Lemp and Hamill 1973). To view the tear film, fluorescein dye is instilled, e.g. by wetting a dry fluorescein impregnated paper strip with a drop of saline and placing it on the bulbar cornea for a brief moment. The dye readily mixes in the tear fluid and after 1 or 2 blinks the tear film takes on a uniform fluorescent appearance. Ask the patient to refrain from blinking and in most cases within 60 seconds dark spots or streaks will form within the tear film. These discontinuities in fluorescence are indicate breaks in the continuity of the tear film. The time elapsing between a complete blink, and the appearance of the first "dark spot or streak" is measured and taken to be the break up time. Five successive measures are routinely taken, and the mean value calculated. In dry eyes break up time is usually less than 10 seconds.[27]

Several workers have suggested this invasive break up time assessment to be of poor repeatability and questionable validity,[28] probably due to:

i. The destabilising effect of fluorescein on the tear film itself
ii. The volume of fluorescein added is uncontrolled and relatively large compared with the natural tear reservoir
iii. Contact with the ocular surface will initiate some reflex lacrimation.

For these reasons many doctors have turned to the non-invasive tear film stability assessment techniques, however, the majority of doctors do still perform TBUT as their standard assessment of tear stability. The usefulness of the TBUT test can be increased by minimizing the amount of fluorescein used. This has two clear advantages:

1. This prevents "quenching" of fluorescence
2. This minimizes the destabilising effects of fluorescein, so should give more valid assessment results.

A much smaller amount of fluorescein can be instilled using a new fluorescein impregnated paper strip with a tapered tip (the Dry Eye test or DET®, Ocular Research Boston, Boston, USA).

NonInvasive tests of tear film stability: The fundamental principles common to these techniques are based on the reflective properties of the smooth, stable tear film. As the film distorts (as it thins), its ability to reflect, undistorted, a regular optical array of pattern diminishes. The time elapsing between a complete blink, and the appearance of the first distortion is measured and taken to be the tear thinning time (TTT). Five successive measures are routinely taken, and the mean value calculated. In essence, non-invasive tests of tear stability are based on observing the quality and stability of the first Purkinje image.[29]

The Bausch and Lomb keratometer can be used to measure the TTT, using the standard mires as a light pattern source (Patel, et al, 1985). However, the mires cover a smaller total area of the cornea, and so may be more difficult to accurately use.

Corneal topographers based on the Placido disc can also be used to assess tear stability. The video monitor in most computerized photokeratoscopes is used to align the instrument and record the Purkinje images when crisp and sharp. By asking the patient to blink and observe the time taken for part of the reflected image to break down in clarity, the tear stability is measured and widen the the potential of the videokeratoscope.

The various noninvasive tear film stability assessment techniques can be considered in terms of those which measure the tear thinning time (TTT), and those which measure the non-invasive break-up time (NIBUT). NIBUT is believed to be a measure of the time taken for a discontinuity in the superficial lipid layer of the tear film to occur following a blink, whereas, TTT is a measure of the time taken for the tear film to thin, following a blink. Tear thinning is believed to occur just prior to tear break up. For this reason, TTT and NIBUT are taken to be similar parameters, not interchangeable or synonymous, but both indicative of tear film stability.

Tear Volume Tests

Estimates for the volume of tears covering the ocular surface range from b2.74+ – 2μL (Mathers et al, 1996) to 7μL (Mishima, et al 1966). The bulk of this volume is made of fluid secreted by the main (primary) and secondary lacrimal glands. When reading, tears are passively secreted and flowing onto the ocular surfaces and in a few seconds there will be a blink. This will force tear fluid towards the lacrimal puncta and via these, the tears will pass from the ocular surface and into the lacrimal canalicuae. Intuitively, a dry eye is one with with low tear volume. Tests for tear volume could either be invasive or non-invasive.

Invasive Tests

Schirmer test: This is a strip of filter paper, (45 mm long and 5 mm wide) which is hooked over the lower eyelid. The hook is 5 mm with a rounded edge. On contact with the ocular surface the paper absorbs tears. The length of paper wetted over a set time of 5 minutes is an indication of tear volume. The paper can irritate the ocular surface initiating a reflex action whereby the volume of tears secreted by the lacrimal glands increases. Thus, Schirmer test is measuring both a basal and reflex tearing. By anesthetizing the ocular surface, it is claimed the reflex stimualtion is prevented and a true measure of basal tear secretion can be made (Jones, 1966, Lamberts, et al 1979, Jordan and Baum 1980, Clinch, et al 1983). The Schirmer strip comes into contact with not only the ocular surface but also the lid margin and lashes. This suggests that, maybe the lid margins should also be anesthetised if the aim is to measure basal tear secretion. Many investigators conclude, the Schirmer test measures the flow of tears rather than volume and the fact that it irritates the ocular surface is a useful adjunct. If the Schirmer score is still low after irritating the ocular surface then clearly there is a dry eye present as opposed to a marginally dry eye. Low Schirmer test results are encountered when corneal sensitivity is reduced in severe dry eyes. (Xu, et al 196). Furthermore, Schirmer test results are low after refractive surgery presumably because corneal sensitivity has been reduced (Ozdamar, et al 1999, Aras, et al 2000). The Schirmer test has been criticized for its low reproducability, it is time consuming, it is irritating and has poor diagnostic value especially when attempting to investigate the marginal dry eye (Feldman and Wood 1979, Patel, et al 1987, Cho and Yap 1993). A dry-normal cut off value of 5 mm of wetting in 5 minutes has been used for many years but this is not reliable because, 17% of normal eyes have a Schirmer wetting of less than 5 mm (Wright and Meger, 1962) and 32% of dry eyes have a Schirmer wetting of more than 5 mm (Farrell, et al 1992). The true value of the Schirmer test in the modern setting is questionable even though it is still one of the most popular tests used by clinicians.[30-33]

Cotton Thread test: Cotton can soak up tear fluid by capillary action. The cotton thread (Kurihashi 1978, Hamano, et al 1982) is dyed with a pH sensitive phenol red which changes from yellow-orange to red-orange with contact with tears. This is useful for quickly checking the length of the wetted thread. The volume of tears taken up ny the thread depends upon the exact type of cotton and the duration of the insertion. The Hamano thread is inserted for 15 seconds. This thread is 70 mm long with a 3 mm hook at one end (Zone-Quick™). The lower lid is gently depressed and the 3 mm is placed over the lower lid margin, on to the conjunctiva about half the distance from the center towards the outer canthus. The patient is asked to relax and keep looking straight ahead. Alternatively, the patient could just keep the eyes closed. After removing the thread from the ocular surface, the soaked up tears continue to flow along the thread. It is good paractice to measure the length of weeting as soon as the thread is removed to reduce this effect of systemic error. The soft thin cotton is less irritating compared with the stiffer Schirmer test and more likely to infer basal tear volume (Hamano, et al 1982). Using the thread, dry eyes tend to wet below 10 mm, averaging at 6.9 mm (Mainstone, et al 1996). Wetting values for normal eyes range from 15.4 mm (Cho and Kwang 1996) to 27.4 mm (Little and Bruce 1994). It appears that within normals, differences in thread wetting values are related to ethnic variations.

Does the thread measure tear flow or volume? A correlation between tear flow and thread wetting has not been substantiated (Tomlinson et al 2001). It could be, the tear fluid present at the ocular is absorbed by when the thread is first inserted and once this is depleted to a critical mass, reflex lacrimation is stimulated and the subsequent tears soaked up by the thread represents the tear flow at that point in time. Exactly what the thread measures at any moment during use is still open to question.[34-37]

Fluorophotometry: Fluorophotometry is a laboratory based system used to measure tear flow and turnover rates. A controlled measure of fluorescein is instilled in the eye and the fluorescense is gauged over time. The rate of decay in fluorescense indicates tear flow of fluorescein instillation. Fluorophotometric data indicates that the measurement of tears using the phenol red cotton test is not related to tear flow (Tomlinson, et al 2001). It must be remembered, both tests are invasive and this in itself can effect the parameter under investigation.[38]

Noninvasive Tests

Tear meniscus height and curvature: The tear meniscus is bound between the ocular surface, lid margin and air. The surface exposed to the air is concave and cylindrical. The distance from the lid margin to the boundary between the ocular surface and the edge of the tear rivulus is the tear meniscus height (TMH). It is claimed 75-90% of the total fluid covering the ocular surface is contained within the upper and lower tear menisci. (Holly 1986). The volume of fluid contained in the lower meniscus is the product of length and area if a cross section. In turn the area of the cross section is dependant on the TMH and the curvature of the meniscus (TMC). It follows, the height and/or curvature of either the lower or upper tear meniscus is proportional to tear volume. In clinical practice TMH can be measured quickly and reliably at a magnification of 30x or more using a graduated eyepiece. The resolution can be improved by increasing the magnification for example using a video capture system.

Further, measurement of TMH is a useful non-invasive technique for investigating not only the OSS but also when the patient is complaining of epiphoria. If the TMH is consistently high there may be a partial blockage of the naso-lacrimal drainage system.

The subjective measure of TMH is relative, not an absolute measurement because it depends on the observer´s interpretation of where the base of the tear meniscus starts and where the top of the tear meniscus ends. Mainstone, et al (1996) instilled fluorescein as an aid to view the tear meniscus and reported mean values of 0.46 mm (s.d. + – 0.17 mm) in normals and 0.24 mm (s.d. + –0.09 mm) in dry eyes.

Armed with a good slitlamp, an image recording system or eyepiece graticule, tear volume can be clinically assessed, non-invasively and reliably, on condition magnification is greater than 30x.[39-41]

Other Tests

Impression Cytology

Conjunctival impression cytology (CIC) is a minimally invasive technique allowing for the investigation of of conjunctival changes at the cellular level (Egbert, et al 1977, Tseng 1985, Nelson 1988, Knop and Brewett 1992). This technique involves pressing a piece of material, cellulose-acetate filters being commonly used, onto the bulbar or tarsal conjunctiva. The action of application and removal of the filter results in a fine sheet of superficial conjunctival tissue remaining adhered to the filter. The adhered tissue can then be fixed and stained, and the visualised cells observed directly (light microscopy). It has been suggested, that CIC may be useful in predicting failure of contact lens wear (Hirji and Larke 1981), too little is yet know for the prediction on refractive surgery. However, using CIC, the goblet cell count in the OSS is definitely reduced.

The sensation felt when the filter is applied is similar to that experienced on the first fitting of a contact lens (due to the presence of a foreign body and the inability to blink), and slight irritation is felt as the filter is removed. Topical anesthetic can be used to minimize the discomfort. The key to good subject tolerance of this technique lies in a confident and rapid cell collection following a full explanation of the technique.

Goblet cell population density can be assessed by impression cytology if the goblet cell contents are stained specifically. Alow goblet cell population density is thought to indicate inability to produce a sufficient mucus phase of the tear film, as the major proportion of this layer is produced by goblet cells.

Because the ocular surface and tear film are intrinsically related, ocular surface assessment must not be forgotten. Currently accepted techniques of ocular surface staining assessment are quick and easy. In the future, clinicians could routinely assess ocular surface changes at the cellular level, if impression cytology can be adapted for clinical utility. [42-45]

Corneal Topography in Combination with Confocal Biomicroscopy

"The frying pan theory"

1. *Examining the corneal topography carefully is a necessity for a successful lasik procedure.*
2. *However it must be understood that when performing a corneal topography we are not measuring the superficial surface of the cornea but the anterior surface of the tear film.*

In the topography below one of the authors´ corneal topography was taken just after blink and then 20 seconds after blink.

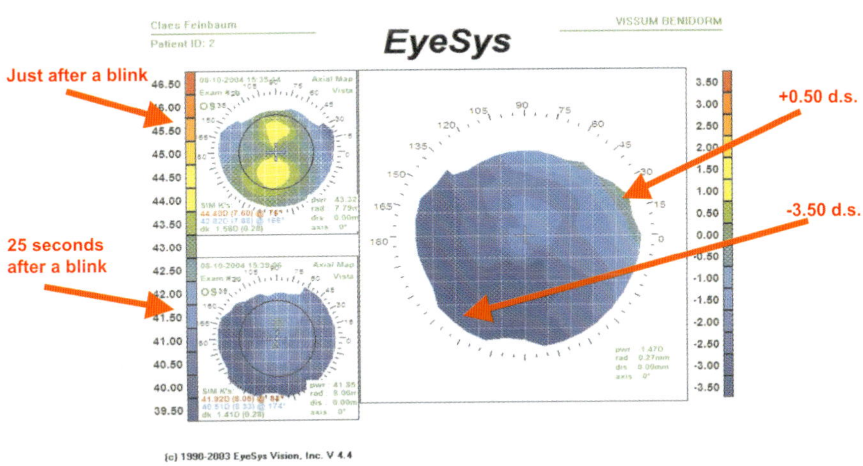

Fig. 40.4

If there is a big change from a wet cornea to a dry cornea performing corneal topography, then an alternative refractive surgical procedure should be a signal of contemplating a different stategy. The following problems could occur:

1. HOA.
2. Dry eye or OSS.

With the confocal microscope these changes on the corneal surface will look like this: These are so called steep pitts.

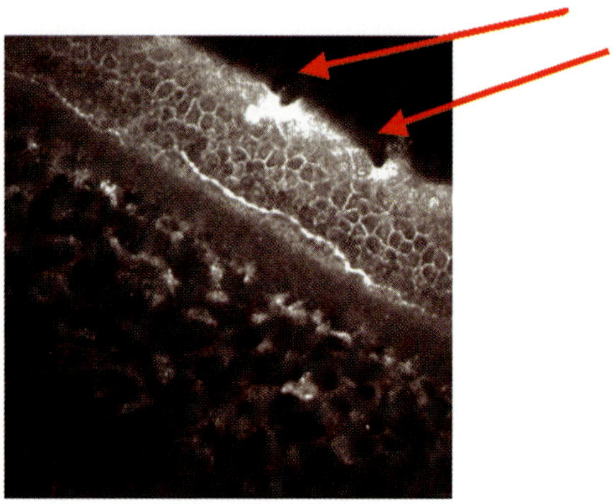

Fig. 40.4

Like the teflon frying pan surface there is no possibility for above surface to be wetted like an undisturbed surface since these so called "pitts" are rather deep. The bottom line with the frying pan theory is that the surface will not be wetted properly and this could happen after refractive surgery, especially after the LASIK procedure.

Management of the Ocular Surface Syndrome

Stepwise determination of the minimum intervention required to achieve results will help ensure a balance of patient compliance, long-term success and cost-effectiveness. The management of OSS is designed to reduce symptoms and inflammation and to re-establish a normal ocular surface. Efforts should be aimed at maintaining or restoring the preocular tear film and ridding the lids of potential sources of tear film destabilization. Whenever possible, environmental factors contributing to dry eye should be identified and either modified or eliminated. When associated medical conditions are identified, consultation with or referral to the patient´s primary care physician or other health care provider may be indicated.

Attempts to relieve dry eye symptoms and re-establish a normal ocular surface have produced a myriad of possible remedies. Traditional approaches include both tear supplementation and tear conservation measures. Several alternatives have been used with varying degrees of clinical success:

- Ocular hygiene
- Topical treatment with tear supplements, ointments, and soluble polymeric inserts
- Punctal occlusion

  Alternative methods for relieving symptoms specific to ocular surface disorders include:
  - Hydrophilic bandage lenses
  - Moisture chamber goggles
  - Tarsorraphy
  - Estrogen replacement
  - Salivary gland transplant
  - Limbal grafts.

Blepharitis

Acute sequelae to blepharitis are usually the direct result of infection of the lipid-producing glands that open to the lid margin. Their clinical presentation includes internal and external hordeola. The treatment is relatively straightforward. Though essential, lid hygiene alone may not resolve the problem. Depending upon the clinical findings, an appropriate anti-infective drug can be administered topically, systemically, or in combination. On the other hand, chronic blepharitis is a disease for which there is no complete cure. Aggressive therapy should initially include a minimum of 6 weeks of lid hygiene and appropriate anti-infective medications to gain control of the condition, followed by continuing treatment to maintain control of the chronic blepharitis.

Because each category of blepharitis is actually a separate condition, each has to be adressed individually:

- Staphylococcal blepharitis
- Seborrheic blepharitis

- Seborrheic/staphylococcal blepharitis
- Meibomian seborrheic blepharitis
- Seborrheic blepharitis with secondary meibomianitis
- Meibomian keratoconjunctivitis
- Angular blepharitis
- Demodicosis.

When topical treatment for OSS is prescribed, the patient should be given the rationale for the treatment, along with specific dosages, frequency, and duration. The patient should be made aware of the expected results and given instructions to follow in case of adverse effects. A follow-up examination of the patient should be scheduled to assess effectiveness.

The treatment of blepharitis require close, ongoing cooperation between the patient and the practitioner. Thorough discussion of the causes, the rationale for treatment and the expected results is essential in the managing of this condition. Most patients with blepharitis have a significant improvement in their symptoms when the appropriate hygiene, topical, and/or systemic treatments are instituted. Since there is no cure for the chronic forms of blepharitis, patients must actively participate in steps to control the inflammatory process. Thorough explanation of both the chronicity of the disease and the rationale for the therapy helps encourage patient compliance. Specific instructions and realistic expectations for the abatement of symptoms should be reinforced by scheduled follow-ups.[46]

Frequency and Composition of Evaluation and Management Visits for OSS

Mild Induced OSS

Frequency of examination: Annual or as necessary

History: Yes

Slit Lamp Biomicroscopy: Yes

Supplementary tests: Fluorescein, rose bengal or lissamine green, TBUT

Management: Unpreserved tear supplements daily.

Moderate OSS

Frequency of examination: Every 6-12 months or as necessary

History: Yes

Slit Lamp Biomicroscopy: Yes

Supplementary tests: Fluorescein, rose bengal or lissamine green, TBUT, Schirmer test

Management: Unpreserved tear supplements 4-5 times a day.

Severe OSS

Frequency of examination: Every 3-6 months

History: Yes

Slit Lamp Biomicroscopy: Yes

Supplementary tests: Fluorescein, rose bengal or lissamine green, TBUT, Schirmer test

Management: Unpreserved tear supplements at liberty, ointment at bedtime, punctal occlusion.

In More Detail

Artificial Tears

There are several artificial tear substitutes (ATS) formulations designed to compensate for either lacrimal or mucous insufficiency. Most ATSs act as tear substiutes. Inter-nation variations in legislation has lead to the situation whereby, in some countries some substitutes are on prescription only and in others they can be sold over the counter. Most drops contain preservatives and in many cases the drops increase symptoms because of patient hypersensitivity to the preservatives. Single dose preservative free drops appear as a more expensive option, however, this is not always the case. Most preserved drops should be discarded 28 days after opening. If the dry eye problem is occasional, say 2 or 3 times per week, then a 20 or 30 dose pack would last a lot longer and offer a much better cost-effective choice to the patient. The value of artificial tears can be assessed very rapidly using one or more of the simple tests described above for investigating the OSS.

When a single drop is instilled onto the ocular surface the bulk of its volume rapidly drains away via the naso-lacrimal duct. In effect, only a minute amount of the initial drop is of real value in terms of ocular surface wetting and lubrication. When using a single dose sachet, ask the patient to tilt the head back, instill a drop on one eye, wait a few moments, and then instill on the other eye. There will still be fluid remaining in the sachet, wait a few moments more and repeat the procedure. This way is a useful way of making maximum use of the drops.[47]

With most ATSs the increase in tear stability peaks approximately 15 minutes after instillation. Thereafter, the tear stability reduces and reaches baseline about 90 minutes later. Many investigations claim, persistent use of drops can produce a longer lasting improved baseline in tear stability. This could be mediated by either:

i. A healing effect
ii. Return of the epithelial to a more natural state or,
iii. Gradual repopulation of active conjunctival cells.[48]

On instillation, ATSs can momentarily blur the patient´s vision. If the drop has a refractive index radically different from the refractive index of natural tears and the drop mixes poorly with the tears, the instilled drop will scatter light in the direction towards the retina. In turn this affects the quality of the retinal image hence visual disturbances. Some patients find this disturbing at critical viewing times. Highly viscous drops and ointments are the worse offenders. The refractive index values of some popular ATSs are listed in the Table 40.1. Clearly, some are more likely to affect vision than others. In common with most other eye drops, artificial tears are buffered to maintain a pH close to the pH of natural tears. Depending on the concentration of the instilled drop the eye can tolerate comfortably, a pH range from 6.6 to 7.8 is advisable.[49] Thus, the pH of artificial tears should fall within these limits. In the Table 40.2, the measured pH of various ATSs were taken under masked randomised conditions. In theory, some ATSs will be more acceptable in terms of comfort compared with others. (Patel 2001).

Table 40.1: Refractive Index and pH of some artificial tears

Substitute	*Refractive index*	*pH*
Viva-Drops	1.3354	6.7
Hypromellose	1.3347	8.2
SNO-Tears	1.3357	5.3
Tears Naturelle	1.3339	6.5
Isopto-Plain	1.3351	7.4
Hypo-tears (UK)	1.3391	5.9
Celluvisc	1.3351	6.4
Refresh	1.3342	6.2
Visco-Tears	1.3376	7.1
Clerz	1.3352	7.4
Genteal	1.3332	6.7
Ocucoat	1.3346	7.2
Hypotears (USA)	1.3393	5.5
Optifree re-wetting drops	1.3337	6.9

1. Refractive Index measured using S-10 refractometer (Atago, Japan)
2. pH measured using pH Meter model 10 (Corning-Eel Scientific Instruments)
3. All samples were fresh, previously unused and measured at room temperature (25 degrees).

Oral Antioxidants

The lacrimal glands, conjunctivae and meibomian glands obtain nutrients from the vascular system. A number of quintessential anti-oxidants are prominent in the biochemical processes leading to manufacture and secretion of essential tear constituents. Vitamins A, C, E, zinc, selenium and molybdenum together with other key nutrients prominently feature in tear metabolism.

It has been shown, within a "normal, healthy, symptom-free" population group, the blood plasma levels of essential antioxidants such as Vitamin C can be so low, that they reach near pathological levels.[50]

Other than injecting nutrients directly into the blood stream we could reach these tissues via the digestive tract. Within a "normal, allegedly healthy, symptom-free" population group, either Vitamin C (1000 mgm/day), or Vitamin A (2250 µgm/day), or an anti-oxidant mixture (1 tablet/day of Redoxan™, La Roche) can substantially improve tear stability after 7-10 days of treatment.[51] In a controlled study featuring placebo and cross-over design, oral ingestion of the antioxidant mixture VisionACE™ (Vitabiotics, UK) for 1 month can substantially improve both tear stability and goblet cell count in symptomatic marginal dry eyes.[52]

Tear substitutes and ointments containing vitamin A (or its analogues) are available for direct application to the ocular surface. Vitamin A is fat soluble and therefore, it should be supplied in a suitable non-aqueous medium. Aqueous tear drops containing vitamin A have such a low vitamin A content that it is difficult to believe these preparations do any good other than act as a placebo. If these drops do improve ocular surface health then the cause is probably the lubricant vehicle not the vitamin A.

Punctal Occlusion

When the OSS is due to insufficient aqueous production and other, less obtrusive methods have been tried and found to be insufficient, then punctal occlusion should be attempted. Aimed at preserving the tears, several plugs are available in various sizes, materials, construction, and they are often supplied with an intricate method for insertion. For example the Herrick plug is fabricated from flexible silicone rubber, it is peg shaped and supplied with a thin flexible wire inserter. The Freeman plug is made from a harder polymer, is capstan shaped and has an intricate assembly which facilitates insertion. Punctal plugs wider than the actual puncta are normally fitted to rest tight in the lacrimal canals. If the plug is too narrow, it would simply pass down the canals by the massaging effects produced by the lid muscles by constant blinking and natural eye movement.

To insert a plug, simply dilate the punctum using a Foster dilator. The sterile dilator is a tapered blunt pin. Passing it down the punctum and rotating with the hand and gently pushing from side to side will widen the punctum. Topical anesthesia and a drop of lubricant can be useful. The Freeman plug fitting assembly has a plug dilator incorporated in its design. The plug is pushed down the punctum and turned through 90 degrees passing the apex of the L shaped canal. When using the Freeman plug, the plug release assembly is pressed between the fingers, this frees the plug and the applicator assembly is gently withdrawn from the canal. For the Herrick plug, once it is inside the canal, the wire is gently rotated and pulled back. The fluted end of the Herrick plug in contact with the walls of the canal is held in place by friction as the wire is gently withdrawn.

Temporary collagen plugs should be used initially as a provocative test which allows the clinician to assess the value of a more prolonged punctal therapy and allows the patient a chance to experience the benefits or otherwise. These temporary plugs are manufactured from porcine collagen and some patients may decline these plugs on religious or other grounds. The plug should be the same or one step wider than the punctum. The punctum is widened as described above, the prepared sterile plugged is gripped between the pincers of sterilized fine jeweller´s forceps, the eyelid is pulled back to reveal a gaping punctum and the plug is inserted into the punctum. Once the plug touches the lid margin, it soaks up tears and expands. A swelling plug will become difficult to insert, hence it is advised to get the plug in as a "hole-in-one". Once inserted, the plug should be gently pushed down into the canal until it is no longer visible to the clinician. The swelling of the inserted plug keeps it in place and prevents extrusion. Tear stability and meniscus height should be measured prior to punctal plugging. The collagen plug will dissolve within a week or so, it is useful to check the patient within 48 hours. Both tear stability and meniscus height should be re-evaluated. Patients very quickly realise if the plug is doing any good. If the patient complains of epiphoria, then rest assured the plug will dissolve away in a few days. Ideally, if the plug is working, patient symptoms and tear characteristics will initially improve and fall back towards baseline as the plug gradually dissolves.

Some clinicians prefer occluding all 4 puncta. However, in the author´s opinion, plugging the lower puncta is sufficient in most cases because the bulk of tears drain away to the naso-lacrimal duct via this route. Occasionally, plugs can end up ejected from the canaliculi. After 6-14 months, in about 1% of cases the plug may pass out the punctum.[53] It could be lost by passing into the nasal cavity. In extreme cases, the puncta may be sealed with cautery or cyanoacrylate adhesives.

Other Treatment Alternatives

Ointments and lubricants either prevent ocular surface friction damage, retain fluid or maintain surface hydration. If the patient tends to sleep with the eyes partially open, an ointment at bedtime is called for. Similarly, ointments are useful in superficial ocualr surface damage.

Lid scrubs are useful for cleaning the lid margin at the junction between the skin and palpebral conjunctiva, unblocking meibomian gland openings, removing environmental debris (pollution), make-up, dry skin, denatured skin and mucosal secretions. Scrubs are useful in cases of mild blepharitis or meibomitis. Also, lid massaging forces fresh meibomian secretions to pass through the duct openings.

Liposomal sprays are calimed by the manufacturers, to enhance the skin and mucous membranes. The spary is made up microvesicles consisting of an inner aqueous phase and outer phospholipid bilayer floating in an aqueous outer phase. Their use produces a refreshing sensation. No clinical trials have been performed and the authors´have no experience of this product.

Lipid therapy is suitable when the OSS symptoms are of environmental origin. Gently pinching the lower or upper lid margin will squeeze meibomian oils out onto the ocular surface. After a few blinks, the extra lipid is spread over the precorneal tear film, thickening the lipid layer (Craig, et al 1995) and this should in turn reduce the evaporation of tears from the ocular surface. In cases where the meibomian secretions which are insufficiently soft and viscous, hot compresses or hot spoon presses can soften secretions by raising the temperature. This eases the passage of the meibomian oils to the surface.

When the OSS is severe leading to painful ocular surface damage and recurrent surface erosion, bandage lenses (preferably silicone-hydrogel lenses) worn on an extended wear basis could be considered. Bandage lenses protect the ocular surface in cases where either, blinking causes more harm to the corneal epithelium or, the corneal epithelium is weakly fixed to the basement membrane.

If all else fails, the patient should be referred for tarsorraphy.

PRIMUN NON NOCERE

(Firstly do no ha)

REFERENCES

1. Stulting RD, Carr JD, Thompson KP, et al.Complications of laser in situ keratomileusis for the correction of myopia. Ophthalmology 1999;106:13-20.
2. Jabbur NS, Sakatani K, O´Brien P. Survey of complications and recommendations for management in dissatisfied patients seeking a consultation after refarctive surgery. J Cataract Refract Surg Vol 30 Sep 2004;1867-74.
3. Holly FJ, Lemp MA. Wettability and wetting of corneal epithelium. Exp Eye Res 1971;11:239-50.
4. Lemp MA. Report of the National Eye Institute/Industry workshop On Clinical Trials in Drye eyes. CLAO 1995 J;21:221-32.
5. Muller LJ, Marfurt CF, Kruse F, Tervo TMT. Corneal nerves: structure, contents and function. Exp Eye Res 2003;76:521-42.
6. Holly FJ, Lemp MA. Exp Eye Res 1971;11:239.
7. Holly FJ, Lemp MA. Exp Eye Res 1973;15:515
8. Zisman WA. Contact angle, Wettability and Adhesion. Advances in Chemistry Series No. 43 Am. Chem. Soc Washington DC 1964;1.
9. van Oss CJ, Chaudhury MK, Good RJ. Adv. Colloid Interface Sci 1987;28:35.
10. van Oss CJ, Chaudhury MK, Good RJ. Chem. Rev 1988; 88:927.
11. van Oss CJ. Cell Biophys 1989;14:1.
12. van Oss CJ in Biophysics of the cell surface R Glaser and D. Gingell eds, Springer verlag 1990;131.
13. Sharma A. In Biophys Chem 1993;47:87.

14. Tiffany JM. Lacrimal gland, tear film and dry eye syndromes. D.A. Sullivan, ed. Plenum Press, New York, 1994;231.
15. Gipson IK, Inatomi T. Paper presented at Second International Conference on the Lacrimal Gland, tear Film and Dry Eye syndromes; Basic Science and clinical relevance, Bermuda, 1996.
16. See ref. 14.
17. See ref. 15.
18. See ref.14.
19. See ref.15.
20. Bron AJ, Tiffany JM. The lacrimal system. OP. van Bijstervald, M.A.Lemp and D. Spinelli, eds. <kugler and Ghedini Amsterdam 1991;27.
21. Tiffany JM, Winter N, Bliss G. Curr. Eye Res 1989;8:507.
22. Tiffany JM. Acta Ophthalmol 1990;68:175.
23. Tiffany JM. Acta Ophthalmol 1990;68:182.
24. Tseng CG, Maumenee AE, Stark WJ, et al. Ophthalmology 1985;92:717.
25. Sharma A. Acid-base interactions in the cornea-tear film system; surface chemistry of corneal wetting, cleaning, lubrication, hydration and defense. J.Dispersion Science and technology 1998;19(6 and 7):1031-68.
26. American Optometric Association. Care of the patient with ocular disorders. St. Louis (MO): American Optometric Association 2002;59.
27. Patel S, Murray D, McKenzie A, Shearer DS, McGrath BD. Effects of fluorescein on tear break-up time and on tear thinning time. Am J Optom Physiol Opt 1985;62: 188-90.
28. Lemp MA, Hamill JR. Factors affecting tear film breakup in normal eyes. Arch Ophthalmol 1973;89:103-05.
29. Blades KJ, Murphy PJ, Patel S. Tear thinning time and topical anaesthesia as assesses using the HIRCAL grid and the NCCA. Optom Vis Sci 1999;76:164-69.
30. Cho P, Yap M. Schirmer test I. A review. Optom Vis Sci 1993;70:152-56.
31. Cho P, Yap M. Schirmer test II. A clinical study of its repeatability. Optom Vis Sci 1993;70:157-59.
32. Schirmer O. Studies of the physiology and pathology of the secretion and drainage of tears. Arch Ophthalmol 1903;56:197-291.
33. Wright JC, Meger GE. A review of the Schirmer test for tear production. Arch Ophthalmol 1962;67:564-65.
34. Blades KJ, Patel S, Murphy PJ, Pearce EI. Is there a reflex component of phenol read thread wetting? Optom Vis Sci 1999;76(Suppl):228.
35. Blades KJ, Patel S. The dynamics of tear flow within a phenol red impregnated thread. Ophthal and Physiol Opt 1996;16:409-15.
36. Cho P, Kwong YM. A pilot study of the comparative performance of two cotton thread tests for tear volume. J Br Contact Lens Ass 1996;19:77-82.
37. Little SA, Bruce AS. Repeatability of the phenol-red thread and tear thinning time tests for tear function. Clin Exp Optom 1994;77:64-68.
38. Tomlinson A, Blades KJ, Pearce EI. What does the phenol red thread test actually measure? Optom and Vis Sci 2001;78:142-46.
39. Hamano H, Hori M, Mitsunaga S, Kojima S, Maeshima J Tear secretion test (a preliminary test) Jap J Clin Ophthalmol 1982;32:103-07.
40. Mainstone JC, Bruce AS, Golding TR. Tear meniscus measurement in the diagnosis of dry eye. Curr Eye Res 1996;15:653-661.
41. Oguz H, Yokoi N, Kinoshita S. The height and radius of tear meniscus and methods of examining these parameters. Cornea 2000;19:497-500.
42. Van Bijisterveld OP. Diagnostic tests in the sicca syndrome. Arch Ophthalmol 1969;82:10-14.
43. Hirji NK, Larke JR. Conjunctival impression cytology in contact lens practice. J Brit Cont Lens Assoc 1981;4: 159-61.
44. Egbert PR, Lauber S, Maurice DM. A simple conjunctival biopsy. Am J Ophthalmol 1977;84:798-801.
45. Nelson JD, Wright JC. Impression cytology of the ocular surface in keatoconjunctivitis sicca. In the preocular tear film in health, disease and contact lens wear 1986. Ed: Holly FJ, Dry Eye Inst, Lubbock, Yx 140-156.
46. American Optometric Association. Care of the patient with ocular surface disorders. St Louis (MO): American Optometric Association 2002;59.
47. Stevenson D, Tauber J, Reis BL. The Cyclosporin A phase 2 study group; Efficacy and safety of cyclosporin A ophthalmic emulsion in the treatment of moderate-to-severe dry eye disease. A dose-ranging, randomized trial. Ophthalmology 2000;107:967-74.
48. Milder B. The lacrimal apparatus. In Adler´s Physiology of the eye 1975 (ed: RA Moses). St Louis, CV Mosby.
49. Carney LG, Fullard RJ. Ocular irritation and environmental pH. Aust J Optom 1979;62:335-36.
50. Johnston CS, Thompson LL. Vitamin C status of an outpatient population. J Am Coll Nutr 1998;17:366-70.
51. Patel S, Plaskow J, Ferrier C. The influence of vitamins and trace element supplements on the stability of the precorneal tear film. Acta Ophthalmol 1993;71:825-829.
52. Blades KJ, Patel S, Aidoo KE. Oral antioxidant therapy for marginal dry eye. Eur J Clin Nutrition 2001;55: 589-97.
53. Fayat B, Assouline M, Hanush S, et al. Silicone punctal plug extrusion resulting from spontaneous dissection of canalicular mucosa. Ophthalmology 2001;108:405-09.

LASIK Hinge Location and Dry Eye

41

David T Vroman, Luis E Fernández de Castro
Kerry D Solomon (USA)

Normal tear function is essential for maintaining corneal function and structure. As the popularity of LASIK has grown, the number of patients experiencing dry eye symptoms has grown as well. According to the 2004 Refractive Surgery Survey,[1] dry eye symptoms are the most common problem encountered after LASIK and occur in 15 to 25% of patients. The dry eye symptoms range from a mild irritation and foreign body sensation to pain, photophobia and decreased visual acuity with visual fluctuation. There may be several factors that influence these symptoms, but decreased corneal sensation may play a major role.

The cornea is innervated by sensory nerve fibers originating from the ophthalmic division of the trigeminal nerve, and by sympathetic nerves. It is the tissue most densely innervated in the body. Corneal sensation is essential to maintaining the integrity of the ocular surface. Neurotrophic keratitis can result from common ocular disorders such as herpes simplex or herpes zoster infections or from uncommon insults affecting the fifth cranial nerve such as tumor, irradiation, or strokes.[2] In its early stages, neurotrophic keratopathy can manifest as an interpalpebral punctate keratitis and visual fluctuation and can progress to loss of epithelial integrity and corneal stromal melting.[3] Experimental and clinical studies have demonstrated that corneal nerve damage alters the metabolism and vitality of the epithelium, impairs epithelial healing, and is responsible for trophic ulceration.[4] Corneal surgical procedures may disrupt the normal organization of corneal innervation, including refractive surgery, which has been shown to cause decreased corneal sensation. This has been documented after epikeratophakia,[5] radial keratotomy,[6] photorefractive keratectomy (PRK),[7] and laser in situ keratomileusis (LASIK).[8-11] A number of possible etiologies explaining the appearance of dry eye following LASIK have been proposed. These include damage of the globlet cells by the pressure generated by the suction ring, alteration of the corneal curvature affecting tear stability, and medications that can induce transient dry eye symptoms.[12] More significant is the transection of a significant number of afferent sensory nerves in the cornea during the formation of the flap and, therefore, interruption of the cornea-trigeminal nerve-brain stem-facial nerve-lacrimal gland reflex arc that influences both basal and stimulated tear production.[8,13-18]

Damage to the corneal nerves has a direct effect on the health of the epithelium. In diseases where the trigeminal nerve has been damaged, a non-healing epithelial defect can occur. This epithelial breakdown may be due to poor blinking, decreased tear production, or by loss of direct neurotrophic effects on the epithelium. In some patients with dry eye after LASIK, there are signs of dryness with relatively few symptoms and ample tear production. These patients may be suffering from the loss of the direct effects that the corneal nerves may have in maintaining a healthy epithelium.

The subject of corneal innervation has gained importance in recent years due to the observation that corneal nerves are routinely injured following modern refractive surgical procedures. An example is LASIK surgery where a microkeratome is used to create a hinged lamellar corneal flap, disrupting the normal organization of corneal innervation. This damage can lead to transient or chronic neurotrophic deficits.[12,13] Some authors suggest the corneal nerves predominantly enter the cornea at the 9- and 3-o'clock position. Thus, creating a LASIK flap with a hinge provides a potential conduit for superficial innervation. A vertical flap (superior hinge) would transect both of the major areas of corneal innervation, while a horizontal flap (nasal hinge) would transect only one of these areas.[14] This suggests that a nasally hinged corneal flap may cause less loss of sensation than a superior hinge.[14-16,19] Descriptions of the anatomy of the mammalian corneal innervation are numerous; nevertheless many aspects of corneal nerve architecture remain incompletely understood. The true distribution of corneal nerves is controversial and it is still being elucidated.

To determine whether patients undergoing LASIK might actually have dry eye, we conducted a prospective, randomized, masked study to determine the effects of hinge position (superior vs. nasal hinge) on corneal sensation and dry eye signs and symptoms after LASIK.[20] The study included 47 patients undergoing bilateral myopic LASIK surgery. The first eye was randomly assigned to have a nasal or superior hinge flap; the fellow eye had the alternate location. Visual acuity, contrast sensitivity, corneal sensation, basic secretion test (BST), tear film break up time (TBUT), conjunctival and corneal staining, and a subjective questionnaire were evaluated preoperatively and postoperatively at 1 week, 1, 3 and 6 months. We observed a decrease in central corneal sensation at all time point in both eyes compared to baseline (Fig. 41.1). The improved nasal sensation did not seem to change the clinical outcome (Fig. 41.2). Dry eye occurred with the same frequency and there were no differences in the questionnaire. We observed a decrease in BST at the first week visit in our patients. We also established that dry eye and decreased corneal sensitivity affect many LASIK patients postoperatively and that even six months following surgery, corneal sensitivity was significantly decreased compared to preoperative measurements.

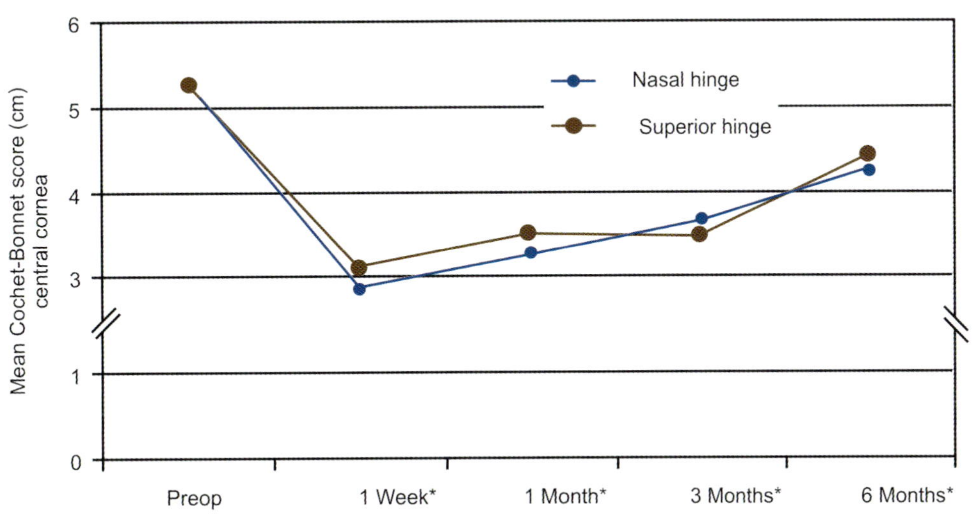

Fig. 41.1: Illustrates the mean central corneal sensation (Cochet-Bonnet) in nasal and superior hinge groups when compared to preoperative values (*P <.01)

Our study showed that central corneal sensation was significantly depressed in both groups for the entire six month duration of the study as illustrated in Figure 41.1. This is compatible with results from several other studies.[15,16,18,21] Figure 41.3 demonstrates a decrease in tear production at one week that increased to normal levels at one month. The tear breakup time was also reduced at the one week and one month visits (Fig. 41.3). These alterations were shown to be subjectively important as patients reported increased dryness using the subjective questionnaire at 1, 3 and 6 month postoperative visits.

Differences between nasal and superior hinge in corneal sensation and dry eye have been previously studied,[14,19] showing nerve fibers oriented in a 9-3 hour (temporal-to-medial) orientation. Our study demonstrated an improved nasal corneal sensation at one month in the nasal hinge group but found no

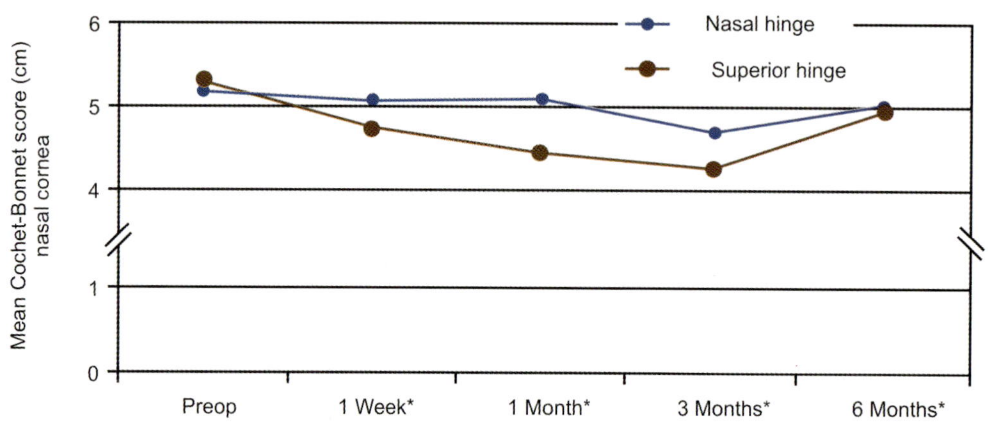

Fig. 41.2: Illustrates the mean nasal corneal sensation (Cochet-Bonnet) in eyes with the nasal hinge when compared to those with the superior hinge (*P <.01)

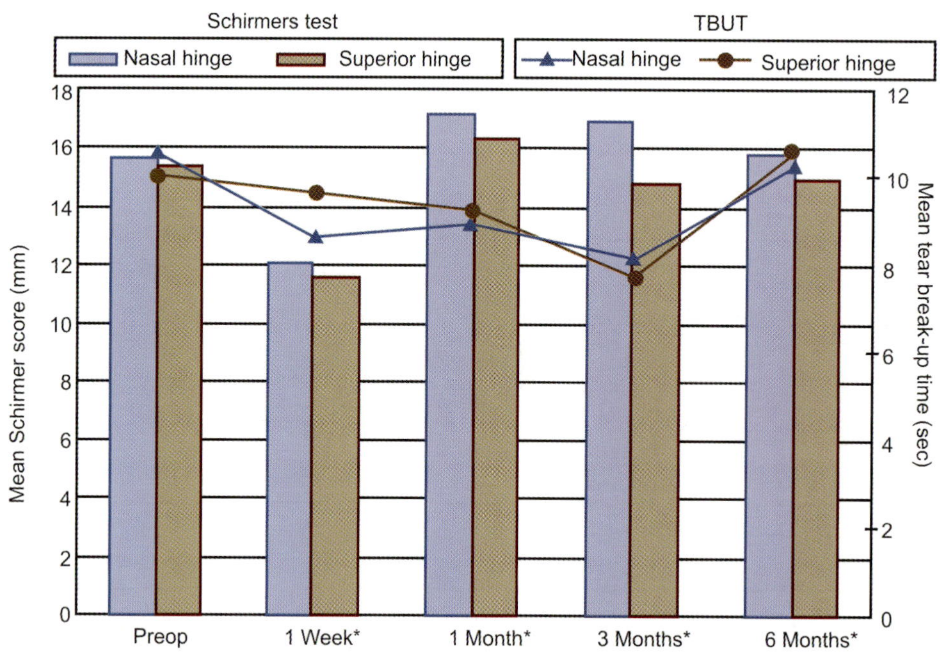

Fig. 41.3: Illustrates the mean basal secretion test and tear break up time scores, in nasal and superior hinge groups when compared to preoperative values (*P <.05)

difference in dry eye. This agrees with recent studies using in vivo confocal microscopy that show that subbasal nerve fibers run in a 6-12 hour (superior-to-inferior) orientation. Müller et al.[22] reported finding that leashes extend across the corneal apex preferentially in the 6-12 direction while other leashes approach the apex in the 5-11, 7-1, 9-3, 2-8 and 4-10 hour direction.

The current description is that nerve bundles enter the cornea at the periphery in a radial fashion parallel to the corneal surface. The majority of the stromal nerve fibers are located in the anterior third of the stroma; however, thick stromal nerve trunks move from the periphery towards the center below the anterior third of the stroma due to the organization of the collagen lamellae.[22] Eventually the stromal nerve fibers turn abruptly 90° and proceed toward the corneal surface. The nerves penetrate Bowman's layer throughout the peripheral and central cornea.[23] After penetrating the Bowman's layer, the large nerve bundles divide into several smaller ones. Each small nerve bundle then turns abruptly once more at 90° and continues parallel to the cornea surface. The exact orientation and the depth of the deep nerve fiber bundles is not entirely known and may be variable between patients.[22-25]

There is also a question as to how the nerves regenerate. Will nerve fibers re-innervate the central cornea by growing up from underlying stroma, or will peripheral nerves grow centrally? The pattern of regrowth could affect the speed of re-innervation as well as our understanding of the potential benefits of certain hinge locations. A potential important feature of LASIK is that it spares the epithelium, the Bowman layer, a considerable proportion of the anterior stromal nerve plexus and the corneal nerves in the hinge region. Furthermore, the flap contains the original Schwann cell pathways, which might facilitate the process of nerve recovery. Examination of the regeneration of the subepithelial nerve plexus after LASIK has showed that regenerating fibers appears first as short sub-basal leaches. Then by 3 months they are elongated, but interconnections are not observed before the sixth postoperative month.[26] A prospective 5-year study demonstrated that sub-basal nerve density in the central cornea, measured by confocal microscopy, did not recover to near preoperative densities until 5 years after LASIK.[27]

Factors such as flap size, hinge width and depth of the flap play an important role in the health of the corneal surface. Lamellar cutting of the cornea during LASIK impairs corneal sensitivity and depth of the corneal ablation affects the extent of loss of corneal sensitivity and recovery.[26] Furthermore, the diameter of the flap and the ablation area may also have an effect on the degree of corneal sensation loss and time for its recovery. Deeper and wider ablation as well as a wider flap may cause a greater reduction in corneal sensation.

CONCLUSION

It is important that surgeons avoid inducing dry eye after LASIK. To do this, the entire corneal surface must be evaluated preoperatively including tear secretion, mucous layer, and the meibomian glands. Each of these components is essential for a healthy tear film and must be maximized prior to surgery. Therefore, any treatment available for dry eye should be used preoperatively to minimize this common finding postoperatively.

Successful surgery is dependent on not only the measured postoperative visual acuity or quality of vision, but also the preoperative expectations of the patient as determinants of overall satisfaction. It is therefore crucial that every refractive surgeon discuss the indications, methods, possible risks, limitations, and potential alternatives with his/her patient in advance of a planned elective refractive procedure to accurately gauge the expectations of the patient and recommend the best course, including possibly choosing an alternative or deferring surgery.[28]

REFERENCES

1. Sandoval HP, Fernández de Castro LE, Vroman DT, Solomon KD. Refractive surgery survey 2003. J Cataract Refract Surg 2005;31:221-33.
2. Martin X, Safran AB. Corneal hypoesthesia. Surv Ophthalmol 1988;33:28-40.

3. Lambiase A, Rama P, Aloe L, Bonini S. Management of neurotrophic keratopathy. Curr Opin Ophthalmol 1999;10:270-76.
4. Joo MJ, Yuhan KR, Hyon JY, et al. The effect of nerve growth factor on corneal sensitivity after laser in situ keratomileusis. Arch Ophthalmol 2004;122:1338-41.
5. Koenig SB, Berkowitz RA, Beuerman RW, et al. Corneal sensitivity after epikeratophakia. Ophthalmology 1983;90:1213-18.
6. Shivitz IA, Arrowsmith PN. Corneal sensitivity after radial keratotomy. Ophthalmology 1988;95:827-32.
7. Kanellopoulos AJ, Pallikaris IG, Donnenfeld ED, et al. Comparison of corneal sensation following photorefractive keratectomy in laser in situ keratomileusis. J Cataract Refract Surg 1997;23:34-38.
8. Matsui H, Kumano Y, Zushi I, et al. Corneal sensation after correction of myopia by photorefractive keratectomy and laser in situ keratomileusis. J Cataract Refract Surg 2001;27:370-73.
9. Patel S, Perez-Santonja JJ, Alio JL, et al. Corneal sensitivity and some properties of the tear film after laser in situ keratomileusis. J Refract Surg 2001;17:17-24.
10. Benitez-del-Castillo JM, del Rio T, Iradier T, et al. Decrease in tear secretion and corneal sensitivity after laser in situ keratomileusis. Cornea 2001;20:30-32.
11. Chuck RS, Quiros PA, Perez AC, et al. Corneal sensation after laser in situ keratomileusis. J Cataract Refract Surg 2000;26:337-39.
12. Wilson SE, Ambrosio R. Laser in situ keratomileusis-induced neurotrophic epitheliopathy. Am J Ophthalmol. 2001;132:405-06.
13. Wilson SE. Laser in situ keratomileusis-induced (presumed) neurotrophic epitheliopathy. Ophthalmology 2001;108:1082-87.
14. Donnenfeld ED, Solomon KD, Perry HD, et al. The effect of hinge position on corneal sensation and dry eye after LASIK. Ophthalmology 2003;110:1023-30.
15. Kumano Y, Matsui H, Zushi I, et al. Recovery of corneal sensation after myopic correction by laser in situ keratomileusis with nasal or superior hinge. J Cataract Refract Surg 2003;29:757-61.
16. Nassaralla BA, McLeod SD, Nassaralla JJ. Effect of myopic LASIK on human corneal sensitivity. Ophthalmology 2003;110:497-502.
17. Lemp MA. Report of the National Eye Institute/ Industry workshop on clinical trials in dry eyes. CLAO J 1995;21:221-32.
18. Battat L, Macri A, Dursun D, et al. Effects of laser in situ keratomileusis on tear production, clearance, and the ocular surface. Ophthalmology 2001;108:1230-35.
19. Lee KW, Joo CK. Clinical results of laser in situ keratomileusis with superior and nasal hinges. J Cataract Refract Surg 2003;29:457-61.
20. Vroman DT, Sandoval HP, Fernández de Castro LE, et al. Effect of hinge location on corneal sensation and dry eye alter laser in situ keratomileusis for myopia. J Cataract Refract Surg 2005;31:1881-87.
21. Toda I, Asano-Kato N, Komai-Hori Y, et al. Dry eye after laser in situ keratomileusis. Am J Ophthalmol 2001;132:1-7.
22. Muller LJ, Marfurt CF, Kruse F, et al. Corneal nerves: structure, contents and function. Exp Eye Res 2003; 76:521-42.
23. Müller LJ, Pels L, VrensenGF. Ultrastructural organization of human corneal nerves. Invest Ophthalmol Vis Sci 1996;37:476-88.
24. Kim J, Foulks GN. Evaluation of the effect of lissamine green and rose Bengal on human corneal epithelial cells. Cornea 1999;18:328-32.
25. Müller LJ, Vrensen GF, Pels L, et al. Architecture of human corneal nerves. Invest Ophthalmol Vis Sci 1997;38:985-94.
26. Bragheeth MA, Dua HS. Corneal sensation after myopic and hyperopic LASIK: clinical and confocal microscopic study. Br J Ophthalmol 2005;89:580-85.
27. Erie JC, McLaren JW, Hodge DO, Bourne WM. Recovery of corneal subbasal nerve density after PRK and LASIK. Am J Ophthalmol 2005;140:1059-64.
28. Jabbur NS, Sakatani K, O'Brien TP. Survey of complications and recommendations for management in dissatisfied patients seeking a consultation after refractive surgery. J Cataract Refract Surg 2004;30:1867-74.

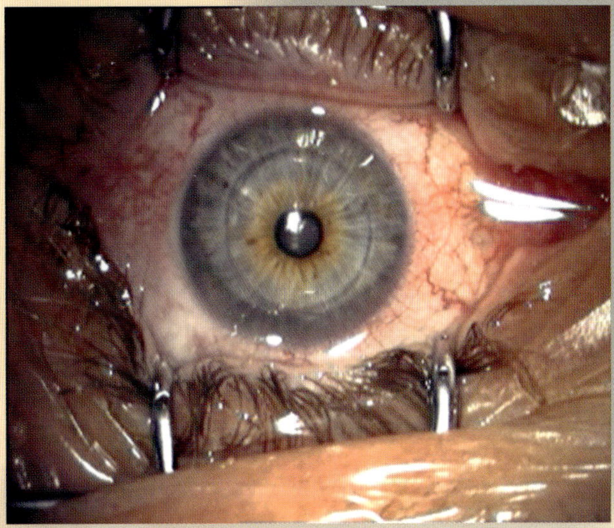

Recent Advances and Future Prospects

SECTION FOUR

ReLASIK (LASIK Enhancement)

42

Guillermo Avalos-Urzua, Ariadna Silva-Lepe (Mexico)

INTRODUCTION

LASIK(laser *in situ* keratomileusis) is, nowaday, probably the safest and most predictable refractive surgery available.

Patients believe that the procedure will permanently and completely eliminate their refractive defect.

It is the refractive surgeon's responsibility to inform the patient that the procedure is intended to eliminate their dependency on glasses or contact lenses, and that the degree of correction obtained will depend on several variables as the diopters the patient has, as well as the combination of different types of refractive errors (myopia with astigmatism, hyperopia with astigmatism, etc). The sum of all factors will have an impact on the final corrective results.

Inevitable sometimes we'll have to "redo" some eyes. Depending on the postoperative characteristics of the cornea, it may be necessary and useful to do an enhancement in order to improve the results obtained during the first surgery. Enhancement rates in USA range from 6 to 15%; with millions of people undergoing LASIK, this translates into hundreds of thousands of enhancements being performed annually.[1]

LASIK surgery is performed intrastromally, allowing the surgeon to perform a second ablation to correct any under or overcorrection. Furthermore it allows us to do retreatment (enhancement of the first procedure, of any defect which may have occurred during the first surgery, such as the inducement of astigmatism or the production of irregular astigmatism, or the presence of regression, which is common in the majority of refractive procedures.

Regression has been reported by many authors. Guell and Muller[2] report higher rate of regression after LASIK for high myopias in comparison to moderate myopias. Chayet et al[3] observed early postoperative regression that stabilized between 3 and 6 months after treatment in myopias with MSE – 14.02 D. One regression mechanism is the proliferation of keratocytes in the corneal stoma, while another possible mechanism is epithelial hyperplasia.

The majority of refractive surgeons are in agreement that the limit of myopic correction with LASIK is – 12.00 D since the corneal flatness in high myopias is excessive and generates poor optic quality corneas.

As the degree of myopia increases, the amount of regression and the subsequent need for enhancement procedures increase as well. The typical maximal regression occurs between two and four weeks postoperative, after which relative stability is achieved. A smaller amount of regression is generally noted one, two, three months postoperatively.

Qi et al[4] evaluated the results of excimer retreatment for undercorrection or regression after LASIK. They studied 2, 149 eyes that were divided into two groups according to their degrees of pre-first LASIK myopia spherical equivalents. Group I was $\leq$ 10.00 diopters (D) (41 eyes); group II was > 10.00 D (47 eyes). The retreatment ratio was 4.1% among the 2,149 eyes. In group II, the ratio was 2.3 times that of the group I. In the comparison with other eyes, the eyes received retreatment no difference in sex, laterality and age. Over 50.0% had pre first LASIK diopters $\geq$ 10.00 D, and 73.9% had astigmatism correction in first LASIK. After retreatment, no undercorrection or regression occurred in group I, but there was undercorrection in group II. The ratio within +/– 1.00 D of emmetropia after 1 year was 68.3% in group I and 51.1% in group II. The UCVA above 0.5 was over 90.0% in all eyes. Eight eyes (9.0%) lost two or more lines of BCVA. The serious complication after retreatment was keratoconus of 3 eyes in group II. They concluded that the risk factors which lead to retreatment after first LASIK are high myopia with astigmatism before first LASIK and the reaction to the operation.

In this study, retreatment was safe, effective, predictable and accurate for </= –10.00 D correction in first LASIK. But, to prevent the occurrence of serious complication such as keratoconus, it is better not to perform retreatment for > – 10.00 D in first LASIK.

Other factors that increase chances of LASIK retreatment are higher initial corrections, astigmatism and older age of patients, as shown by Hersh et al[5] in their study that included 2,485 eyes (1,306 patients) who underwent LASIK surgery for myopia, hyperopia or astigmatism. Of the 2,485 patients, 288 eyes of 233 patients underwent one retreatment, and 3 eyes of 3 patients required two retreatment procedures.

They stated that the overall 1-year incidence of retreatment was 10.5%. They concluded that higher initial corrections and residual astigmatism were associated with a significantly higher rate of retreatment. Patients older than 40 years were at greater risk for retreatment. No gender difference was evident.

All of the previously discussed was also emphasized by Perlman and Reinert.[6] In their paper these authors tried to confirm that enhancements after primary LASIK are effective in dealing with residual refractive errors, and to determine if any variables prior to or during the primary LASIK procedure predisposed eyes to require subsequent enhancement. They concluded that enhancements were an effective way of dealing with residual refractive errors after primary LASIK. Age greater than 45 years or a history of recent rigid contact lens use was significantly associated with the need for enhancement in patients with myopia or myopic astigmatism.

Factors Associated to LASIK Enhancements

A. *Patient dissatisfaction:* While some patients may be happy with 20/25 or 20/35 corrected vision, others won't be as content. Durrie[7] strives for "20/happy" for his patients, maintaining that it's all right to enhance a patient at 20/25 or even 20/20 if the patient has stable refraction and topography that can be corrected with current technology. Regarding patient perceptions, "The rule of thumb is that there is no rule of thumb" enhancements depend on the patient's needs.

   Speaker[1] gives the patient a contact lens to simulate the intended result. He postulates that particularly in pre-presbyopic or presbyopic patients, sometimes the effect cannot be anticipated unless the patient tries out the contact first.

B. *Patient age:* When evaluating the patient's request for an enhancement, take his or her age into consideration. It is said that a younger patient who is undercorrected will generally be more inclined to be persistent about the enhancement, while undercorrected patients who are pre-presbyopic and presbyopic may find it advantageous to have a broad range of vision preserved so that the only time they would need glasses would be to drive at night.

   On the other hand, people in their 20s and 30s can still see well if they are slightly overcorrected, but in presbyopic patients who are overcorrected, they do not see well either distance or close, and they are persistent in wanting the correction.

C. *Effect of environmental factors:* Walter KA, Stevenson AW[8], determined whether environmental factors affect LASIK enhancement rates. They found that the 2-week-preoperative mean outdoor relative humidity, procedure room relative humidity, outdoor temperature, and procedure room temperature may have to be considered during LASIK planning. The effect of these environmental variables on LASIK outcomes warrants further evaluation.

D. *Other:* Some authors have designed formulas to predict the probability of LASIK enhancement as Hu et al[9]. They developed a formula to predict a patient's need for LASIK enhancement. Multivariate logistic regression analysis was used to determine a formula for the probability of enhancement surgery. Age ($P < .0001$), preoperative cycloplegic sphere ($P < .0001$), and surgeon ($P < .0001$) were the statistically significant factors for predicting retreatment. The predictive formula derived from these factors had a sensitivity of 79%, a specificity of 61%, and positive and negative predictive values of 31 and 93%, respectively. Older age, higher preoperative cycloplegic sphere, and surgeon significantly influenced a patient's likelihood for LASIK retreatment. A formula based on these predisposing factors helps to more accurately predict the need for retreatment.

INDICATIONS

Clinical indications[1] for retreatment include residual or induced astigmatism and under- and overcorrection. It is very important that surgeons and ophthalmologists evaluate patients with induced astigmatism and who may have lost a line of best-corrected visual acuity to make sure the induced astigmatism is not caused by striae, or wrinkles in the flap. If astigmatism is caused by striae, and the ophthalmologist plans to do an enhancement by lifting the flap, the result is unpredictable. One should be careful not to lead patients to believe that a small amount of laser correction will restore a quality of vision as it may not.

The amount of residual defect recommendable for treatment for a second ablation is greater than 0.75D.

EVALUATION

All patients who undergo enhancement should first have their cycloplegic refraction evaluated as well as an ultrasonic pachymetry and a corneal topography.

Pachymetry

The primary factor that determines whether or not to do an enhancement is the result of the pachymetry, which can differ if you are doing an enhancement in a patient with a preoperative correction greater or lower than –6.00 D. As a safety measure, the surgeon should always leave 250 microns of stroma plus an average of 160 microns of thickness of the corneal flap, leaving us with a total of 410 microns. As a basic principle, reablations should not be performed if the cornea shows a total pachymetry of less than 410 microns. If the preoperative correction in the original surgery is less than –6.00 D, the undercorrection is usually between –0.5 and –1.50 D. Since first ablations are usually less than 80 microns, surely a second ablation of 20 microns can be performed without any inconvenience. If we have a cornea of 530 microns and remove 160 microns the flap plus an additional 80 microns of the ablation, we are left with a stroma under the flap of 290 microns, leaving us with 40 microns for the second ablation.

In myopias greater than –6.00 D, for example with –11.0 D, also with a cornea of 530 microns, we do a first ablation of approximately 130 microns which leaves us with a residual stroma of 240 microns and a total pachymetry of only 400 microns.

In this case an enhancement is not an option since the surgeon needs to recognize the potential risk of creating corneal ectasia.

In their paper Muallem et al[10] evaluated whether flap thickness changes after the primary LASIK procedure and assessed the accuracy of intraoperative pachymetry and ablation depth measurements in predicting stromal bed thickness before enhancement in eyes that have had primary myopic LASIK. They concluded that the flap thickness tended to be thicker at enhancement than at primary LASIK. Intraoperative pachymetry and ablation depth measurements proved to be precise tools to predict stromal bed thickness before enhancement in eyes that had primary myopic LASIK. They suggested that this information may help in planning LASIK enhancements.

Two methods were compared for estimating residual stromal bed thickness before repeat LASIK, by Randleman et al.[11]

They compared 2 methods of calculating residual stromal bed (RSB) thickness after repeat LASIK, to determine which method generates more conservative RSB thickness estimates, and to determine any factors related to the discrepancy between these 2 calculation methods. This group compared calculated RSB thickness after second and third LASIK using either original corneal thickness (CT) minus flap thickness and all ablations (original CT method) or pre-enhancement CT minus flap thickness and enhancement ablation (repeat CT method). They conclude that using original preoperative CT measurements provides a more conservative and thus safer approach than using CT measurements obtained before repeat LASIK to calculate RSB thickness after repeat LASIK.

Topography

Another important factor is the topography. Kanellopoulos[1] referred in his publication that topography-guided LASIK enhancement using the *Allegretto Wave system* appears to be safe and effective for improving poor quality of vision associated with small, eccentric ablations and irregular astigmatism after previous refractive surgery.

Based on data collected of 17 consecutive eyes during a mean follow-up period of 6.5 months, he concluded the topography-guided enhancement resulted in improved topography accompanied by a reduction in the mean asphericity value toward a more desirable level. There was good cylinder correction and reasonable spherical adjustment, accompanied by marked improvement in night vision quality. Patients eligible for the procedure had to present with a small optical zone, decentered ablation, irregular astigmatism, or night vision problems and have a residual SE ±1.50 D. In addition, they were required to have estimated post-enhancement thicknesses of 280 μm in the stromal bed and 400 μm for the total cornea. As an additional criterion, patients needed to have highly reproducible topography maps. Only topographies with ≥ 75% of the corneal surface mapped were included. Retreatment was performed with flap lifting, not cutting, and ultrasonic pachymetry measurements were obtained preoperatively and after flap lifting to verify that patients fulfilled the criteria for residual stromal and corneal thickness.

TIMMING

Stability is imperative before an enhancement can be considered. Stability of postoperative refraction in LASIK, when you have treated myopias lower than –6.00 D, is two months. For this reason, with this group of patients it is appropriate to do the enhancement after two months. When treating myopias greater than –6.0 D the stability of the postoperative refraction can prolong itself up two 6 months, and any intent of reablation should be done after this time. If you are going to do a retreatment due to an overcorrection of a myopic LASIK, you should wait at least 6 months, since in the first few weeks post-LASIK there may exist overcorrections that progressively diminish in the first two months. Before this time, if overcorrections exist we should manage them with medication (pilocarpine 0.5 or 1%) for several months in order to induce myopia or with the application of soft contact lenses since this stimulates the epithelial hyperplasia and in some cases we can obtain regression of the overcorrection. After six months, if the overcorrection persists we should think of doing hyperopic LASIK. Hersh et al[5] found that the average length of time between initial treatment and enhancement was 7.3 +/– 6.4 months; 85% of retreatments took place within 1 year.

CONTRAINDICATIONS

Contraindications for enhancement include the thickness of the cornea. Simon[1] cited 250 microns as the minimal bed thickness in order to perform either the primary surgery or an enhancement. Durrie[17] considers the total corneal thickness, which includes 160 microns for the flap and 250 microns for the bed.

As for other contraindications, it has been cited[10] uncontrolled blepharitis, dry eye and epithelial basement membrane dystrophy.

REOPERATION TECHNIQUE

The best option for correcting residual defects induced during the first LASIK surgery is a second LASIK procedure. One of the primary advantages of LASIK is its adjustability, which allows for the possibility of a future reablation (enhancement).

The original surgeon should have the characteristics of the cut registered such as de diameter, thickness, hinge, size or free cap and if the cut was regular or irregular as well as the reason for the complication of the cut.

Diameter: It is important to know the diameter of the cut in order to avoid making an error in lifting a flap that was partial or insufficient in diameter; especially if the reablation is going to be hyperopic to treat an overcorrection.

Thickness: Thin flaps (130 microns or less) shrink easily when being lifted, producing striae or folds, which result in visual postoperative defects.

Hinge: When doing a hyperopic retreatment with a large hinge you will obtain an appropriate ablation since the hinge will be blocking the treatment zone.

Free cap: The greatest of care is required when lifting the flap in order to avoid a second free cap and the future risk of displacement.

Regular or Irregular surfaces: It is preferable to treat whatever irregularity of the cut on the same level in order to obtain a better result in your retreatment. If the original procedure was done by another surgeon, it is necessary to do a careful study of the corneal disk with the slit lamp. The best way of doing this is to install a drop of anesthesia and with a round instrument 4 to 5 mm in diameter (the author uses the Caro/Avalos Flap Smoother) apply pressure to the center of the cornea which makes the cut in the cornea evident. In this way you can evaluate the diameter of the cut while having a good idea of the size of the hinge. It is very difficult to visually appreciate the thickness of the cut with the slit- lamp, if it is 130 or 160 microns; this is a personal judgment call. With the slit-lamp (biomicroscopic examination) it is very difficult to know if the cut was partial or not, we can only visualize the border of the cut and attempt to appreciate its limits. Regularity or irregularity of the cut is preferably observed with the topography since the flap makes it impossible to see irregular areas in the stroma. The LASIK surgeon generally achieves good exactitude in the correction of the refractive problem. When there is an undercorrection it could be due to an insufficient ablation or to regression. In low myopias (less than –6 D) if a significant undercorrection is present and we did not do the original surgery, we should assume that probably problems existed in the cut. Irregular astigmatism in the topography or haze in the interface can confirm that it was not a good quality cut and in this case a retreatment should be performed by means of a second cut.

There are two options for performing the reablation:

A. a second cut,

B. relifting the flap.

Second Cut

It has been mentioned that 6 months after the original procedure the process of healing between the flap and the stroma is complete, making it difficult to lift the flap. Lifting the flap increases the risk of producing epithelial ingrowths in the interface. A new cut can be made at the same depth of the anterior cut or it can be deeper (180 or 200 microns).

A second cut could produce a free lamellar tissue that could cause disastrous refractive conditions that are not easily resolved. As well, a second cut causes a double interface, which can produce diminution of the BCVA and ghosts in vision. If the first cut had irregularities in the corneal stroma doing a second cut on another depth will not correct this stromal abnormalities, since they need to be treated on the same level in which they occurred.

In my opinion, one of the fundamental aspects of doing a retreatment is to know if I performed the original LASIK procedure or if it was performed by another surgeon.

Relifting the Flap

It is generally believed that it is easer to lift the flap six months after the original procedure, it has also been mentioned that you can lift the flap even after three years.[12] In our clinic it has be done after three years without difficult, by using an appropriated technique. Other motives for recommending the management of the original flap is that the intrinsic risk of the microkeratome (thin flap, free cap, holes, etc.) are not present.

Domniz et al[13] compared enhancement techniques following LASIK. Recutting was performed on 263 eyes and the flap was lifted in 55 eyes that had LASIK for simple myopia or myopic astigmatism. The time interval between LASIK and retreatment was 340 ± 46 days in the recutting group and 215 ± 36 days in the flap lifting group. In the recutting group, mean spherical equivalent refraction improved from –1.48 ± 1.25 D to –0.49 ± 0.88 D at 6 months. In the flap lifting group, mean spherical equivalent refraction improved from –1.05 ± 1.49 D to –0.45 ± 0.39 D at 6 months. Refractive cylinder did not change significantly in either group.

There was a significant increase in uncorrected visual acuity UCVA of 6/6 in each group. In the recutting group, UCVA of 6/6 increased from 3.8 to 65.2% at 6 months, and in the lifting group from 3.6 to 71.1% at 6 months. In the recutting group, seven free flaps and three macerated flaps that required removal occurred. One eye in the recutting group and two in the lifting group developed significant epithelial ingrowth. No patient lost more than one line of BSCVA. Their conclusion was that procedures were safe, effective, and highly predictable for enhancements, but flap complications may be more likely with recutting.

In Hersh et al[5] study nearly all (285) of the 288 retreatments performed, were accomplished using a manual flap lift approach; 3 eyes required a repeat microkeratome cut.

Netto et al[14] at The Cole Eye Institute analyzed the results achieved with LASIK retreatment after lifting the original flap in a large series of patients. LASIK retreatment was performed in 334 eyes, and the mean time between initial procedure and retreatment was 8.2 ± 6.2 months. The mean spherical equivalent (SE) improved from –1.2 ± 0.6 diopters (D) (range, –4.2 to +1.2 D) before retreatment to +0.2 ± 0.4 D (range, –3.1 to +1.1 D) after the retreatment. The uncorrected visual acuity (UCVA) after retreatment was 20/20 or better in 58% and 20/40 or better in 92% of eyes. The mean SE was within ±1.0 D in 96% of the patients and within ±0.5 D in 80.5% after retreatment. Eighteen eyes (5%) lost 1 line of best-corrected visual acuity, and 4 eyes (1%) lost 2 lines. In this study, LASIK retreatment surgery performed by relifting the flap was a useful procedure for correcting residual refractive errors after the primary LASIK procedure. It provided good uncorrected visual acuity, predictable results, good refractive stability, and few complications.

SURGICAL TECHNIQUE

Enhancements should be treated the same way as the first LASIK procedure; the same rules of the asepsis are applied to the second treatment. During surgical cleaning, the patient face is washed with betadine solution and they are given their first dose of anesthetic (proparacaine). This is followed by drops of ciprofloxacin. They are then placed on a stretcher where a drape is placed over their face in order to isolate the eyelids and eyelashes from the ocular globe. Once on the stretcher, a second dose of anesthetic is applied and the speculum is placed. A mark is made in the corneal epithelium whith the side of a 25 G needle followed by the application of a gentian violet color mark, this mark is radial and is extended from the border of the pupil to the limbus. Once this has been done, excess color should then be cleaned away with a wet sponge.

With a round instrument, pressure is apply to the center of the cornea, in order to observe the border of the corneal disk cut or flap through the microscope, for this purpose I use a glass rod or I recommend using the Caro/Avalos compressor instrument. Occasionally in light colored iris this can be difficult to observe. In both eyes, the easiest zone of the flap to observe is the temporal inferior sector of the cornea. Once this has been located, use a thin slightly curve spatula and attempt to insert it under the edge of the corneal disk in a parallel movement, without withdrawing the round instrument that is applying pressure to the eye. This will help to overcome epithelial resistance. Once the point of the spatula is under the corneal flap, steer it towards the center of the pupil. Then, in a rotating movement while maintaining the instrument in a fixed position in the center of the pupil, rotate above and below trying to loosen it at least 180 degrees. During this movement the spatula should not be withdrawn or reinserted, in order to avoid inserting epithelial cells in the interface. Once it has been loosened 180 degrees, withdraw the spatula and with a nontoothed forceps lift the corneal flap in a semicircular movement (upwards and downwards) in order to finish loosening the corneal flap until you arrive at the hinge, then fold the disk back over the conjunctiva. One should be careful when lifting the flap to be sure to withdraw the tag of the epithelium in order to avoid inserting it under the flap toward the interface. With a dry sponge clean the entire length of the stromal border of the cornea while making sure that the sponge does not pass toward the stroma. I recommend dampening the stromal face of the flap to avoid dryness caused by exposure to the environment, which will form striae and folds. I do not recommend the use of saline solution to separate the disk from the stroma since it modifies the hydration of the stroma and consequently the ablation as well as the adhesion between the flap and the posterior stroma.

Perez-Santonja et al[15] in their paper describe a refinement technique for LASIK retreatment called circular flap rhexis, based on a careful flap edge identification, linear epithelial tear for minimizing epithelial irregularities and defects, and a delicate flap replacement to promote a strong adhesion between the flap edge and the stromal bed. Their LASIK retreatment with this flap rhexis technique was performed in 43 eyes at 3 or 6 months after the primary LASIK. After a 12 months follow-up, the epithelial ingrowth and flap melting rates were recorded. Epithelial growth was found in 9.3% of the cases (4 out of 43 eyes) and flap melting in 2.3% of the cases (1 out of 43) at 12 months after LASIK retreatment by circular flap rhexis. These disorders were always peripheral and did not affect visual acuity or corneal astigmatism.

They concluded that LASIK retreatment using circular flap rhexis is an effective technique to decrease the epithelium related complications after LASIK retreatment.

Once the stroma is exposed, align the eye with the lasers aiming beam in order to proceed with your retreatment in regards to the quantity of the ablation, it should be performed the total amount correction for patients between 20 and 35 years old. From 35 to 45 years decrease 10% of the correction and from 45 years onwards decrease by 20% of the total amount to be corrected.

When finalizing the ablation you should irrigate the stroma to eliminate all the debris from both the previous and current ablation. Clean the flap especially around the edge in order to avoid leaving epithelial remains. Once the flap has been collocated in its correct position and is properly aligned, dry the border with a wet sponge and use the Caro compressor in the central portion of the flap, applying pressure for 15 seconds, which would produce good adhesion between the flap and the stroma and avoids its posterior displacement if, when lifting the flap, you produce a significant epithelial defect you should apply a soft contact lens for 3 to 5 days which allows complete healing. If there are not epithelial defects, the postoperative indications should be the same as in the original procedure, apply drops containing dexamethasone and antibiotics (fluoroquinolones), add nonsteroidal drops if you choose in order to decrease postoperative sensation. It is the surgeon's decision whether or not to use a patch for several hours.

The postoperative regimen is normal, including the use of steroids and antibiotics for 8 days and artificial tears for a month.

After an enhancement, the patient needs to be treated with steroids and antibiotics to prevent against infection or diffuse lamellar keratitis, which occurs in the interface between the flap and the stromal. Suresh and Rootman[16] reported a case of bilateral infectious keratitis occurring as a complication of bilateral simultaneous LASIK enhancement procedures. Corneal scraping from the interface of both eyes grew *Staphylococcus aureus*. The infection cleared after treatment with fluoroquinolones. The patient was left with bilateral paracentral corneal scars.

They concluded that when bilateral surgery is performed, bilateral infection may occur as a rare complication.

Therefore, the patient should be seen by their surgeon frequently, with special attention been paid to epithelial healing at the edge of the flap as well as periodic follow-up each month to observe the possibility of the appearance of epithelial ingrowth. If epithelial ingrowth appears at some postoperative stage, you can apply laser YAG (yttrium-aluminum-garned) on the area in order to destroy epithelial cells and to avoid relifting the flap.

I have been doing this procedure for the past 10 years with very successful results (Figs 42.1 to 42.5).

Rubinfeld et al[17] reported serious complications caused by recutting LASIK flaps for enhancement and reconsider the current preferred method of LASIK enhancement. In this retrospective noncomparative nonconsecutive case series comprised LASIK patients in the private practices of 9 experienced refractive surgeons and those reported in a survey of refractive surgeons. Case histories, refractions, corneal topographies, slit-lamp photographs, and measurements of uncorrected and best corrected (BCVA) visual acuity after recutting LASIK flaps were collected. Surveys of refractive surgeons and an

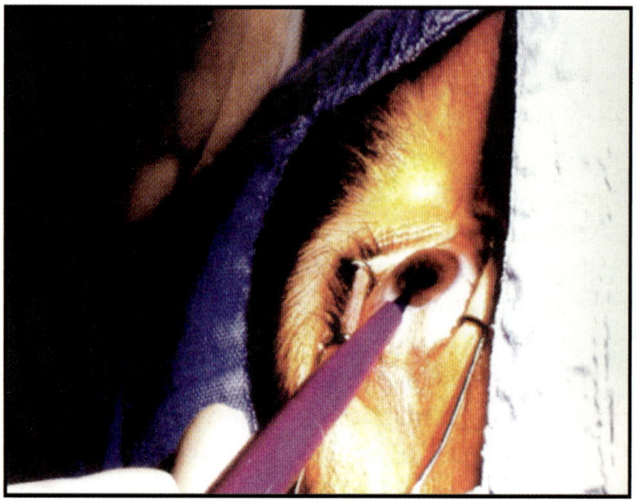

Fig. 42.1: Reference mark

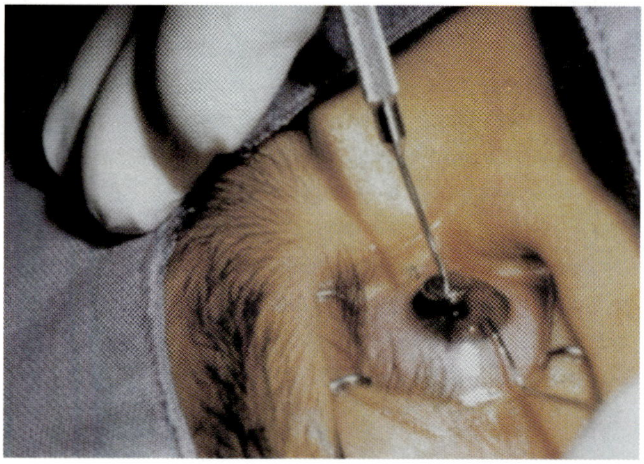

Fig. 42.2

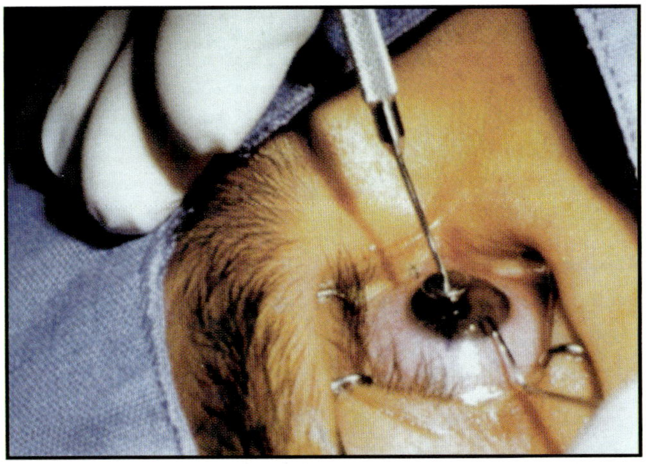

Fig. 42.3: Use a thin slightly curve spatula, attempt to insert

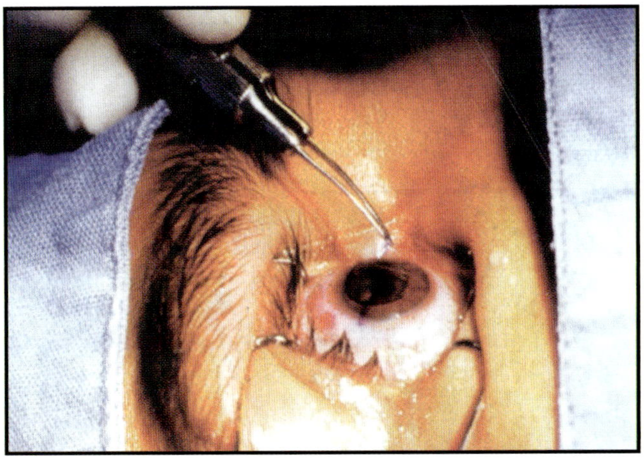

Fig. 42.4: Lift the flap with a fine forceps

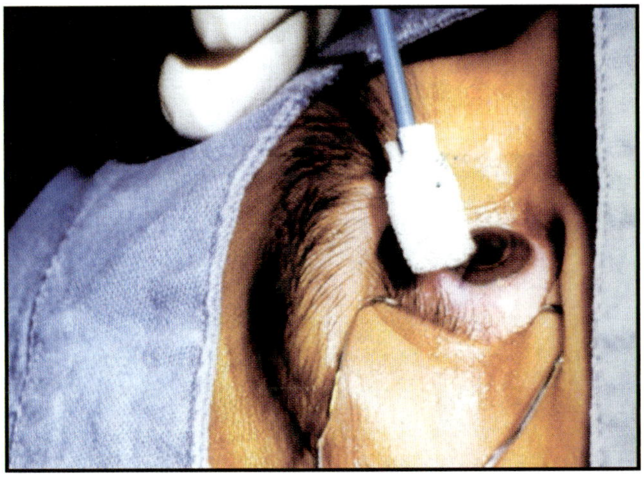

Fig. 42.5: Recollocate the flap and dry the border with a wet sponge

analysis of changing practice trends among the authors and these surgeons were assessed. In 12 cases, significant loss of BCVA and subjective visual difficulties resulted from recutting LASIK flaps. Most surveyed surgeons had changed their practice from recutting to lifting flaps even 9 to 10 years postoperatively with good results. They concluded that recutting flaps for enhancement should be avoided unless other alternatives are unavailable.

We can establish various principles or rules before doing our retreatment:

- Do a corneal topography and ultrasonic pachymetry.
- If the characteristics of the original cut are known and it was a normal cut, always lift the flap.
- The time since the original surgery is not important. In this respect, you should be cautious if a cut of a large diameter appears near the limbus. In this zone scarring is very pronounced due to the perilimbic vessels which make it difficult to find the edge of the flap and to lift it.
- In this particular case I do recommend a second cut. If the characteristics of the first cut are unknown, and the cornea studies do not give enough information about the initial cut, you can opt to do a second cut.
- Do a second cut if you find irregular astigmatism in the topography, haze or multiple metallic particles in the interface, since this tells us that there were problems with the cut.
- Do not do a retreatment in high myopias if the total pachymetry is less 460 microns.
- Wait six months to do a second cut.
- Be careful whith flat corneas (less than 39 D) because of the risk of a thin cut, small diameter cut and free cap when doing a second cut.
- Do not irrigate below the flap when lifting it, this hydrates the stroma and the ablation is not properly performed.
- Carefully study the cornea doing topography and pachymetry revision on several occasions since some cases of progressive regression can mean ectasia.

COMPLICATIONS

- Flap dehydration and shrinkage
- Laminated cut with a loose lamellar stromal tissue
- Epithelial ingrowth
- Striae
- Haze in the interface
- Dislodged flap
- Ectasia

Two of the complications previously mentioned produce very significant visual defects, the loss of stromal tissue during a second cut and ectasia post-LASIK.

Fortunately I have no experienced the loss of stromal tissue during a second cut after LASIK. However, I have had a case when doing LASIK on a patient who previously had had lamellar keratectomy.

I would like to exemplify a complication (ectasia) with the following pictures (Figs 42.6 to 42.13).

Outcomes After Laser *in situ* Keratomileusis Retreatment

Alka et al[18] evaluated the refractive and visual performance after (LASIK) retreatment. They studied 33 eyes of 23 patients who underwent LASIK retreatment for residual myopia with or without astigmatism. The mean spherical equivalent refraction was –2.85 ± 2.17 D. They found that ablation zones following retreatment should be ≥5.00 mm and remain unchanged to improve visual performance.

Like much of medicine, there are no hard-and-fast rules to LASIK enhancement. Each surgeon has his or her own guidelines on why, when and how to re-treat. Many times, the need for enhancement is based purely on patient perception; but in some circumstances, there may be a clinical indication. In any case, LASIK enhancement is an integral part of the refractive surgeon's practice.[19]

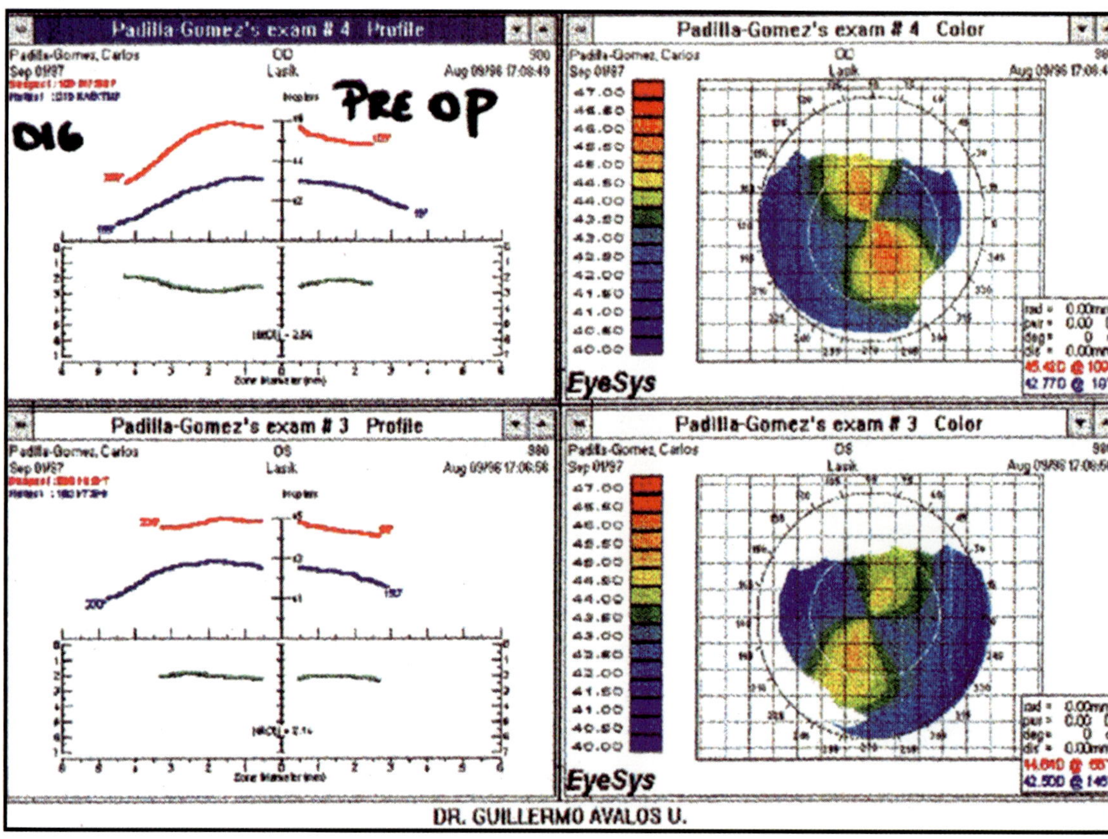

Fig. 42.6: Patient 1 preoperative

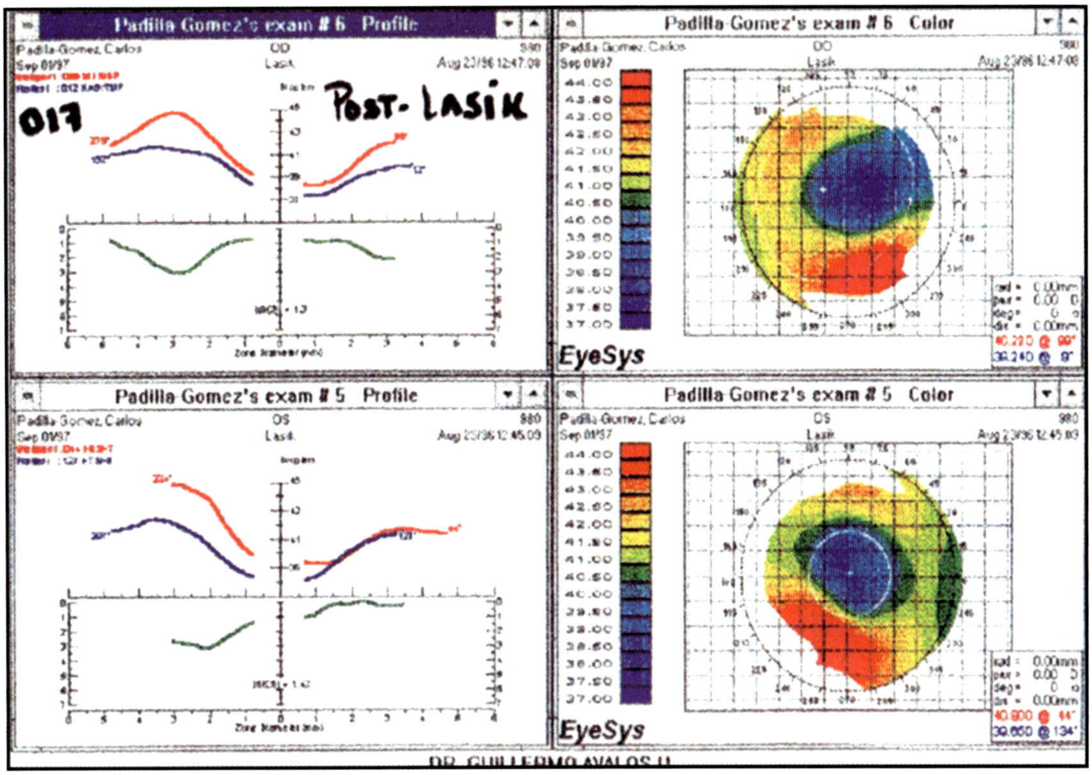

Fig. 42.7: Patient 1 Post-LASIK

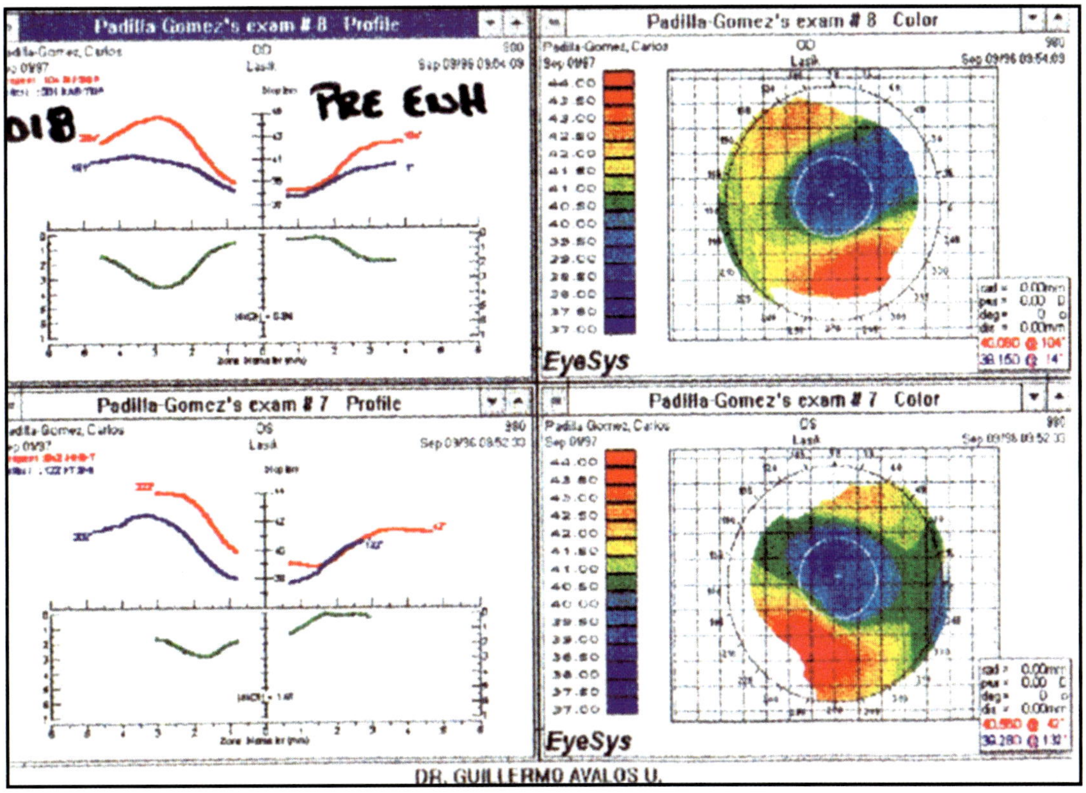

Fig. 42.8: Patient 1 Pre-enhancement (undercorrection)

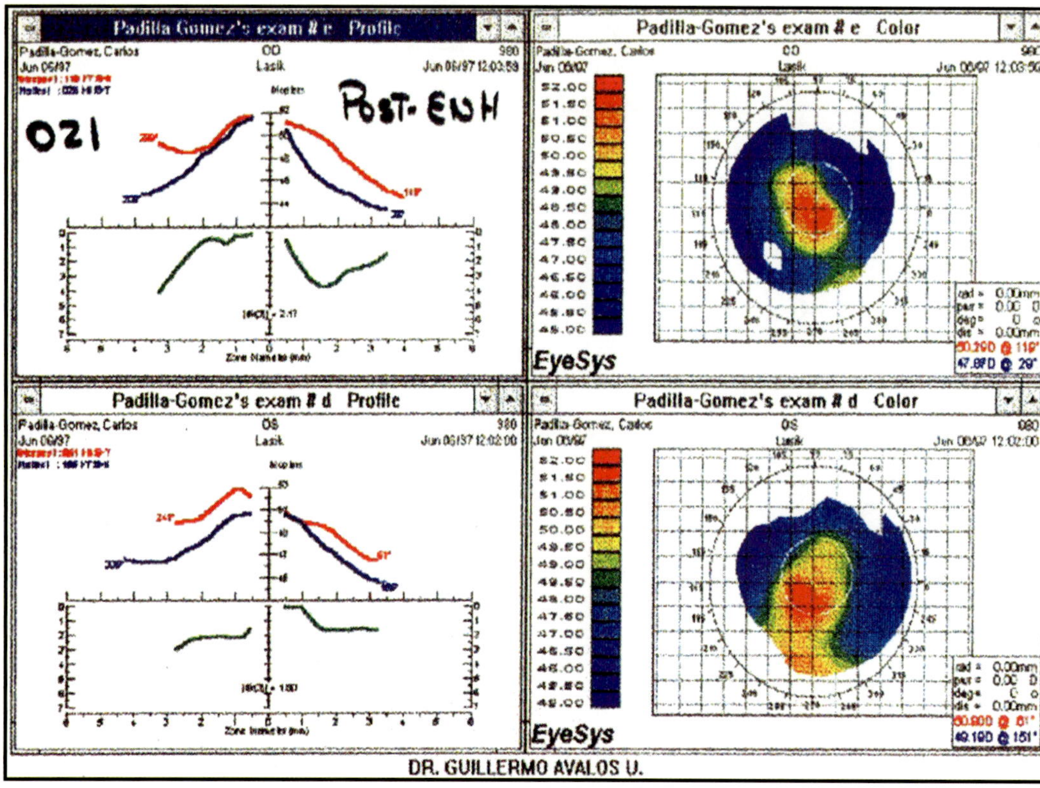

Fig. 42.9: Patient 1 post-enhancement (9 months later)

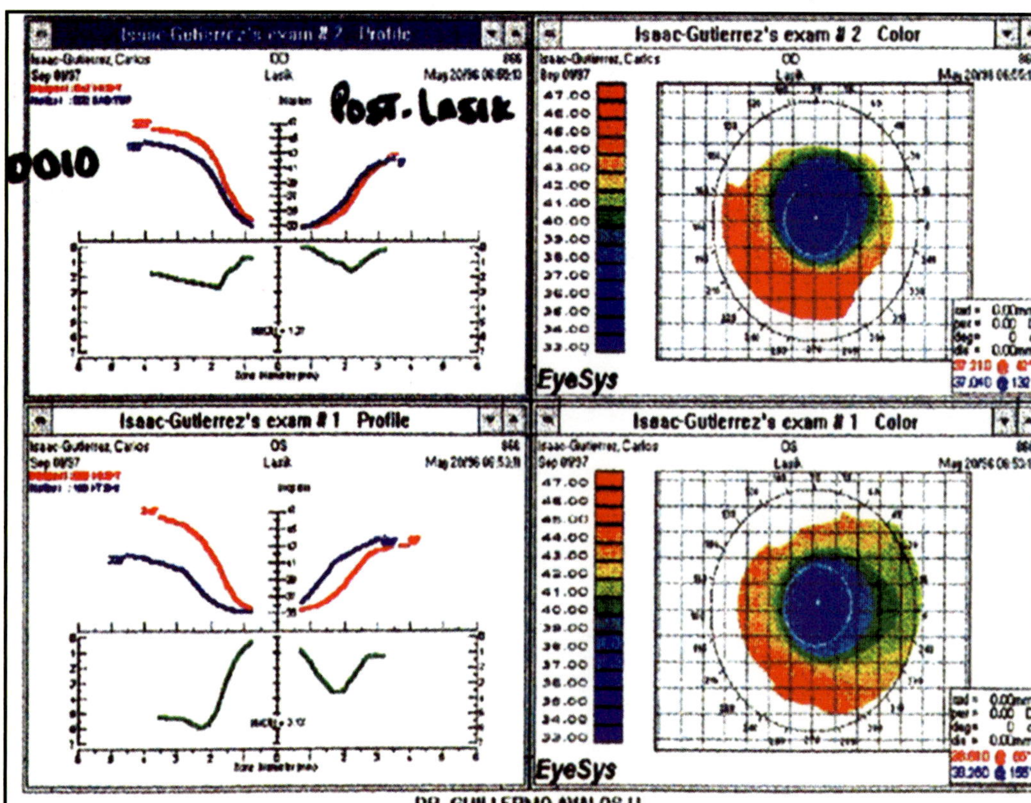

Fig. 42.10: Patient 2 post-LASIK

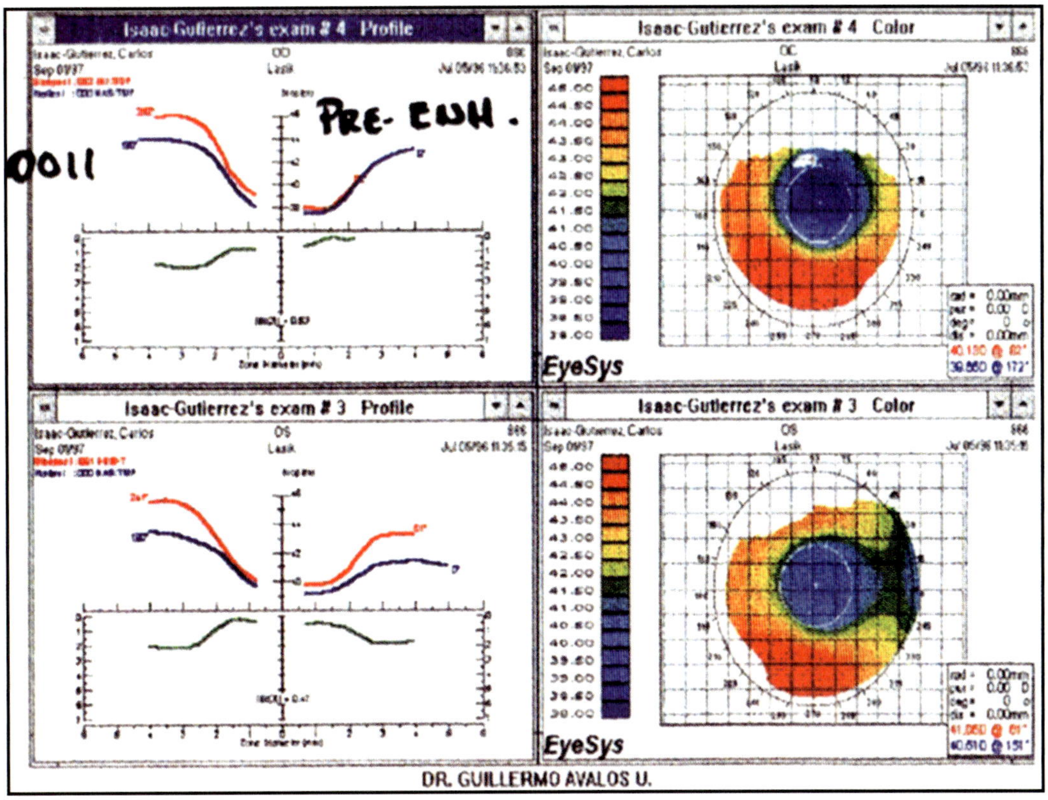

Fig. 42.11: Patient 2, pre-enhancement (undercorrection)

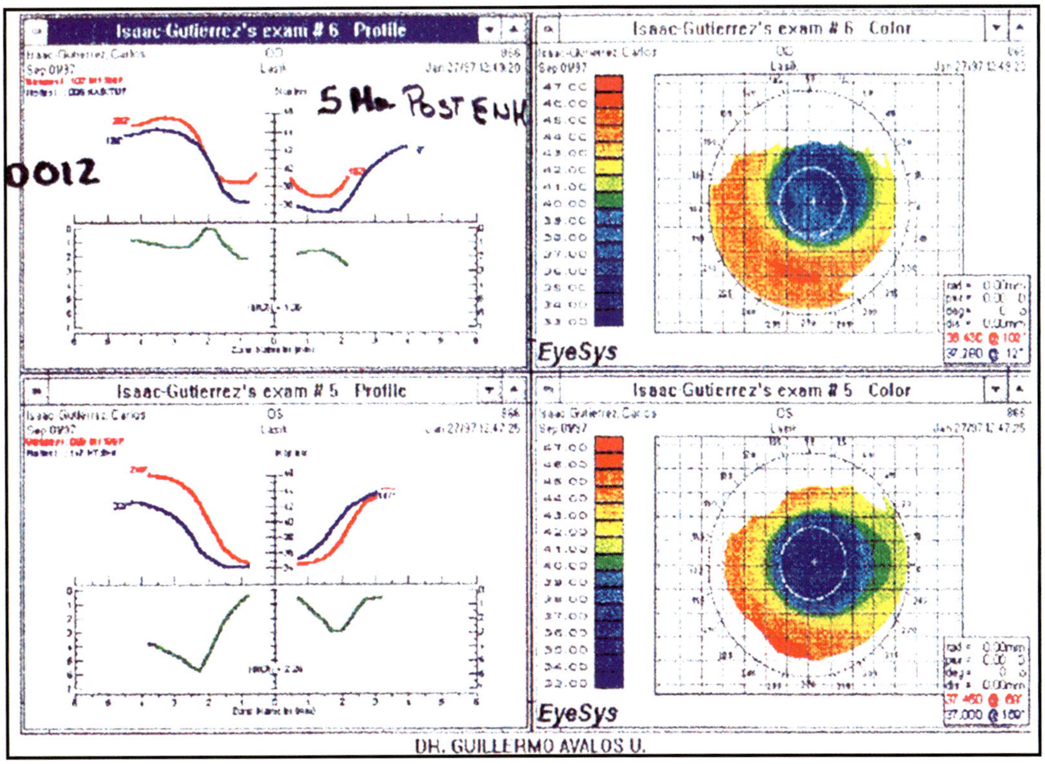

Fig. 42.12: Patient 2, 5 months post-enhancement

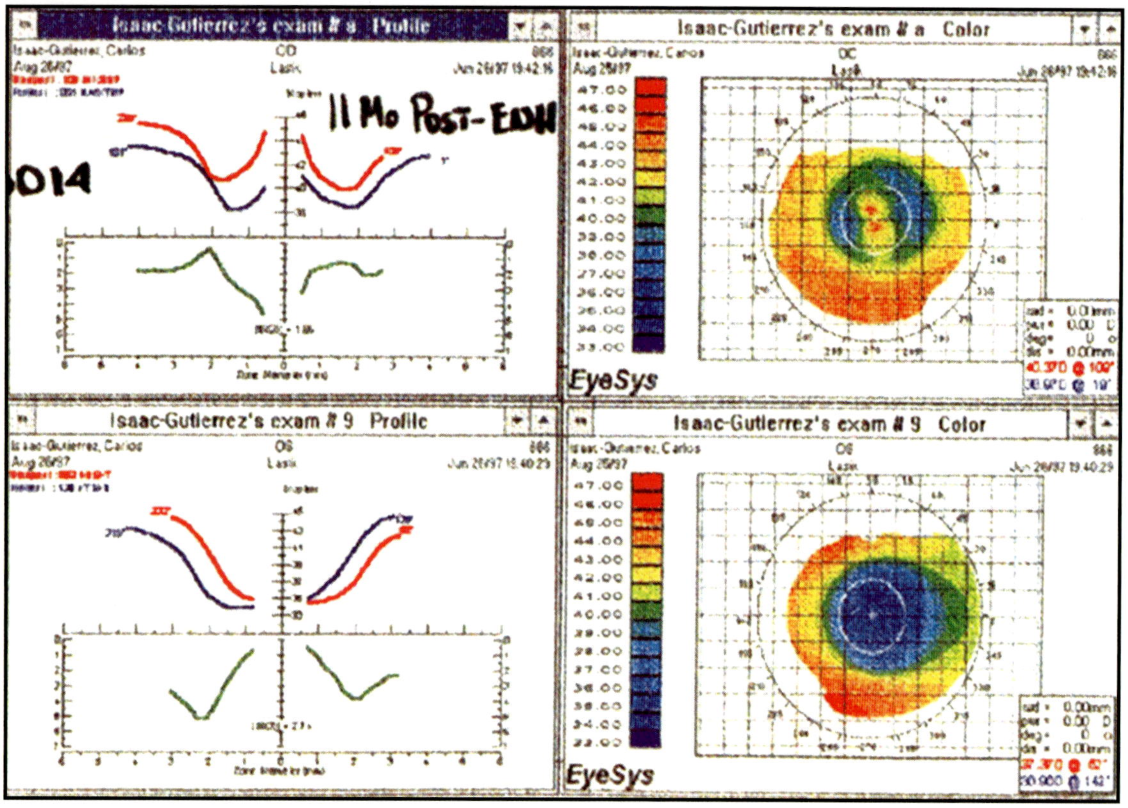

Fig. 42.13: Patient 2, 11 months post-enhancement

SUMMARY

LASIK improves refractive predictability, since the residual defects can be improved or corrected, simply by lifting the flap and applying a new ablation. If this procedure is done following the correct parameters of time and technique, we can be assured of obtaining excellent optical and surgical results.

REFERENCES

1. Guttman C. Topography-guided LASIK enhancement advantageous. Quality of vision enhanced in eyes with small eccentric ablations, irregular astigmatism. Ophthalmology Times Apr 1, 2005. Available at http://Laser ot.adv100.com/ophthalmologytimes/article/articleDetail.jsp?id=153461. Accessed April 22, 2005.
2. Guell JL, Muller A. LASER *in situ* keratomileusis (LASIK) for myopia from –7.00 to –28.00 diopters. J Refractive Surgery 1996;12:228-38.
3. Chayet A, Assil K, Montes, et al. Regression and its mechanism after laser *in situ* keratomileusis in moderate and high myopia. Ophthalmology 1998;105:1194-99.
4. Qi H, et al. Excimer retreatment for undercorrection or regression after laser *in situ* keratomileusis. Zhonghua Yan Ke Za Zhi 2002;38(2):72-75.
5. Hersh PS, Fry KL, Bishop DS. Incidence and associations of retreatment after LASIK. Ophthalmol 2003;110(4):748-54.
6. Perlman EM, Reinert SE. Factors influencing the need for enhancement after laser in situ keratomileusis. J Refract Surg. 2004;20(6):783-89.
7. Durrie DS, Vande Garde TL. LASIK enhancements. Int Ophthalmol Clin. 2000;40(3):103-10
8. Walter KA, Stevenson AW. Effect of environmental factors on myopic LASIK enhancement rates. J Cataract Refract Surg. 2004;30(4):798-803.
9. Hu DJ, et al. Predictive formula for calculating the probability of LASIK enhancement. J Cataract Refract Surg. 2004;30(2):363-68.
10. Muallem MS, et al. Flap and stromal bed thickness in laser in situ keratomileusis enhancement. J Cataract Refract Surg. 2004;30(11):2295-302.
11. Randleman JB, et al. A comparison of 2 methods for estimating residual stromal bed thickness before repeat LASIK. Ophthalmology. 2005;112(1):98-103.

12. Suarez E. KMSG Hotline 1999.
13. Domniz Y, et al. Recutting the cornea versus lifting the flap: comparison of two enhancement techniques following laser *in situ* keratomileusis. J Refract Surg 2001;17(5):505-10.
14. Netto MV, Wilson SE. Flap lift for LASIK retreatment in eyes with myopia. Ophthalmology 2004;111(7): 1362-67.
15. Perez-Santonja JJ, et al. Circular flap rhexis: a refinement technique for LASIK retreatment. Arch Soc Esp Oftalmol 2001;76(5):303-08.
16. Suresh PS, Rootman DS. Bilateral infectious keratitis after a laser *in situ* keratomileusis enhancement procedure. Cataract Refract Surg. 2002;28(4):720-21.
17. Rubinfeld RS, et al. To lift or recut: changing trends in LASIK enhancement. J Cataract Refract Surg. 2003;29(12):2306-17.
18. Alka R, Ramamurthy B, Namrata S, et al. Outcomes After Laser in situ Keratomileusis Retreatment in High Myopes. J Refract Surg 2003;19:159-64.
19. Schena L. LASIK Enhancement: Why, When and How. EyeNet Magazine. Available at http://www.aao.org/aao/news/eyenet/archive/06_01/refract.html. Accessed April 22,2005.

Solid-state Lasers for Refractive Surgery

43

MATTEO PIOVELLA, FABRIZIO I CAMESASCA,
BARBARA KUSA (ITALY)

INTRODUCTION

Laser technology for refractive surgery advanced with unrelentless pace during the past 20 years. The introduction of concepts such as wavefront analysis and customized ablation required manifold developments dealing with an increased, outmost precision of treatment.

Solid-state lasers in ophthalmic surgery have meant increased energy efficiency, as well as reduced size and costs. Presently, a new generation of UV-generating solid-state lasers is becoming available even for refractive surgery, including lasers such as the LaserSoft and the CustomVis.[1, 2]

Katana, Solid-state UV Laser for Refractive Surgery Since 2003

A good example of solid-state laser for refractive surgery, LaserSoft, is a continuous wave-diode pumped all-solid-state UV laser for refractive surgery recently introduced by Katana Technologies GmbH. A solid-state is not an excimer laser, since the UV laser ablation radiation is generated by nonlinear frequency conversion of infrared laser light in a laser crystal. A sequential frequency conversion with nonlinear crystals shifts the wavelength of the laser radiation into the range of 208 to210 nm. The resonator structure and the beam delivery ensure an emission of the laser radiation with a TEM_{oo} transversal mode, as well as an emission of laser radiation with a true Gaussian beam. The continuous wave-diode pumping provides a very stable shot-to-shot UV output with impressive long-term stability.

A Gaussian beam means excellent UV light spot distribution on the cornea. In fact, differently from the usual excimer laser, the solid-state laser does not need beam-forming elements, i.e. mirrors—in the beam path. Thus, energy at the corneal surface—fluency—is very stable. The laser beam is highly collimated, providing an increased beam precision and the technical features adequate to a fast scanning. Furthermore, the ablation pattern utilized in LaserSoft ensures an extremely homogenous cornea surface due to the accurate overlap made possible by true Gaussian spots. Differently from an excimer laser, in a solid-state laser there is no gas exchange and gas discharge involved, with the related instabilities in output radiation, due to the physical nature of the discharge process. The solid-state approach reduces the requirements for maintenance and costs, providing high stability and long lifetime.

This device generates a flying spot of 0.2 mm in diameter, operating at repetition rate of 1 kHz. Thanks to this high repetition rate, the energy per pulse is lower then in standard excimer treatments. Ablation has strongly reduced shock waves, and to no audible sound due to ablation or laser firing. The whole procedure takes place in a silent environment, much reassuring to the patient, without the risk of noise-induced abrupt motion.

To fully exploit the opportunities provided by custom ablation, a very fast laser like LaserSoft requires a fast eye-tracker. The LaserSoft eye-tracker has a latency of 1 ms and controls ablation centration at very high repetition rates. This very fast eye-tracker ensures a reliable, high repetition centration of ablation on the x-y axes as well as well as the ocular rotation.

All these features makes the solid-state laser an ideal device for accurate custom ablation (Figs 43.1 and 43.2).

The ablation profiles currently adopted by this laser are designed to preserve the strongly aspherical physiological corneal curvature, as well as to minimize the induced spherical aberration.

Different reflection losses and fluence values for different angles of incidence of the ablating laser radiation during surgery are also taken into account in the ablation algorithm.

Clinical Experience

We hereafter illustrate our clinical experience with a solid-state laser. Patients were treated at two different centers: Messina (PRK) and Campobasso (LASIK), Italy. The results were gathered after one year and were analyzed with the software Datagraph, using graphs recommended by GO Waring III.[3,4] After signing a specific informed consent, 37 eyes, were treated with LASIK and PRK procedures with LaserSoft ablation. Preoperative refractive data are reported in Table 43.1. Preoperative BSCVA of all eyes was between 0.3 and 1.0. LASIK was performed with the Hansatome microkeratome, choosing a flap thickness of 180 micrometer. Treatment diameters ranged between 6 and 7 mm, and transition zones between 8 and 9 mm.

One-year results were well within the current standards provided by normal excimer lasers (Table 43.1). Figure 43.3 shows the scattergram of the attempted versus the achieved refractive change for each eye. Figure 43.4 shows the spherical equivalent refractive outcome with the corresponding numbers. At one year, 100% of the eyes were in the so called happiness zone of ± 1D, 94% were within ± 0.5 D, and 87% were within ± 0.25 D. Figure 43.5 shows stability of refraction. The mean achieved change of spherical equivalent with time is also given. Table 43.2 provides the refractive and BSCVA results at one-year.

Efficacy consists of two components: component 1 is the spectacle corrected visual acuity at baseline (BSCVA); component 2 is the cumulative graph of uncorrected visual acuities after refractive surgery (UCVA). In our study, 45% of the eyes show a postoperative UCVA better then 20/20 from a cohort with 41% being preoperatively at 20/20 with best correction. The preoperative BSCVA of all eyes was between 1.0 and 0.3.

Solid-state Lasers vs Excimer Lasers

Table 43.3 presents the differences between common excimer lasers and solid-state laser. Presently, solid-

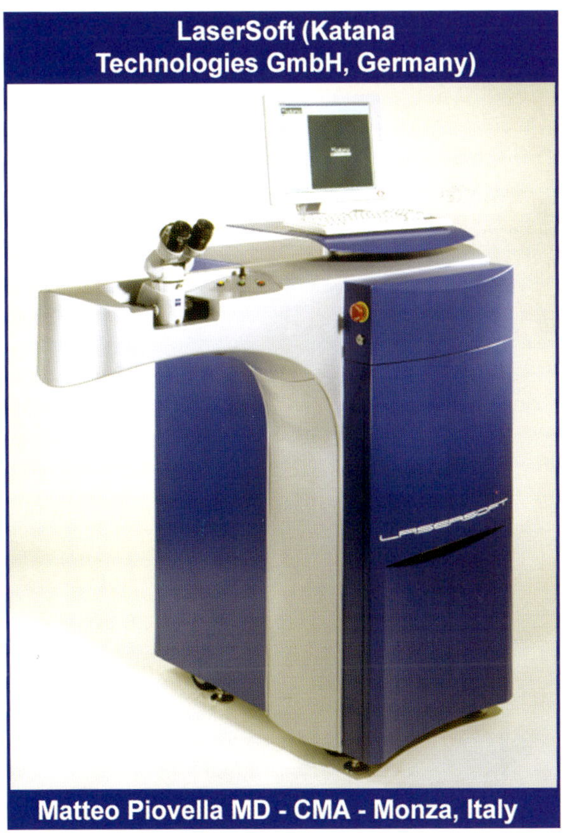

Fig. 43.1: LaserSoft solid-state laser

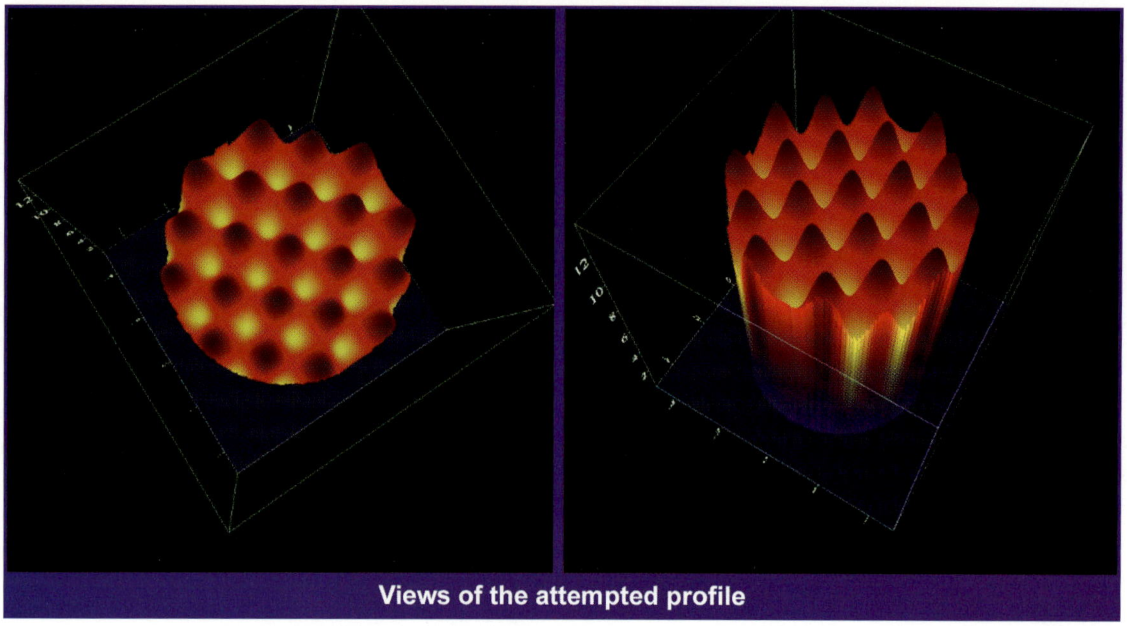

Fig. 43.2: Experimental model, possibilities for custom ablation offered by small spot size. Views of the attempted profile

Table 43.1: Preoperative vs one-month data, 37 eyes

	SE refractive defect (mean ± SD)	*Sphere (mean ± SD)*	*Cylinder (mean ± SD)*	*SE refractive defect, range*	*BSCVA*
Preoperative	–1.71 D ± 3.71 D	–1.46 D ± 3.32 D	– 0.51 D ± 1.97 D	– 8.00 D to +6.75 D	0.80 ± 0.23
One year	–0.03 D ± 0.13 D	–0.03 D ± 0.19 D	–0.01 D ± 0.19 D	–0.50 D to +0.25 D	0.83 ± 0.23

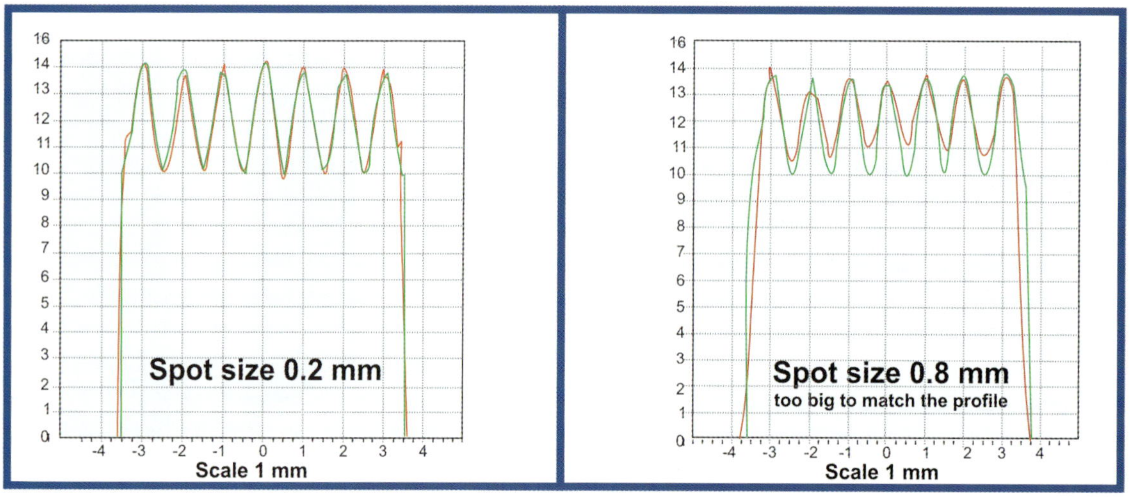

Fig. 43.3: Experimental model, small spot size and custom ablation. Views of the attempted profile with a 0.2 mm spot size solid-state laser vs. that of a 0.8 mm spot size

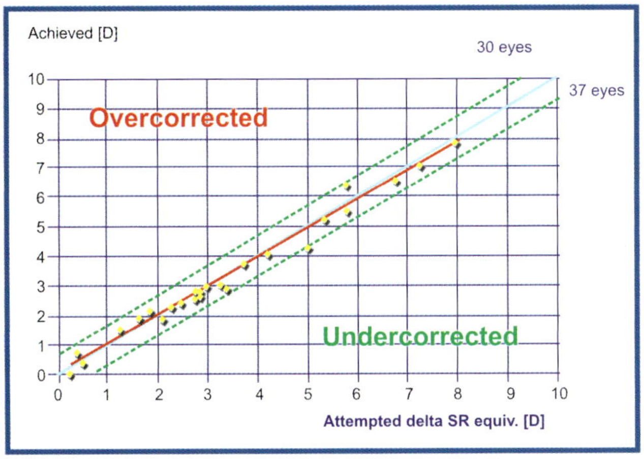

Fig. 43.4: Show the scattergram and therefore an impression of the spread of cases of the attempted versus the achieved refractive change for each eye for LASIK

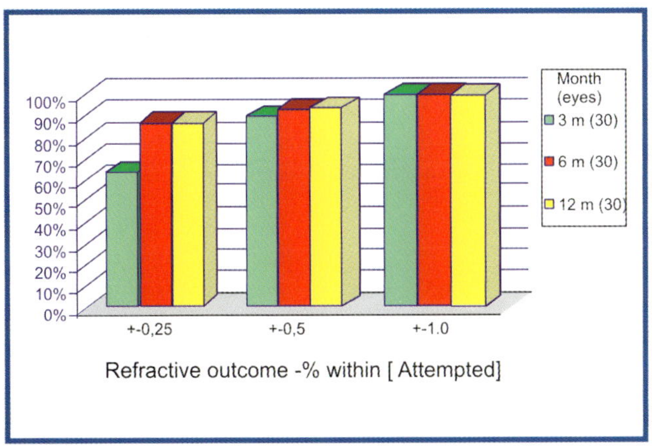

Fig. 43.5: Spherical equivalent refractive outcome at one year. Of all eyes, 100% are in the so-called happiness zone of ± D, 94% are within ± 0.5 D, and 87% are within ± 0.25 D

state laser presents several significant examples of technical evolution in refractive surgery lasers. The solid-state laser features a tiny flying spot with a diameter of 0.2 mm and it operates at repetition rate of 1 kHz. Its very small spot size fits the present requirements for effective custom ablation.

The vast majority of excimer lasers commonly available on the market features a 1 mm flying spot, and they never have spots smaller than 0.65 mm, thus with a much wider spot ablation area than a solid-state laser (Fig. 43.6). There is a technical limit in decreasing the spot size of an excimer laser, as

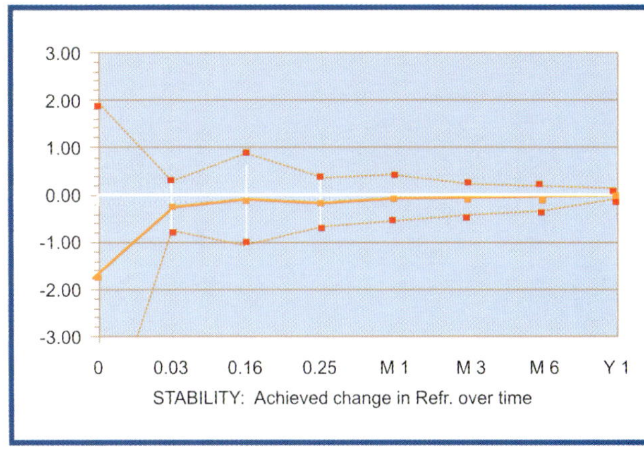

Fig. 43.6: Refractive stability of the study group, at one year

smaller spots would have a less homogeneous beam. Utilizing the usual excimer laser repetition rates, a 0.2 spot size would mean a very long treatment time, with the entire precision problem related to eye motion. To maintain ablation time within acceptable limits, and thanks to its technical features, the repetition rate of a solid-state laser is much higher in the solid-state than in excimer lasers.

The mirrors in a solid-state laser transmit the UV light without further elaborating it, unlike an excimer

Table 43.2: Refractive and BSCVA results at one-year follow-up, 37 eyes

SE refractive defect, Attempted vs obtained	*BSCVA preoperative vs one-year*
–0.03 D ± 0.20 D	0.0 ± 0.2

Table 43.3: Excimer vs solid-state lasers for refractive surgery

	Common excimer laser	*LaserSoft solid-state laser*
Spot size (mm)	0.8 – 1.0	0.2
Beam quality	Multimode (additional optics for clearing the excimer beam)	Single mode (Gaussian)
Repetition rate	50 – 500 Hz	1 kHz
Eye-tracker speed	Approximately 150 Hz	More than 1 kHz

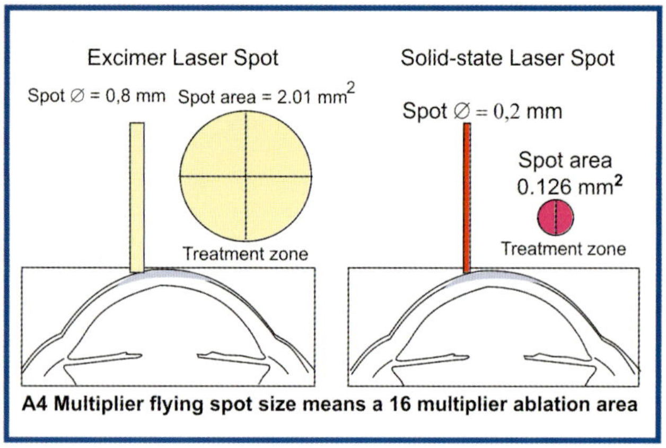

Fig. 43.7: Solid-state vs excimer laser spot size

laser. This thanks to the true Gaussian profile of the beam.

Solid-state lasers appear to be easier to use lasers for refractive surgery, requiring less maintenance. The fast eyetracking ensures a reliable centration of ablation for x-y directions as well as the rotation of the eye at high repetition rates.

CONCLUSION

Solid-state lasers appear to be a promising solution for a refractive surgery, applying less energy to the cornea and using a small flying spot of 0.2 mm, thus with the theoretical potential of inducing less scarring.

LaserSoft and solid-state UV lasers in general appear as a safe, reliable, stable, more compact as well as less costly alternative to gas-operating excimer lasers for refractive surgery.

REFERENCES

1. Personal Communications, 2003 Meeting of the ISRS/AAO, November 14-15, 2003, Anaheim, CA. Syllabus, pp 289.
2. Personal Communication, 2004 Meeting of the ISRS/AAO, October 22-23, 2004, New Orleans, LA. Syllabus, pp 10.
3. Datagraph Med (Medical Data Analysis Software) Ingenieurbüro Pieger, Germany.
4. Waring G. Standard Graphs for Reporting Refractive Surgery. J Refract Surg 2000;16:459.

Corneal Biomechanics—Customization

44

DIPAN DESAI (INDIA)

A thorough understanding of corneal biomechanics—a relatively new subject—is essential if one is to achieve optimal results in refractive surgery. The last two decades have seen drastic changes in the field of refractive surgery, and most of the successes achieved are through the cornea. Hence today, it is extremely relevant to understand corneal biomechanics before attempting laser refractive procedures such as PRK, LASIK Custom LASIK, LASEK and Epil-LASIK; non-ablative procedures such as CK or incisional procedures such as RK, AK and LRI. Comprehensive knowledge of biomechanical factors alone can translate into excellent visual outcome.

It was on Munnerlyn's Shape Substraction model, that laser refractive surgery had evolved for all these years. It was based on sphere as the ideal shape. Algorithms were drawn from many procedures and adjusted as the mean responses of central cornea.

Customization

In the early days, eyes were assessed with subjective and objective refraction measured in sphere and cylinder and visual acuity. All factors assessed and considered only the central cornea. Thus the outcome of the laser refractive procedures was based only on spheres, cylinders and visual acuity of the center of the cornea.

With the advent of wave-front analysis, one was now able to measure higher order aberrations from a larger region of the cornea, giving the optical performance of the entire eye. The laser is now programmed to correct sphere, cylinder and all aberrations. However, as it does so while ablating, it induces significant higher order aberrations. These aberrations are a result of the response of the cornea to the changes in structure—both anatomical and pathophysiological—produced by the ablation pattern and flap creation.

Biomechanical Model

Biomechanics deals with these altered and induced aberrations due to flap-making, cutting of Bowman's membrane and corneal fibrils. The cornea is a layered structure having 300 to 500 fibrils or lamellae with cross-linking. This cross-linking is more in the superior and peripheral layers. When the lamellar bands of cornea are cut from the center by laser, they have less tension in the periphery and are relaxed (Fig. 44.1). This peripheral corneal stroma now takes up fluid, expands and becomes steeper. Also, because of the cross-linking in the corneal fibrils, which is more in the peripheral and superficial cornea, there is a peripheral centrifugal force exerted by the severed collagen fibrils. This leads to further flattening of the central cornea. This flattening causes overcorrection in myopic and undercorrection in hypermetropic eyes. This is known as the hyperopic shift. Studies have demonstrated that the curvature outside the

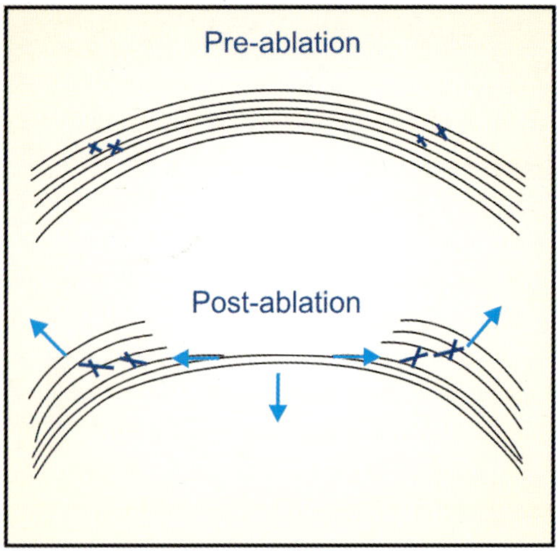

Fig. 44.1

optical zone is increased with increasing level of correction (greater ablation). The elevated zone also had with-the-rule peripheral astigmatism pattern. Also with increasing correction there is peripheral thickening in the transition zone where ablation occurred and increased pachymetry was observed in the outer area. These findings suggest that by performing laser surgery, one changes corneal biomechanics, leading to unaccounted aberrations by wave-front analysis. These issues have to be assessed with new models.

Clinical Deductions from Biomechanical Studies

1. Flap thickness does not influence higher order aberrations. This is affected by the stromal bed. The flap only mirrors the bed.
2. The smaller the flap diameter, the greater the response and vice versa.
3. The thicker the cornea, the greater the response.
4. Hinge placement has no significant difference in regional values.
5. Nasal and superior regions of the flap tend to be thicker, while temporal and inferior regions tend to be thinner.
6. Mechanical flaps tend to be thinner in the center than in the periphery.
7. The greater the central flattening, the greater the higher order aberrations (increasing coma)
8. Femtosecond laser flaps cause minimum higher order aberrations, and are more uniform and consistent than mechanical flaps. Second order aberrations are seen in both.
9. Studies by Vinciguerra et al demonstrate that in ultra-thin corneas, the critically important concept is not only residual stromal bed thickness for mechanical stability (preventing ectasia). Very large (10 mm) diameter PTK ablations were carried out with over five years of stability; with compelling evidence that the large optical zone may protect against ectasia, even in the presence of thin cornea. With this the stress is evenly distributed over a larger zone and thus less mechanical stress is imposed on a smaller zone. This rationale may be important for newly developing treatments of keratoconus, Intacs placement, or use of conductive keratoplasty (Alio et al). The smaller diameter and steep zone of the keratoconus is expanded to redistribute stress over a larger zone, thus leading to a more regular corneal shape and stability.

Why the Need for Devices to Measure Corneal Biomechanical Properties?

In corneal refractive surgery it is essential to understand the link between corneal microstructure and biomechanics as the shape of the cornea changes during a surgical procedure and will most certainly change after the procedure as a passive response to changed mechanical properties. We also know that biomechanical properties of cornea are important to assess individual variations that influence treatment response. However, without the ability to measure these properties *in vivo*, these influences cannot be predicted or controlled.

1. Biomechanical assessment, along with topography, pachymetry and wave-front analysis will lead to better preoperative assessment and postoperative results.
2. A better understanding of laser refractive surgery and non-ablative refractive correction (CK) can be achieved.

3. These devices help to determine factors for iatrogenic keratectasia.
4. Devices to measure intra-ocular pressure accurately can now be researched and manufactured, keeping in mind individual corneal characteristics.
5. Subclinical keratoconus can be diagnosed early.
6. Selective suture removal in penetrating keratoplasty is facilitated.
7. They will help in newer treatment modalities such as the cross-linking induced by riboflavin/ultraviolet A to treat early keratoconus by stabilizing the corneal structure.

New Devices to Measure Corneal Biomechanics

At present three new devices are being developed to measure biomechanical properties as a function of altered corneal stability and elasticity due to surgical intervention or pathology such as keratoconus.

1. Reichert's Ocular Response Analyzer devised by David Luce. This helps to determine the biomechanical properties of the cornea and their relationship to intra-ocular pressure.[3]
2. Dynamic Corneal Imaging deviced by G Grabner et al. This assesses the elastic properties, *in vivo*, of normal and abnormal human eyes and eyes after refractive surgery.[8]
3. Interferometric Techniques (Electronic Speckle Pattern Interferometry). This helps to quantify biomechanical changes in the cornea after microkeratome incisions as would be performed in LASIK.[17]

The Future

Several advances have been made in terms of developing machines for *in vivo* and *in vitro* measurements of elasticity, intra-ocular pressure and biomechanical properties of the cornea.

In future, customized LASIK will not only take into consideration corneal topography and wavefront analysis. Newer devices to measure biomechanical properties will help to integrate biomechanical customizations and this will improve the quality of vision and patient outcomes by leaps and bounds.

REFERENCES

1. DA Luce, inventor. Leica Microsystems Inc, assignee. US patent 2002;419:631.
2. Daniel S, Durrie MD, Guy M, Kezirian MD. Femtosecond laser versus mechanical keratome flaps in wavefront-guided laser *in situ* kertomileusis: Prospective contralateral eye study. JCRS 2005;31: 120-26.
3. David A Luce. Determining in vivo biomechanical properties of the cornea with an ocular analyzer. JCRS 2005;31:156-62.
4. Doughty MJ, Zaman ML. Human corneal thickness and its impact on intraocular pressure measures: a review and meta-analysis approach. Surv Ophthalmol 2000;44:367-408.
5. Dupps WJ Jr, Roberts C. Effect of acute biomechanical change on corneal curvature after photokeratectomy. J Refract Surg 2001;17:658-69.
6. Ehlers N, Bramsen T, Sperling S. Applanation tonometry and central corneal thickness. Acta Ophthalmol 1975;53:34-43.
7. Fredrik J, Potgieter FRCSE, Cynthia Roberts, Ian G Cox, Ashraf M. Mahmoud, Edward Eherderich, Marlize Roctz, Wouter Steenkamp. Prediction of flap reponse. JCRS 2005;31:106-14
8. Gunther Grabner MD, Reinbard Eilmsteiner, Christian Steindl Dipl-Ing, Josef Ruckhofer, Renzo Mattioli Dipl-Ing, Wolfgang Husinsky. Dynamic corneal imaging JCRS 2005;31:163-74.
9. Gunvant P, Broadway DC, Watkins RJ. Repeatability and reproducibility of the BVI, ultrasonic pachymeter. Eye 2003;17:825-28.
10. Hjortdal JO, Erdmann L, Bek T. Fourier analysis of video-keratographic data; a tool for separation of spherical, regular astigmatic and irregular astigmatic corneal power components. Ophthalmic Physiol Opt 1995;15:171-85.
11. Jose L, Guell, Fortino Velasco, Cynthia Roberts, Maria Teresa Sisquella, Ashraf M. Malnnoud. Corneal flap thickness and topography changes induced by flap creation during laser in situ keratomileusis. JCRS 2005;31:115-19.
12. Jun Liu, Cynthia J Roberts. Influence of corneal biomechanical properties on intraocular pressure measurements: Quantitative analysis. JCRS 2005;31: 146-55.
13. Kaufmann C, Bachmann LM, Thiel MA. Intraocular pressure measurements using dynamic contour

tonometry after laser *in situ* keratomileusis. Invest Ophthalmol Vis Sci 2003;44:3790-94.

14. Kezirian GM, Stonecipher KG, Comparison of the IntraLase femtosecond laser and mechanical keratomes for laser *in situ* keratomileusis. J Cataract Refract Surg 2004;30:804-11.
15. Marshall J, Trokel S, Rothery S, Krueger RR. Photoablative reprofiling of the cornea using an excimer laser: photorefractive keratectomy. Laser Ophthalmol 1986; 1:21-48.
16. Munnerlyn CR, Koons SJ, Marshall J. Photoreactive keratectomy: a technique for laser refractive surgery. J Cataract Refract Surg 1988;14:46-52.
17. Philip David Jaycock, MRCOphth, Leon Lobo, Jamal Ibrahim, MEng, John Tyrer, John Marshall. Interferometric technique to measure biomechanical changes in the cornea induced by refractive surgery. JCRS 2005;31:175-84.
18. Pinsky PM, Datye DV. A microstructurally-based finite element model of the incised human cornea. J Biomech 1991;24:907-22.
19. Pinsky PM, Datye DV. Numerical modeling of radial, astigmatic, and hexagonal keratotomy. Refract Corneal Surg 1991;8:164-72.
20. Roberts C. The cornea is not a piece of plastic [editorial]. J Refract Surg 2000;16:407-13.
21. Soergel F, Jean B, Seiler T, et al. Dynamic mechanical spectroscopy of the cornea for measurement of its viscoelastic properties *in vitro*. Ger J Ophthalmol 1995; 151-56.
22. Velinsky SA, Bryant MR. On the computer-aided and optimal design of keratorefractive surgery. Refract Corneal Surg 1992;8:173-82.
23. Whitacre MM, Stein R. Sources of error with use of Goldmann-type tonometers. Surv Ophthalmol 1993;38:1-30.

Thermal Keratoplasty for Hyperopic Correction using a Focused Diode Laser

45

JT Lin (USA), Vivek Kadambi (India)

INTRODUCTION

Corneal reshaping procedures, such as photorefractive keratectomy (PRK) and laser assisted *in situ* keratomileusis (LASIK) have been performed by lasers in the ultraviolet (UV) wavelength of 193-213 nm. The commercial UV refractive lasers include ArF excimer laser (at 193 nm) in US Pat. No. 4,773,414 of L'Esperance, et al and other non-excimer, solid-state lasers such as those proposed by Lin in 1992 (US pat. No. 5,144,630) and in 1996 (US pat. No. 5,520,679). The above-described systems using lasers to reshape the corneal surface curvature, however, are limited to the corrections of myopia, hyperopia and astigmatism (Table 45.1). They do not significantly contribute to the treatments of presbyopia or glaucoma.

Refractive surgery using a scanning device and lasers in the mid-infrared (mid-IR) wavelength was first proposed by Lin in US Pat. No. 5,144,630 and 5,520,679 and later proposed by Telfair et al in US Pat. No. 5,782,822. These inventions disclosed the generation of mid-IR wavelength of 2.5 to 3.2 microns, by various methods including, but not limited to, the Er:YAG laser (at 2.94 microns), the Raman-shifted solid-state lasers (at 2.7-3.2 microns) and the optical parametric oscillation (OPO) lasers (at 2.7-3.2 microns).

Hyperopia may be surgically corrected by LASIK which involves corneal tissue removal. Alternatively, minimally invasive techniques may be employed using Ho:YAG laser (at 2070-2120 nm) or the diode laser (at 1885 nm), through thermal keratoplasty procedures known as Holmium Laser Thermokeratoplasty (Ho: LTK) and Diode Laser Thermokeratoplasty (DTK), respectively. Radiofrequency (RF) wave can also be used to create the same effect by a procedure known as conductive keratoplasty (CK).[1-4] Procedures of LASIK, Ho:LTK, DTK and CK have also been recently used for the correction of presbyopia which is limited to monovision treatment by inducing myopia in the non-dominant eye. This is in contrast to the laser scleral ablation (LASA) procedure which normally treats both eyes and does not result in any myopic shift.[5,6]

HYPEROPIA CORRECTION (TABLE 45.2)

The recent paper of Rehany and Landa[3] reported results of DTK using a diode laser having a focusing optics for contact mode with deeper penetration of the laser thermal energy in the corneal stroma. However, their data still showed significant six-month postoperative regression of about 0.7 diopter. Papadopauls et al[2] using non-contact Ho:LTK in 50 hyperopic eyes showed that 32 cases reached refraction stability within 1 to 3 months follow-up, 5 cases within 3 to 6 months and 3 cases within 12 months. Their data also showed a similar regression as that of DTK. The major factor responsible for post-

Table 45.1: Summary of technologies for vision corrections (laser and non-laser methods)

1.	PRK, LASEK, EPILASIK	Corneal surface ablation with laser (epithelium removed or preserved); suitable for low diopter corrections (< 3.5 D) or high diopter with thin cornea; simple procedure
2.	LASIK	Stroma ablation by laser after a "flap" is prepared by microkeratome; (less pain, fast recovery, epithelium intact, less haze); potential keratome failure, thin cornea, flap complication
3.	LASA, LACA	Presbyopia treatment by laser scleral ablation (LASA) to increase accommodation via ciliary body contraction; combining effects of change in scleral elasticity, lens curvature change and anterior chamber shift. Efficiency may be improved by deeper laser ciliary-body ablation (LACA)
4.	LZT, LCT	Laser zonules thermal (LZT) stimulation for presbyopia: non-invasive method using gona lens and focused laser. Laser ciliary-body thermal shrinkage (LCT) for presbyopia
5.	SEB	Scleral expansion band implanted in scleral layer to cause near vision improvement; major regression
6.	ACS	Anterior ciliary sclerotomy by diamond knife incision; major regression which may be reduced by silicon expansion plug
7.	CK	Conductive keratoplasty using radio frequency wave for hyperopia and monovision correction; treated eye to see near but losing its far vision; non-surgical, corneal curvature changed via thermal shrinkage
8.	LTK and DTK	Laser thermal keratoplasty (LTK) using Ho:YAG (at 2.1 μm) or diode laser (1.45-2.1 micron) (DTK)
9.	MFCR	Multi-focal corneal reshaping by excimer LASIK
10.	AIOL	Accommodative IOL implanted to lens capsule; forward movement for accommodation; good for post-cataract eyes; loop, thin plates, human optics
11.	MIOL	Multi-focal IOL implanted for patient with high refraction errors
12.	Super Vision	Customized LASIK combined with wave-front technology; flying-spot scanning laser with eye tracking is required for customized and irregular corneal reshaping

**Major technologies (inventors):* Broad-beam Excimer (L'Esperance, Blum, Taboada); LTK (Sand); SEB (Schachar); Flying-spot LASIK (Lin); LAPR and LACA (Lin), LZT (Lin, Martinez); Eye-tracking (Lai); Solid-state UV Laser for LASIK (Lin, Lai); MFCR (Ruitz). Most of the above technologies have been patented (1988-2004) and greater details may be found in their patents by online searching of "US Patent" files or by the following US pat. No: 4718418, 5484432, 5520679, 5144630, 6263879, 6258082, 5533997, 5354331

operative regression with Ho:LTK and DTK, is the cone-shaped laser power profile (or temperature profile) within the corneal stroma, where the penetration depth (d) is limited by the strong tissue absorption of the laser energy. While the existing DTK system with a tightly focused beam within the stroma may have successfully improved the penetration depth, it did not improve the effective tissue volume (ETV) for collagen shrinkage. The non-focused Ho:LTK has its majority of laser energy absorbed by superficial stromal layer of about 0.15

Table 45.2: Comparison of technologies for hyperopia correction

Method	*Features*
LASIK	ArF excimer laser corneal surface ablation
Ho:LTK	Ho:YAG laser (at 2.1 micron) non-focused beam, shallow penetration
DTK	Diode-laser (at 1.88 micron), focused CW beam
DTK-Plus	Diode-laser (at 1.4-1.9 micron), optimal focused beam
CK	Penetration depth controlled by electrode length

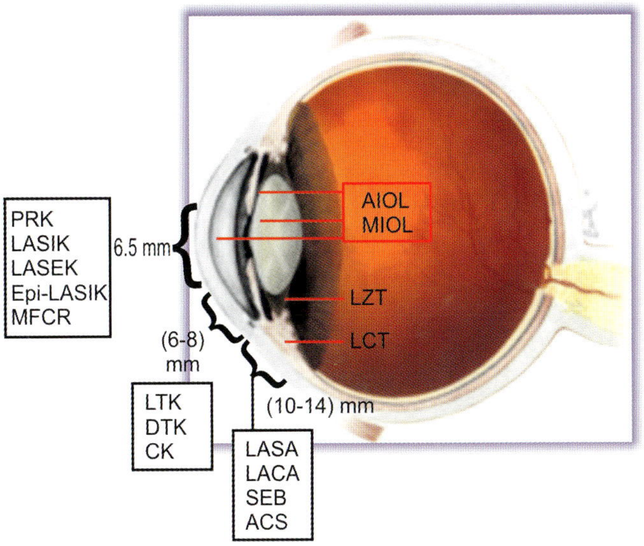

Fig. 45.1: Summary of various technologies for vision correction (referred to Table 45.1 for notations)

mm. To overcome the limitation of penetration depth and maximize the ETV for thermal shrinkage, we propose a new concept based on an optimized focusing beam which was used in a system called DTK-plus by New Vision, Inc. (patent pending).

PENETRATION DEPTH

The laser power density profile (or irradiance/ transmittance profile) of a focused laser inside an absorbing medium, in this case, ocular tissue, may be calculated by a revised Beer's law:

$$P = B\exp(-dA) \quad \text{(Eq. 1)}$$
$$B = [f / (f-d)]^2 \quad \text{(Eq. 2)}$$

where A is the absorption coefficient of the cornea tissue at a given laser spectrum; B is a focusing factor which is inversely proportional to the focused beam spot size (derived from simple geometry); f is the focal length of the optics and d is the penetration depth or position away from the corneal surface, which in case of contact mode equals zero. It should be noted that when d approaches f, B is calculated by the square of the ratio between the initial beam spot size (at d = 0) and the beam waist (a diffraction-limited finite size at d = f) to avoid the singularity of formula (2). From above formula, one may readily see that the laser irradiance has a fast exponential decrease due to its absorption in ocular tissue, which is competing with the increasing factor B in a focused beam. The net result of power absorption and beam spot decrease (or increase of power density) produces a peak value (P*) of the laser irradiance profile located at the focal point or position of minimal beam spot. For example, given a laser spot size (diameter) of 1.0 mm on the corneal surface (or d = 0) which is focused to a minimal spot of 0.25 mm (at d = f), one may easily calculate, from Eq. 2, B = (1, 4, 16, 4, 1) at d/f = (0, 0.5, 1.0, 1.5, 2.0).

Using the published transmittance data (Atchinson and Smith, "Optics of human eye, p. 108) to calculate the absorption coefficient[7] (A) to be about 20 to 70 cm^{-1} for laser wavelength at about 1.4 to 2.1 micron, the absorption term exp(-dA) may be calculated at various penetration depth (d).

Several important features may be addressed based on the above calculated profiles. The peak irradiance (P*) of a focused laser is inversely proportional to the absorption coefficient (A), i.e. a laser having a larger A value has a lower P* than that having a smaller A value. However, this peak power effect from focusing factor (B) may be totally suppressed by the exponentially decreasing term by an appropriate choice of the focal length (f). Mathematically, a perfect flat-top (PFT) profile would be possible under the condition of B=exp (+dA) for all depth (d). For A = 55 cm^{-1} as an example, the PFT condition is given by B = (1.0, 3.96, 7.9, 15.7) at depth position of d = (0, 0.25, 0.375, 0.5) mm. This PFT condition is fundamentally impossible to meet under a typical lens design having B = (1, 4, 7.1, 16) for spot size of (1, 0.5, 0.37, 0.25) R, R being the spot size on the corneal surface which produces an almost flat-top (AFT) oscillating function. These AFT profiles require a deeper focal point (f) at 1.0 mm (or two times of the corneal thickness) for the case of A=30 cm^{-1}. In general, the condition for AFT profile is given by B*=exp (f*A), therefore, f*= (0.92, 0.7, 0.62, 0.55, 0.46) mm, for A= (30, 40, 45, 55, 60) cm^{-1}.

The laser irradiance profile is almost flat in the vertical (depth), the laser footprint (spot size) is conical in shape in a focused beam. Therefore, no homogeneous laser irradiance profile exists in both vertical and horizontal directions. The most one may achieve is an approximate flat-top (AFT) profile in the depth direction and under the condition defined above. To achieve maximal thermal shrinkage tissue volume (MTTV), the preferred focal length includes: $f = f^* +/- 0.2$ mm for small $A = (20 \text{ to } 35)\ cm^{-1}$, and $f = f^* +/- 0.05$ mm for large $A = (40 \text{ to } 70)\ cm^{-1}$.

TEMPERATURE PROFILE

For RF devices, the penetration depth is controlled by the configuration of the electrode tip. For IR laser of 1.4 to 2.2 microns, the absorption (0.5 mm path) in cornea, sclera or conjunctival tissue is about 60% (at 1.4 micron), 75% (at 1.45, 1.87 and 2.1 micron), 50% (at 1.8 micron), 95% (at about 1.89 micron) and over 99% (at about 1.92 microns) for non-focused beam.[7] These are the criteria for the selected IR lasers in addition to the focusing factor (B) discussed earlier. The absorption depth at various laser spectra for various ocular tissues is one of the critical elements in defining system parameters of this invention. Given value of "A" with respect to the treated tissue, we may predict the penetration depth (d) by the revised Beer's law, Bexp ($-A \times d$) discussed earlier. However, the penetration depth is also an increasing function of the power of the thermal energy beam.

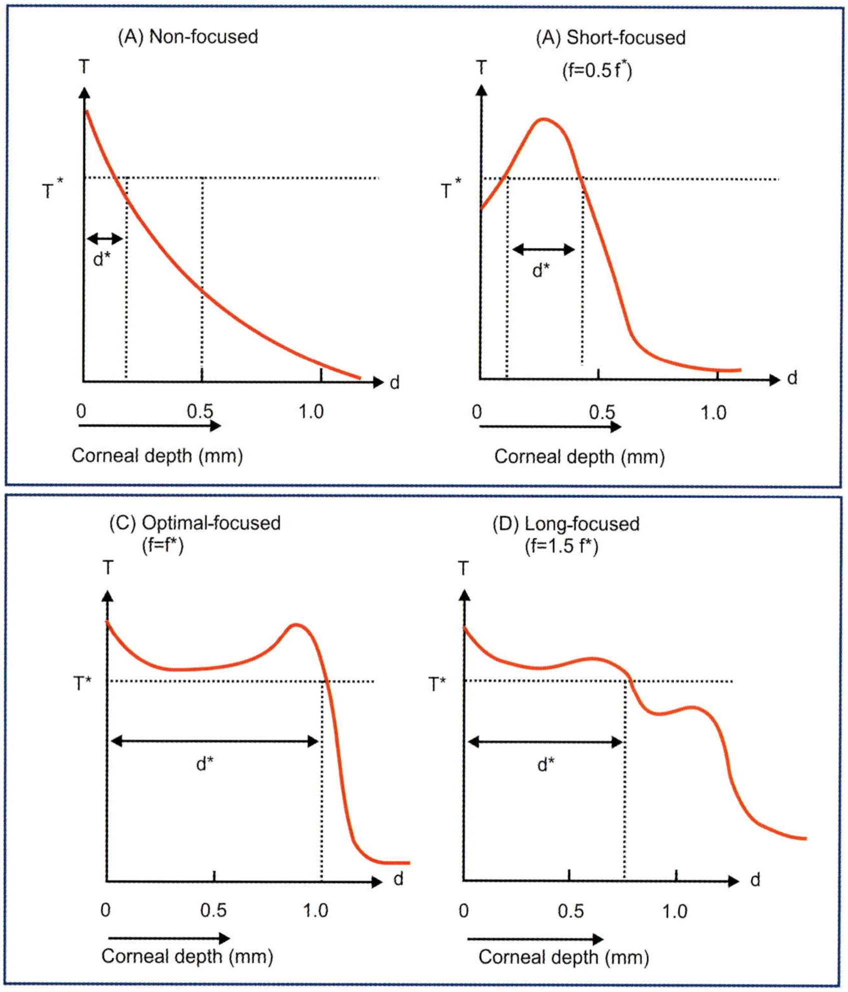

Figs 45.2A to D: Temperature profiles for non-focused and focused laser, where the threshold temperature (T*=58°C) defines the penetration depth (d*)

As shown earlier, higher "A" values tend to move the temperature peak profile forward towards the corneal epithelium. Therefore, to avoid cornea epithelial damage while achieving significant deep thermal penetration, the laser wavelength and the focal length must be carefully specified.

Figure 45.2 schematically shows the temperature profile of the treated tissue relative to the surface temperature "Ts" based on the calculated laser power density profiles. Figures 45.2A to D, respectively represents temperature profiles for non-focused, short-focused ($f < f^*$), optimally-focused (with $f = f^*$) and long-focused ($f > f^*$) cases, where f^* is defined by $B^*=\exp(f^*A)$, or $f^*= (\ln B^*/A)$, and where $B^*= (7\text{-}16)$ is the value at focal point.

It was known (Stringer HPT, Nature, vol. 204, p.1307, 1964) that stroma collagen shrinkage temperature is 58°C (defined as the threshold temperature "T*") to 75°C. Given the T*, we may evaluate the effective penetration depth (d*), the depth where tissue thermal shrinkage starts to effectively occur. As shown by Figures 45.2A to D, d* increases with f upto about $f = f^*$, then it starts to decrease after f* and approaches to the non-focused value.

The significance of Figure 45.2 may be summarized as follows:

a. Non-focused laser has the shortest effective penetration, d* = (0.1-0.2) mm depending on A and T*.
b. Short-focused case with $f < f^*$ has lower temperature on the treated surface, and therefore less risk of surface damage. However, this scenario results in a higher temperature in the vicinity of the endothelial (about 0.5 mm for the case of cornea) and hence the concern of endothelial damage increases.
c. At the optimal focusing case ($f = f^*$), the temperature profile is almost flat-top, similar to that of laser power profile shown in Figure 45.2, therefore it has the maximal d* whereas the risk of epithelial or endothelial layers may be reduced under controlled laser power and treatment time, typically about 1 to 5 seconds.
d. For long-focused beam ($f > f^*$), the value of d* decreases. To keep d* at least 80% of the corneal stroma thickness (0.5 mm), as an example, the preferred parameters of this invention includes f is about (0.8-1.5) and most preferable (0.9-1.1) times of f*, where f* is about 0.4 to 1.4 mm, for B*=16. The preferred range selection of focal length also significantly reduces the risk of overheating on the epithelial or endothelial tissue of the cornea.

SAFETY AND EFFICACY

Non-focused LTK used in Ho:YAG laser (by Sunrise Technologies, Inc.) suffers the disadvantages of shallow penetration, typically less than 1/3 of the cornea stroma thickness. In order to increase the effective penetration depth (d*), defined by the region where stroma temperature is higher than the shrinkage threshold (T*), one needs to use a higher laser power which causes excessive injury to the epithelial layer. Using a focused laser will improve d* and reduce the risk of epithelial damage. However, for short focal length case, used in the conventional DTK system (ProLaser), as shown in Figure 45.2(B), with the focal point inside the stroma increases the risk of endothelial layer damage because of the peak-power profile may be too close to the layer. DTK-Plus system (New Vision, Inc.) using an optimal focal length (f*) about 0.8 to 1.2 mm, longer than the corneal thickness, has a minimal risk of epithelial or endothelial damage, while offering a much deeper d*, in the range of about 0.4 to 0.6 mm.

Conductive keratoplasty (CK) using RF wave electrode may offer a rather deep thermal penetration, controlled by the length of the conductor tip, however, it has been shown to cause scaring and postoperative regression. Regression and poor predictability are the two major drawbacks of existing systems of the CK device, Ho:YAG, LTK and conventional DTK. These problems are mainly caused by epithelial or stroma tissue healing and poor control over the temperature profile produced by the thermal energy beam, which may be laser induced or RF wave generated. The conventional-DTK (ProLaser) uses a diode laser at about 1885 nm and having a tolerance of 5 nm which causes the absorption coefficient (A) to change from 40 to 55 cm^{-1}. This uncertainty in A value and the rather long exposure time (about 4 seconds in each treated spot) may result in the change of d* and temperature profile which leads to poor predictability. The new DTK-Plus system (New Vision, Inc.) uses a lower and narrower "A" value at a proprietary wavelength. This not only offers a deeper d*, which is controlled by the optimal local length given by f*= (ln B*)/A, with B* about 16, but also repeatable temperature profiles from spot to spot at a shorter exposure time of about 2 to 3 seconds. Therefore, it offers better predictability of refractive outcomes with less regression due to less damage to epithelial or endothelial layer. In addition, a smaller spot size of about 200 micron in DTK-Plus versus about 50 micron in conventional DTK system, reduces the stromal overheating caused by the hot-spot of small laser spot size at the focal point.

Both conventional-DTK and DTK-Plus produce a conical temperature profile, however, DTK-Plus, by virtue of its energy focal length, has a horizontal profile about two times wider than that of conventional DTK. It is important to note that the hyperopic refractive change at a given laser power exposed to the treated spot is proportional to d*W, which is equal to (effective penetration depth) × (mean width of the conical profile). Therefore deeper "d*" and wider width "W" will result in higher diopter hyperopia correction, even when a lower laser power is used. In the CK device, a cylindered temperature profile and deep d* are achievable by the length of conductor tip (about 450 micron). However, a typical tip diameter is only about 90 micron which limits the width (W) of the temperature profile to about 200 micron or less, in comparison to about 200 to 600 micron width in DTK-Plus, and about 50 to 150 micron width in conventional DTK.

The currently used Ho:LTK, DTK devices still suffer instability and postoperative regression which may be significantly reduced by choosing an optimal focusing depth associated to the absorption coefficient (A) at a given laser spectrum.

The threshold temperature (T*) for permanent thermal shrinkage (PTT) of the treated tissue is about 58°C. It is important to note that PTT occurs near the surface layer of the treated area in a collimated beam, whereas it penetrates deeply into the area defined by the focal point (or focal length f) in a focused beam. Deep penetration is one of the critical elements for efficacy and postoperative stability presented in this new system. The Ho:LTK system of Sand suffers major regression due to its non-contact, non-focused superficial laser heating. The new system of DTK-Plus in focused mode overcomes the drawback of prior systems and also provides other advantages including less damage to the corneal epithelial and endothelial layers. It creates sufficient coagulation in almost the entire stroma versus only less than 30% in non-focused cases. The prior system of Sunrise Technologies using a non-focused short-pulsed Ho: YAG laser results in epithelial damage since the laser power peaks on the surface and causes insufficient coagulation in deep stroma. The currently used conventional DTK using tightly focused CW diode laser (with f about 0.3-0.5 mm) improves the penetration depth, however, it still has a narrow peak profile which results in postoperative regression and a low initial efficacy, of less than 2.0 diopter of correction. The broader laser profile under the AFT condition introduced in this chapter not only provides better efficacy for higher hyperopic correction of upto +4 diopter, but also reduces the postoperative regression.

CONCLUSION

Thermal keratoplasty using either CK, non-focused, pulsed Ho:YAG laser (Ho:LTK) or focused CW diode lasers (conventional DTK and DTK-Plus) offer the advantages of being minimally invasive with reduced risk of complication in comparison with LASIK for hyperopia or mono-vision presbyopia treatment. CK, Ho:LTK and DTK also have the advantage of low system cost. However, the refractive predictability and postoperative regression are the major drawbacks when compared to LASIK. The new DTK-Plus system, with better predictability and higher refractive correction capability than the conventional-DTK and CK, therefore, may be a better alternative for hyperopia correction. Furthermore, a combined procedure (JT Lin, unpublished, pending patent) for thermal shrinkage of corneal stroma and ocular tissues located outside the limbus would have futuristic applications in the treatment of presbyopia.

REFERENCES

1. Alio JL, Ismail MM, Sanchez-Pego JL. Correction of hyperopia with non-contact Ho:YAG laser thermal keratoplasty. J Refract Surg 1997;13:17-22.
2. Papadopauls NT, Balidis M, Brajitikos PD, et al. Non-contact Ho:YAG laser thermal keratoplasty for hyperopia: two-year follow-up. J Refract Surg 2005; 21:82-86.
3. Rehany U, Landa F. Diode laser thermal keratoplasty to correct hyperopia. J Refract Surg 2004;20:53-61.
4. Pallikaris IG, Nroumidi TL, Pangopoulou SI, Alegakis AK, Astyrakakis NI. Conductive keratoplasty for low moderate hyperopia: 1-year results. J Refract Surg 2003;19:496-506.
5. Lin JT, Mallo O. Treatment of presbyopia by infrared laser radial sclerotomy. J Refract Surg 2003;19:465-7.
6. Lin, JT, Kadambi V. The new mechanism for laser presbyopia reversal and accommodation: Presbyopia, A Surgical Textbook. Thorofare, NJ: SLACK Inc; 2002; 63-70.
7. Atchison and Smith. Optics of the Human Eye, Butterworth-Heinemann, 2000;110.

Recent Update on Lasik Techniques

46

BOJAN PAJIC (SWITZERLAND)

I. FEMTOSECOND LASER

In future new femtosecond laser systems will be developed with a higher pulsfrequency, a lower energy application per effect and a shorter treatment time. So the bubble formation caused by photodisruption will be much smaller and the cutting surface smoother. The next developing steps are already done by IntraLase with a pulsfreqeuncy of 30 KHz and 60 KHz. The treatment time reduces with the 60 KHz below 30 seconds. Up to now, advantage of IntraLase femtosecond laser is comparing with other systems, that there is customize treatment possible, not only in the refractive but also in cornea surgery, e.g. for cornea grafting.

DaVinci femtosecond laser with a pulsfrequency in a MHz range is very fast, stable and precise. The first outcomes shows nearly no bubbles with very smooth surface in the interface. The all overall treatment, cutting time is below 20 seconds. The results will be reported.

II. PATTERN OF ELEVATED, IRREGULAR ASTIGMATISM AND ABERRATION HIGHER ORDER AFTER PERFORMING A LAMELLAR KERATOTOMY WITH AN AMADEUS SIS KERATOM IN KERATOPLASTY EYES

Aim

The aim was to investigate if there is a decrease of the corneal astigmatism power, irregularity and a reduction of a higher order aberration.

Patients and Methods

Five perforated keratoplasty eyes with an astigmatism of more than 5 dpt, a corneal irregularity of more than 4 dpt in the 5 mm zone and a substantial aberration of higher order undergo keratectomies with an Amadeus Sis microkeratom (Fig. 46.1). The best preoperative visual acuity range was in all cases beneath 0.125. A 8.5 mm suction ring with a hinge of 0.7 mm was used in all cases performin a lamellar LASIK cut (Figs 46.1 to 46.7). Standard ophthalmological examination, inclusive visual acuity examination, a corneal topography and wavefront measuring were performed before and 6 week after treatment. For purposes of statistical data analysis the SPSS program was used.

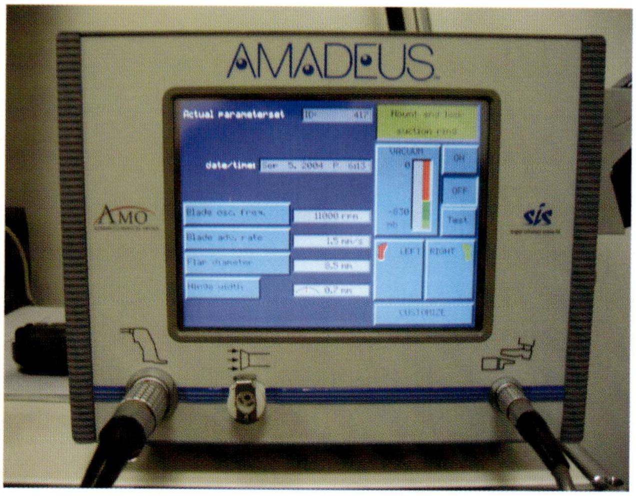

Fig. 46.1: Amadeus SIS Keratom

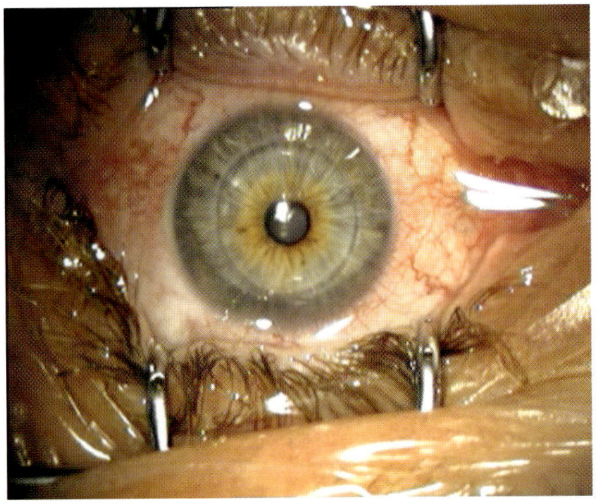

Fig. 46.2: PKP cornea

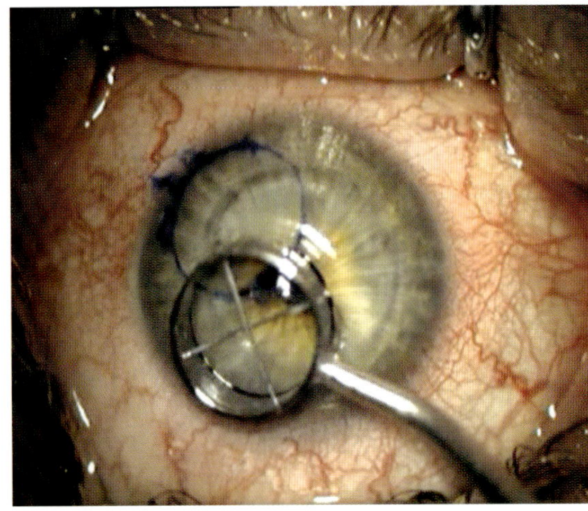

Fig. 46.3: Marking

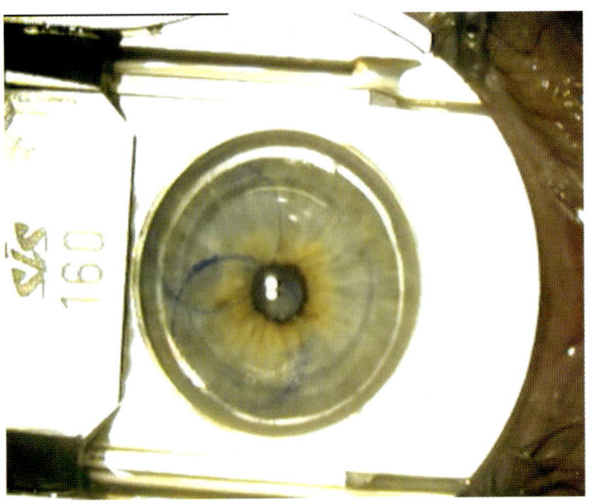

Fig. 46.4: Centring of cutting device

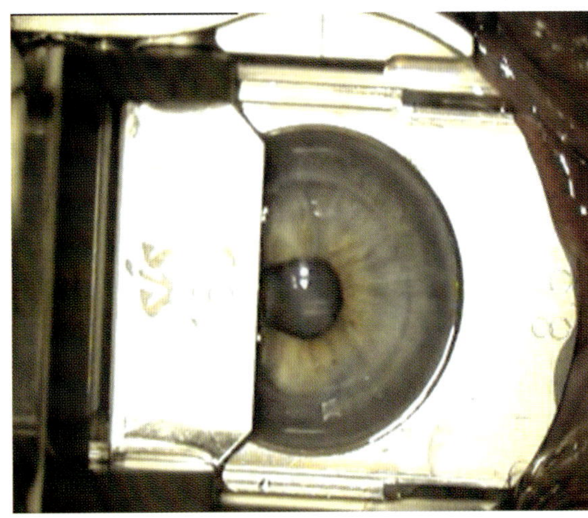

Fig. 46.5: Cut

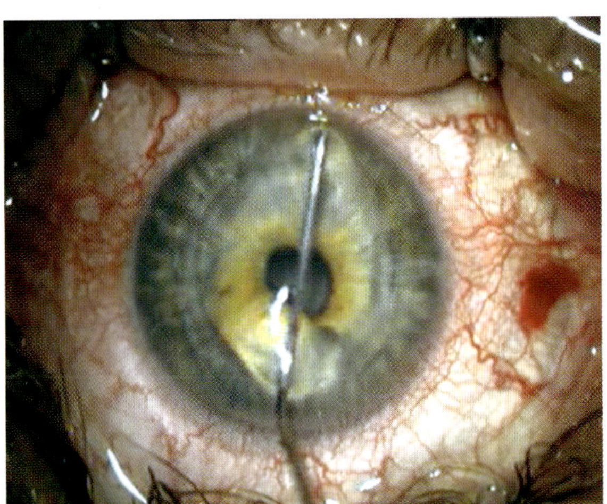

Fig. 46.6: Flap readaptation

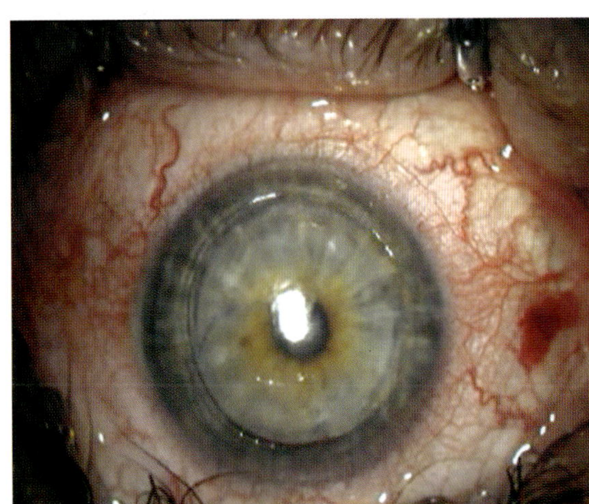

Fig. 46.7: Repositioning

Figs 46.2 to 46.7: Technique of keratotomy

Results

After performing a lamellar keratotomy and readaptation of the corneal flap there was a significant corneal-irregularity-index decrease in mean of – 0.33 ± 0.42 dpt in the 5 mm zone (Table 46.1). At the same time the corneal astigmatism reduction of – 2.83±2.14 dpt was not significant, whereas the axis position changed 13.66 ± 2.08 degree. The high significant decrease of aberration of higher order was detected. Thus as an important visual acuity improvement of 3 up to 7 lines, mean 5 ± 1.41, was acquired and is highly significant (Table 46.2).

CONCLUSION

The tissue tension power of the scar formation after penetrating keratoplasty could bias the optical characteristics of the corneal centre. A lamellar keratotomy in the anterior third of the cornea leads already to a relevant tissue relaxation with a decrease of the corneal irregularity and aberration (Figs 46.8 to 46.11).

III. ROTATIONAL EYETRACKER SYSTEM

By introducing the dynamic rotational eye tracker the already approved X/Y tracker which compensates actively for transversal movements of the eye will be upgraded to compensate misalignments in rotation.

Table 46.1: Topographical corneal parameters

	MW	*SD*
Δ corneal-irregularity-index	– 0.33	0.42
Δ astigmatism power	– 2.83	2.14
Δ astigmatism axis change	13.66	2.08

Table 46.2: Subjective refraction parameters

	MW	*SD*
Δ spherical power	0.66	1.7
Δ astigmatism power	0.92	0.88
Δ axis	33.87	5.82
Δ visual acuity improvement	5 lines	1.41 lines

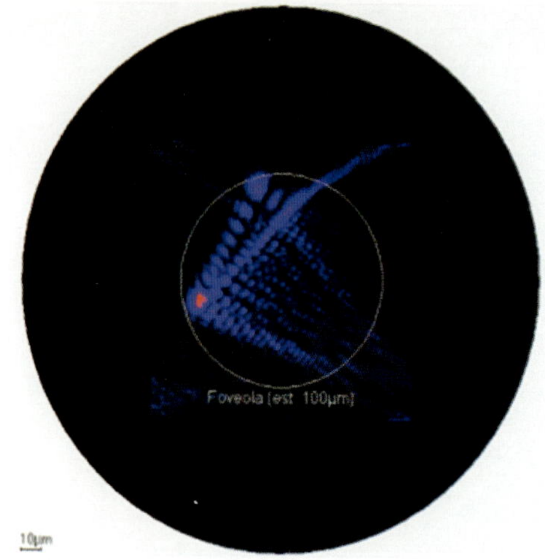

Fig. 46.8: Aberration higher order PSF before keratotomy

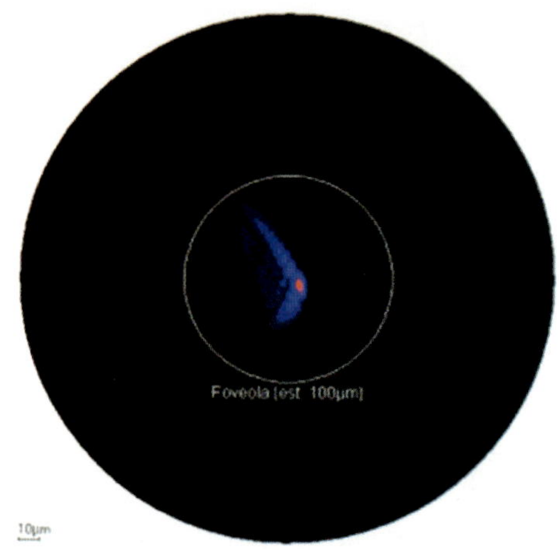

Fig. 46.9: Aberration higher order PSF after keratotomy

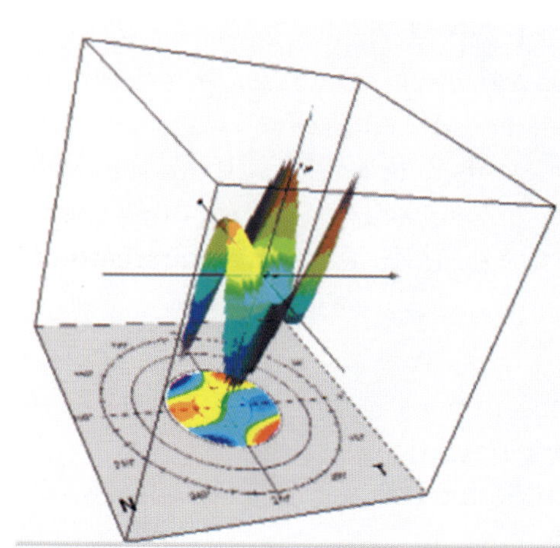

Fig. 46.10: Aberration higher order 3D before keratotomy; ampl.: 13.28 µm

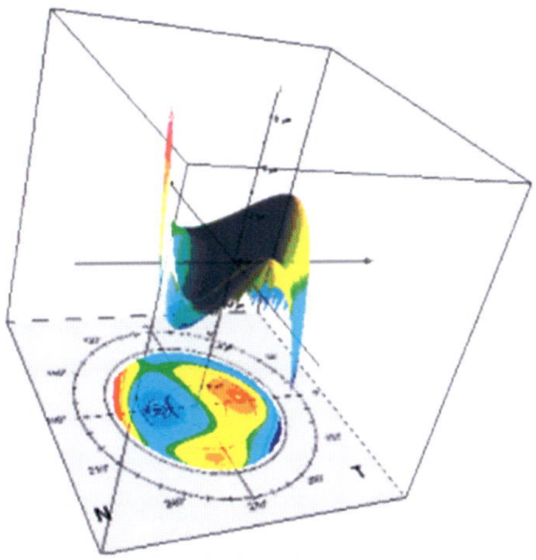

Fig. 46.11: Aberration higher order 3D after keratotomy; ampl.: 1.82 μm

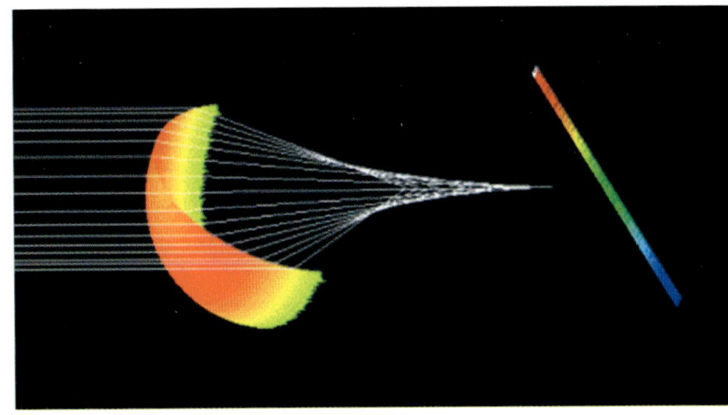

Fig. 46.12: Positive spherical aberration

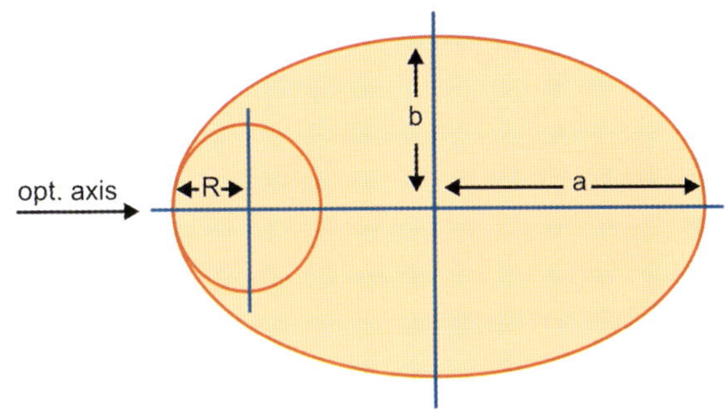

Fig. 46.13: Definition of the asphericity

While the uses of the acquired pupil images only, additional objectively acquired information is needed to provide a rotational tracking capability. B and L's H.EYE.TECH rotational tracker module is based on the iris pattern recognition technology. It is well known that iris patterns are similar to finger prints unique biometric properties of an individium. By using the appropriate technology not only the individual eye can be recognized (which is a safety feature for itself), but also specific match parameters such as rotational misalignment between two images of the same iris can be obtained. Almost all diagnostic examinations such as objective measures like wavefront and topography as well as subjective refraction are measured while the patients are seated. However the LASIK treatment is performed on the supine patients. During the surgery the cyclotorsion is a dynamic phenomena, it is said that the angle can change up to 15 degrees within the treatment.

IV. ASPHERIC ABLATION ALGORITHMS

Spherical aberration describes the rotational symmetric deviation of the refraction of light rays if compared to the perfect refracting surface. Spherical aberration can be expressed in the μm of Zernike aberration. Standard Algorithms induce positive spherical aberration and create too oblate corneal shapes (Fig. 46.12). The asphericity parameter Q is a measure for the ellipticity of a surface if compared to perfect circle/sphere (Fig. 46.13). It can be described with the following formula:

If $Q = 0$ then there is a spherical shape. If $Q > 0$ then there is a oblat shape and if $Q < 0$ then the shape is prolat (Fig. 46.14). The mean Q value of the population is at – 0.3, those of the perfect asphericity at – 0.5 and perfect sphericity at 0.0 (Fig. 46.15). Photorefractive procedures induce besides of the intended correction a mix of high order aberrations. This mix is mainly dominated by spherical aberration. Reasons could be a biodynamical response of the cornea to a significant volumetric tissue removal (Fig. 46.16) and a laser efficacy variation on curved surfaces due to cosine effect and increased reflectivity (Fig. 46.17). Determination of the amount of postoperatively observed spherical aberration have been done. Zyoptix FDA data have been processed to evaluate potential correlations between

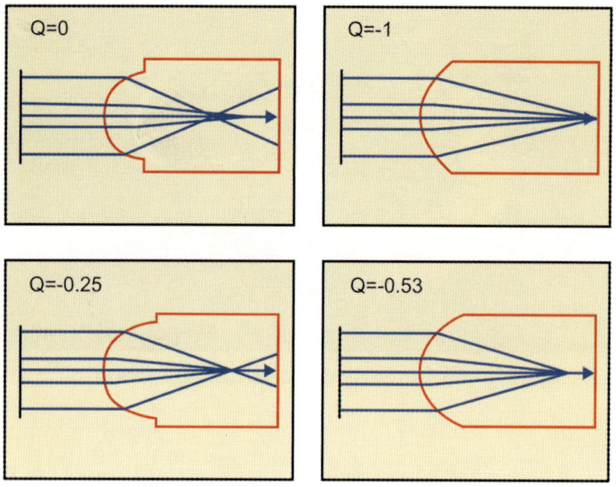

Fig. 46.14: Q depending shapes

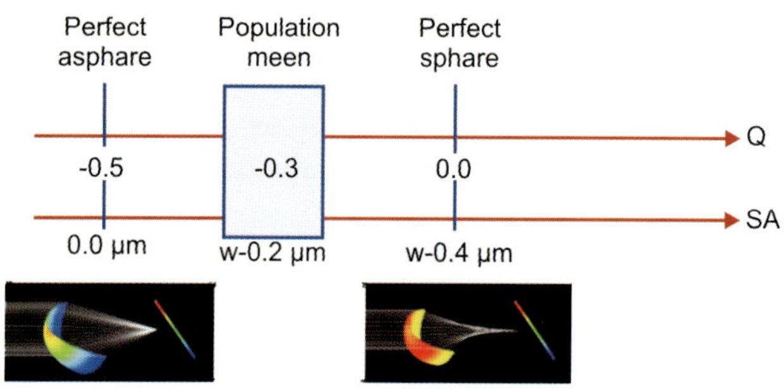

Fig. 46.15: Q value at perfect asphericity, sphericity and mean population

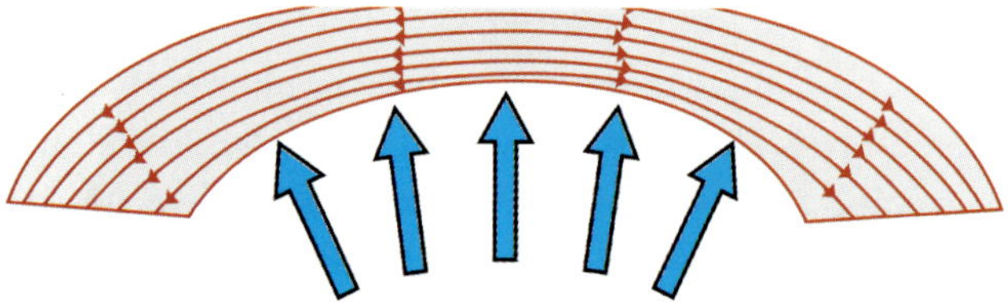

Fig. 46.16: Corneal biodynamic response

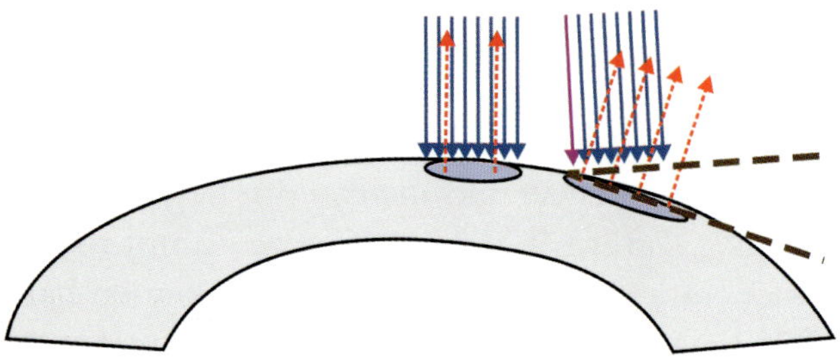

Fig. 46.17: Laser efficacy variation

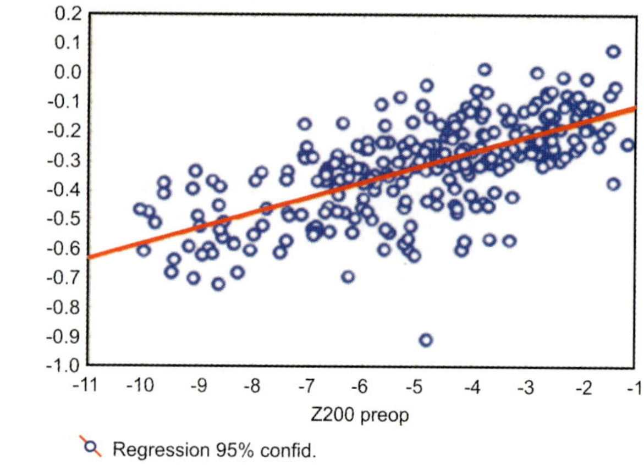

Fig. 46.18: Determination of the amount of postoperatively observed spherical aberration

postoperatively observed aberrations and preoperative parameters. Most significant driving factor is spherical equivalent and second important driving factor preoperative existing spherical aberration. Based on these findings, a mathematical model has been created, which calculates the amount of induced spherical aberration (Fig. 46.18). Spherocylindrical correction mainly induce spherical aberration. The higher the treatment value is the higher is the induction of spherical aberration. Thus that leeds to the following treatment strategy. The final Zyoptix aspheric treatment is a combination of two main ablation components, it is said a basic ablation component to correct the classical refractive error by using 2 mm and 1 mm Zyoptix laser spots and an aspheric ablation component to correct the surgically induced spherical aberration. The total ablation profile is the sum of the two components (Fig. 46.19).

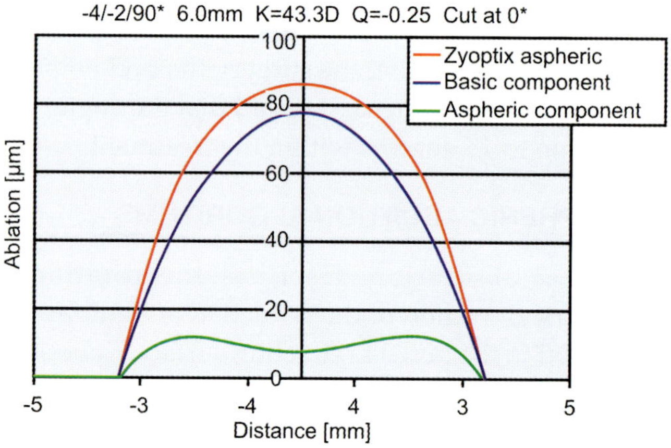

Fig. 46.19: Simulation of zyoptix aspheric treatment profile

Compared to the already known Tissue Saving mode the Zyoptix Aspheric Algorithm utilizes a more general analytical model (elliptical surfaces instead of spherical surfaces), corneal asphericity parameter (Q-Value), a model for the surgically induced spherical aberration which generates an additional ablation component. The next step in the development of aspheric algorithms is the integration of the Zyoptix aspheric mode and the wavefront driven mode into one single algorithm. The first clinical results show, treated with Zyoptix Aspheric Algorithm, a spherical aberration neutral algorithm (No clinically significant induction of SA over a 6.0mm pupil), significantly less induced postoperative higher-order aberrations (HORMS), better preservation of corneal asphericity, better low contrast visual acuity.

V. WAVEFRONT DRIVEN PROCEDURES WITHOUT PHARMACOLOGICAL PUPIL DILATION

One of the recommendations on optical zones is to plan an optical zone which is 0.2 mm to 0.5 mm larger than the mesopic pupil. A wavefront measurement does not provide sufficient data to meet this recommendation in all cases (Fig. 46.20). To generate sufficient data a pharmacological pupil dilation has been recommended (Fig. 46.21). The main reasons for elimination of pharmacological pupil dilation are to remove the need for standardized dilation protocol, to take out the extreme pupil shift issues, to take away sources of variation caused by dilation process, to open the possibility for a one day procedure. To achieve these benefits it's necessary to expand the data map to provide the option for creating an optical zone 0.2 mm-0.5 mm larger than the acquisition pupil. We like to demonstrate problems of a Zernicke polynomials wavefront map extrapolation (Fig. 46.22) and a possible solution.

Fig. 46.23

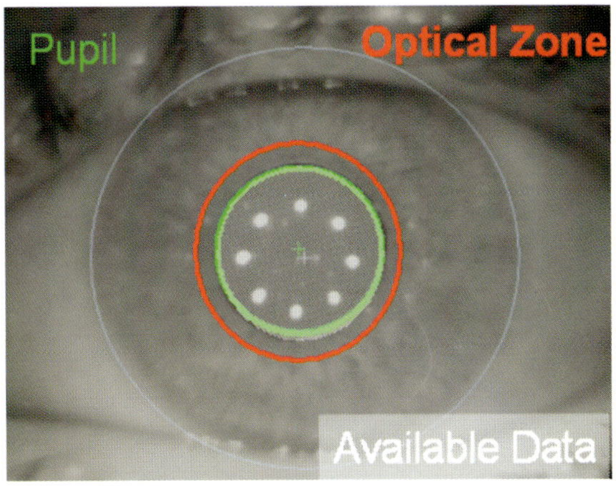

Fig. 46.20

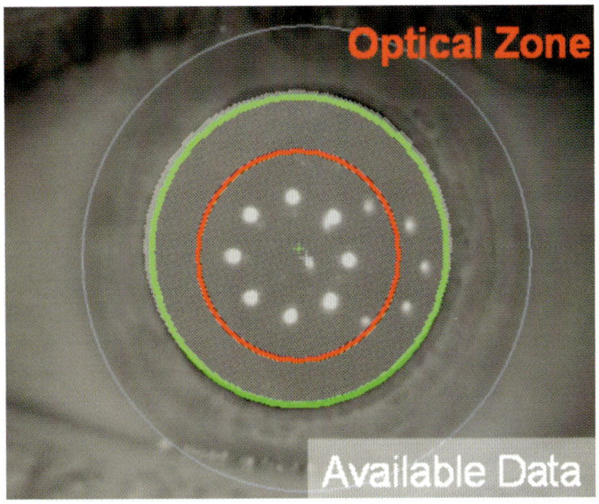

Fig. 46.21

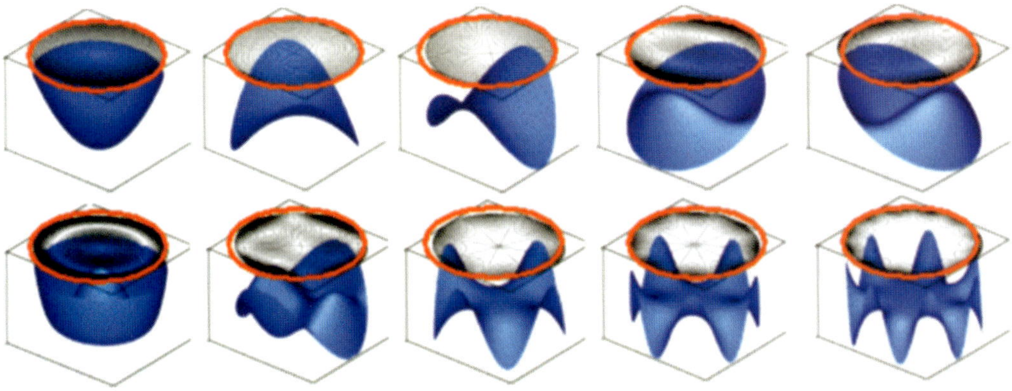

Fig. 46.22

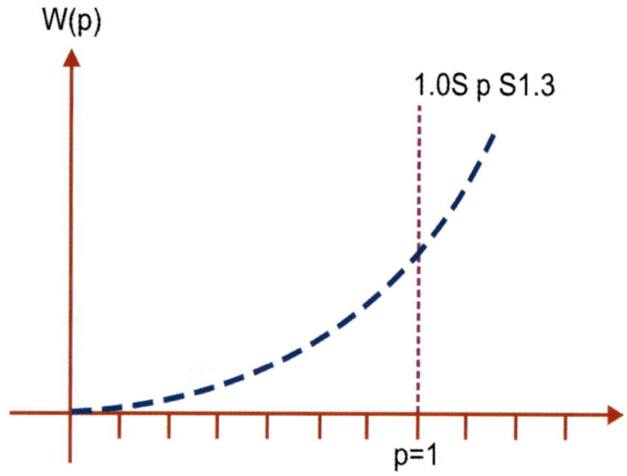

Fig. 46.23: Mathematical dependency between ρ

$$W(\rho,\varphi) = \sum_{n,m\,\pi} A^{\pi}_{n,m}\, x Z^{\pi}_{n,m}\,(\rho,\varphi)$$

for

$$0 \le \rho \ge 1$$

$$Z^{\pi}_{n,m}(\rho,\varphi) = \sqrt{2(n+1)} x R^{m}_{n}\,(\rho)\, x \cos\,(m\varphi) \quad \text{for m} \neq 0 \text{ and } \pi = \text{even}$$

$$Z^{\pi}_{n,m}(\rho,\varphi) = \sqrt{2(n+1)} x R^{m}_{n}\,(\rho)\, x \sin\,(m\varphi) \quad \text{for m} \neq 0 \text{ and } \pi = \text{odd}$$

$$Z^{\pi}_{n,m}(\rho,\varphi) = \sqrt{(n+1)} x\, R^{m=0}_{n}\,(\rho) \quad \text{for m=0}$$

and:

$$R^{m}_{n}(\rho) = \sum_{s=0}^{(n-m)/2} \frac{(-1)^{s}\,(n-s)!}{s![(n+m)/2-s]![(n-m/2-s]!}\,\rho^{n-2s}$$

$$W(\rho) = 1.0 \times \rho^{2} \qquad 0 \le \rho \le 1$$

Here are different ways to manipulate the wavefront map, the first to pretend that the actual pupil was larger when the Zernikes are determined and push the border or the second to ignore $p \le 1$ criterion and move beyond the border. If the first mode is used than data outside the pupil have been generated, but the wavefront shape inside the pupil has been modified (Fig. 46.24). The second mode is to ignore $p \le 1$ criterion and move beyond the border, it is said to attack the border mode. The wavefront shap inside the pupil remains stable but outside the border the function do not correlate to empirical clinical datas (Fig. 46.25). Both straight forward methods of using mathematical tools for extrapolating the wavefront do not provide feasible output if this is compared to clinical reality (Fig. 46.26). Learning from the data mode a controlled extension of the map, using the available mathematical tools and the available clinical information will be the right strategy. Data from the Zyoptix FDA study have been used to develop the algorithm for a 10% extrapolation of the original pupil size. More than 3000 wavefront exams have been used in an iterative development process to verify the performance of the expansion strategy. A variety of pupils sizes was used as the base for this verification covering the range between 5.0 mm and 7.0 mm diameters. Finally an independent data set from 5 globally distributed sites (Asia and Europe) has been analyzed to confirm and validate the outcomes. An Algorithm has been developed using mathematical transformations and basic clinical data which expands

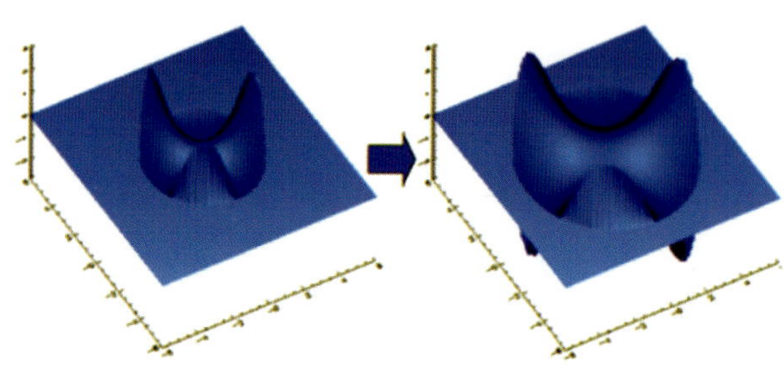

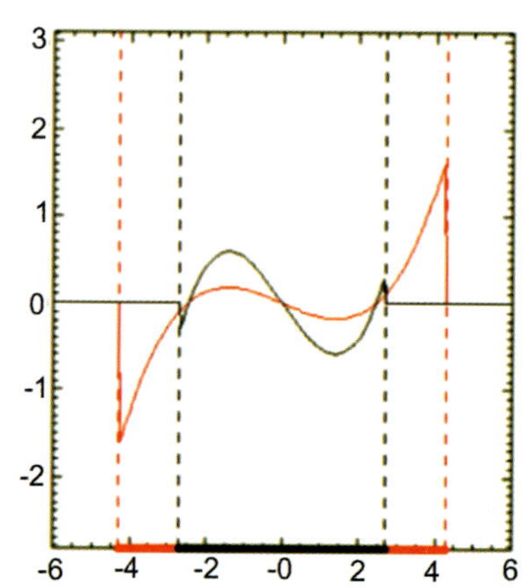

Fig. 46.24: First mode wavefront extrapolation

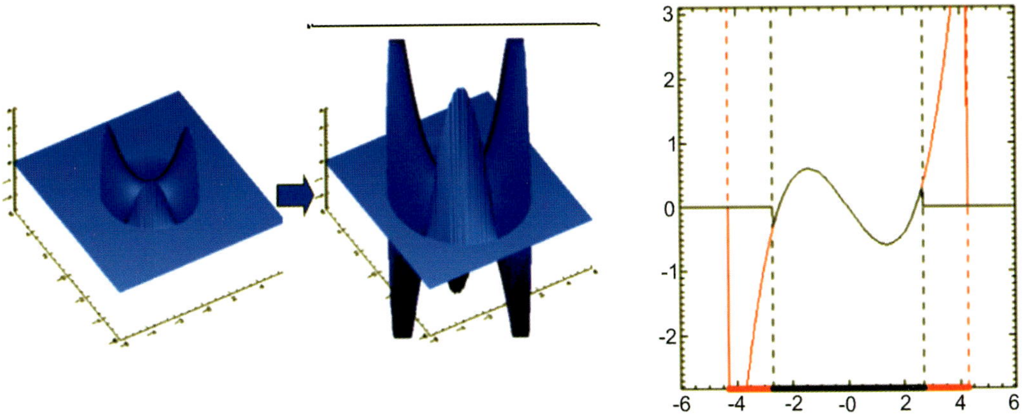

Fig. 46.25: Second mode wavefront extrapolation

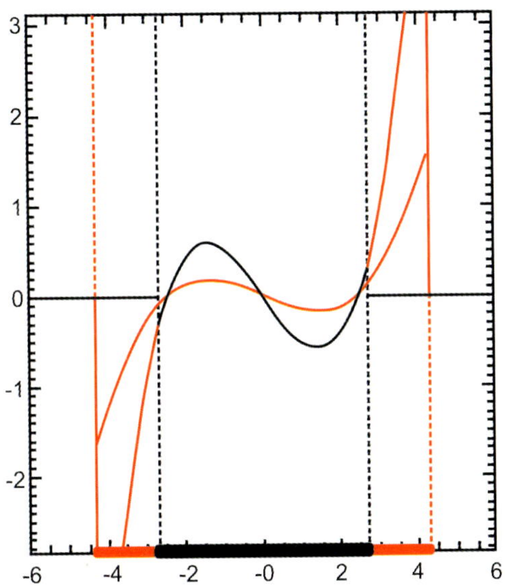

Fig. 46.26: Compare both modes

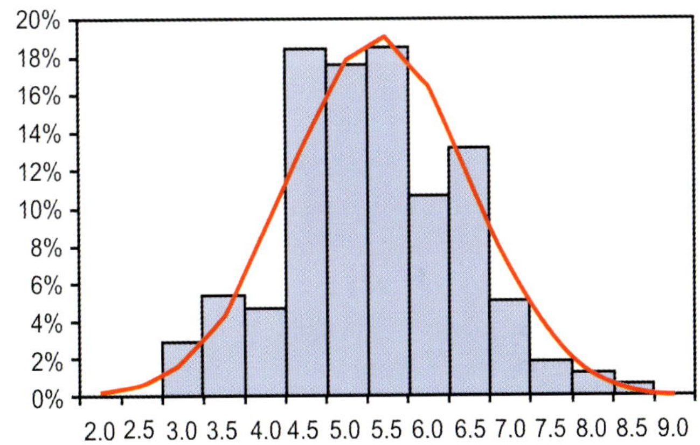

Fig. 46.27: Clinical mesopic pupil data

myopic wavefront maps. The maps are expanded by 10% using the NoDilationZyoptix Algorithm. Mesopic pupil data have been collected to derive a pupil size distribution model. (N = 329) (Fig. 46.27). A best fit normal distribution has been derived as the analytical distribution model for the estimation of the potential of NoDilationZyoptix (Fig. 46.28). Mesopic pupils smaller than 4.5 mm do not benefit significantly from personalized procedures. A fraction of 85% remains within the range: [4.5 mm; 9.0 mm]. Eyes with Zywave pupils larger 7.0 mm are in the most of the cases not subject to dilation. A residual fraction of

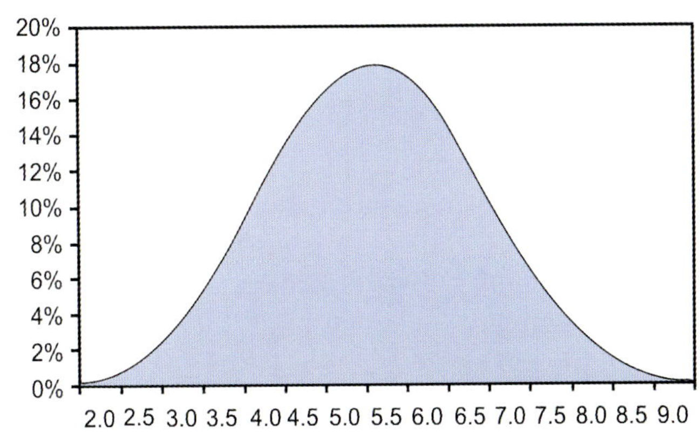

Fig. 46.28: Analytical pupil size distribution model

78% remains in the range: [4.5 mm; 7.0 mm] (Fig. 46.29). In theory every body in [4.5 mm; 9.0 mm] range can be treated using NoDiZy. 10% extrapolation provides for almost all cases an offset of 0.5 mm (3% at 4.5 mm do not reach 0.5 mm). In the case of a minimal tolerated OZ, the number of cases which will benefit is decreased. The final number depends on the individual OZ minimum and can be modelled (Fig. 46.30).

A new strategy has been developed to extend myopic wavefront maps by 10% of their original size. By implementing this Algorithm into the Zywave software the number of patients who benefit from a nondilation procedure can be increased significantly.

Zernicke polynomials wavefront map calculation

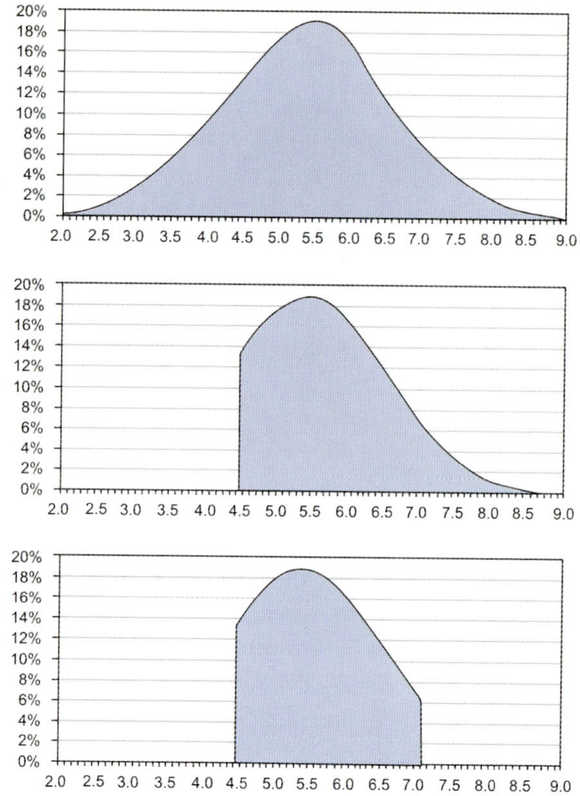

Fig. 46.29: Pupil size distribution and the related optical zone

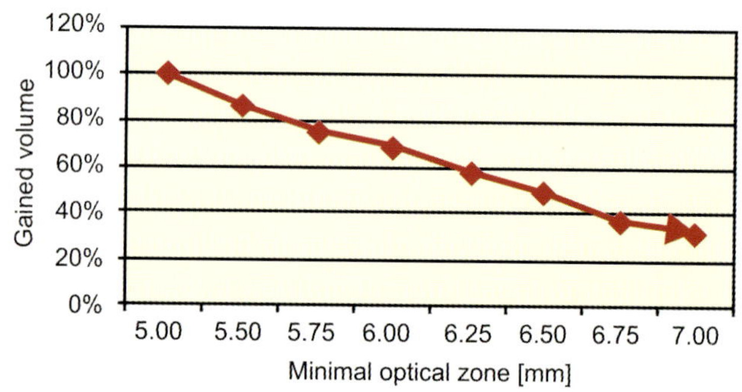

Fig. 46.30: Gained volume by No Dilation Zyoptix for a given minimal OZ size

VI. OPTICAL COHERENCE TOMOGRAPHY—INTEGRATED ONLINE PACHYMETRY (OCP)

OCT is a noncontact technique that acquires pachymetry measurements based on optical interferometry. It has also been demonstrated to be able to acquire measurements not possible by traditional ultrasound techniques.[1-3] OLCR is a continuous version of OCT that can measure corneal thickness at the rate of 18 Hz using light in the infrared range. It has been incorporated into an excimer laser platform and can perform measurements during corneal ablation.[4-6]

The integrated online pachymetry is based on the OCT principle. the interference capability of light rays is used to measure distances critical components are accuracy of defining the length defines also the accuracy of the measurement. Total achievable DL defines dynamic range of the pachymetry measurement. Speed of moving achieving DL defines the time scale for the measurement. Quality of data processing defines signal/noise ratio and speed of data processing defines final acquisition rate (Fig. 46.31).

First feasibility data using a fully intergrated OCP platform is a B and L's H.EYE.TECH Excimerlaser. Contact free measurement of flapthickness is possible with a online ablation depth monitoring. The wavelength range at λ : 1300 nm with a output: of less than 200 μW. Current goal regarding the OCP is a measurement of flap thickness before ablation as a safety feature for the surgeon. Future goal is to improve current technology to a level, at which the ablation procedure can be monitored in realtime (Fig. 46.32A and B, 46.33). (Fig. 46.34, 46.35).

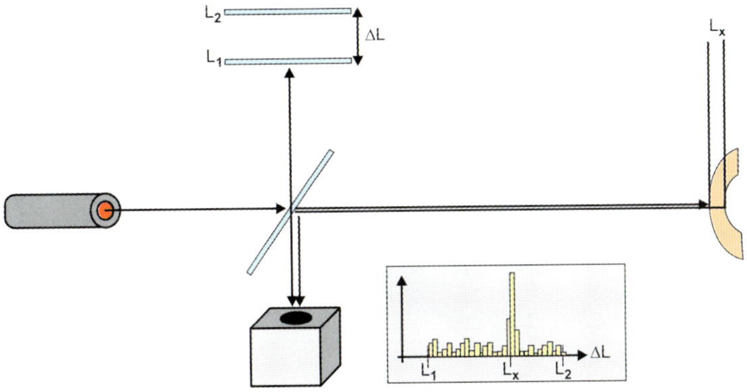

Fig. 46.31: Concept of OCP

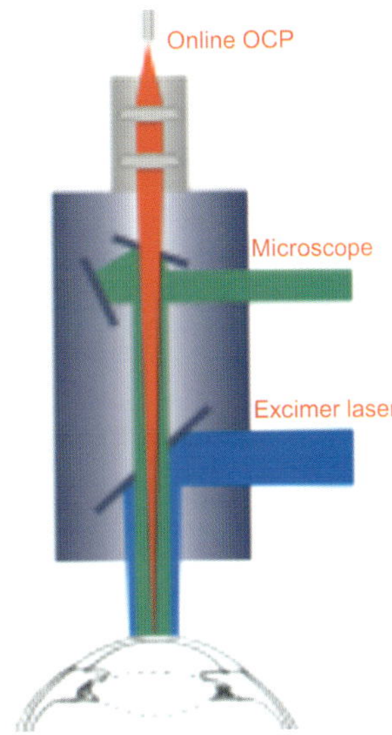

Fig. 46.32A: Noncontact online pachymetry in B and L's H.EYE.TECH Excimerlaser

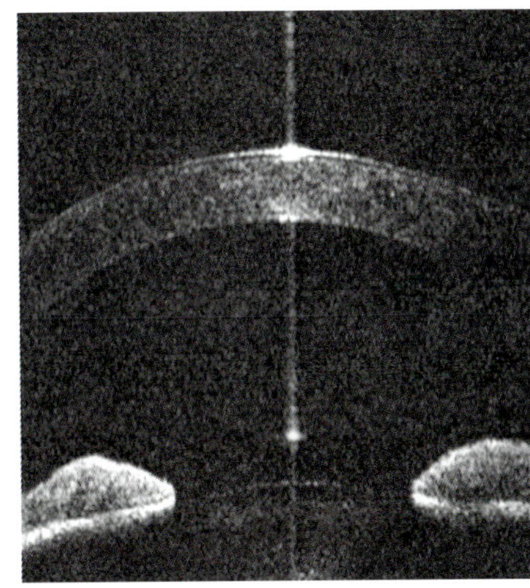

Fig. 46.32B: Ultrasound image of pachymetry measurement

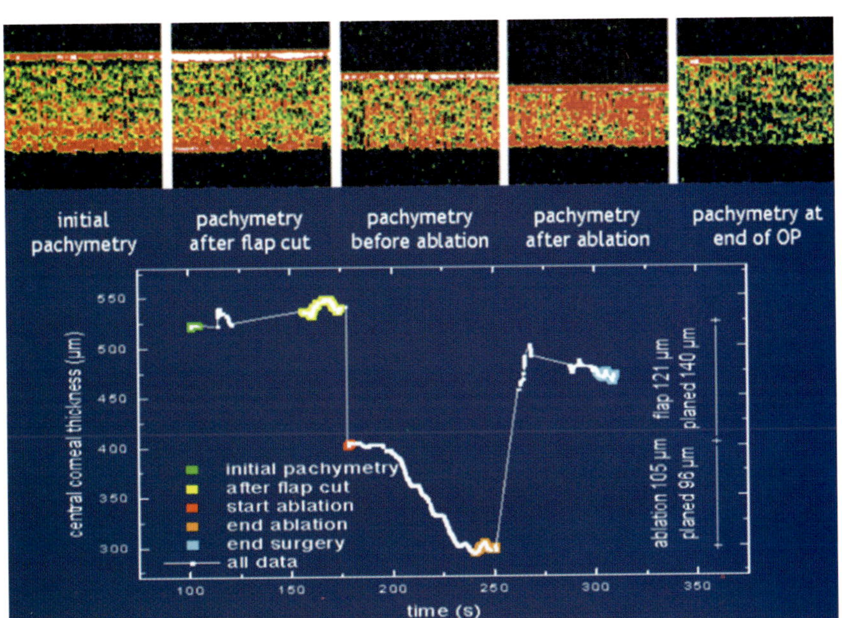

Fig. 46.33: Monitoring of realtime, online pachymetry

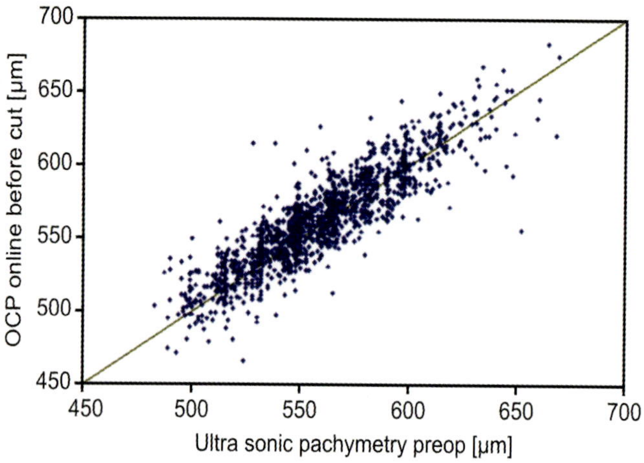

Fig. 46.34: Ultra sonic versus OCP online pachymetry

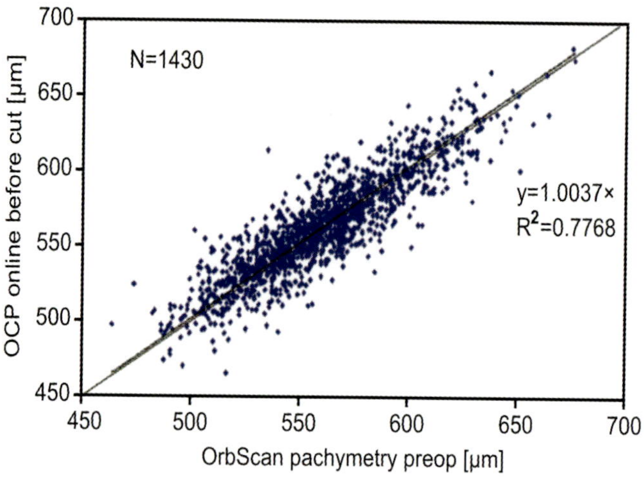

Fig. 46.35

CONCLUSION

Feasibility data show that the OCP data are consistent to the ultrasound and Orbscan measurements. Flap thickness data do not show any variation to the known other studies. Postoperative Pachymetry data are consistent to the laser ablation data research activities on extended future applications ongoing. Future potential is to install an online tracking tool and a closed loop ablation process monitor in the Excimerlaser delivered datas from the real-time OCP.

REFERENCES

1. Bechmann M, Thiel MJ, Neubauer AS, et al. Central corneal thickness measurement with a retinal optical coherence tomography device versus standard ultrasonic pachymetry. Cornea 2001;20:50-54.
2. Wang J, Fonn D, Simpson TL, et al. Relation between opticalcoherence tomography and optical pachymetry measurements of corneal swelling induced by hypoxia. Am J Ophthalmol 2002;134:93-98.
3. Wong AC, Wong CC, Yuen NS, et al. Correlational study of central corneal thickness measurements on Hong Kong Chinese using optical coherence tomography, Orbscan and ultrasound pachymetry. Eye 2002;16: 715-21.
4. Genth U, Mrochen M, Waiti R, et al. Optical low coherence reflectometry for noncontact measurements of flap thickness during laser in situ keratomileusis. Ophthalmology 2002;109:973-78.
5. Bohnke M, Widmer S, Waiti R. Real-time pachymetry during photorefractive keratectomy using optical low-coherence reflectometry/Biomed Opt 2001;6:412-17.
6. Wirbelauer C, Pham DT. Intraoperative optical coherence pachymetry during laser in situ keratomileusis: first clinical experience. J Refract Surg 2003;19:372-77.

ACKNOWLEDGEMENTS

The authors thank for distinct support of Dr. Gerhard Youssefi and Anton Hilger (Technolas) for personal and technical advice.

Index

A

B

C

D

E

F

H

I

K

L

M

N

O